1 MONTH OF
FREE
READING

at

www.ForgottenBooks.com

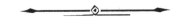

By purchasing this book you are eligible for one month membership to ForgottenBooks.com, giving you unlimited access to our entire collection of over 1,000,000 titles via our web site and mobile apps.

To claim your free month visit:

www.forgottenbooks.com/free1238410

ISBN 978-0-332-74787-3
PIBN 11238410

PSYCHOPHARMACOLOGY ABSTRACTS is a publication of the
National Clearinghouse for Mental Health Information
of the National Institute of Mental Health. It is a
specialized information medium designed to assist the
Institute in meeting its obligation to foster and support laboratory and clinical research into the nature
and causes of mental disorders and methods of treatment and prevention. Specifically, this information
service is designed to meet the needs of investigators in the field of psychopharmacology for rapid and
comprehensive information about new developments and
research results.

PSYCHOPHARMACOLOGY ABSTRACTS is distributed gratis to
investigators doing research in psychopharmacology. It
is not available on a subscription basis. Requests
to receive the ABSTRACTS should be accompanied by a
brief statement of the research interests and scientific specialty of the investigator. Requests to receive the ABSTRACTS, address changes, and other communications should be addressed to:

>Psychopharmacology Abstracts
>National Clearinghouse for Mental
> Health Information
>National Institute of Mental Health
>Bethesda 14, Maryland

(The text of PSYCHOPHARMACOLOGY ABSTRACTS is prepared
under contract with the Literary Division of Biological and Medical Services, Philadelphia, Penna.)

U. S. DEPARTMENT OF HEALTH, EDUCATION AND WELFARE
Public Health Service
National Institutes of Health
National Institute of Mental Health
Bethesda 14, Maryland

PSYCHOPHARMACOLOGY ABSTRACTS

Volume 2, Number 7

1369 Laborit, H. Mechanismen
biologischer Regelung von Stoffwechsel-
vorgängen unter dem Einfluss der Umwelt
und pharmakologischer Stoffe. [Mechanisms
of the biological regulation of metabolic
processes under the influence of the
environment and drugs.] Ärztliche
Forschung, 1962, 16, 383-402.

A broad general discussion is given on
the regulatory role of DPN and TPN in
carbohydrate metabolism, in which the
author maintains that disruption of oxidative phosphorylation forms a common basis
for a wide variety of pathological conditions,
and that the basic mechanism of action of a
wide variety of drugs is either an oxidative
or reductive effect with respect to TPN.
Thus, drugs which oxidize TPN, such as
the phenothiazine derivatives, favor the
entry of glucose into the pentose phosphate
shunt and exert hypnotic, hypokalemic,
lipidogenic, galactorrheic, hypotensive
and hyperthermic effects, while drugs
which reduce TPN, such as the MAO
inhibitors, favor the Embden-Meyerhoff
scheme and have analeptic, hypertensive
and antiketogenic properties. This theory
is supported by a review of the literature
on the effects of drugs on blood pressure,
the physiology of sleep, anesthesia and
analgesia, including EEG studies, the
biochemistry of fatigue, shock, mental
illness and diabetes, age and arteriosclerosis, artificial hibernation and the
biology of cancer. (47 refs.)

Hôpital Boucicaut
78 Rue de la Convertion
Paris 15, France

1370 Capparell, Homer V. Drug therapy
in mental illness. Pennsylvania Medical
Journal, 1962, 65, 899-905.

Agents used as adjuvants in the care of
disturbed patients include the following:
reserpine, phenothiazine derivatives
(chlorpromazine, promethazine, promazine,
trifluoperazine, etc.) and antidepressants
(iproniazid, isocarboxazid, phenelzine,
imipramine, nialamide, tranylcypromine,
etryptamine, etc.). Side effects from
phenothiazines include extrapyramidal
reactions and jaundice, while antidepressants

may cause hypotension or hepatotoxicity.
The physician must exercise judicious
judgement in selecting drugs, due to the
notorious lack of drug specificity for a
given complex of symptoms. Such
tranquilizers as meprobamate or
chlordiazepoxide are very valuable in
office practice in treating minor emotional
disorders. (No refs.)

[No address]

1371 Nettleship, A., & Lair, Charles V.
Time and disease. Journal of Clinical
and Experimental Psychopathology and
Quarterly Review of Psychiatry and
Neurology, 1962, 23, 106-115.

The perception of time and its relationships
to disease processes are reviewed. Topics
include theoretical considerations, medical
and psychiatric contributions to time
perception, modifications of the sense of
time by neuropsychological conditions and
the assessment of ambiguity in the passage
of time. Hashish and alcohol effects are
mentioned. Four areas of psychological
research that have contributed to an
understanding of the concept of time (either
directly or indirectly) are discussed, i.e.,
maturation, learning, perception and
sensory deprivation. The intact neural
mechanism is considered basic to man's
interpretation of time. (32 refs.)

Laboratory Service
VA Hospital
Fayetteville, Ark.

1372 Gilbert, Gordon J. Reaction to
glutethimide. New England Journal of
Medicine, 1962, 266, 1119. [Letter]

A physician questions the proper classification of 3 previously reported cases of
prolonged glutethimide administration
(Zivin and Shalowitz, 1962). These
patients may have really shown withdrawal
symptoms, although they were purportedly
still receiving the medication. Similar
symptoms (grand mal seizure, fever,
delirium, confusion and hallucinosis)
have been noted in patients suffering
from phenobarbital, meprobamate or

alcohol withdrawal.

Neurology Service
U.S. Air Force Hospital (MATS)
Travis Air Force Base, Calif.

1373 Ross, Paul. A.P.C. as a cause of renal disease. Medical Journal of Australia, 1962, 2, 539-543.

This is a review of the evidence linking phenacetin abuse to renal damage. Topics discussed include: the fate of phenacetin in the body, toxic effects on red cells, toxic effects on the kidney, prevalence, diagnosis, prognosis and treatment. Deleterious effects due to analgesics may be a consequence of a preexisting renal disease. Some contaminating ingredient in the analgesic may be responsible for causing renal damage. How much phenacetin is likely to cause renal damage and what amount is likely to be fatal? There seems to be a sufficiently probable causal relationship between phenacetin and renal disease, even in the absence of unequivocal experimental proof, to warrant the recommendation that this drug be made available only on a prescription basis. (36 refs.)

[No address]

1374 Berblinger, Klaus W. Psychiatric perspectives in medicine. Psychosomatics, 1962, 3, 106-119.

Psychiatric treatment routinely revolves around initial referral to the psychiatrist followed by hospitalization with subsequent psychotherapy, including directive therapy (advice and counseling, hypnosis and hypnotherapy) and nondirective techniques (medical psychotherapy, analytically oriented psychotherapy and psychoanalysis). Psychopharmacological treatment encompasses utilization of the major tranquilizers (phenothiazine derivatives, e.g., chlorpromazine), rauwolfia alkaloids, minor tranquilizers (meprobamate), barbiturates, sedatives and hypnotics, bromides, nonbarbiturate sedatives and hypnotics (glutethimide) and stimulants (amphetamines and hydrazines). Admoni-

tions are given for the care and handling or suicidal patients (evaluation of suicidal risk, general assessment, criteria for imminent suicide and prevention of impending suicide), homicidal patients (those with impaired control, i.e., epileptics, paranoids, and severely depressed patients) and addicted patients. Posttraumatic psychiatric reactions and iatrogenic illness are also discussed. (24 refs.)

[No address]

1375 Stokvis, B. Psychotherapie und Psychopharmakologie bei Psycho- und Somatoneurotikern. Heil-Erfolge oder Schein-Erfolge? [Psychotherapy and psychopharmacology in psychoneurotic and psychosomatic diseases. Therapeutic response or placebo response?] Acta Psychotherapia, 1962, 10, 246-264.

A brief, critical discussion of the excessive use of psychotropic drugs for neurotic complaints under the influence of mass publicity, and a review of the criteria for establishing the existence of a placebo response, are followed by a report of a study on the possible "placebo effect" of psychotherapy. The techniques of individual and group psychotherapy are reviewed and the requirements for a study of its true effectiveness are outlined. A comparison of the results in 105 neurotic patients given either supportive or analytical psychotherapy, and a follow-up study of 245 patients with psychosomatic disorders, 113 of whom received psychotherapy, indicated that there is little difference in effectiveness between various types of psychotherapy and that psychotherapy did not seem to alter the prognosis in psychosomatic illness. The author warns, however, against the premature drawing of unfavorable conclusions with regard to psychotherapy. (27 refs.)

Psychosomatic Center
University of Leiden
Leiden, The Netherlands

1376 Impastato, David J. Effect of drug therapy on the frequency of EST. American

Journal of Psychotherapy, 1962, 16, 387-396.

The following topics are included in a discussion of the merits of ECT (EST) as opposed to drug therapy: frequency of ECT, deleterious effects of ECT (fractures, memory changes, the aura of fear, tension and anxiety, decreased mortality), disadvantages of drug therapy (delayed therapeutic response to antidepressant drugs, inferior therapeutic results with drug therapy, toxic effects), advantages of ECT (rapid response, increased efficacy, increased safety, less time and expenditure required) and advantages of drug therapy (greater familial acceptability, no loss of working time, no memory disturbances). ECT is used 25-50% less since the institution of the antidepressants. ECT is classified as being ultimately superior to drug therapy. Drug treatment is contraindicated in suicidal patients.

Department of Psychiatry
New York University School of Medicine
New York, N. Y.

1377 Moe, Robert, Bagdon, Robert E., & Zbinden, Gerhard. The effect of tranquilizers on myocardial metabolism. Angiology, 1962, 13, 4-12.

A series of studies on the effects of tranquilizers on myocardial metabolism in various animals in vivo and in vitro is reviewed. Topics discussed included the following: the typical peripheral mode of action, effect of these tranquilizers on heart and brain bioamines, the rate of O_2 uptake in in vitro preparations of rat heart slices, lactic acid content in total heart muscle and contractile responses of electrically driven auricles; in vivo effects on myocardial necrosis induced by isoproterenol, CNS and autonomic function. Drugs mentioned include chlorpromazine, chlordiazepoxide and meprobamate. Direct effects of chlordiazepoxide and chlorpromazine upon the myocardium and associated vascular system appeared to be of a transitory antiadrenergic nature. (17 refs.)

Department of Cardiovascular Pharmacology
Hoffmann-LaRoche, Inc.
Nutley 10, N. J.

1378 Paget, G. E. Limitations of animal tests to detect sensitization reactions in man. Proceedings of the Royal Society of Medicine, 1962, 55, 9-11.

The limitations of animal tests to detect sensitization reactions in man are discussed. The principles upon which screening tests are usually based are analyzed. Extrapolation of meaningful results to human therapeutics is often handicapped by species differences in the absorption, metabolism and transport of a particular drug, as well as inherent differences in disease processes. Opinions on sensitization phenomena, e. g., chlorpromazine-induced cholestatic jaundice, and conventional side effects are elucidated. The probability of truly effective animal screening at human sensitivity levels in view of our inadequate present knowledge of important related processes, is viewed pessimistically for the immediate future. (2 refs.)

[No address]

1379 Medical Times. A plea for the placebo. Medical Times, 1962, 90, 161-162.

The use of the placebo in the typical double-blind trial situation is contrasted with its therapeutic utility in medical practice. The placebo can be, under certain circumstances, more powerful than the active drug in alleviating the patient's symptoms and becomes a true therapeutic agent. (No refs.)

Manhassett, L. Is., N. Y.

1380 Krauss, Stephen. Insulin therapy. Lancet, 1962, 2, 382. [Letter]

A combination of insulin and a ganglion-blocking hexamethonium derivative [no details] decreased the coma induction period to less than one half and also the dose required to produce the 1st coma to one third in 147 patients treated with modified insulin shock from 1956-1960 at the University of Vienna Psychiatric Hospital (Hift 1961). The method was safe, with an occasional case of orthostatic collapse from hypotension constituting the only detriment. Neither clinical results nor criteria for selection of suitable cases has been forthcoming. Prior to the initiation of this combination, hyaluronidase was substituted for the hexamethonium derivative, but clinical results were variable and not very significant. (4 refs.)

[No address]

1381 Scocchera, Licia Fides. Un nuovo derivato fenotiazinico: la dixirazina. [A new phenothiazine derivative, dixyrazine.] Clinica Terapeutica, 1962, 23, 375-382.

Dixyrazine inhibition of CR's in rats, effects on reducing benzadrine mortality, its antiapomorphine and antihistamine activities are outlined. Dixyrazine potentiation of hexabarbital, hypotensive effects, behavioral effects and psychomotor activity are given in comparison to promazine and chlorpromazine. Its action is somewhat similar to these latter compounds but its toxicity is less. Its low toxicity makes it valuable for long-term therapy and the agent has been used clinically for dyspepsia and similar conditions, cardiovascular pathological states, pyrosis, spasms, vomiting, colitis, asthma with a nervous component, psychoneurosis, especially anxiety, insomnia and depression. In man the average dosage which produces tranquility is 20-150 mg per day. (8 refs.)

[No address]

1382 Symmers, W. St. C. The occurrence of angiitis and of other generalized diseases of connective tissues as a consequence of the administration of drugs. Proceedings of the Royal Society of Medicine, 1962, 55, 2-28.

The occurrence of angiitis and connective tissue disease as a consequence of drug administration is reviewed and analyzed.

Topics discussed include the relationship between angiitis, anaphylactoid purpura, thrombotic purpura and other collagen diseases, sensitization to drugs, and 2 "collagen-disease-like" syndromes that occur in association to drugs. Promazine and chlorpromazine were mentioned, among others, as possibly responsible for some of these conditions. The possibility of a drug-induced condition should be considered, even though there does not seem to be a clearly established relationship between drug allergy and collagen disease. (4 refs.)

[No address]

1383 Berblinger, Klaus W. Psychiatric perspectives in medicine—Part II. Psychosomatics, 1962, 3, 42-52.

The full gamut of psychiatric classification is presented in an attempt to redefine and stabilize current nomenclature. Neurotic reactions are categorized as follows: simple nervousness, acute anxiety state, tension state, anxiety neurosis, hysterical disorders (conversion reaction), phobicobsessive states, obsessive-compulsive reactions, neurasthenia and hypochondriasis. Reactions designated as psychotic include: acute organic brain syndromes, subacute and/or chronic organic brain syndromes, the schizophrenias, pseudoneurotic schizophrenia and depressive reactions, encompassing immediate, delayed and anticipatory grief reactions, reactive depressions, depressions of nebulous genesis, involutional depression, overtly psychotic depressions, cyclic depressions and depression/masking inchoate schizophrenia. Psychophysiological stress reactions and the sociopathic disorders are also discussed. Parenteral use of thorazine is indicated during manifestation of considerable excitation or agitation. (No refs.)

[No address]

1384 London, D.R., & Milne, M.D. Dangers of monoamine oxidase inhibitors. British Medical Journal, 1962, No. 5321, 1752. [Letter]

Potentiation of pethidine by MAO inhibitors

with serious consequences has been reported in 14 different cases (including 3 deaths) culled from the literature. This drug combination may be administered accidentally. Prompt acidification of the urine coupled with increased diuresis increases the chances of recovery. Urinary excretory levels of unchanged pethidine must be elevated from 1 to 4% to exclude massive toxicity, and acidification of urine is 1 method of facilitating such excretion. The basic mechanism for pethidine potentiation involves a reduction in the rate of metabolic inactivation of pethidine by microsomal enzyme systems within liver cells, resulting in the accumulation of highly toxic metabolites. (11 refs.)

Westminster Medical School
London S.W. 1, Great Britain

1385 Ström-Olsen, Rolf. Insulin therapy. Lancet, 1962, 2, 47. [Letter]

Deep insulin therapy is advocated, and a physician explains the special department at Runwell Hospital which was constructed in the treatment block primarily to facilitate such therapy. Reduction of the number of attending nurses is accomplished by employing beds with padded sides, thus requiring only 2-3 nurses for every 6-8 patients undergoing treatment. (No refs.)

Runwell Hospital
Wickford, Essex
Great Britain

1386 Israels, M.C.G. Drug agranulo-cytosis and marrow aplasia. Proceedings of the Royal Society of Medicine, 1962, 55, 36-38.

Drug-induced agranulocytosis and marrow aplasia is reviewed in relation to many different types of drugs. The former condition was caused on occasion by tranquilizers, i.e., chlorpromazine [dosage unspecified], promazine (150-600 mg/day), imipramine (225 mg/day), meprobamate [dosage unspecified] and pecazine (75-150 mg/day). Most cases were not fatal and recovery often resulted after withdrawal; in other instances

antibiotics, transfusions and corticoid therapy were used. (18 refs.)

Royal Infirmary
Manchester, Great Britain

1387 British Medical Journal. Today's drugs. British Medical Journal, 1962, No. 5321, 1751. [Editorial]

Anileridine, a potent synthetic analgesic, resembles pethidine and, to a lesser extent, morphine. It is 2 1/2 times more potent than pethidine, remains active when administered orally and exerts a far less profoundly depressant effect upon the respiratory system and blood pressure than does morphine. It possesses a weak sedative effect and transient action. Caution is indicated in patients with impaired hepatic function. The tendency toward addiction is doubtlessly comparable to that evinced by other potent analgesics. The drug should be widely useful in treating chronic pain, postoperative pain, biliary and renal colic and may be of value in obstetrics. (No refs.)

British Medical Association
Tavistock Square
London W.C. 1, Great Britain

1388 Braceland, Francis J. Modern trends in psychiatry. Virginia Medical Monthly, 1962, 89, 75-82.

The role of psychiatry in society is discussed, from its initial relegation to the position of medicine's stepchild to its present all-pervading influence. Early psychiatry emphasized patient isolation, but even Kraepelin's concepts afforded a means of restoring order to the welter of doubt and confusion that cloaked mental illness. World War II precipitated increased rapprochement between psychiatry and medicine. Undifferentiated and paranoid schizophrenia, depression and character disorders predominate in psychiatric practice today. Rehabilitation procedures will eventually stem from community recognition of a common need. A comprehensive plan encompassing community service clinics, guidance centers, general hospital inpatient and outpatient facilities will do much to diminish the chronicity of severe mental illness. Familial acceptance is an important factor in rehabilitation procedures. (2 refs.)

200 Retreat Avenue
Hartford, Conn.

1389 Lebensohn, Zigmond M. American psychiatry— retrospect and prospect. Georgetown Medical Bulletin, 1962, 16, 3-19.

A comprehensive report on American psychiatry includes the following topics: early foundations of American psychiatry, moral treatment, indifference preceded by a morass of dirt, filth, overcrowding and isolation from medicine, the 4 cornerstones of modern psychiatry (i.e., neuropathology, neurophysiology, psychology and psychodynamics) , the somatic therapies including insulin, metrazol, ECT and the tranquilizers, the influence of psychoanalysis on American psychiatry, and, conversely the influence of American psychiatry on psychoanalysis, research in psychiatry, American psychiatry, American attitudes and the law and the ultimate outlook for American psychiatry. (18 refs.)

Department of Psychiatry
Georgetown University School of Medicine
Washington, D.C.

1390 McBride, W.G. Teratogenic effects of drugs. Medical Journal of Australia, 1962, 2, 1001. [Letter]

Cautious and careful, objective evaluation is urged before ascribing teratogenic effects to a drug. Issue was taken with certain authors who had attributed possible congenital malformations to the maternal intake of phenmetrazine or ancoloxin (meclozine and pyridoxine) during pregnancy. The 2.5% incidence of such malformations in patients taking ferrous salts, and 2-3% in patients receiving no drugs, were cited. Unfavorable observations should be reported, but incrimination in causing congenital abnormalities should

be the result of a critical analysis; patients should not be alarmed unnecessarily by uncritical accusations against drugs. (2 refs.)

143 Macquarie Street
Sydney, Australia

1391 McCutcheon, A.D. Phenacetin. Medical Journal of Australia, 1962, 2, 976-977. [Letter]

Shaw's (1962) opinion that evidence concerned with phenacetin toxicity is "poor" is contradicted. The affirmative evidence from Scandinavia, Switzerland and Germany was considered extensive and convincing; the small amount of contradictory evidence in experimental animals may not even be applicable to humans. Although only a few Australian papers have called attention to this type of toxicity, it was expected to become more apparent to the now alerted medical community. (2 refs.)

Baker Medical Research Institute
Melbourne, Australia

1392 Neil, W.H. Influence of drugs on driving. Texas State Journal of Medicine, 1962, 58, 92-97.

This detailed analysis of the effects of drugs on driving stresses the scarcity of statistical data on this important topic. Areas and drugs discussed include alcohol, narcotics (morphine, codeine and pethidine), hypnotics and sedatives (pentobarbital, amobarbital, secobarbital and thiopental) , tranquilizers (chlorpromazine and meprobamate) , antihistamines, CNS stimulants (amphetamines and caffeine) , antibiotics, hallucinogens (marihuana) , drugs impairing visual acuity (atropine), other drugs (insulin, phenytoin, primidone, trianethadione and paramethadione and drug synergism (alcohol plus barbiturates). Except for alcohol, legislative action probably is not indicated until the influence of these medications on the accident rate can be shown to be significant, but patients should be warned of the possible dangers. (16 refs.)

1217 West Cannon
Fort Worth, Tex.

1393 Lefever, Harry. The exploration of inner space. Medical Times, 1962, 90, 625-631.

This is an appeal for greater emphasis on research in the realm of the mind and mental disease. Topics discussed include the characteristics and symptoms of certain psychotomimetic agents, the metabolism and properties of serotonin, a historical survey, trends in basic research and contemporary theory. Among the agents mentioned were LSD, Cannabis extracts, bufotenin, harmine, mescaline, alcohol, barbiturates, narcotics and ataractics. The complexity and importance of this field is illustrated. (21 refs.)

Chestnut Lodge
Rockville, Md.

1394 Murti Rao, D.L.N. Drug addiction in India. Journal of the Indian Medical Association, 1962, 38, 152-153. [Editorial]

The status of drug addiction in India is detailed. Drugs mentioned include opium, morphine, heroin, ganja, cocaine, barbiturates, tranquilizers and alcohol. Among the topics discussed were incidence of addiction, the medicosocial problem, the psychological and psychopathic aspects, institutionalized treatment, legal needs, education and proposal of a governmental study committee. (8 refs.)

[No address]

1395 Cawte, J.E. Neurosis in general practice: the everyday use (or non-use) of tranquilizers. Medical Journal of Australia, 1962, 2, 378-379.

In relation to the everyday prescription of tranquilizers, patterns of prescription, the matching game (symptom to drug), the expectations of the patient and physician and the skillfulness of the physician as an interviewer are discussed. (1 ref.)

[No address]

1396 Laurence, D.R., & Webster, R.A.

Pathologic physiology, pharmacology, and therapeutics of tetanus. Clinical Pharmacology and Therapeutics, 1962, 4, 36-72.

Tetanus as a disease entity is fully described and explanations of the entire disease process are given. The convulsions and spasticity which characterize tetanus result from an exaggerated reflex response to afferent stimuli due to the suppression of balanced cerebral inhibition. Control of spasticity may be maintained by drugs which act at various sites along the reflex pathway: hypnotics and sedatives, general anesthetics, centrally-acting muscle relaxants and neuromuscular blocking agents. Agents currently used to ameliorate the effects of tetanus include mephenesin, 2-amino-6-methyl-benzthiazole, dicyclopropylhetoxime, meprobamate, phenothiazine derivatives, antitoxin, phenobarbital, paraldehyde, curare, etc. (412 refs.)

Department of Pharmacology
University College Hospital Medical School
London, Great Britain

1397 Cobb, Sanford. Muscle relaxants and consciousness. World Neurology, 1962, 3, 72-77.

The mechanisms of dulling perception, the use of curare in preventing reflex response, the use of EEG's and the processes of deafferentation and hyperventilation of patients are discussed. Factors which help patients become amnestic in relation to surgical experience are elucidated. Mechanisms of protection from perception and memory of operative experience under the conditions of very light anesthesia and complete muscular paralysis are outlined. An incidence of surgical memory as low as 1 in 1000 is reasonable justification for the plea for a little more anesthesia and a little less relaxant. (7 refs.)

Department of Anesthesiology
University of Miami School of Medicine
Miami, Fla.

1398 Adams, Henry B. Is mental illness on the increase? Virginia Medical Monthly, 1962, 89, 124-130.

Statistics on admissions to public mental institutions are analyzed and discussed with regard to: consistency of admission rates from year to year, range of differences between states, relationships among admission rates, rates of discharge, and other indices of patient movement in hospitals, the influence of sociological factors, the effects of tranquilizing drugs on rates of admission and discharge and a comparison of patient movement rates in various types of mental institutions. Effects of tranquilizers are evaluated by comparison of changes from 1950 to 1955, and it is concluded that the numerical increase in discharges has been almost identical with the increase in admissions, both figures being about 28,000. If it is legitimate to attribute the increase in discharges to the tranquilizers, it would be equally legitimate to state that the increase in admission rates was also at least indirectly attributable to the tranquilizers. Thus it is fallacious to interpret the number of persons admitted for hospital treatment as a measure of the incidence of mental illness. Finally, the author concludes that most patients are hospitalized for their maladaptive, faulty, socially disapproved patterns of personal conduct which provoke rejection from other people. Until the essential properties of the many varieties of conduct labelled as mental illness are defined, it is impossible to measure the frequency of behavioral disorders in the general population. (11 refs.)

[No address]

1399 Himwich, Harold E. Problem of specific factors in psychopharmacology. Some specific effects of psychoactive drugs. In: Rinkel, Max [Ed.] Specific and non-specific factors in psychopharmacology. New York: Philosophical Library, 1962, 3-71.

The in vitro effects of psychoactive drugs are detailed, with emphasis on reserpine and analogous amine-liberating drugs, as well as iproniazid and amine-augmenting drugs. The drug effect relationships of decarboxylase and MAO are elucidated in

relation to intracellular cerebral metabolism, i.e., a discussion of possible mechanisms of drug action. (157 refs.)

Research Division
Galesburg State Research Hospital
Galesburg, Ill.

1400 Wagner, John G. Manually sorted punched card system for pharmaceutical literature. Journal of Pharmaceutical Sciences, 1962, 51, 481-484.

The use of 5 by 8 inch Royal McBee cards and direct coding in a hand system for pharmaceutical literature was described and illustrated. Although originally designed for use in a department of product research and development in a pharmaceutical house, the cards may be valuable for the faculty of a college of pharmacy or for processing psychological data. Use of this system for a cooperative literature searching system and a separate complete article file are discussed. (12 refs.)

Pharmacy Research Section
Product Research and Development Unit
The Upjohn Co.
Kalamazoo, Mich.

1401 Malitz, Sidney. Problems of non-specific factors in psychopharmacology. Personality. Variables and drug effectiveness. In: Rinkel, Max [Ed.] Specific and non-specific factors in psychopharmacology. New York: Philosophical Library, 1962, 141-148.

Specific and nonspecific factors in psycho-pharmacology are discussed, beginning with the formula $E = (P \times T) \pm E_n \pm g + h + i + j$ where E equals drug effects, p - physiologic characteristics of the drug, T - target symptoms, e - ego strength of patient, En - environment of patient, g - dose and route of drug, h - personality characteristics of patient, i - expectations of the patient and j - expectations of the therapist. Ego strength can be characterized by N = T-e, where N is the need for drug treatment, T - severity of target symptoms and e - ego strength of subject. Many such variables must be taken into account in determining the overall effect of drugs (6 refs.)

Department of Experimental Psychiatry
N. Y. State Psychiatric Institute
New York, N. Y.

1402 Katz, Martin M., & Cole, Jonathan O. Research on drugs and community care. Archives of General Psychiatry, 1962, 7, 345-359.

This review and analysis on drugs and community care encompasses home versus hospital care for schizophrenics, a study of ataractic drugs, drugs and social therapy in chronic schizophrenia, the effect of ataractic drugs on hospital release rates, predictor variables (clinical history, sociological variables and the role of personality), data collection and analytical methods, the summation of clinical results, problems in meeting requirements of research design and recommendations on methodological issues.

NIMH
Bethesda, Md.

1403 Myerson, Ralph M. Enzymes and the central nervous system. Pennsylvania Medical Journal, 1962, 65, 803-806.

Compatibility of various enzyme systems promotes facilitation of intermediary metabolism at the cellular level of the CNS. Congenital metabolic disorders result when discrepancies occur in normal metabolic pathways due to the absence of a single enzyme. Phenylketonuria and galactosemia are typical examples of enzyme deficiencies, the enzymes in question being phenylalanine hydroxylase and galactose-1-phosphate uridyl transferase, respectively. CSF elevation of some CNS enzymes is frequently indicative of various syndromes. In relation to the biochemistry of mental dysfunction, it is theorized that an abnormality in indole metabolism (in the breakdown of epinephrine or its precursors) may be present in schizophrenia. (No refs.)

VA Hospital
Philadelphia, Pa.

1404 Sachtleben, P. Tagung der Deutschen Gesellschaft für Kinderheilkunde in Heidelberg vom 11. bis 13. September 1961 unter dem Vorsitz von Prof. Dr. Ph. Bamberger, Heidelberg. Zerebrale Anfälle. [60th Meeting of the German Pediatrics Society in Heidelberg, Sept. 11-13, 1961 under the chairmanship of Prof. Dr. Ph. Bamberger, Heidelberg. Cerebral Attacks.] Deutsche Medizinische Wochenschrift, 1962, 87, 49-51.

The papers reviewed include 1 on the clinical characteristics of childhood epilepsy, 1 on the value of the EEG in the diagnosis of cerebral attacks, several on other types of childhood convulsions, and 1 on the treatment of childhood epilepsy, by Groh, in which the speaker refers to symptomatic treatment with anticonvulsive agents, vitamin B_6 and ACTH, and mentions the use of meprobamate, phenothiazine, or nialamide in the presence of accompanying emotional disorders. The importance of proper dosage and environment is emphasized. (No refs.)

Universitäts-Kinderklinik
Homburg/Saar, Germany

1405 Ippen, H. Lichtbeeinflusste Arzneimittel-Nebenwirkungen an der Haut. [Photosensitive dermatological side effects of drugs.] Deutsche Medizinische Wochenschrift, 1962, 87, 480-488; 544-548.

A discussion of the etiology and clinical characteristics of photosensitive skin reactions, with a comparison between photodynamic and photoallergic reactions, is followed by a review of all the drugs for which such reactions have been reported. These include drugs for both external and internal use, 1 section being devoted to phenothiazine derivatives. The author then discusses the diagnosis, prophylaxis and treatment of photosensitive drug reactions on the basis of a detailed discussion of their mechanism of action. (196 refs.)

Hautklinik der Medizinischen Akademie
Düsseldorf, Germany

1406 Vandierendonck, R. Proeve ener
Synthese van het Stotterprobleem (gericht
op de therapie). [Testing some theories
concerned with stuttering (with guidelines
for therapy).] Belgisch Tijdschrift voor
Geneeskunde, 1962, 18, 225-244.

As part of an extensive review on the
etiology and treatment of stuttering, based
both on the literature and on the author's
general experiences, he mentions that
the treatment of stuttering should include
psychotherapy, drugs and speech therapy,
complemented by rhythmic exercises and
unilateral kinesitherapy. Anticonvulsive
agents such as barbiturates, hydantoins or
oxazolidines should be used only in the
presence of a hereditary epileptic trait,
which is rather common in stutterers. In
other cases, tranquilizers are recommended,
particularly meprobamate, which may
even be preferable to anticonvulsants in all
cases. Favorable preliminary experiences
with chlordiazepoxide are also mentioned.
(28 refs.)

Dienst voor Spraaktherapie
Brugge, Belgium

1407 Hargrave, Michael A. Renal damage
and phenacetin. Medical Journal of
Australia, 1962, 2, 648. [Letter]

The suggestion is made that the relatively
high incidence of peptic ulcers in patients
suffering from chronic renal disease may
be due to chronic self-medication with analgesics containing salicylates, particularly
phenacetin. Another thought was the possible value of a routine renal investigation
in ulcer patients. These patients might be
harboring latent renal insufficiency.
(No refs.)

Flat 4
1 Marne Street
Vaucluse, N.S.W.
Australia

1408 British Medical Journal. Mental
subnormality. British Medical Journal,
1963, No. 5324,177-178.

The first of 4 symposia on mental subnormality, held at the Institution of
Child Health, University of Birmingham
on November 3, 1962, encompassed the
following topics: the biochemistry of
mental subnormality (phenylketonuria,
maple-sugar disease, galactosemia, etc.),
genetically determined disorders of
cerebration (chromosomal aberrations,
including mongolism, Turner's syndrome
trisomy 21 or 22, etc. detected by
buccal smears) fetal environment (peri-
natal brain damage, kernicterus, meningitis,
encephalitis, lead poisoning, etc.)
diagnosis (thorough physical and mental
evaluation can preclude development of
permanent deleterious sequelas), and
developmental assessment (a 4-point
scale for determining proficiency in
locomotion, hearing, speech, hand
and eye coordination, and a personal-
social rating). (No refs.)

British Medical Association
Tavistock Square
London, Great Britain

1409 British Medical Journal. Amphetamines.
British Medical Journal, 1963, No.
5324, 173.

Amphetamines (amphetamine, tranylcypromine and methamphetamine), hydrazines
(phenelzine, nialamide and isocarboxazid)
and iminodibenzyl derivatives (amitriptyline and imipramine), are fully discussed
in their current role as antidepressants along
with principles of treatment and problems
of drug assessment. These drugs should
be tested for possible teratogenic effects.
Side effects from the above drugs are
fully enumerated. (7 refs.)

British Medical Association
Tavistock Square
London, Great Britain

1410 Keberle, H., Hoffmann, K., &
Bernhard, K. The metabolism of glutethimide (Doriden). Experientia, 1962, 18, 105-111

Metabolic studies on glutethimide, a mild hypnotic, are reviewed. In dogs, glutethimide is excreted almost entirely (92-94%) in the form of metabolites conjugated with glucuronic acid with the remainder in nonconjugated form. Two pathways are involved: dextrorotatory α-phenyl-α-ethyl glutarimide is hydroxylated in the glutarimide ring while the levorotatory form is hydroxylated at the side chain. When rats were given 6 mg of glutethimide p. o. and sacrificed 50 minutes later specific radioactivity ratios for the CNS were: cerebrum 226, diencephalon 300, cerebellum 281, mesencephalon 285 and spinal cord 249. Lack of cumulative effects through complete inactivation, and rapid complete elimination of its metabolites are cited as reasons for the absence of after effects and the virtual absence of side effects. (10 refs)

Forschungslaboratorien
CIBA Aktiengesellschaft
Basel, Switzerland

1411 Knoblogh, Hilda, & Pasamanick, Benjamin. Mental subnormality. New England Journal of Medicine, 1962, 266, 1045-1052.

Topics presented in relation to mental subnormality include genetic abnormalities, metabolic disorders, chromosomal aberrations including abnormalities of the sex chromosomes, autosomal aberrations, prenatal factors and maternal infection. Abnormalities mentioned included those of protein metabolism (phenylketonuria, Hartnup disease and Wilson's disease), carbohydrate disorders (galactosemia, idiopathic hypoglycemia, sucrosuria and lipochondrodystrophy), lipid disorders (infantile amaurosis, Niemann-Pick disease and the infantile form of Gaucher's disease), certain types of nonendemic goitrous cretinism, hypercalcemia, cerebro-ocular-renal disease of Lowe, nephrogenic diabetes insipidus, maple-sugar disease and congenital nonhemolytic jaundice with kernicterus. Pare et al. (1959) have suggested that 5HT decarboxylase may be

inhibited in cases of phenylketonuria. Further biochemical data are reviewed. (73 refs.)

Department of Pediatrics
Ohio State University College of Medicine
Columbus, Ohio

1412 Delay, Jean. Psychotropic drugs and experimental psychiatry. In: Wortis, Joseph [Ed.] Recent advances in Biological Psychiatry. New York: Plenum Press, 1962, 4, 111-132.

The following topics are expounded in an address emphasizing psychiatry from a historical perspective: variations in psychological "tonus", the neuroleptic syndromes, experimentally-induced states of abnormal behavior and psychodysleptic drugs as aids in treatment and diagnosis. Psycholeptic drugs are categorized as hypnotics, tranquilizers or psychic energizers, with elucidation of numerous compounds. Drug-induced psychoses manifest diverse symptomatology varying with both the drug and the individual. Psilocybin offers new avenues of therapeutic approach. A combination of chemotherapy and psychotherapy provides the most effective means of alleviating mental illness. (No refs.)

University of Paris
Paris, France

1413 Feldman, Paul E. Problems of non-specific factors in psychopharmacology. Personality. Non-drug parameters of psychopharmacotherapy. The role of the physician. In: Rinkel, Max [Ed.] Specific and non-specific factors in psychopharmacology. New York: Philosophical Library, 1962, 149-158.

The role of the physician (i.e., types of therapists) is detailed. Perusal of the drug-treatment-success-records of various staff members suggested that therapists can be classified in 3 principal types: type 1 those who are outstandingly successful, type 2 those who are moderately successful, and type 3 those who are relatively unsuccessful. The hospital population involved is fairly homogeneous, consisting primarily of patients with schizophrenic disorders and depressive syndromes. The population of therapists consisted of 21% type 1, 41% type 2 and 38% type 3. Type 1 averages significant improvement in 90% of the drug trials, type 2 in 44% and type 3 in but 4%. In spite of ample psychological data on therapists, no personality correlations in relation to success could be made. The misconception that therapeutic success with drugs is equated with lack of sophistication in dynamic psychiatry is discredited and the need for clearer delineation of the characteristics of investigators stressed. (No refs.)

Topeka State Hospital
Topeka, Kan.

1414 Beecher, Henry K. Problems of non-specific factors in psychopharmacology. Methodology. A quantitative approach to psychopharmacology. In: Rinkel, Max [Ed.] Specific and non-specific factors in psychopharmacology. New York: Philosophical Library, 1962, 85-93.

The historical origins of the quantitative approach to psychopharmacology are traced, with particular regard to the need for recognition and precise development of tools for measurement and techniques in the quantitative analysis of obtained data. Indications for increased quantification prevail in studies on schizophrenia and for the determination of psychotomimetic drug effects. Progress in the realm of behavioral science necessitates development of a system which will ultimately validate predictability. Accuracy in psychopharmacology may only be achieved through a quantitative approach to sensation. (8 refs.)

Anesthesia Laboratory
Harvard Medical School
Cambridge, Mass.

1415 Hoagland, Hudson. Problems of specific factors in psychopharmacology. Discussion. In: Rinkel, Max [Ed.] Specific and non-specific factors in psychopharmacology. New York: Philosophical Library, 1962, 72-82.

The work done on psychoactive drugs in relation to amine metabolism by Himwich (Abstract 1399) is discussed. The stock piling of serotonin by MAO inhibitors and its release by serotonin play a far more important role than levarterenol. Released serotonin has a striking sedative and parasympathetic effect. Schizophrenics show marked excitement and sympathetic overactivity with increased 5HIAA excretion after the administration of MAO inhibitors followed by reserpine. Enhancement of brain serotonin may have induced some reversal of drug effects. Similar experiments have been performed utilizing cats, dogs, rats and rabbits as subjects. (9 refs.)

Worcester Foundation for Experimental Biology
Shrewsbury, Mass.

1416 Rinkel, Max [Ed.] Specific and non-specific factors in psychopharmacology. New York: Philosophical Library, 1962, Pp. 174.

This book is a compilation of papers given at the Third World Congress of Psychiatry held in Montreal, Canada from June 4-10, 1961 under the chairmanship of Jean J. Delay. Nonspecific factors which interfere with a comprehensive and more accurate evaluation of the therapeutic efficacy of psychoactive drugs are discussed. Amobarbital amphetamine, chlorpromazine, ethotrimeprazine, imipramine, isocarboxazid, chlordiazepoxide, tranylcypromine, reserpine and some hallucinogens are among the prominent drugs detailed.

Research Division
Massachusetts Mental Health Center
Boston, Mass.

1417 New York State Journal of Medicine. Dystonic reactions produced by tranquilizers, New York State Journal of Medicine, 1962, 62, 559. [Editorial]

Dystonic reactions produced by the phenothiazines include tonic contractions, myoclonic unilateral of bilateral twitches in any muscle group, hyperextension of the neck and trunk, speech difficulties, perioral tremors, mandibular tics, impaired swallowing ability and oculogyric crisis. Marked fear usually accompanies the sudden onset of dystonic symptoms, which fortunately are brief in duration and occasionally under partial voluntary control. (No refs.)

[No address]

1418 Journal of the Indian Medical Association. Treatment of psychiatric disorders of different categories. Journal of the Indian Medical Association, 1962, 38, 234-235. [Editorial]

Insulin shock treatment, ECT and tranquilizing drugs (phenothiazine derivatives, Rauwolfia preparations, meprobamate, isocarboxazid and imipramine) are used to ameliorate acute exacerbations of psychotic behavior. Psychotherapy and occupational therapy are essential to prevent recurrences. Family attitudes must also undergo modification to the extent that the patient is exposed to the beneficial effects of affection and understanding. Mental disorders are classified as organic psychoses (acute and chronic brain disorders) and psychogenic disorders (functional psychoses including affective reactions and personality disorders, psychoneurotic disorders such as anxiety, hysteria, dissociation and obsessive-compulsive neuroses, psychophysiological disorders, personality disorders and mental deficiency). The role of the mentally defective child in society is fully elucidated. Socially maladjusted individuals such as psychopaths, drug addicts and sexual deviates are discussed from a social standpoint. (7 refs.)

Indian Medical Association
Bombay, India

1419 Journal of the Indian Medical Association. MAO inhibitors in clinical practice. Journal of the Indian Medical Association, 1962, 38, 611-612. [Editorial]

MAO inhibitors which are currently in use as psychic stimulants include iproniazid, pheniprazine, isocarboxazid, nialamide and phenelzine. Postulates are promulgated for mechanisms of drug action. These drugs augment rapport and increase insight in instances of neurotic depression. Some amelioration of psychotic symptoms may be achieved. Angina pectoris also responds favorably to treatment with MAO inhibitors, especially nialamide (50-75 mg/day) which apparently exerts the least toxic effects. Side effects include over-excitement, nervousness, muscle twitching, dry mouth, constipation, bladder disturbances, orthostatic hypotension, respiratory difficulties, etc. MAO inhibitors greatly diminish the body's ability to detoxify drugs, therefore, the following drugs are contraindicated during MAO inhibitor administration: barbiturates, amphetamine, aminopyrine, acetanilid, cocaine, procaine, meperidine, alcohol, ether and phenephrine. Antihypertensives should also be prescribed with caution. Fatal cardiovascular complications have followed phenelzine and isocarboxazid therapy. (13 refs.)

Indian Medical Association
Bombay, India

1420 Lancet. Thalidomide: Part 2. Lancet, 1962, 2, 3363-337. [Editorial]

The Invalid Children's Aid Association of Britain plans to offer coordinated services to aid all parents whose babies have been maimed by thalidomide. Personalized instructions should facilitate parental acceptance and further rehabilitation. All efforts will be made to correlate learning procedures with the normal childhood developmental pattern. Greater powers of control must be allotted to the Food and Drug Administration to diminish the possibility of exposing the public to the effects of toxic drugs. Only drugs adjudged safe beyond any doubt should be administered during pregnancy. Stringent supervisory regulations are urgently needed to control drug distribution. (17 refs.)

7, Adam Street
Adelphi
London, W.C. 2, Great Britain

1421 Herford, Mary. Thalidomide defects. Lancet, 1962, 2. [Letter]

In an effort to mitigate the effects of the thalidomide disaster, a physician suggests that the pharmaceutical house responsible for developing thalidomide contribute ; 500,000 pounds toward training personnel to deal with problems unique to thalidomide babies and to facilitate similar endeavors related to the tragedy. Coordination of the medical profession and auxiliary services is absolutely essential for any degree of efficacy. (No refs.)

Farnam Royal
Buckshire, Great Britain

1422 Journal of the American Medical Association. Double-blind studies on obstetrical analgesia. Journal of the American Medical Association, 1962, 181, 333-334. [Editorial]

Drugs used as obstetrical analgesics are evaluated. The paper by Powe et al 1962 was cited as providing evidence for the importance of using a double-blind study and doing all possible to minimize bias in order to achieve a more objective and meaningful conclusion. The possible need for differentiation of sedation and analgesia when evaluating a drug is also mentioned. (3 refs.)

American Medical Association
Chicago, Ill.

1423 Lagae, J. Singultus. [Hiccough.] Belgisch Tijdschrift voor Geneeskunde, 1962, 18, 31-33.

The etiology, prognosis and treatment of different types of hiccoughs are reviewed. Among the therapeutic techniques suggested are various types of causal treatment and symptomatic treatment with chlor-promazine, promazine, chloralhydrate, procainamide, calcium gluconate and anesthesia of the gastric mucosa with lidocaine. (No refs.)

[No address]

1424 Walter, Kurt. Zur modernen Pharmakotherapie psychischer Störungen und Erkrankungen. [The modern drug therapy of mental disturbances and diseases.] Deutsches Medizinisches Journal, 1962, 13, 179-185.

As part of a post-graduate course in physical medicine, the author presents an historical review of the development of psychotropic drugs and their role in the treatment of mental illness, from the hallucinogens and early sedatives to reserpine, phenothiazines and energizers. Implications for the etiology of neurosis and psychosis and the interrelationships between mind and body are pointed out, with special emphasis on the question of the symptomatic nature of drug effects. Side effects, the relationship between side effects and therapeutic activity, and the problem of abuse are also discussed. (No refs.)

[No address]

1425 Hofmeister, A. Neodorm—ein neues Schlafmittel. [Neodorm—a new hypnotic.] Hippokrates, 1962, 33, 434-435.

This is a brief review of the chemical and pharmacological properties, side effects, clinical indications, dosage and general effects of pentobarbital (Neodorm) in man and animals. In addition to its analgesic and anticonvulsive properties, the principal indication for the drug is insomnia; the only contraindication is liver damage. (12 refs.)

Rodenbeckerstrasse 40
495 Minden/Westphalia
Germany

1426 Sattes. Symposion über die Pharmakotherapie der Schizophrenie. [Symposium
on the drug therapy of schizophrenia.]
Deutsches Medizinisches Journal, 1962,
13, 471-472.

The central themes of a 2-day symposium
held in Germany in March of 1962 are
discussed and brief abstracts are given of
some of the important contributions from
the approximately 80 participants. Particular
attention was paid to the therapy-resistant
schizophrenias and to residual defects
remaining after successful drug treatments,
as well as to the problem of maintenance
therapy. A monograph is promised.
(No refs.)

[No address]

1427 Rundle, A. T. Etiological factors in
mental retardation. I. Biochemical.
American Journal of Mental Deficiency,
1962, 67, 61-68.

Biochemical anomalies associated with
mental deficiency can be divided into 3
groups: those involving abnormal carbohydrate metabolism or storage, those
involving amino acid or protein metabolism
and those in which a range of lipoid material
is known to be defective. Galactosemia,

idiopathic hypoglycemia, sucrosuria,
phenylketonuria, Hartnup's syndrome,
hepato-lenticular degeneration (Wilson's
disease), arginino-succinuria, cystathio-
nuria, organoaciduria (Lowe's syndrome),
congenital methemoglobinemia, maple sugar
disease, and the neurolipidoses are reviewed. (44 refs.)

St. Lawrence's Hospital
Surrey, Great Britain

1428. Rundle, A. T. Etiological factors in
mental retardation. 2. Endocrinological.
American Journal of Mental Deficiency,
1962, 67, 69-77.

Mental retardation based on thyroid,
parathyroid or insulin insufficiency is
reviewed. Hypoparathyroidism, the effects
of the various sex chromosome aberrations,
including the presence of supernumerary
chromosomes, Turner's syndrome,
Klinefelter's syndrome, nephrogenic
diabetes insipidus, hypoglycemia, dwarfism,
microcephalic dwarfism, cachectic
dwarfism, sexual infantilism associated
with mental retardation and mongolism.
(87 refs.)

St. Lawrence's Hospital
Surrey, Great Britain

See also 1444, 1478, 1497

1429 Gwynne, Peter H., Hundziak, Marcel, Kavtschitsch, Joseph, Lefton, Mark & Pasamanick, Benjamin. Efficacy of trifluoperazine on withdrawal in chronic schizophrenia. Journal of Nervous and Mental Disease, 1962, 134, 5, 451-455.

Seventy-eight chronic withdrawn schizophrenics (mean age - 49; mean hospitalization time - 20 years) were randomly divided into 3 groups, equally apportioned as to sex, and treated with total daily doses of trifluoperazine (10 - 40 mg) , chlorpromazine (100 - 400 mg) or inert placebo. Drugs were administered p.o., b.i.d. for 4 months. Benztropine methanesulfonate (2 mg. daily) was occasionally given to control side effects. Five independent evaluations, using the MSRPP Scale, were made on each patient by 3 attendants and 2 physicians in a double-blind study before the start of therapy, 2 months after the onset and at its termination. The Mann-Whitney U Test was applied to the data, i.e., significance p $<$ 0.05. After 4 months of treatment, a significant decrease in withdrawal was observed between trifluoperazine and placebo (p = 0.03) and between trifluoperazine and chlorpromazine (p = 0.02). No significant differences in other behavioral areas were noted.

Research Division
Department of Psychiatry
Ohio State University
Columbus, Ohio

1430 Bradley, William F. Adjunctive use of prozine in somatic illness. Ohio State Medical Journal, 1962, 58, 765-768.

A group of 97 patients with organic disorders complicated by superimposed psychological stress manifested as anxiety, tension or apprehension were selected from a general internal medicine practice. Forty-seven patients aged 30-65 years received Prozine (25 mg promazine plus 200 mg meprobamate b.i.d. or t.i.d.) and 50 patients of corresponding age received inert placebo for 12 weeks. Seventy-four percent of the Prozine-treated group and 18% of the placebo group became calmer. Excessive drowsiness was observed in 8 treated and 5 placebo patients, 17 and 10% respectively.

Dosage was reduced to half a tablet to combat drowsiness, and 75% of the Prozine-treated group experienced continued serenity undisturbed by drowsiness, while 20% of placebo patients experienced similar results. Minor additional side effects included nausea, weakness, insomnia and dry throat which were not ameliorated by a reduction in drug dosage. After 2 weeks on Prozine, 67% of the patients obtained 7 or more hours of sleep per night, whereas only 44% had obtained that amount of sleep prior to medication.

Central Ohio Medical Clinic
Columbus, Ohio

1431 Myrianthopoulos, Ntinos C., Kurland, Albert A., & Kurland, Leonard T. Hereditary predisposition in drug-induced parkinsonism. Archives of Neurology, 1962, 6, 5-9.

A survey was made of 728 relatives of 59 psychiatric patients (schizophrenia 47, psychosis with mental deficiency 6, manic-depressive psychosis 1 and miscellaneous 5) all over 40 years of age who received phenothiazine derivatives p.o. (600 mg chlorpromazine/day in 16 patients, 75 mg prochlorperazine/day in 14, 100 mg triflupromazine/day in 5, 12 mg perphenazine/day in 13, 100 mg promazine/day in 1 control patient, 8 mg thioproperazine/day in 3, 5 mg fluphenazine/day in 8) for 6 weeks - 6 months during which they developed parkinsonian manifestations. The survey also included 777 relatives of 67 controls who proved resistant to the potential parkinsonian effects of the above drugs. Relatives of those manifesting parkinsonian side effects yielded 13 cases of Parkinson's disease, while relatives of the controls exhibited only 3 cases. Differences were not statistically significant and further studies are necessary to determine the existence of genetic predisposition to parkinsonism precipitated by phenothiazine derivatives.

Epidemiology Branch
National Institute of Neurological Diseases
    and Blindness
NIH
Bethesda, Md.

1432 Wickstrom, Jack, and Haddad, Ray. An evaluation of the muscle relaxant properties of chlordiazepoxide: A double-blind study. The American Journal of the Medical Sciences, 1962, 244, 23-29.

The value of chlordiazepoxide (10 mg t. i. d. p. o.) as a muscle relaxant was assessed in a double-blind study of 70 patients with painful spastic disorders associated with fractures, bone disease and musculoskeletal trauma. The patients were divided into 2 equal groups: group A received the drug and rest, heat, traction, etc.; group B received a placebo and physical therapy. Ninety-five percent of group A and 48% of group B obtained adequate relief. Four unresponsive patients from group A did not respond to further chlordiazepoxide therapy; 9 out of 19 nonresponders from group B obtained definitely superior results with the known drug. Side effects (drowsiness, dizziness and ataxia) occurred in both groups; decreasing the dosage controlled these effects in group A only. Chlordiazepoxide (25-75 mg i. m.) was also tested in 11 severe, emergency orthopedic cases; the lower dosages were used with an adjunctive opiate or strong analgesics (morphine, demerol and xylocaine). Good results were obtained in 6 patients and fair in 4; a double-blind study was not used in this case.

Division of Orthopedic Surgery
Tulane University School of Medicine
New Orleans, La.

1433 Lasagna, Louis. Personality. The relation of drug-induced changes to personality. In: Rinkel, Max [Ed.] Specific and non-specific factors in psychopharmacology. New York: Philosophical Library, 1962, 114-129.

Rorschach and interview data revealed an unusually high degree of psychological maladjustment in 56 young male volunteers. Three psychotics were present in the group and 2 were hospitalized either before or after the studies. Also, postoperative patients were interviewed and assessed for Rorschach signs, and the characteristics of 54 chronically ill patients classified according to placebo reaction. The nondrug variables were often as important or more

important than the drug in contributing to the net "drug reaction." The personality of patients and their attitudes were more important determinants of the response to medication (placebo in this instance) and possible direct drug effects.

Johns Hopkins University School of
    Medicine
Baltimore, Md.

1434 Rebhun, Joseph. Long-term use of amine oxidase inhibitor (isocarboxazid) in hypertension. Journal of American Geriatrics Society, 1962, 10, 440-446.

Ten outpatients, aged 62-91 years, with refractory hypertension and depression (plus concomitant organic disease) were given isocarboxazid (10 mg/day increased to 10 mg t. i. d.) for 30-36 months. Other hypotensive agents were also administered (reserpine and chlorothiazid). Extensive laboratory tests were performed (urinalysis, cephalin flocculation, bromsulfalein, serum transaminase and nonprotein nitrogen, etc.) and blood pressure readings were determined on a weekly or bi-weekly basis. After 3 weeks of treatment, some decrease in blood pressure was noted in all patients, and a safe level was maintained in 7 for the duration of the study. Two patients gained excessive weight, manifested increased hypertension and displayed euphoric behavior. Laboratory tests remained within normal limits, with no evident hepatotoxicity. Mental depression was alleviated in all cases, as were chest pains, nausea and dizziness. Minimal transient side effects included constipation, weakness and insomnia. The hypotensive action of MAO inhibitors in general is also discussed.

205 West Pearl Street
Pomona, Calif.

1435 Gomirato, G., & Gandini, S. Considerazioni sulla dinamica del delirio primario dedotte dal trattamento con uno psicofarmaco (1, 1, 3-triciano-2-amino-1-propene). [Considerations on the dynamics of primary delirium following its treatment with a psychoactive drug - 1, 1, 3-tricyano-2-

amino-1-propene.] Giornale di Psichiatrie e di Neuropatologia, 1962, 15, 1-15.

Two cases, treated with 1, 1, 3-tricyano-2-amino-1-propene, were detailed. Both were paranoid-schizophrenics having a delirium component. Dosage was 0. 5 g t. i. d. given orally. The agent was successful in suppressing the hallucinatory and delusional factors.

Clinica delle Malattie Nervose e Mentali
Università di Siena
Siena, Italy

1436 Morrison, Benjamin O., Laburdette, Leo, & Rogers, James. Method of testing cerebral stimulant drugs for improvement in cerebration or mentation. Medical Times, 1962, 90, 269-274.

A method was described for testing an analeptic cited as Product 5032. It was tested on 18 patients with CBS (arteriosclerosis and cerebral arteriosclerosis with senile psychosis, cerebral thrombosis and cerebral vascular accidents with hemiplegia) for 6-17 weeks. Patients were evaluated objectively according to mental status work sheets for sensorium and intellect. Included were orientation, digit span, work paths, simple calculation, proverbs, the cowboy or donkey story, general knowledge and absurdities. Increases in memory and digit span should show the greatest and intelligence the least improvement. Subjectively, 48% of the patients improved. However, when evaluated objectively no improvement was demonstrable. The value of such objective testing was stressed.

Department of Medicine
Louisiana State University School of
    Medicine
New Orleans, La.

1437 Oettinger, Leon, & Simonds, Robert. The use of thioridazine in the office management of children's behavior disorders. Medical Times, 1962, 90, 596-604.

Thioridazine (0. 2 to more than 3. 0 mg/kg/ day) was administered to 279 ambulatory children aged 5-16 years in 4 diagnostic categories: hyperkinetic behavior syndrome (hyperactivity, hyperirritability and short attention span) ; retarded with associated behavioral disturbances (IQ below 75), epilepsy (grand mal, petit mal and epileptic equivalents) and miscellaneous conditions. Patients were usually studied for at least 3 months and followed up for 24 months. Where possible, the Bender-Gestalt, Goodenough Draw-A-Man and/or Ruettgers tests were utilized; evaluation was also made by parents, teachers and physicians. A partial-blind study was performed, with neither patients nor parents aware of whether drug or placebo was being used in any given case. Results obtained were good in 82 patients, fair in 87, unchanged in 72 and worse in 38. The drug was somewhat more effective in 132 patients with marked hyperactivity. Side effects (drowsiness in 16 patients, increased irritability in 6, increased hyperactivity in 6 and deteriorated behavior in 5, etc.) occurred in 38 patients, but were not of sufficient severity to require marked concern.

1405 San Marino Avenue
San Marino, Calif.

1438 Gelder, M. G., & Vane, J. R. Interaction of the effects of tyramine, amphetamine and reserpine in man. Psychopharmacologia, 1962, 3, 231-241.

The interaction of tyramine, amphetamine and reserpine was studied in 2 groups of patients: normal patients recovering from an acute psychiatric illness (usually affective) and chronic schizophrenics receiving reserpine for many months. Blood pressure response to i. v. tyramine (10 mg in 15 seconds) was used to measure the extent of peripheral depletion of levarterenol, and presumably contral stores as well, by reserpine (4-15 mg/day). The effects of i. v. amphetamine (10 mg in 15 seconds) on reserpine side effects were noted. The effects of chlorpromazine (50 fold higher than reserpine) on the central actions of amphetamine were also noted. The amphetamine effect was estimated by the patient's mood, optimism, self-confidence, well-being, talkativeness and energy; the evaluation of reserpine was based on mood, wakefulness, energy, nausea, dizziness, tremor and stuffiness of the nose. Reserpine produced a significant reduction in the pressor effect of tyramine. Amphetamine continued to produce euphoria and alerting after treatment with reserpine, but its effects were reduced by large doses of chlorpromazine. Amphetamine i.v. rapidly abolished symptoms produced by large doses of reserpine.

Maudsley Hospital
London, Great Britain

1439 Williams, Graham, & Cope, Ian. An evaluation of a combination of pethidine and levallorphan ("Pethilorfan") in labour. Medical Journal of Australia, 1962, 2, 499-503.

Pethidine (usually 100 mg in primiparas) and a mixture of 100 mg pethidine and 1.25 mg of the narcotic antagonist levallorphan were compared for their value during labor in 475 women; 205 received pethidine, 189 the mixture and 81 neither drug (ether or trichloroethylene was usually used.). The neonatal state was evaluated by Apgar ratings, the time taken for the establishment of sustained spontaneous respiration and the respiratory minute volume 4-6 hours after delivery. The extent of maternal analgesia was assessed on the state of consciousness and emotional state of the mother at the end of the 1st stage of labor, the degree of analgesia (judged by the nurse and patient) and toxicity. The addition of levallorphan to pethidine did not impair the degree of maternal analgesia. The state of the newborn was slightly better (82% with an Apgar rating of 7) where mothers had received levallorphan rather than pethidine (70% with 7).

Royal Hospital for Women
Sydney, Australia

1440 Leitch, Alexander., Cullen, William, & Robertson, Duncan. The treatment of mania by thioproperazine (Majeptil). Psychopharmacologia, 1962, 3, 307-315.

The use of thioproperazine (15-22.5 mg/day i.m., then p.o., usually 5-10 mg t.i.d., then 1-2 mg t.i.d.) was studied in 17 hospitalized patients, 22-66 years old, with mania and hypomania, in an uncontrolled

study, for a period of up to 546 days. Some patients had received prior treatment, i.e., trifluoperazine and chlorpromazine (both i.m. and p.o.) and ECT, without any favorable response. In most cases excitement, rapid continuous talking or singing and interference with other patients was greatly reduced and brought within easy control within 24 hours. Most patients seemed normal within a few days, except for some garrulousness and mild euphoria, which persisted for 1-4 weeks but did not require any restriction of activity or special observation. Virtually all treated patients were considered much improved or recovered upon discharge (17-546 days of hospitalized treatment). There were few side effects, primarily controllable (with benzhexol, benztropine or promethazine) parkinsonism in 10 patients. Most patients continued to receive 1-2 mg thioproperazine t.i.d. after discharge.

Glenside Hospital
Bristol, Great Britain

1441 Burt, C.G., Gordon, W.F., Holt, N.F., & Hordern, Anthony. Amitriptyline in depressive states: a controlled trial. Journal of Mental Science, 1962, 108, 711-730.

Amitriptyline and imipramine (150-200 mg/day p.o. for 4-6 weeks) were administered to 73 hospitalized female depressive patients (30-70 years old), divided into 4 groups (old severe, young severe, old mild, and young mild, those below 50 years of age being considered young). Evaluation in this double-blind controlled trial was based on a rating scale for depression, an overall clinical assessment and an occupational therapy rating scale; side effects were also recorded. Amitriptyline (78%) was better than imipramine (58%) in alleviating most of the symptoms of depression, especially in the old severe group of patients. Mild side effects, tremor, dry mouth, agitation, etc., were equally prevalent for both drugs.

Royal Park Psychiatric Hospital
Victoria, Australia

1442 Seager, C.P., & Bird, R.L. Imipramine with electrical treatment in depression-controlled trial. Journal of Mental Science, 1962, 108, 704-707.

A controlled, double-blind study of the effect of imipramine (25-50 mg t.i.d.) and placebo on ECT was performed on 43 hospitalized patients (40 females, 28-71 years old) with moderate to severe depression, retardation or agitation. A number of these patients were followed for 6 months as outpatients, while continuing to receive imipramine or placebo. Imipramine caused neither a reduction in the number of ECT treatments required nor any potentiation. However, the drug did markedly reduce the rate of relapse.

Barrow Hospital
Bristol, Great Britain

1443 Fox, Richard. Safe sedation? A controlled trial of "megimated" amylobarbitone. Journal of Mental Science, 1962, 108, 731-734.

Fifty-two psychiatric patients were studied who required amylobarbital, usually 200 mg/day; included were depressives, neurotics and schizophrenics. Three identical-appearing tablets were administered in a blind study: 1 contained only 100 mg amylobarbital, a 2nd had both 100 mg amylobarbital and 10 mg bemegride (megimide) and a 3rd had a placebo. Dosage was 2 tablets at night, repeated once if required; each patient received a given tablet for 3 nights. Sleep, difficulty in waking, drowsiness the following morning and side effects were noted; the patient and night nurse completed questionnaires. The bemegride did not detract from the hypnotic action of the amylobarbital nor did it cause any toxic effects. Bemegride slightly lessened the hangover effect and appeared to add to the safe use of amylobarbital.

Bethlem Royal Hospital
London, Great Britain

1444 Parnell, R.W., & Skottowe, Ian. The significance of somatotype and other signs in psychiatric prognosis. Part I & II. Proceedings of the Royal Society of Medicine, 1962, 55, 707-716.

In a lengthy discussion of medical, social and physiographic factors in mental disease, statistical comparisons of the effectiveness of chlorpromazine treatment, ECT, deep insulin coma therapy, the use of reserpine and other tranquilizers are drawn. Two-hundred-and-three male schizophrenics taken from a global population of over 3,000 were analyzed in relation to those that did not. Insulin therapy results were poor, and some of the successes in the insulin group may have been influenced by the frequency of chlorpromazine treatment. Findings in women schizophrenics were similar. Comparisons were also made of therapy with and without chlorpromazine. In each case groups treated by chlorpromazine came out best and insulin therapy worst, with reserpine and ECT occupying intermediate positions.

Warneford Hospital, Oxfordshire
Great Britain

1445 Hankoff, Leon D., Heller, Boris, & Galvin, John W. The setting in psychopharmacological treatment. Psychosomatics, 1962, 3, 201-208.

A private psychiatric clinic and a city hospital clinic each contributed a caseload of 10 ambulatory depressed females (10 involutional depression, 4 reactive depression and 6 schizophrenic depression), aged 17-59 years, to a crossover study designed to assess the effects of isocarboxazid (10 mg, t.i.d. decreased as necessary) alternated with placebo for 2 months. Psychiatric evaluation, a self-administered adjective checklist, a blood-pressure reading and a clinical rating scale comprised assessment of clinical status. A 3rd group of 10 patients acted as controls. Global psychiatric evaluation with a 5-point scale was undertaken at the close of the study. To insure greater reliability, a 4th group of 30 female schizophrenics (mean age 42.2 years) were also treated with isocarboxazid as above. Significantly better treatment response was obtained in both office and clinic groups in comparison with a clinic placebo group. A marked hiatus was observed in the timing of improvement, however, with office patients improving in about 3 weeks and clinic patients in about 6 weeks (with Wilcoxon's Test for paired replicates, p<0.01). Profuse, minor side effects were prevalent, including various somatic complaints in placebo-treated groups and insomnia, constipation, pedal edema and dizziness characterizing isocarboxazid-treated groups. Comparable results were obtained in office and clinic patients with isocarboxazid in early depression.

Department of Psychiatry
State University of New York
Downstate Medical Center
Brooklyn, N. Y.

1446 Feinblatt, Theodore M., & Ferguson, Edgar A. Phenobarbital idiosyncrasy: avoidance by use of phenobarbital-niacin. New York State Journal of Medicine, 1962, 62, 221-223.

Phenobarbital idiosyncracy, iodism and brominism result from a common mechanism, namely that of poisoning oxidative coenzymes I and II. Niacin supplies the essential portion of the pyridine nucleus necessary to reconstitute both of these coenzymes. Forty-four patients (neurosis 30, hypertension 3, insomnia 3, menopausal syndrome 2, male climacteric 2, and 4 with organic illness), aged 23-66 years with demonstrated phenobarbital idiosyncrasy (neurologic 23, cutaneous 15 and bizarre 6) received phenobarbital-niacin (average 76 mg/day, comparable to previous doses of phenobarbital) for an average of 5 weeks. In 91% of the patients, idiosyncratic reactions previously elicited by phenobarbital were completely absent when the combination was substituted. In 9%, lassitude, depression, irritability and daydreaming were equally severe on either drug. In 29 cases, symptoms of phenobarbital idiosyncrasy (depression, lassitude, pruritis, skin rash, irritability, daydreams and panic) disappeared during continued administration of phenobarbital-niacin at equivalent dosage levels.

Kings County Hospital
Brooklyn, N. Y.

1447 Maerz, John C., Lee, Howard G., & Hunter, Harry H. Psychosomatic disorders treated with trifluoperazine. Psychosomatics, 1962, 3, 220-222.

Sixty-six patients with various psychosomatic disorders (epigastric distress, bowel disorders, vasomotor disturbances, etc.), aged 18-88 years, received trifluoperazine (1-2 mg p.o., b.i.d. or t.i.d.) for 2 weeks to 3 months. Reassurance, counseling and other supportive measures contributed adjunctive therapy. The addition of antispasmodics or anticholinergics produced excellent remissions in those with gastrointestinal problems complicated by anxiety. Patients with rigid personality structures responded least favorably. No overt side effects could be detected. Anxiety was reduced and tension states were effectively controlled in 46 patients (70%) treated with trifluoperazine. Also some antidepressant effect was observed in menopausal patients.

Oaks Medical Clinic
Perkiomen and Highland Avenues
Oaks, Pa.

1448 Jones, Thomas H. Chlordiazepoxide (Librium) and the geriatric patient. Journal of the American Geriatric Society, 1962, 10, 259-263.

Chlordiazepoxide (10-25 mg t.i.d. initially, then adjusted as necessary) was administered p.o. to 25 elderly patients (aged 52-92 years) with medical or surgical disorders who had been unresponsive to phenobarbital or chloral hydrate. Many patients [number unspecified] had moderately advanced arteriosclerosis with some degree of cardiac failure which required the constant use of digitalis preparations, and many suffered from forms of recent myocardial infarctions. Chlordiazepoxide was uniformly successful in relieving anxiety, tension and depression, in resolving emotional and behavioral crises and even in ameliorating severe personality problems. There were no serious side effects, and drowsiness related to dosage was relieved by decreased dosage or drug discontinuation. Medication was beneficial to patients with serious cardiac disorders,

Clinical studies
Abstracts 1449-1451

by preventing overexertion and producing
a generally placating effect. Chlordiazepoxide is trustworthy and effective in treating
geriatric patients whose illnesses necessitate treatment in nursing homes.
Several case histories served as detailed
examples attesting to drug efficacy.

2713 Argonne Road
Millwood, Washington

1449 Bertucelli, L. Esperienze
terapeutiche con un derivato fenotiazinico:
la mepazina. [Therapeutic experiences
with a phenothiazine derivative, pecazine
(Mepazine)]. Giornale di Psichiatria e di
Neuropatologia, 1962, 15, 495-517.

The antidepressive and anxyolitic effects of
pecazine (average daily oral dose 150-
400 mg) were detailed in 32 psychiatric
case histories. Diagnoses included depression, hypomania, neurosis, confusional and psychomotor agitational syndromes,
chronic alcoholism, etc. Chlorpromazine
was also used in some cases. Pecazine
had efficient sedative action and definite
antihallucinatory activity. Antianxiety
effects were consistent and some amelioration of depression was obtained. Best
results occurred in the control of psychomotor agitation, confusional excitement
and aggression. Poor results were obtained
with endogenous depression. Side effects,
e.g., slight tachycardia, modest arterial
hypotension, slight drowsiness and asthenia,
were infrequent and negligible.

Clinica delle Malattie Nervose e Mentali
Università di Modena
Modena, Italy

1450. Brick, Harry. Use of meprobamate
in Virginia State Penitentiary - an abstract.
Virginia Medical Monthly, 1962, 89, 480-
482.

Approximately 60 male prison patients received meprobamate (400 mg/day p.o.) or
placebo for 8 weeks in a double-blind study.
Each man received the Rorschach Test
before and after 8 weeks of medication.
Posttreatment Rorschach results implied
that medication reduced neurotic tension

and anxiety factors up to 30%, while 5%
reduction occurred in the placebo group.
Medication produced a positive result
in 80% of the drug group and 27% of the
placebo group. No adverse effects or
allergic reactions were noted and no
indication of addiction appeared. At half
the recommended dosage meprobamate
reduced anxiety and tension as well as
neurotic patterns in the penitentiary.
Further research in this area is indicated.
Previously published pilot studies provided
the impetus for the present work.

Department of Mental Hygiene and
Hospitals
Richmond, Va.

1451 Jones, Carroll C. Clinical results
with a new hypnotic (chlorhexadol).
Current Therapeutic Research, 1962, 4,
327-329.

Chlorhexadol [dosage unspecified] and a
placebo were used in a double-blind
study in 40 hospitalized patients with an
average age of 43 years, 13 of whom also
received chloral hydrate (1 g/day) for
several days and some of whom had gastrointestinal complaints. Each patient served
as his own control in a crossover experiment,
usually after 7 days. Observations were
made 1-2 hours after drug administration
for sleep, apparent depth of sleep (rated
1 to 4 on ease of arousal, respiration and
body movements), disturbances of sleep,
complaints and side effects. In 59% of
the observations the patients was asleep
after chlorhexadol, compared to 53% for
chloral hydrate and 41% for placebo.
Chlorhexadol was rated as excellent in
16 patients and good to very good in 13 in
effecting sleep, compared with 10 on the
placebo. Chlorhexadol had no effect in
6 patients while placebo had no effect in
15. In the 13 patients who also received
chloral hydrate (11 rated excellent to good),
chlorhexadol was rated excellent to good
in 10. Side effects (nausea and vomiting)
were noted in 1 patient receiving chlorhexadol.

John Sealy Hospital
Galveston, Tex.

1452 Stanley, W. J., & Fleming, H. A clinical comparison of phenelzine and elec-tro-convulsive therapy in the treatment of depressive illness. Journal of Mental Science, 1962, 108, 708-710.

Thirty-eight hospitalized depressed females, 18 treated with ECT and 20 with phenelzine (15-30 mg t. i. d.), were clinically evaluated on the basis of a 9-point rating scale for depression before and after 1 month of treatment. This rating scale was based on the work of Foulds and Caine (1958) and McCall's (1958) breakdown of the Minnesota Depression Scale. Phenelzine was inferior to ECT. Side effects of ECT included transient headache, confusion and memory impairment, but there were no serious side effects. Three patients on phenelzine developed marked pedal edema on higher dosage, which responded to a reduction in phenelzine dosage and chloro-thiazide [dosage unspecified]. Also 1 patient on phenelzine developed mild postural hypotension and 1 developed a tran-sient skin rash.

Winwick Hospital
Warrinton, Lancashire
Great Britain

1453 Heaton-Ward, W. A. Inference and suggestion in a clinical trial. Journal of Mental Science, 1962, 108, 865-870.

Nialamide (25 mg b. i. d.) was tested in 51 mongoloid patients in a double-blind study, to assess its possible influence on their mental age and behavior over a 26-week period. Evaluation was based on the Revised Stanford-Binet Intelligence Scale (form L) and a behavior questionn-aire completed by the nurses. Chronologi-cal ages of these patients were 6 years 8 months to 36 years 5 months and mental ages were 1 year 7 months to 4 years 9 months. Favorable results were obtained during the 1st 13 weeks of the experiment and unfavorable results during the 2nd 13 weeks upon statistical analysis. In view of this incongruity, the data was considered inconclusive. After 20 weeks of nialamide treatment, 1 patient (the only side effect noted) developed a mild neutropenia.

Stoke Park Hospital Group
Stapleton, Bristol
Great Britain

1454 Howard, Fred J., & DeVere, Warren. Intramuscular meprobamate in the treat-ment of tetanus in infants and children. Journal of Pediatrics, 1962, 60, 421-429.

Moderately severe or severe tetanus with spastic activity constituted the presenting symptom in 15 pediatric patients 5 days to 4 years of age treated with meprobamate (80-100 mg i. m. every 3 hours) in addition to antitoxin (i. v.) and phenobarbital (4-8 mg) alternating with chlorpromazine (3-6 mg i. m.) every 3 hours. For comparison, 26 out of a series of 76 simi-larly afflicted pediatric patients received the same medication with the exclusion of meprobamate from the regimen. Seizures were better controlled with meprobamate than with the phenobarbital-chlorpromazine combination. Mild spasms were precipitated by injections early in the disease. Apnea required resuscitation in 3 patients. Many babies remained semicomatose for several days between spasms. Patients treated with meprobamate experienced spasms on less than half the number of days than those who did not receive the drug. Duration of hospi-tal stay was definitely reduced in those receiving meprobamate, and less nursing care was required. Requisite amounts of phenobarbital and chlorpromazine were decreased when meprobamate was administered, thus diminishing the risk of profound respiratory depression and spastic activity. Case histories of 3 patients were presented in full to exemplify typical improvement wrought by meproba-mate. A higher degree of relaxation was obtained with the drug, but the mortality rate was unaffected.

Dhahran Health Center
Dhahran, Saudi Arabia

1455 Meirsman-Roobroeck, G. C., Rolly, G., Lateur, J., & Geirnaert, G. Metho-hexital. Nieuw en ultra-kort werkend intraveneus barbituraat. [Methohexital. A new and ultra-short acting intravenous

barbiturate.] Belgisch Tijdschrift voor
Geneeskunde, 1962, 18, 200-209.

A review of the chemical and pharmacological properties of methohexital is followed
by a brief report of a clinical trial of a 1%
solution of this barbiturate for the induction
of anesthesia in 258 surgical patients.
Excellent results were obtained with doses
of 10-100 mg i. v. (0.9 mg/kg) in a wide
variety of surgical procedures, including
41 simple operations for which methohexital was used alone and a large number
of serious operations in which methohexital
was followed by nitrous oxide, muscle
relaxants and controlled respiration.
Given alone, the drug produced unconscious-
ness in 20-90 seconds, lasting 3-4 minutes.
It had no effect on the EEG, and mild side
effects such as apnea or respiratory depression, cough, hiccough, laryngeal spasm,
muscular twitch, mild hypotension and
tachycardia appeared in less than 10% of
the cases.

Universiteit te Gent
Ghent, Belgium

1456 Tölle, Rainer. Zur Behandlung
akuter Erregungszustände bei endogenen
Psychosen. [The treatment of states
of acute excitation in patients with endogenous psychoses.] Archiv für Psychiatrie und
Zeitschrift für die Gesamte Neurologie,
1962, 203, 85-100.

Convulsive therapy (ECT or cardiazol
convulsions) was compared with chlorpromazine (150-300 mg/day i. m. or 400-600
mg/day p. o.), levomepromazine
(75-300 mg/day i. m. or 150-500 mg/day
p. o.), perazine (150-450 mg/day i. m. or
300-800 mg/day p. o.) and thioproperazine
(30-90 mg/day i. m. or 60-140 mg/day
p. o.) in 76 severely agitated female psychotics suffering from catatonic schizophrenia
(42 cases), agitated depression, euphoria
and restlessness, mania and manic-depressive reaction. Of the 76 patients, 29 were
initially treated with convulsions, usually
followed by neuroleptic therapy, while 47
received neuroleptics initially. Clinical
evaluation by psychiatrists and nurses
indicated that agitated and stuporous
catatonics responded well to both types of

therapy; neuroleptics were also effective
in pernicious catatonia, and were more
effective than convulsions in the presence
of marked changes in affect. Convulsive
therapy, however, was more effective
in restless, euphoric schizophrenics
and severely depressed manic-depressives.
In general, the effect of neuroleptics was
more rapid and more complete than that
of convulsions. The piperazine derivatives
were preferred in catatonia and paranoia,
but levomepromazine was superior to the
other drugs in affective disorders.
Combinations of levomepromazine and one
of the piperazine phenothiazines were
effective in many cases, with a minimum
of side effects. Only 2 of the 76 patients
did not respond at all, and 1 of these
responded to insulin shock. Of the 47
treated with neuroleptics, 10 failed to
respond immediately, but 2 responded
when the drug was withdrawn and 6 of the
8 others responded to ECT.

Universitäts-Nervenklinik
Tübingen, Germany

1457 Osmond, H., & Hoffer, A.
Massive niacin treatment in schizophrenia.
Review of a nine-year study. Lancet,
1962, 2, 316-319.

Trials of nicotinic acid (niacin) in the
treatment of schizophrenia from 1952
through 1961 are reviewed. Treatment
with niacin is based on the adrenaline
metabolite theory of schizophrenia. For
example, of all patients treated for
schizophrenia in Saskatchewan from 1952
to 1955, 73 received nicotinic acid and
98 had other treatment. The nicotinic
acid group showed a distinct advantage
over the others, e. g. patients who had
never had nicotinic acid spent 2/5 of a
year in hospital, while those who received
it spent an average of 1/6 of a year.
Although the vitamin has an effect even
after patients stop taking it, it should be
taken for a year in early schizophrenia
(3-6 g/day for outpatients) and it may
then be discontinued. It should be taken
again as soon as symptoms return, for
a duration of 5 years, continuously or
intermittently. When patients in hospital
do not respond to nicotinic acid or its
amide, a course of 8-20 ECT's combined with

the agent often precipitates much improvement. It does not seem to affect the more
chronic illnesses and even in acute illness
its action is often less impressive than
that of the phenothiazines. However it is a
useful adjunct in the treatment of schizophrenia, both for acute cases and for the
reduction of relapse rate.

Saskatchewan Hospital
Weyburn, Saskatchewan
Canada

1458 Khonchak, M. & Viktor, A. Opyt
primeneniya preparata meprobamate (An-
daksina) pri lechenii predmenstrual'nogo
simptomokompleska. [Experimental use of
a meprobamate preparation (Andaxin) in the
treatment of the premenstrual symptom
complex.] Akusherstvo i Ginekologiya, 1962,
1 , 29-31.

Meprobamate (400 mg t. i. d. or 200 mg
t. i. d. plus 400 mg at bedtime, p. o.) was
used in 86 cases of premenstrual tension.
Treatment was usually begun 6-8 days before onset of menstruation and continued
for 11 days thereafter, but in some cases a
5-day treatment period was given around
the time of ovulation. Symptoms disappeared completely in 42 cases, with considerable
improvement in 16, improvement in 19 and
failure in 7. A particularly good response
was seen in patients with symptoms of
hyperexcitability. Side effects were severe
in 1, moderate in 1 and mild in 7 cases, the
most severe being in allergic skin reaction
and fever.

Janos Hospital
Budapest City Council
Budapest, Hungary

1459 Aronson, Philip R., & Hosbach,
Richard E. Chronic hyperventilation syndrome clinical results, electrocardiographic
findings with chlordiazepoxide. Angiology,
1962, 13, 23-31.

Eleven patients with chronic hyperventilation syndrome, 4 adolescent females ages
11 to 14 and 7 adults (3 male and 4 female)
aged 18 to 52 years, were treated in a
double-blind study. All patients were seen

every 1-3 weeks and medication frequently
changed so that either placebo or chlordiazepoxide (15-40 mg daily was administered. An alkalemia after hyperventilation,
both with and without chlordiazepoxide, was
consistently produced and the chloride and
sodium levels were unaltered after over-
breathing. Chlordiazepoxide did not affect
CO_2 combining powers which tended to fall
after 2 minutes of hyperpnea. Five out of
the 11 were symptomatically relieved by
chlordiazepoxide hyperventilation and the
less common ST segment depression,
appeared to be inhibited by the medication.
This resulted in a normal ECG and therefore
less confusion with "false positive" Master
two-step exercise tests and so-called "non-
specific borderline" patterns. The changes
in serum potassium levels or heart rate
(sympathetic effect) do not seem to explain
these findings. A direct myocardial or,
more likely, CNS effect is possible.

Medical Arts Building
Norwich, N. Y.

1460 Williams, Meyer, Niebel, Harold H.,
& McGee, Thomas F. Effects of oxanamide
on anxiety during oral surgery. Journal of
Oral Surgery, Anesthesia, and Hospital
Dental Service, 1962, 20, 101-107.

The effect of oxanamide (Quiactin; 400 mg
p. o.) on preoperative anxiety was tested in
a double-blind placebo-controlled study involving 300 male veterans awaiting dental
surgery. Evaluation was by means of the
Taylor Manifest Anxiety Scale, filled out 1
hour before tooth extraction (just before
administration of either the drug, a placebo
or nothing). Also a special anxiety scale
was filled out by the dentist post-operatively.
Neither oxanamide nor placebo had any
significant effect on the degree of preoperative anxiety as measured by the Anxiety
Scale; both, however, produced improvement
in subjective well-being and most patients
seemed overtly less anxious. Dentists
were unable to distinguish between oxanamide
and placebo-treated patients.

Dental Service
West Side VA Hospital
Chicago, Ill.

i

1461 Nahunek, Karel, Rodova, Alena, Hosak, Ladislav, Jaros, Milos & Hadlik, Josef. Nialamid und seine Kombinationen mit Stoffen von Reserpincharakter (Fenoharman, Reserpin) bei der Therapie endogener Depressionen. [Nialamide and its combinations with reserpine-like substances (fenoharmane, reserpine) in the treatment of endogenous depressions.] Deutsches Medizinisches Journal, 1962, 13, 424-425.

Nialamide (increasing doses up to 200-400 mg/day for 7-60 days) was first tried alone in 25 patients with various types of endogenous depression. Cure or marked improvement was obtained in 8, usually within 2 weeks, partial improvement in 3, no effect in 10 and aggravation in 4. Patients with anxious depression failed to respond. Nine of the patients who did not reapone were then treated with nialamide (up to 150 mg/day) plus fenoharmane (up to 200-300 mg/day) for 7 days, followed by nialamide plus reserpine (up to 2-3 mg/day) for 7-21 days. No improvement was observed with fenoharmane, and only 1 case responded to nialamide plus reserpine. There were no serious complications, the only side effects being migraine headache, insomnia, hypomania, confusion, and nausea and vomiting. Preliminary studies on the effect of 75 mg of nialamide on psychomotor function in 10 patients showed a stimulatory effect on reaction time, tapping rate, free association and arithmetic ability, which could not, however, always be correlated with subsequent clinical improvement.

Psychiatric Clinic
J. E. Purkinje University
Brno, Czechoslovakia

1462 Kieser, Jürgen. Zur Methodik der kontrollierten Hypothermie in der psychiatrischen Klinik. [The technique of controlled hypothermia in the psychiatric clinic.] Archiv für Psychiatrie und Zeitschrift für die Gesamte Neurologie, 1962, 203, 185-195.

In order to prevent injurious effects from the intensity of the body's own defense mechanisms, the author recommends partial neuroplegia and hypothermia in certain diseases of the nervous system, particularly encephalitis, meningo-encephalitis, meningitis, acute exacerbations of cerebral forms of thromboangitis obliterans, and infective-toxic psychoses. Treatment, presented in schematic form, consists of premedication with a lytic cocktail (50 mg each of chlorpromazine and promethazine, and 2 cc each of pethidine and hydergin). Subsequent infusion during artificial cooling include diethazine (250 mg and 125 mg), chlorpromazine and promethazine (each 50 and 100 mg), pethidine (1 cc) and hydergin (1 cc and 1 ampule), all in suitable media containing sugars, vitamins, etc. Rapid cooling and subsequent rapid reheating of the body is stressed, since both transtional phases are fraught with danger. Proper care must be taken with respect to nutrition, hormonal substitution, mineral balance, and circulation.

Psychiatrische und Neurologische Klinik
Universität des Saarlandes
Homburg/Saar, Germany

1463 Birkmayer, W., & Neumayer, E. Die Normalisierung des affektiv-vegetativen Pegelstandes. [Normalization of the level of the affective-automatic nervous system.] Deutsches Medizinisches Journal, 1962, 13, 433-437.

On the basis of experience with fluphenazine (initially 1 mg t. i. d. p. o., doubled in case of need) in 110 patients with affective-autonomic arousal reactions due either to sensory or mental stimuli or organic disease, as well as a theoretical review of neurophysiology and the etiology and treatment of vegetative dystonia and autonomic lability, the authors conclude that fluphenazine is the best available regulator of the reticular formation, increasing its sensitivity threshold without entailing side reactions such as lassitude, exhaustion, or general depressive symptoms. However, the authors caution against the higher dosages, since only the rapidity, but not the effectiveness of its action, is increased. EEG studies in 20 patients showed a general increase in the alpha effect and inhibition of the arousal reaction. In organic disease, the drug should be combined with specific therapy.

Neurologische Abteilung
Versorgungsheimplatz 1
Vienna, Austria

1464 Deleanu, M., Sirbu, A., & Asgian, B.
Luftionen in der Behandlung von Schlaflo-
sigkeit bei psychogenen, neurotischen
Zuständen. [Ionized air in the treatment
of insomnia in psychogenic, neurotic cases.]
Deutsche Gesundheitswesen, 1962, 17,
1329-1331.

The results of treating 100 cases of
psychogenic insomnia by means of ionized
air are reported. Treatment consisted of
daily sessions during which the patients
inhaled negatively ionized air having
300-12000 ions/ml, depending on the
patient's respiratory rate, initially for
15 minutes, increasing to 40 minutes over
10-20 days. Results were favorable in
65 cases, the duration, depth, and onset of
the sleep being such as to cause the
patients to feel rested. A recheck of 47
of these patients 3-15 months later showed
persistence of the favorable effects. In
13 patients, temporary improvement
occurred, but insomnia recurred after
physical trauma, intellectual overwork, or
illness. In some cases, resumption of
treatment again had favorable results. In
the remaining cases, improvement was at
best transitory. In no case did serious side
effects arise, and the occasional headaches
and restlessness were only temporary.

Institutul de Igiena
Cluj, Romania

1465 Kronberger, Leo. Über die Verwendung eines Langzeit-Sedativums in der
präoperativen Zeit und dessen Einfluss auf
die Blutgerinnung. [On the use of a long-
acting sedative during the preoperative
period and its influence on coagulation.]
Deutsches Medizinisches Journal, 1962,
13, 14-16.

Doscalun, a long-acting sedative containing
0.1 g atropine-N-n-octyl-bromide and
0.075 g phenobarbital, was administered
in the form of gelatin sustained-release

capsules to 47 patients, including 35
surgical patients who were treated with
the drug 6 days before and 8 days after
the operation. All seemed markedly
more relaxed and even-tempered.
Functional disturbances common to the
operations either vanished or else were
prevented. Determinations of the
antithrombin-time and heparin-time in
12 of these patients showed significant
effect against thrombosis. This effect
was not comparable to that of anticoagulants.
An additional 12 patients, who were subjected
to endoscopies only and were treated 2 days
before and on the day of this procedure,
showed no significant change in antithrombin-
and heparin- times.

Chirurgische Universitätsklinik
Graz, Austria

1466 Gutzmann, Hermann. Über die
Möglichkeit bzw. Notwendigkeit der
medikamentösen Behandlung des Stotterns.
[The possibility and necessity of drug
treatment of stuttering.] Deutsches
Medizinisches Journal, 1962, 13, 467-469.

The author reports his experience with
methylpentynol for the treatment of
stuttering in approximately 40 patients.
The drug is available in 0.25 g capsule
form or as drops (30 drops = 1 ml = 0.15 g).
Ten patients showed no improvement or
retrogressed. Another 12 patients showed
partial improvement under treatment which
was, for other reasons, suspended before
completion. Finally, 15 patients responded favorably. Dosages are stated
to be very variable, but are not given
except in a few cases. The drug appears
highly promising in cases uncomplicated
by cerebral disorders.

Poliklinik für Stimm- und Sprachkranke
Freie Universität zu Berlin
Berlin, Germany

1467 Finke, H. Über die Behandlung der
Depression mit Nardil (Phenelzin) in der
ambulanten Praxis. [Ambulatory treatment
of depression with Nardil (phenelzine).]
Hippokrates, 1962, 33, 312-316.

Phenelzine (average 4 tablets/day) was used over a 2 1/2-year period in 72 ambulatory patients falling into 4 groups: endogenous depression; reactive, neurotic depression and collapse conditions with depressive symptomatology; involutional and climacteric depression; and schizophrenia with depressive symptoms. Out of 25 patients in the first group, 15 were cured, 4 greatly improved, and 6 somewhat improved. In the second group, 23 were cured or greatly helped and 7 showed moderate improvement. In the third group, 3 showed no change and 11 either considerable improvement or total cure. In the fourth group (3 patients), there were no cures. Maintenance therapy was given at 1 tablet/day. The only side effects noted were orthostatic hypotension, headaches, dizziness, and respiratory difficulty, all of which could be eliminated by reducing the dosage or, in cases of hypotension, by administration of vasopressor drugs.

Wilhelmstrasse 5
Kassel 35, Germany

1468 Klein, Donald F., & Fink, Max. Behavioral reaction patterns with phenothiazines. Archives of General Psychiatry, 1962, 7, 449-459.

Two-hundred-and-seven hospitalized patients received psychotherapy and drugs; chlorpromazine (600-2000 mg/day), promazine (600-1000 mg/day), prochlorperazine (30-90 mg/day) or imipramine [dosage unspecified] were used. Evaluation was made essentially on patterns of changes in 8 target symptoms, i.e., suppressive denial, reduction of anger, affective stability, autistic compliance, decreased agitated depression, somatizing, unaffected episodic agitation, unaffected episodic anxiety and miscellaneous. Improvement was general in all categories except unaffected episodic agitation and anxiety. Extrapyramidal side effects were controlled by trihexyphenidyl, orphenadrine or procyclidine, the latter being favored (dosage 10-15 mg daily). A discussion relating to current psychopharmacological research, patient population descriptions, medication effects, target symptoms and modes of drug action is also included.

Department of Experimental Psychiatry
Hillside Hospital
Glen Oaks, N. Y.

1469 Carrier, J., Hamoneau, G., Plassat, & Bernes, J. Contribution à l'étude des thérapeutiques antialcooliques. [Contribution to the study of antialcoholic therapies.] Journal de Médecine de Lyon, 1962, No. 1008, 647.

A total of 189 treatments was carried out, 145 with apomorphine [no dosage specified] and 43 with disulfiram [dosage unspecified]. On the basis of sobriety for at least a year 10.6% were improved with apomorphine and 37.2% with disulfiram.

Hôpital Psychiatrique de Saint-Jean-de-Dieu
Lyon, France

1470 Broussolle, P., Achaintre, A., Tiebaut, & Barbier. Etudes évolutives et comparatives à l'aide du test de comportements de Fergus Falls. [Developmental and comparative studies on behavior using the Fergus Falls test.] Journal de Médecine de Lyon, 1962, No. 1008, 644.

In a brief note, the Fergus Falls test was found to be restricted to banal components of behavior and insufficiently centered on the psychopathology of the subject. A hospitalized group of geriatric patients was studied weekly for several months. The test did allow more objective judgement when coupled with the personal impressions of the therapist.

[No address]

1471 Miribel, J., & Ferreno, E. Le P.M. 671 en dehors du Petit Mal Epileptique. [P.M. 671 aside from petit mal epileptic seizures.] Journal de Médecine de Lyon, 1962, No. 1008, 651.

Ethosuximide (P.M. 671) was used in treatment of 80 patients, most with petit mal epilepsy but 10 with other conditions, e.g., Ramsay-Hurt syndrome,

infantile encephalopathies and other
conditions with abnormal EEG's. The
drug [dosage unspecified] was found as
efficacious in these conditions as it is in
petit mal epilepsy.

[No address]

1472 Oltman, Jane E., & Friedman,
Samuel. Comparison of temporal factors
in depressive psychoses treated by EST
and antidepressant drugs. American
Journal of Psychiatry, 1962, 119, 579-580.

A statistical comparison was made between
manic-depressive female patients, 119
in the depressive phase who received ECT
(EST) for 3 years and 72 comparable
patients who received antidepressant drugs
for a similar period of time. Follow-up
studies were maintained for 2 years.
(The 2nd period of study was prorated to
equal the initial time span.) A 46% overall
rise in hospital admissions accompanied
a 37% increase in depressive psychoses.
Six percent of the drug-treated patients
received some ECT during the initial
portion of the study. Patients in the drug
group enjoyed a diminished period of
hospitalization. With ECT, 60% of the
patients were hospitalized for more than
3 months as compared with 31% in the
drug group. Individual hospitalization in
excess of 6 months totaled 24% with ECT
and 10% with drugs. Average length of
total hospitalization during the drug era
was 37% of that observed during ECT.
After 2 years, 20% of the ECT group and
6% of the drug group were still hospitalized.
One drug-treated patient committed suicide.
Readmissions were slightly in favor of
the ECT group.

Fairfield State Hospital
Newtown, Conn.

1473 Thorn, Ingrid. Primidone and
chlordiazepoxide in cerebral palsy. Developmental Medicine and Child Neurology,
1962, 4, 325-327.

Chlordiazepoxide (0.25-1 mg/kg p.o.) or
primidone [dosage unspecified] were administered for 1 month to 1 year to 50 patients

aged 1-15 years with athetosis or quad-
riplegia due to cerebral palsy. The drugs
reduced muscular hypertonicity, improved
performance of voluntary movements, partially reduced hyperkinetic movements,
diminished sleep disturbance due to muscular activity and crying but exerted no
definite effects on emotional reactions.
Drug effects were often observable within
24 hours, and were optimal in cases of
athetosis or rigidity. Twenty patients
responded favorably, 16 moderately, 10
not at all and 4 poorly. Side effects included drowsiness in 23, irritability and
depression in 6 and enuresis and encopre-
sis in 1. Individual patients often reacted
differently to primidone and to chlordiazepoxide. Combined results were about
equally efficacious. Work is contemplated
with diazepam. Drug therapy is a valuable
adjunct to the standard therapeutic regimen utilized in cerebral palsy.

University Clinic of Pediatrics
Rigshospitalet
Copenhagen, Denmark

1474 Keats, Sidney, Kambin, Parviz, &
Nordlund, Thora. Clinical experiences
with chlordiazepoxide (Librium) in infantile cerebral palsy. Developmental Medicine and Child Neurology, 1962, 4, 336-
337.

Chlordiazepoxide (5-40 mg/day p.o.) was
administered for 1 1/2 - 7 months to 86
children with cerebral palsy who had undergone treatment for an average of 3 years.
Using absences of side-effects and improvement in physical and emotional status as
criteria for evaluation, 16 children were
rated as good, 25 as fair, 35 without
change and 10 as poor. Chlordiazepoxide
was tolerated best by spastic cerebral
palsy patients. Athetoid and ataxic patients
could not tolerate high doses. Emotional
status was improved and progress was observed in the physical therapy schedule.
A muscle relaxant effect was exerted in the
rigidity group. Further studies are indicated, particularly in patients whose progress is hampered by anxiety and tension.

Clinical studies
Abstracts 1475-1478

Cerebral Palsy Treatment Center
New Jersey Orthopedic Hospital
179 Lincoln Avenue
Orange, N. J.

1475 Green, Carl L. Manic depressive
psychosis,responded favorably to ECT and
medication, particularly chlorpromazine.
A 51-year-old male patient evidencing the
manic phase of manic depressive psychosis
received ECT and tranquilizers [unspecified]
which precipitated a return to an apparently
normal functional status. Extensive discussion of the cas followed presentation of
the history.

Louisville General Hospital
Louisville, Ky.

1476 Gruber, Charles M., Jr., & Baptisti,
Arthur, Jr. Effectiveness and acceptability
of single oral doses of morphine in postpartum patients. Journal of Laboratory and
Clinical Medicine, 1962, 60, 879.

In a double-blind study, capsules containing
placebo or 15-120 mg of morphine were
administered to groups of 6-200 postpartum
patients after which drug effectiveness,
acceptability and safety were determined
from 1-6 hours after drug administration.
Frequency and intensity of symptoms were
also evaluated 6 hours after drug administration. Since changes in pain intensity were
directly proportional and relief of pain inversely proportional to the initial pain, drug
efficacy comprised a summation of these 2
estimates of analgesia. Thus, the effective-
ness/acceptability ratio of dose-response
was calculated for morphine. This assay
technique will be evaluated by comparing
results with those obtained from using nor-
acymethadol, and experimental drug.

[No address]

1477 Sanger, Maury D. The use of tranquilizers and antidepressants in allergy. Annals
of Allergy, 1962, 20, 705-709.

After presenting a discussion of the allergic
patient, pointing out that he is frequently
under both physiological and psychological

stress, the general action of the psychotropic drugs is reviewed. A study in which
tranquilizers and/or antidepressants were
administered to 186 patients selected from
a larger group on the basis of a 2 year study
is discussed. These patients had "break-
throughs" although suitable antiallergic
treatment was used. Tranquilizers including meprobamate, prochlorperazine, perphenazine, chlordiazepoxide, phenobarbital,
etc. (dosages not given) administered to
121 patients produced good to excellent results in 60%. Antidepressants including
nialamide, phenelzine, amphetamine,
imipramine, and amitriptyline administered
to 113 patients (including 48 who did not
respond to tranquilizers) produced good to
excellent response in 61%. The most frequent side effect was drowsiness with only 1
severe reaction reported in a 6-year-old
child who had been given 24 mg doses of
perphenazine. Responses to MAO inhibitors
was slower with more side effects. Best
results were obtained with imipramine and
particularly amitriptyline which were
effective in 5-7 days. Three case histories
are given as illustration.

Veterans Administration
Brooklyn Outpatient Clinic
Brooklyn, N. Y.

1478 Bernstein, Arthur, & Simon, Franklin.
Anxiety and angina pectoris. Angiology,
1962, 13, 17-22.

The mechanisms of pain in angina mediated
through catecholamines and renal pathways
are reviewed. Major factors precipitating
angina pectoris are physical effort and
emotional stress. Management of the former
is self-evident and the latter difficult.
Emotional factors also present a problem
in evaluating the therapeutic efficacy of antianginal drugs. Neither supposedly objective
tests, double-blind studies, nor "clinical
impressions" can be depended upon to give
adequate criteria for critical evaluation,
and care must be taken to avoid dependence
upon any single technique. Experience has
shown that papaverine, dioxyline, the
nitrates and MAO inhibitors are effective
antianginal agents. Their efficacy is considerably enganced by the addition of a
sedative. In this respect, the barbiturates

552

and tranquilizers have been of great help, but undesirable side effects, particularly oversedation and habituation, limit their usefulness. The authors have used chlordiazepoxide 5 mg q. i. d in combination with papaverine or dioxyline phosphate in 120 patients with angina for a period of 1-2 years. there has been definite improvement in 90% but reports of drowsiness in 10%. Use of an MAO inhibitor as a single agent in the future shows great promise, as some possible MAO inhibitor mechanisms of action are: coronary dilation through increased 5HT hemic content; blockade of neurohumoral CNS transmission in sympathetic ganglia; decreased levarterenol sensitivity of the heart, and changes in carbohydrate metabolism.

2130 Millburg Avenue
Maplewood, N. J.

1479 Sumner, David. The treatment of parkinsonism with UK 738: a clinical trial. American Journal of Psychiatry, 1962, 119, 534-537.

Twenty patients took part in an open trial with methylbenztropine (UK 738). The dose used ranged from 4-10 mg/day in divided doses. Six mg was found to be th optimal dose. Sixteen of the 20 improved, 1 was unchanged and 3 found intolerant. At this point a double-blind crossover study lasting 3 months was undertaken using 20 patients. Identical tablets contained either 2 mg methylbenztropine, and inert substance or 2, 5 mg benzhexol. Methylbenztropine had only a very slight effect on the symptoms of Parkinson's disease and was not as effective as benzhexol. No side effects were seen with benzhexol but 2 patients complained of lightheadedness with methylbenztropine.

Neurological Registrar's Office
General Infirmary
Leeds, Great Britain

1480 Pearse, J. J., & Reiss, Max. Symposium on psychoendocrinology. II. Psychoendocrine aspects of mental retardation. Canadian Psychiatric Association Journal, 1963, 8, 14-23.

The relationships between mental and physical retardation were studied in 150 subjects. Most were diagnosed as "undifferentiated" and "familial"; all revealed the following indications of endocrine insufficiency: retardation in growth and weight, thyroid hypofunction, adrenocortical hypofunction and retardation in gonadal development. The patients were approximately 9 to 15 years of age. They were treated with thyroid and/or gonadotropic hormone, e. g., 2-3 grains of dried thyroid daily, 1000-5000 of gonadotropic hormone. In mongoloids, I^{131} neck uptake and 24-hour red cell uptake (radioactive triliodothyronine) studies were undertaken. While mongoloids examined showed signs of gonadal underdevelopment, they did not seem to suffer from thyroid deficiencies. Degrees of improvement throughout the caseload were exemplified in 4 case histories, e. g., improvement in behavior and I. Q. in a hypothyroid patient.

Neuro-Endocrine Research Unit
Willowbrook State School
Staten Island 14, N. Y., N. Y.

1481 Woods, Grace E. Preliminary clinical trial of carisoprodol in infantile cerebral palsy. Developmental Medicine and Child Neurology, 1962, 4, 28-34.

Forty-six cases of cerebral palsy (9 athetoid, 25 spastic diplegia and 12 various) were treated with carisoprodol, beginning with 250 mg morning and midday. Readings were made by various staff members, e. g., occupational therapists. Marked improvement was noted in 16, some improvement in 17, no improvement in 11 and the condition was worsened in 2. Athetoids showed the most marked degree of improvement and spastic diplegics also showed improvement. Drowsiness was a prevalent side effect. This was considered a serious impediment to learning in these children. Irritability was also common and, in 1 child, controlled with thioridazine. The latter drug was recommended for controlling this side effect.

Hortham Hospital
Almondsbury, Bristol
Great Britain

1482 Blom, S. Trigeminal neuralgia: its
treatment with a new anticonvulsant drug
(G-32883) . Lancet, 1 , No. 7234, 839-840.

G-32883 (400-800 mg/day p.o.) was
administered to 11 patients with classical
trigeminal neuralgia for 6 months. Six
patients were symptoms free within 24
hours. Slight numbness remained in 4
patients, and 1 feebleminded woman was
only partially aided by the drug (i.e., her
attacks became less frequent) . Slight
giddiness which subsided in a few days
constituted the only side effect in 6, while
exanthema developed in 1 patient. Four
patients who were previously unresponsive
to diphenylhydantoin reacted favorably to
G-32883 without the vertigo which had
precluded diphenylhydantoin administration.
When dosages of G-32883 were lowered
or the drug withdrawn, paroxysmal pain
returned within 24 hours. No conclusions
can be drawn as of yet with respect to
long term drug effects. Prior to the
advent of G-32883, diphenylhydantoin
(300-600 mg/day p.o.) was administered
to 22 patients with trigeminal neuralgia
for 6 months to 3 years. Operations were
performed in 3 cases due to failure of drug
treatment or development of intractable
side-effects. Freedom from pain prevailed
in 8, 9 received considerable amelioration,
1 experienced only slight improvement and
4 were unaffected. Moderate to severe
vertigo occurred in 14, necessitating
cessation of treatment in 2 (who were
vastly improved on G-32883) . Two reacted
well initially to diphenylhydantoin, but
could obtain no real long-term relief until
G-32883 was substituted.

Department of Neurology
University Hospital
Uppsala, Sweden

1483 Tortora, Anthony R. Influence of
acetophenazine (Tindal) upon the attitude
of cardiac patients. Journal of American
Geriatrics Society, 1962, 10, 270-273.

Fifty heart patients, aged 34 to 86 years,
were given acetophenazine (Tindal) , 20 mg
tablets 2-4 times daily. The diagnoses
included 11 hypertensive arteriosclerotic
heart disease, 11 arteriosclerotic heart
disease, 11 postmyocardial infarction,
2 rheumatic heart disease, 2 coronary
insufficiency, 2 essential hypertension,
1 premature ventricular contractions,
1 heart block and 9 cardiac neurosis cases.
Nineteen had definite psychoneuroses and
2 Parkinson's disease. A study of 12
angina pectoris patients was also made,
and these cases were given a coronary
vasodilator for 3 weeks followed by the
addition of 20 mg acetophenazine t.i.d.
for 4 weeks. Then the vasodilator was
replaced with a placebo for 3 more weeks.
The degree of frequency of anginal pain
was recorded during each of the 3 courses
of treatment. There was a definite
reduction in the frequency and severity
of pain in 7 who were emotionally upset
when acetophenazine was added to the
regimen. Four patients who had
concomitant neoplastic disease needed
less analgesics. Improvement in the 50
patient. case load was 27 excellent, 17
good and 6 poor. Twelve of the 50 cases
showed mild and transient side effects:
4 experienced drowsiness which disappeared
with dosage reduction; pruritis was observed
in 3 which persisted in 2 despite dosage
reduction, and 2 patients complained of
mild agitation during the first 4 days of
acetophenazine therapy. Further 1 case
each of heartburn, headache and dry
mouth occurred.

8303 Fourth Avenue
Brooklyn 9, N.Y.

See also 1370, 1375, 1380, 1413, 1498,
1606, 1614, 1651.

1484 Jones, E. B., & Williamson, D. A. J. Thalidomide and congenital abnormalities. Lancet, 1962, 2, 222. [Letter]

Apparently the recent increase in the incidence of congenital limb defects is due to thalidomide and numerous other nonspecific operant factors, the identity of which are presently unknown. Only 1 history of thalidomide administration in early pregnancy was obtained in 8 instances of birth defects.

Royal Hampshire County Hospital
Winchester, Great Britain

1485 Wroblewski, Felix. Follow up of thioridazine administration. American Journal of Psychiatry, 1962, 119, 589. [Letter]

A physician is accused of misrepresentation in a paper entitled "Jaundice follow-up of thioridazine administration" describing subclinical jaundice in a patient with transient minimal elevations in serum bilirubin and serum transaminase activity following administration of thioridazine. Increasing evidence indicates that minimal elevations in serum transaminase concomitant with administration of chemotherapeutic agents may reflect alterations in liver cell permeability or hepatic drug metabolism rather than drug-induced hepatotoxicity. Frequently, continued administration of a drug associated with transient minimal serum transaminase elevation has resulted in a spontaneous return of the serum laboratory test aberrations or hepatotoxic manifestations to normal levels. Drugs should not be classified as hepatotoxic when clinical aspects and liver function tests remain normal.

Memorial Hospital for Cancer and Allied Diseases
New York, N. Y.

1486 Block, Stanley L. Reply to the foregoing. American Journal of Psychiatry, 1962, 119, 590. [Letter]

In reply to queries about his previously published article "Jaundice following thioridazine administration", a physician reaffirms that hepatotoxicity may occur from thioridazine administration, and substantiates this viewpoint with a case history. The transient changes in serum bilirubin and transaminase which began after 9 months of drug administration returned to normal limits upon discontinuation of therapy. The jaundice described was subclinical and classified as such. Despite concomitant metastatic carcinoma, the patient presently remains in good health with no evidence of hepatic malfunction.

[No address]

1487 Luke, Elizabeth. Addiction to mentholated cigarettes. Lancet, 1962, 2, 110-111.

A case of a 58-year-old woman, who became addicted to mentholated cigarettes (up to 80 per day), is described. She developed toxic acute psychosis and was hospitalized as an emergency because of bizarre overactivity which became unmanageable. She had gastrointestinal upset with occasional vomiting; she became oversensitive, irritable and quarrelsome. Her speech was slow and slurred and her gait ataxic. Laboratory and other diagnostic studies were negative. When she stopped smoking the mentholated cigarettes, symptoms disappeared; a brief test with 1 grain menthol t. i. d. reproduced the symptoms.

Royal Mental Hospital
Aberdeen, Great Britain

1488 Jacobziner, Harold, & Raybin, Harry W. Accidental chemical poisonings. New York State Journal of Medicine, 1962, 62, 550-553.

Two fatalities are presented, 1 due to an overdose of glutethimide (20 g) in a 47-year-old suicidally depressed male and the other due to a ruptured duodenal ulcer complicated by elevated urine and plasma barbiturate levels in an 8-month-old female admitted in coma. A 3rd case was also described; dry-ice dissolved in water ingested by a 3-year-old female produced no untoward effects.

Poison Control Center
The City of New York Department of Health
New York, N. Y.

1489 Garretson, Harvey F., Jr., & Moffitt, Ellis M. Imipramine hydrochloride intoxication. Journal of the American Medical Association, 1962, 179, 456-458.

Nonfatal imipramine intoxication occurred in a 22-month-old male following ingestion of imipramine (25 mg). Drowsiness was followed by severe continuous convulsions, opisthotonos, profound respiratory depression, circulatory collapse, hypotension unresponsive to vasopressors and cardiac arrhythmias. Therapy consisted of controlling seizures, maintaining respiration and administering fluids. Several cases from the literature were cited, with full elucidation of symptomatology and subsequent treatment.

Mississippi Baptist Hospital
Jackson, Miss.

1490 Baldridge, Eugene T., Miller, Leona V., Haverback, Bernard J., & Brunhes, Shannon. Amine metabolism after an overdose of a monoamine oxidase inhibitor. New England Journal of Medicine, 1962, 267, 421-426.

A 30-year-old woman with a manic-depressive psychosis, attempted suicide by ingesting large quantities of MAO inhibitors, i.e., tranylcypromine and isocarboxazid. The induced MAO inhibition caused changes in the levels of pharmacologically active amines and a marked increase in blood serotonin, a slight increase in blood histamine, a marked increase in urinary tryptamine, metanephrine and normetanephrine and a decrease in urinary 5HIAA, indole-3-acetic acid and vanillylmandelic acid. The clinical picture, although due to MAO inhibition, could not be related to changes in the level of any single amine. When 1st seen, the patient was conscious but had gross and uncoordinated movements, incoherent speech and involuntary motions of the jaw and tongue; 6 hours later she became comatose with a temperature of $105^{\circ}F$. She recovered gradually over a 16 day period, after treatment with i.v. fluids, cooling and antibiotics.

Department of Medicine
University of Southern California
Los Angeles, Calif.

1494 British Medical Journal. Ether Sniffing. British Medical Journal, 1963, No. 5324, 198.

A verdict of accidental death was returned at an inquest where a 27-year-old man explained how his 24-year-old wife's death was accidentally caused by ether sniffing. The couple returned home from a drinking bout, and each took a pint bottle of ether to bed. The husband took one sniff and passed out, only to awake the following morning with his wife dead beside him. Both were previously addicted to ether sniffing, and consumed about 1 pint (0.6 l) per day.

British Medical Association
Tavistock Square
London, Great Britain

1495 Dacie, J. V. Haemolytic reaction to drugs. Proceedings of the Royal Society of Medicine, 1962, 55, 28-30.

A case of hemolytic anemia followed nightly administration of 2-3 sleeping pills containing 3 1/2 g of phenacetin for 2 months. Drug withdrawal preceeded rapid return to normality. A 38-year-old woman experienced jaundice and oliguria secondary to hemolytic anemia after taking phenacetin for several months. Phenacetin produced hemolytic anemia in normal therapeutic dosages in normal subjects, in small dosages in glucose-6-phosphate dehydrogenase deficient subjects, and rarely by an auto-immune mechanism. Hemolytic anemias have been attributed to the following drugs: antipyretics and sedatives, sulphonamides, antileprotics, antimalarials, anticonvulsants, urinary antiseptics, antihistamines, antihelminthics and miscellaneous drugs (chlorpromazine, chloramphenicol, etc.). Drug-induced hemolytic anemia occurs by regular mechanisms or is precipitated by some individual idiosyncrasy or hypersensitivity. Racial susceptibility to drugs is predicated on the existence of a deficiency in erythrocytic glucose-6-phosphate dehydrogenase, in not only Negroes, but also Sephardic Jews and certain Mediterranean peoples.

[No address]

1496 Rosen, Carl S., & Lechner, Michael. Jimson-weed intoxication. New England Journal of Medicine, 1962, 267, 448-450.

Two cases of Jimson weed (Datura stramonium) intoxication are described. All parts of this plant contain belladonna alkaloids (hyoscyamine, atropine, scopolamine and hyoscine). In 1 case, a 3-year old boy, symptoms were noted 2-3 hours after ingestion of the seeds; in another case, his 6-year-old sister, 5-6 hours elapsed before symptoms appeared. The boy became markedly confused, disoriented, feverish, displayed muscular incoordination and had convulsions. The girl displayed similar symptoms, except for the absence of convulsions. Treatment was by alcohol sponging and amobarbital [dose unspecified] in the 1st case and by gastric lavage, sodium phosphate and amobarbital in the girl. Both children recovered in 8-12 hours.

Grasslands Hospital
Valhalla, N. Y.

1497 Jacobs, Lionel A., & Morris, John G. Renal papillary necrosis and the abuse of phenacetin. Medical Journal of Australia, 1962, 2, 531-538.

Fifty deceased persons 23-75 years old), 3.7% of those autopsied during 1959-1962 at this hospital, had macroscopic renal papillary necrosis. These cases were analyzed in considerable detail and questionnaires sent to relatives or friends. Forty-seven of these people had been in the habit of taking phenacetin preparations daily and 60% consumed large quantities of phenacetin-containing analgesics for a long period of time before the onset of symptoms of renal disease. Nearly all these people had suffered from marked urinary infections; diabetes mellitus and obstructive uropathies were of minor significance. On final admission, nearly all showed many urinary leukocytes; only 4 persons had a specific gravity above 1.014; the BUN was high in 43 out of 44 and hemoglobin was less than 10 g in 34 out of 46. Diagnosis of such renal disease depends largely on radiological changes and the passing of papillary fragments in the urine for confirmation; a history of phenacetin abuse is also significant. The role of phenacetin in causing chronic interstitial nephritis is discussed; three case histories are given as examples.

Prince Henry Hospital
Sydney, Australia

1498 Morgenstern, G. F. Trihexyphenidyl (Artane) intoxication due to overdosage with suicidal intent. Canadian Medical Association Journal, 1962, 87, 79-81.

A case of trihexyphenidyl intoxication, due to overdosage (180 mg) with suicidal intent, is described in a 29-year-old chronic hebephrenic schizophrenic male, with a history of 4 hospital admissions since the age of 17. He had previously responded well to 200 mg chlorpromazine and 2 mg trihexyphenidyl, each t. i. d. The patient was stuporous upon admission with a fever of 101°F. and respiration somewhat deeper than normal; the skin was dry, flushed and contained liquid blebs. Urinary incontinence was also noted. Treatment was symptomatic, i. e., fluids, aspirin, alcohol sponge, chloramphenicol and penicillin. The intoxication cleared in 5-6 days. Chlorpromazine (300 mg t. i. d.) and trihexyphenidyl (2 mg t. i. d.) were then resumed. Generally, symptoms of this intoxication resembled those of atropine and responded to similar treatment.

Verdun Protestant Hospital
6875 LaSalle Blvd.
Verdun, Quebec
Canada

1499 Mitchell, Hugh G. Chlorpromazine ("Largactil") sensitivity simulating the "acute abdomen." Medical Journal of Australia, 1962, 2, 930. [Letter]

The author describes his own experience with vomiting caused by chlorpromazine [dose unspecified]. He had returned from the Far East with a series of intermittent fevers of unknown etiology. Following attacks of acute pulmonary edema, he was treated with antibiotics, digitalis, acetazolamide and chlorpromazine. He vomited several times a day for months, suffering marked weight loss, in spite of increased doses of chlorpromazine. Contrary to med-ical advice, he ceased taking medication and vomiting stopped. Vomiting recurred briefly only during the few days when chlorpromazine was resumed.

375 Toorak Road
South Yarra, Vic.
Australia

1500 Greene, Bernard L., Liebman, S., & Lustig, Noel. Dangers of using glutethimide: addiction qualities, symptoms of intoxication, and withdrawal convulsions. Illinois Medical Journal, 1962, 121, 139-141.

Glutethimide, ordinarily thought of as innocuous, can be habit-forming and dangerous. Addiction, signs of chronic anxiety and acute withdrawal convulsions have occurred. A 30-year-old woman had been taking this drug for about 3 1/2 years [dose unspecified] before her hospitalization. Neurotic complaints, marital disharmony, occasionally incoherent speech and falling occurred. Hospitalization was advised but refused. Hospitalization was finally required on an emergency basis as a result of acute withdrawal convulsions and related symptoms. Treatment consisted of glutethimide (1 g q. i. d.), dilantin (1 1/2 g t. i. d.) and multiple vitamins (p. o. and parenterally). The glutethimide was gradually eliminated over 8 days and the patient was discharged on the 11th day. It was recommended that prescriptions containing glutethimide be marked "not to be refilled."

[No address]

1501 Im Obersteg, J., & Bäumler, J. Suicid mit dem Psyhopharmakon Tofranil. [Suicide by means of Tofranil.] Archiv für Toxikologie, 1962, 19, 339-344.

A 28-year-old mother with endogenous depression committed suicide by swallowing 5000 mg of imipramine (Tofranil). The similarity in structure and physicochemical properties between imipramine and the phenothiazine derivatives is pointed out and the chromatographic and spectrographic properties of imipramine and its metabolites are presented in tabular form. Whereas in normal usage only its metabolites will be found in the urine, it was possible in this case to demonstrate the presence of un-metabolized imipramine in the blood, urine and organs. Attention is called to the dangers attending the ambulatory use of this drug, since suicide attempts occur in surprising numbers at the point where, while the psychomotor inhibitions are relaxed, the basic endogenous depression still persists.

Gerichtlich-Medizinisches Institut
Universität Basel
Basel, Switzerland

1502 Matiar-Vahar, H., & Schilde, P. Zerebrale Krampfanfälle bei Glutethimid-Abusus. [Cerebral convulsions due to glutethimide abuse.] Deutsche Medizinische Wochenschrift, 1962, 87, 406-408.

After a review of the literature on glutethimide abuse, the authors present 3 cases of their own, 2 male students both 30 years old, and one 45-year-old woman teacher. The first experienced attacks after a continued ingestion of 8 tablets daily, these consisting of loss of consciousness, rigidity, muscular tremors, and frothing at the mouth. Reports on the 3rd case were somewhat more vaguely reported to the physicians but consisted essentially of several attacks similar to those described above. EEG's taken immediately after the attacks showed alpha-type waves and involutional dysrhythmia. Subsequent EEG's were normal, after use of the drug had been stopped. Caution in the use of the drug, as well as placing the drug under the control of doctors, is recommended.

Psychiatrische und Nervenklinik der
    Friedrich-Wilhelm Universität
Kaiser-Karl-Ring 20
Bonn, Germany

1503 von Dittrich, P. Die Behandlung der akuten Vergiftung mit Glutethimid (Doriden) durch extrakorporale Hämodialyse. [Treatment of acute glutethimide intoxication by means of extracorporeal dialysis.] Deutsche Medizinische Wochenschrift, 1962, 87, 357-359.

A 19-year-old male attempted suicide by

ingesting 40 tablets (10 g) of glutethimide. After 3 days of conservative treatment during which no improvement took place, extracorporeal dialysis was resorted to. In 8 hours the patient recovered consciousness, with normalization of reflexes, blood pressure, pulse and respiration. Anuria set in 2 days later, and after 4 days, extracorporeal dialysis was again found necessary. Follow-up 10 weeks later showed normal findings except for some limitation of tubular function and normo-chromic anemia. The authors discuss the triggering mechanism of kidney failure.

Medizinische Universitätsklinik
Allgemeines Krankenhaus
Innsbruck, Austria

1504 Langecker, H., Neuhaus, G., Ibe, K., & Kessel, M. Ein Suicid-Versuch mit Valamin mit einem Beitrag zur Elimination und Therapie. [A suicide attempt by means of Valamin and a contribution to its elimination and therapy.] Archiv für Toxikologie, 1962, 19, 293-301.

The authors report the case of a 21-year-old man who first attempted suicide with a combination of hypnotics, sedatives, and alcohol. A few days later he again attempted suicide by means of 40 g of ethinamate (Valamin) in combination with Coca-cola and alcohol. About 16 hours later he was admitted showing severe intoxication, spontaneous hypothermia of 28.8°C and severe respiratory insufficiency. Treatment consisted of artificial respiration, levar-terenol, extracorporeal dialysis, and suxamethonium. The patient was unconscious for 4 days and then recovered. Chromatographic tests were run on the blood plasma, dialysate, and urine. The methodology is described, and detailed results are presented in chart form. The narcotic limiting concentration in the blood, 17 hours after intake, was about 4 mg%. The presence of 10% metabolites in the urine after 17 hours indicates the great importance of hydroxylation and conjugation in relation to the concentration of urinary metabolites. Extracorporeal dialysis is superfluous in cases of ethinamate poisoning when kidney function is intact.

Hauptlaboratorium Schering AG
Berlin, Germany

Side effects
Abstracts 1505-1509

1505 Grahmann, Hans, & Peters, Uwe H. Über psychotische Erscheinungen bei INH-Entziehung. [Psychotic manifestations after INH-withdrawal.] Archiv für Psychiatrie und Zeitschrift für die Gesamte Neurologie, 1962, 203, 173-177.

A 62-year-old tuberculosis patient arbitrarily suspended treatment with isoniazid (INH) and developed withdrawal symptoms consisting first of insomnia, then extreme vivacity, incessant inconsequent chattering, wild gesticulations, unproductive talk, and evident pressure of a desire, but also inability, to communicate something important to him. There was no clouding of consciousness. The full development of the symptoms took place over a 2-day period, and lasted for about 1 day, with subsequent recovery.

Psychiatrische und Nervenklinik
Universität Kiel
Kiel, Germany

1506 Cramer, Hinrich, & Binet, Jacques-Louis. B₆-Avitaminose und Nervensystem. [B₆-avitaminosis and the nervous system.] Ärztliche-Forschung, 1962, 16, 53-59.

A 61-year-old female tuberculosis patient developed cerebral complications due to vitamin B_6 deficiency following treatment with isoniazid. These consisted of an epileptic-type seizure, followed by severe headaches. Investigation disclosed a disturbance of tryptophane metabolism of the kind described for vitamin B_6 deficiency. Addition of pyridoxine to the treatment over a 3-week period resulted in normal tryptophane metabolism, while the sputum examination remained negative, thus indicating that pyridoxine does not interfere with the antituberculosis effects of isoniazid.

Clinique des Maladies du Système Nerveux
Hôpital de la Salpêtrière
Paris, France

1507 Sours, John A. Peripheral edema and tachycardia during tranylcypromine therapy. American Journal of Psychiatry, 1962, 119, 584-585.

Following administration of chlorpromazine (50-75 mg q.i.d.) and tranylcypromine (10 mg q.i.d.) for 10 days, a 28-year-old male acute schizophrenic with secondary gastrointestinal psychophysiological complications manifested sinus tachycardia and 2+ edema of the ankles, right knee and wrist. Discontinuation of tranylcypromine resulted in dramatic disappearance of symptoms within 24 hours. This constituted the first recorded case of tranylcypromine induced edema and tachycardia occurring simultaneously in a given individual. Drug-induced side effects are directly related to dosage, and quantities in excess of 30 mg q.i.d. increase both the incidence and severity of side effects.

Department of Psychiatry
U.S. Naval School of Aviation Medicine
Pensacola, Fla.

1508 Bacon, G.A. Successful suicide with tranylcypromine sulfate. American Journal of Psychiatry, 1962, 119, 585.

A 17-year-old female received a prescription for tranylcypromine (50- 10 mg tablets) to combat a neurotic depressive reaction. She immediately proceeded to ingest all 50 tablets. Within 2 hours, she became agitated, incoherent and markedly tremulous. Phenobarbital (1 grain i.m.) and secobarbital (2 grains i.m.) were administered over a 4 hour period following hospital admission. (The attending physician was unaware of the number of tablets taken). The patient became comatose and critically ill, with hyperthermia (110°F) and circulatory collapse. Intranasal O_2 and levarterenol bitartrate (3 ampules in 5% glucose over 3 hours), plasma, hydrotherapy and gastric lavage were unable to prevent death from ensuing within 8 hours of drug ingestion. Due to a technical error, gastric lavage was postponed for 5 hours after tablets were taken. Death was essentially an exaggeration of the side effects, which normally occur with tranylcypromine in standard and intensive treatment dosages.

St. Luke's Hospital
Racine, Wisc.

1509   French Devitt, R.E., & Kenny,
Sheila. Lancet, 1962, 2, 430. [Letter]

Within an 8-month period, 3 cases of
phocomelia due to thalidomide were
observed in an area with an 8-year birth
record unmarked by a single case of
phocomelia. Of these 3 patients, 1
received an unknown amount of thalidomide
throughout pregnancy and 2 received
100 mg/day from the 5th to the 11th or
13th week of pregnancy.

South Down Hospital Group
Newry, County Down
Ireland

1510   Calnan, C.D. Contact dermatitis from
drugs. Proceedings of the Royal Society of
Medicine, 1962, 55, 39-42.

The author lists 772 cases of contact dermatitis caused by the following compounds:
antibacterial agents - 220, antibiotics -
124, local anesthetics - 74, antihistamines
- 53, colophony resin - 14, rubefacients, -
8, miscellaneous - 88, all of which are
allergic reactions; he includes cases caused
by occupational contacts: chlorpromazine -
175 and antibiotics - 16. Antibiotics, local
anesthetics and antihistamines are the
major topical sensitizers. Patch test concentrations, differences among countries,
trends in sensitization, e.g., neomycin
sensitivity is steadily increasing with its
extending usage and some effects of legislation are reviewed. Phenothiazine derivatives (particularly promethazine and chlorpromazine) have become prominent in
photocontact dermatitis. The best way to
reduce the incidence of reactions if to use
minimal effective concentration for minimal
periods of time.

[No address]

1511 Chapman, John E., & Lewis, Charles
E. Darvon, Dieldrin and Noludar. Journal
of the Kansas Medical Society, 1962, 63,
228-229.

A 63-year-old woman ingested 780 mg of
dextro propoxyphene hydrochloride (Darvon)
and was admitted with severe hypotension
and dangerously diminished respiratory

rate. Intubation and artificial respiration
precipitated a full return to consciousness
within 18 hours of poisoning. Overdoses
of Darvon lead to CNS depression. The
concomitant respiratory depression may
be alleviated by nalorphine. A 47-year-old
female ingested 4-5 ounces of insecticide
containing dieldrin, followed by 2-3 ounces
of household ammonia, after which she
vomited and experienced 13 grand mal
seizures, which were controlled by i. m.
and i. v. administration of barbiturates
administered following gastric lavage. A
26-year-old colored female took 2700 mg of
Noludar (3, 3-diethyl-5-methyl-2, 4-
piperidinedione) and promptly became semicomatose. Gastric lavage within 1 hour
after drug ingestion was followed by an
uneventful recovery. Psychiatric help
was proffered. Cardiovascular and
respiratory support constituted adequate
treatment in all cases. The Poison Control
Center cases illustrate the need for rapid
evaluation and treatment of patients suffering
from an overdose of poisons common to
most households.

Department of Pharmacology
University of Kansas Medical Center
Kansas City, Kan.

1512 McCawley, Elton L., Brummett,
Robert E., & Dana, George W. Convulsions
from psilocybe mushroom poisoning.
Proceedings of the Western Pharmacology
Society, 1962, 5, 27-34.

Six cases of mushroom poisoning are
reported. There were 2 adults and 4
children, aged 4-9 years. Within 15-30
minutes after eating the cooked mushrooms,
the adults reported a sense of anxiety and
excitement described as a "cheap drunk."
The children were reported variously to
emit a peculiar cry, be dizzy and ataxic,
were weak, disoriented, staring or
incoherent. All exhibited mydriasis with
the pupils widely dilated and fixed. When
tested, however, the pupils responded to
light and accommodation. The mouth was
dry, the skin dry and flushed although some
patients reported a feeling of being cold.
All complained of nausea and stomach
cramps. All the children developed clonic-
tonic type convulsions which were usually

intermittent. One child died. Species identification was possible in 1 case, the mushroom being Psilocybe baeocystis. Paper chromatography was used on a sample and psilocybin identified as the major component with lesser amounts of psilocin present.

Department of Pharmacology
University of Oregon Medical School
Portland, Ore.

1513 Jacobziner, Harold, & Raybin, Harry W. Mixture of tranquilizers, lighter fluid, paint thinner, and iodine poisonings. New York State Journal of Medicine, 1962, 62, 862-864.

Four cases of accidental poisoning included a 21-month-old male who ingested charcoal lighter fluid, a 2-year-old male who swallowed paint thinner, an 11-year-old girl who gargled with an iodine solution, and a 34-year-old female schizoaffective schizophrenic who probably ingested unknown amounts of the following psychoactive drugs: trifluoperazine, imipramine, meprobamate and promazine along with iodine. Marked cerebral depression was evident upon admission, and the initial stupor rapidly progressed to profound coma. Treatment entailed gastric lavage, metaraminol bitartrate infusion and intubation. Rapid recovery ensued. Subsequent psychiatric care included 8 ECT treatments with concomitant psychotherapy.

Poison Control Center
The City of New York Department of
Health
New York, N. Y.

1514 Jacobziner, Harold, & Raybin, Harry W. Glutethimide (Doriden) poisoning. Archives of Pediatrics, 1962, 79, 302-305.

Glutethimide poisoning occurred in 62 individuals, aged 2-70 years, with only 1 fatality (a 64-year-old male who ingested 6 g in a suicidal attempt) . Prominent features of acute poisoning include drowsiness, nausea and vomiting, which precede cerebral edema, hypotension and circulatory collapse. Supportive symptomatic treatment encompasses gastric lavage, fluids, chlorpromazine, caffeine and intubation procedures. A heroin addict who attempted drug withdrawal by ingesting glutethimide (15 0.5 g tablets/day) took an overdose of 12 g in 48 hours and awoke in Bellevue with no ill effects. A complete subjective history of glutethimide addiction was described in a 25-year-old man. Ingestion of more than 1-1/2 g to combat depression resulted in amnesia, a transient psychotic reaction and profound sleep. Drug discontinuation precipitated withdrawal symptoms, including impaired voluntary muscle coordination, general trembling and gastric distress. Toxic reactions attributed to glutethimide mimic those obtained from the barbiturates.

125 Worth Street
New York 13, N. Y.

1515 Smithells, R. W., & Lond, M. G. Thalidomide and malformations in Liverpool. Lancet, 1962, No. 7242, 1270-1273

Fifty-nine mothers gave birth to malformed babies in Liverpool since January 1, 1960. Of the women who had 30 babies evincing ectomelia (gross hypoplasia or aplasia of 1 or more long bones or limbs, including amelia, phocomelia and hemimelia), 12 ingested thalidomide in the 1st trimester of pregnancy. Seven infants had microtia (gross hypoplasia or aplasia of the pinna with or without external auditory meatus) and 3 of their mothers took thalidomide, but thalidomide was ingested by only 2 mothers in a series of 22 infants born with lesser deformities. A group of 40 healthy infants acted as controls. Liverpool instituted a congenital abnormalities registry to facilitate repercussions arising from the thalidomide tragedy. Personal interviews with involved persons indicated the fallibility of retrospective data in attempting to designate which drugs were ingested and dosages of same. Of the 30 babies with ectromelia 11 were still-born, males outnumbered females by 2 to 1, and associated malformations were observed in 12. Other drugs ingested concomitantly with thalidomide include barbiturates, glutethimide and antiemetics. Six mothers of ectromelic infants had clinical influenza and 1 had encephalitis during the 1st trimester of pregnancy. The fact that a history of thalidomide ingestion was obtained from less than half of these mothers may be a reflection of the fallibility of memory and records, or malformations may be virus-induced or precipitated by other drugs with unsuspected teratogenicity. Thalidomide has been responsible for a minimum of 800 fetal malformations in Great Britain

[No address]

1516 Dally, P. J. Fatal reaction associated with tranylcypromine and methylamphetamine. Lancet, 1962, No. 7241, 1235-1236.

A 38-year-old man received methamphetamine [dosage unspecified], and immediately experienced severe hypertension and an excruciating occipital headache. Aspirin and amylobarbital [i. v.] provided relief fairly rapidly. Intravenous methamphetamine administered to patients concomitantly or within 2 weeks of MAO inhibitors (iproniazid, phenelzine, isocarboxazid, phenoxypropazine, pheniprazine, nialamide or tranylcypromine) may result in rapid development of severe occipital headache, chest constriction, tachycardia, palpitations, increased respiratory rate and vomiting. Similar symptoms occur with long-term administration of MAO inhibitors. As such side effects resemble hypertensive paroxysms associated with pheochromocytoma, (thus implicating the adrenal medulla in etiology) the hypertensive crisis may respond favorably to a sustained-action catecholamine inhibitor like dibenamine.

Department of Psychological Medicine
Westminster Hospital
London, S. W. 1, Great Britain

1517 Dubach, U. C. Methyldopa and depression. British Medical Journal, 1963, No. 5325, 261.

A patient with carcinoid syndrome received α-methyldopa (2-2.5 g/day) to control carcinoid flushes. The medication neither controlled diarrhea nor altered blood pressure. The patient evinced marked slowing of motor activity and psychic hallucinations which subsided 24 hours after drug withdrawal. Another patient with carcinoid syndrome also received α-methyldopa (1 g/day) and showed a markedly increased sleeping tendency with some motor retardation during the period of drug administration. Reversal of symptoms has been the rule upon drug withdrawal.

Medizinische Universitätspoliklinik
Basel, Switzerland

1518 Kirman, Brian H. "Ancoloxin" and foetal abnormalities. British Medical Journal, 1963, No. 5325, 265-266.

Ancoloxin (meclozine and pyridoxine) administered to pregnant women 7 1/2-10 weeks after the last menstrual period may, contrary to popular opinion, cause meningocele in the embryo despite the fact that the neural tube closes by the 6th week of gestation, since the excessive variation in ovulation enables fertilization to occur at any time during the cycle. Adequate investigation should be undertaken by scientists who are not affiliated with pharmaceutical companies or financially dependent upon them. Such conditions would indubitably enhance objective interpretation of data.

Carshalton, Surrey
Great Britain

1519 McClure, J. L. Reactions associated with tranylcypromine. Lancet, 1962, No. 7243, 1351.

Tranylcypromine (20-40 mg/day) administered to 3 patients, aged 18-36 years for 5 days to 4 weeks resulted in palpitations, severe occipital headache, vomiting, profuse sweating, hypertension and photophobia. Drug withdrawal resulted in cessation of symptoms within 12-48 hours in 2 patients, but the 3rd died 4 1/2 hours after the onset of symptoms from a ruptured aneurysm of the left posterior communicating artery.

Maudsley Hospital
London, S.E. 5, Great Britain

1520 Mason, Alan. Fatal reaction associated with tranylcypromine and methylamphetamine. Lancet, 1962, No. 7238, 1073.

A 39-year-old man was previously treated for depression with hysteria by ether inhalation and 25 mg i. v. methylamphetamine on 3 occasions. Hysteria was obliterated and tension was reduced by this means. During a 3-week interval, tranylcypromine (10 mg t. i. d. for 2 weeks) was administered, followed by a 25 mg injection of methylamphetamine, which precipitated a severe headache followed by a left hemiparesis (with blood CSF) that culminated before death due to a massive cerebrovascular accident. Autopsy revealed a predisposition to vascular difficulty in the form of considerable atheromatous degeneration of cerebral arteries, which could have reacted similarly to methylamphetamine or tranylcypromine. Timing, however, indicated that death was due to the effects derived from a combination of the 2 drugs.

[No address]

1521 Stark, D. C. C. Effects of giving vasopressors to patients on monoamine-oxidase inhibitors. Lancet, 1962, No. 7244, 1405-1406.

A 33-year-old woman with anxiety received chlordiazepoxide and phenelzine [dosages unspecified] for 1 month prior to bilateral angiography to determine the origin of recurrent headaches. (family history included loss of 3 sisters from subarachnoid hemorrhages due to ruptured aneurysms of the circle of Willis.) Premedication included pethidine (50 mg) and atropine (0.65 mg). Anesthesia included thiopentone (300 mg), suxamethonium (50 mg), and 1% halothane, etc. Hypotension followed manipulation of the left carotid artery, and mephentermine (10 mg i. v.) was administered to facilitate puncture. Gross tachycardia and hypertenstion ensued immediately, but rapid administration of oxygen precipitated a return to normal levels within 15 minutes. A hematoma of the right carotid sheath developed simultaneously with the hypertension and angiography was abandoned. Recovery was uneventful. Effects were apparently due to the combination of a sympathetic amine with a MAO inhibitor, a combination which has proved to be catastrophic at best.

Newcastle General Hospital
Newcastle-upon-Tyne, Great Britain

1522 Quibell, E. P. Thalidomide-damaged infants. Lancet, 1962, No. 7244, 1402.

Effective aid must be provided for a possible total of 500 thalidomide damaged babies in Great Britain (11 of which occurred in a single practice). Difficult individual problems may be partially ameliorated through an initial pediatric assessment to evaluate the problem and ascertain associated defects, early reference (6-8 weeks of age) to a limb-fitting surgeon and early consultation with an orthopedic surgeon. All efforts should be directed toward obtaining an effective functional result. Special prosthetic equipment is indicated and should be instituted as early as possible, in conjunction with the development of understanding parental attitudes. Long range goals should revolve around enabling such children to achieve a reasonable degree of independence since their level of intelligence is essentially unimpaired. Parental attitudes are of the utmost importance and must be sympathetic and understanding at all costs. Coordinated medical endeavors offer the most promising solution to the thalidomide problem.

Chailey Heritage
Craft School and Hospital
Chailey, Sussex
Great Britain

See also 1372, 1373, 1378, 1382, 1384, 1386, 1390, 1391, 1392, 1405, 1407, 1409, 1419, 1420, 1421, 1429, 1446, 1585, 1648, 1649.

1523 Posner, Herbert S., Hearst, Eliot, Taylor, Wilson L., & Cosmides, George J. Model metabolites of chlorpromazine and promazine: relative activities in some pharmacological and behavioral tests. Journal of Pharmacology and Experimental Therapeutics, 1962, 137, 84-90.

NIH general purpose male mice were used in the sleeping time and rotating rod tests, and male Wistar or Osborne-Mendel rats were used in operant behavior tests. The effects of chlorpromazine, chlorpromazine sulfoxide, monomethylchlorpromazine, chlorpromazine-N-oxide, promazine, 2-hydroxypromazine, and 4-hydroxypromazine were studied in relation to potentiation of hexobarbital sleeping time, on stimulated locomotor activity (rotarod test, Kinnard and Carr 1957) and on CR's. In all tests, chlorpromazine sulfoxide was the least active, chlorpromazine-N-oxide though active was less active than chlorpromazine or monomethylchlorpromazine. A lag in the onset of activity was only noted with chlorpromazine-N-oxide in both of the CR tests. Monomethylchlorpromazine was generally only slightly less active than chlorpromazine. 4-Hydroxypromazine was equally or slightly less active than promazine and 2-hydroxypromazine was markedly less active than promazine, except in the sleeping time test when given i.v. In this case it was about as active as promazine, which in turn was less active than chlorpromazine in all tests.

Clinical Neuropharmacology Research Center NIH
Bethesda, Md.

1524 Hurst, Paul M. The effects of d-amphetamine on risk taking. Psychopharmacologia, 1962, 3, 283-290.

The effect of d-amphetamine (10 mg p.o.) on the risk-taking behavior of 29 male prisoners (IQ 104-131; various ages) was investigated, utilizing a gambling situation involving cigarettes. Capsules were ingested 1 1/2 hours before testing. Subjects served as their own controls when receiving placebos. The comparison was done with Wilcoxon's matched pairs rank test to determine the significance of differences between paired observations. The difference was significant in the direction of increased risk-taking under the drug; 19 subjects made more high-risk choices while under the drug and 7 while receiving the placebo, while 3 showed no differences. Apparently d-amphetamine can increase risk-taking. Alternative interpretations were also provided.

The Institute for Research
State College, Pa.

1525 Froelich, Robert E., & Heckel, Robert V. The psychological effects of methylphenidate. Journal of Clinical and Experimental Psychopathology and Quarterly Review of Psychiatry and Neurology, 1962, 23, 91-98.

Experiments were performed on 90 medical students, in order to study the psychoeffects of methylphenidate. Groups of 5-10 subjects were tested in 2 hourly sessions at 24 hour intervals in 9 experimental categories based on 3 variables. Subjects received methylphenidate (20 mg i.v.), drug being used but not of the dosage or the test design. Evaluation was based on learning, recall and relearning of nonsense syllables, performance of motor tasks (Purdue Pegboard) and writing of imaginative responses (Heckel-Steele Sexual Situations Test). The drug had no significant effect on learning, slightly delayed initial learning and augmented facilitation of recall, tended to produce maximum and superior motor performance on the 1st trial and maintained this performance on the 2nd trial. Imaginative productions under influence of the methylphenidate showed decreased inhibition, increased verbal productivity and expression of previously repressed, emotionally charged feelings. Only 1 out of 51 drug-treated subjects withdrew because of side effects (essentially extreme confusion). There was some difficulty in concentrating and mild exhaustion was observed in most subjects, elevation in pulse rate and anxiety level was noted among both treated and placebo subjects.

University of Missouri School of Medicine
Columbia, Mo.

1526 Knight, David A. Problems of non-specific factors in psychopharmacology. Methodology. Test score instability. A source of error in individual drug response. In: Rinkel, Max [Ed.] Specific and non-specific factors in psychopharmacology. New York: Philosophical Library, 1962, 99-113.

Eighteen normal subjects, aged 20-38 years, were tested on 10 successive occasions with the following tests: Flicker Fusion, After-Image Disappearance, Auditory Reaction Time and Tapping Speed. Nine were tested at fixed hours and 9 at randomly varied hours. Fixed and variable scheduling data were pooled for a 2 way analysis of variance. Individual mean discrepancies were significant at the 0.01 probability level, indicating the heterogeneity of the sample.

Verdun Protestant Hospital
Verdun, Quebec
Canada

1527 Miller, James G. Objective measurements of the effects of drugs on driver behavior. Journal of the American Medical Association, 1962, 179, 940-943.

Various combinations of patients and normal subjects received meprobamate (800-1600 mg/day), d-amphetamine, alcohol, prochlorperazine (20 mg), benactyzine, emplcamate (400-800mg), carisoprodol (2100 mg/day), chlordiazepoxide, mebutamate (300 mg), phenobarbital, carbethoxysyringoyl methylreserpate and isothipendyl in order to measure the potentially deleterious effects these drugs have on normal reaction time and judgement as determined by the driver trainer test (American Automobile Association's Auto Trainer), the Whipple Steadiness Test and standard Ortho-rater testing procedures. Most of the tranquilizers did not appear to exert serious behavioral toxicity. Chlordiazepoxide produced diminished accuracy in judgement, some degree of exophoria, and significantly decreased visual acuity. Normal doses of these compounds failed to produce significant behavioral aberrations.

Mental Health Research Institute
University of Michigan
Ann Arbor, Mich.

1528 Thompson, Travis. The effect of two phenothiazines and a barbiturate on extinction-induced rate increase of a free operant. Journal of Comparative and Physiological Psychology, 1962, 55, 714-718.

Phenobarbital (30-120 mg/kg i.p.), thioridazine and chlorpromazine (each 0.75-20.0 mg/kg i.p.) were administered to 9 experimentally naive male Sprague-Dawley rats 30 minutes before they were placed in Skinner boxes, drug effects were determined on the rate of lever pressing for water reinforcement on a regular reinforcement schedule. Dose-response-rate curves indicated that a reduction in lever pressing was produced by successive increments of phenobarbital, chlorpromazine and thioridazine. A 2nd group of 27 rats (experimental conditions same as above) in a 3 x 3 factorial design with triple replication per cell received drugs as above to determine the effects of drug and dosage variation on the extinction inflection ratio (EIR), depression of lever-pressing, and degree of ataxia (rearings, inclined-plane behavior, narrow-walkway beharior, and walking in short alley). Overall analysis of variance yielded a statistically significant F ratio which was attributable to a significant dose effect (p .01), with drug and interaction effects failing to reach significance. An inverse relationship was observed between drug dose and EIR magnitude. Subcomparisons indicated that the difference in drug effects was a reflection of phenobarbital deviation from the phenothiazine group. Ataxia scores for the phenobarbital group were significantly higher than those obtained by the 2 phenothiazines, and were directly related to dosage. No interaction effects were observed in the total ataxia scores, and drug effect was contributed solely by the phenobarbital group. No basic difference was indicated in the effect of the 3 drugs on the EIR increase but the effect on ataxic score was significant.

Laboratory of Psychopharmacology
University of Maryland
College Park, Md.

1529 Bures, J., Bohdanecký Z., & Weiss, T. Physostigmine induced hippocampal theta activity and learning in rats. Psychopharmacologia, 1962, 3, 254-263.

The effect of physostigmine on EEG activity and conditioning was studied in Wistar rats 2-3 months old. Theta activity, which corresponded to the impairment of learning, developed in the hippocampus of curarized or freely-moving, unanesthetized animals for 30-60 minutes after 1 mg/kg i.p., with a maximum after 10 minutes. A 1-trial acquisition of a passive aviodance reaction in an electrified compartment was suppressed 10 minutes after 0.2-1.0 mg/kg physostigimine. No retention of this reaction was found 24 hours after 1-trial learning when 0.5 mg/kg was applied 8 minutes before the retention test; this same dose did not impair the retention of an overtrained (4 times) passive avoidance reaction. An overlearned active avoidance reaction (running to the safe part of the apparatus) was not affected by 0.5 mg/kg of the agent and only partly impaired by 1.0 mg/kg.

Institute of Physiology
Czechoslovak Academy of Sciences
Prague, Czechoslovakia

1530 Kornetsky, Conan, Dawson, Joy, & Pelikan, Edward. A hypothesis based on animal experimentation. Individual animal variation in the effects of pentobarbital and dextro-amphetamine (A comparison). In: Rinkel, Max [Ed.] Specific and non-specific factors in psychopharmacology. New York: Philosophical Library, 1962, 161-171.

Nine male Wistar rats were trained in lever-pressing for food reward (50 presses/reinforcement) in a standard Garson-Stadler box. All drugs were administered in aqueous solution i.p. in the following order: day 1, 5.0 mg/kg pentobarbital; day 2, 5.0 mg/kg pentobarbital; day 3, water; day 4, 10.0 mg/kg pentobarbital; day 5, 10.0 mg/kg pentobarbital; day 6, water; day 7, 1.25 mg/kg d-amphetamine; day 8, 0.75 mg/kg d-amphetamine; day9, water; day 1, 0.5 mg/kg d-amphetamine; day 11, water and day 12, 0.25 mg/kg d-amphetamine. The hypothesis that the degree of response of subjects to one drug was correlated with the degree of the same subjects response to other drugs regardless of dosage was supported. The strength of the relationship between the response tare after saline is inversely related to the dose of the drug used, i.e.,

the higher the dose the lower the correlation at the initial level.

Department of Pharmacology and
Experimental Therapeutics
Boston University School of Medicine
Boston, Mass.

1531 Solle, M., Bauman, R., & Hecht, K. Der Einfluss einer Insulinhypoglykämie auf bedingte Abwehrreflexe der Ratte. [The influence of insulin-induced hypoglycemia on conditioned avoidance reflexes in rats.] Deutsche Gesundheitswesen, 1962, 33, 1381-1388.

In rats treated with 2.0 U/kg Alt-insulin, drowsiness appeared with loss of muscle tone 2-3 hours after injection. Blood glucose levels were measured in relation to injected dosage, as were the various types of inhibition of the avoidance reflex. By means of statistical significance tests, it was found that the induced hypoglycemia was related to increases in the latency period, the duration, and % failures. The differentiation ability remained unchanged. The onset of the inhibitory reactions was not in phase with the onset of hypoglycemia, the latency effect occurring later and lasting longer than the decrease in blood sugar. No statistical relationship between degree of hypoglycemia and strength of inhibition could be established.

Institut für Kortiko-Viszerale Pathologie
und Therapie
Deutsche Akademie der Wissenschaften
zu Berlin
Berlin-Buch, Germany

1532 Liang, H.S., Dodd, R.B., & DeBruine, P.H. A study of the analgesic action of propiomazine and morphine, with a method for assessment of pain in man. Anesthesiology, 1962, 23, 154-155.

In a double-blind study, normal saline, 0.4 mg/cc morphine and 4 mg/cc propiomazine as i.v. infusions were given to normal subjects. Five subjects completed the series of tests: each subject received a different amount of each solution at a different time and an interval of 1 week was allowed between tests. Pain was produced either by electric stimulation of s.c. sensory nerves or through ischemic muscular pain produced by pumping up a pneumatic cuff placed on the upper arm. In the 1st case the current intensity shown on the dial of an electronic stimulator was used to assess pain; in the 2nd instance the subject reported as slight, moderate, etc. Morphine produced significant elevations of both pain thresholds and (0.6-2.0 mg) decreased ischemic pain. Subhypnotic doses of propiomazine neither raised the pain threshold nor diminished ischemic pain.

Division of Anesthesiology
Washington University School of Medicine
St. Louis, Mo.

(0.6-2.0 mg) decreased ischemic pain. Subhypnotic doses of propiomazine neither raised the pain threshold nor diminished ischemic pain.

Division of Anesthesiology
Washington University School of Medicine
St. Louis, Mo.

See also 1433, 1575.

1533 Boehme, Werner R., Siegmund, Estelle A., Scharpf, William G., & Schipper, Edgar. Structure-activity relationships in a series of anticonvulsant bicyclic acylureas, Journal of Medicinal and Pharmaceutical Chemistry, 1962, 5, 769-775.

Anticonvulsant activity against electroshock and pentylenetetrazol-induced convulsions was determined in mice for a series of monocyclic and bicyclic carbonylureas (all administered p.o.) which were synthesized. As well, the procedure of P'an and co-workers (1953) was used to measure hypnotic activity in mice; and dogs were used for 1 compound synthesized. Toxicity and LD_{50} values were calculated following Litchfield and Wilcoxon (1949). The monocyclic carbonylureas containing a hydrogen atom in the alpha position were of no interest as anticonvulsants. 2-Norbornene-5-endo-carbonylurea, however, afforded good protection against both electroshock and pentylenetetrazol-induced convulsions. Introduction of a methyl group alpha to the carbonylurea chain of the monocyclic and bicyclic derivatives markedly enhanced anticonvulsant activity. Cycloalkenyl and bicycloalkenyl derivatives were more active than their saturated congeners. Anticonvulsant activity was abolished by the introduction of carboxyl, carbomethoxy or carboximide groupings. N^3-Acetylation reduced activity slightly but significantly increased the duration of action.

Shulton Inc.
Clifton, N. J.

1534 Rümke, Chr. L., & De Jonge, H. An effect of intraperitoneal saline administration on the duration of hexobarbital narcosis in mice. Acta Physiol. Pharmacol. Neerlandica, 1962, 11, 113-122.

The absorption and concentration effects of SKF 525-A (5 mg/kg s.c. or i.p.) on hexobarbital (60 mg/kg i.v. or 75 mg/kg i.p.) sleeping time in inbred mice (TNO strain N) were assessed, using the spontaneous return of the righting reflex as the criterion for the duration of narcosis. Given 2 hours previous to hexobarbital, the i.p. administration of SKF 525-A prolongs sleeping time. If this pretreatment with SKF 525-A is followed by saline i.p. 1 hour later, the narcosis following i.v. hexobarbital lasts longer than if the saline injection is given s.c. (confirmatory data, Rümke 1962). The narcosis after i.p. hexobarbital lasts longer after an i.p. saline pretreatment than after s.c. saline pretreatment, and the duration of narcosis after i.p. injection of a hexobarbital dose is influenced by the concentration in which it is administered (0.25-0.375 %), i.e., the administration of the weaker solution results in longer narcosis. The local interaction of i.p. administered drugs given a short time after each other, as well as considerations on absorption rates, should be taken into account in studies on the influence of drugs on hexobarbital narcosis and upon other drugs interactions.

Department of Pharmacology
Free University
Amsterdam, The Netherlands

1535 Anderson, Floyd E., Kaminsky, Daniel., Dubnick, Barnard., Klutchko, Sylvester R., Cetenko, Wiaczeslaw A., Gylys, Jonas., & Hart, John A. Chemistry and pharmacology of monoamine oxidase inhibitors: hydrazine derivatives. Journal of Medicinal and Pharmaceutical Chemistry, 1962, 5, 221-230.

Seventy aralkyl and acylated hydrazines were synthesized. Their preparation and chemical properties were described. Some pharmacological testing was done and attempts made to correlate activity with structure. The reserpine-challenge test was used to screen these compounds for MAO inhibition in mice; this test detects MAO inhibition only when it occurs in the brain. Selected successful MAO inhibitors were compared according to their ability to elevate brain-serotonin; they exhibited a dose-response relationship. Generally, the same order of potency prevailed in both tests; monosubstituted hydrazines were more active and more toxic than their acyl derivatives, while the carbamates were slightly less active and less toxic and the acetyl derivatives were the least active and the least toxic. Acute toxicity and activity were not always directly related; i.e., p-phenoxy-amethylbenzylhydrazine was one of the most active and least toxic of these compounds; also, in vitro and in vivo results were not always comparable. Compounds containing bulky para substituents appear to be the most potent and least toxic.

Warner-Lambert Research Institute
Morris Plains, N. J.

1536 McLennan, H. On the action of 3-hydroxytyramine and dichlorisopropylnoradrenaline on spinal reflexes. Experientia, 1962, 18, 278-279.

Chloralose-and urethane-anesthetized cats were studied. The time course of direct inhibition of a monosynaptic reflex arc set up by stimulation of the lateral gastrocnemius nerve was recorded from a ventral root filament. After the administration of 7 mg/kg dichlorisopropyllevarterenol (dichlorisopropylnoradrenalin) i. v., the inhibition of the reflex was completely unaffected, though this dose was sufficient to largely suppress the inhibition of the reflex brought about by reticular formation stimulation. Therefore, the blocking action of the agent on the latter inhibitory process is not exerted at the level of the mononeuron. Further, the firing pattern of inhibitory Renshaw interneurons of the anterior horn was found to be unaffected by the application to the cord of 5% 3-hydroxytyramine. 3-Hydroxytyramine application may lead to excitation of inhibitory interneurons which make synaptic contact with the motoneurons of the cord.

Department of Physiology
University of British Columbia
Vancouver, British Columbia
Canada

1537 Pustrom, Einar, Prange, Arthue J. Jr., & Cochrane, Carl M. Epinephrine blocking and WY-3041 (5,6, diacetoxy N-methyl indole); a comment on the measurement of blood pressure reactivity. Journal of Clinical and Experimental Psychopharmacology and Quarterly Review of Psychiatry and Neurology, 1962, 23, 99-105.

A new drug, 5,6-diacetoxy-N-methyl indole

(WY-3041, 80 mg/day p.o.), was studied in 12 healthy male medical students, aged 23-30 years by the double-blind technique, for its capacity to protect against the systolic hypertensive effects of exogenous epinephrine. Each subject was tested on 3 occasions at 48 hour intervals once with WY-3041, once with a placebo and once with nothing, prior to receiving an i. v. injection of epinephrine (0.0125 mg). The drug exerted no blocking effects on blood pressure reactivity. No significant differences in blood pressure were observed among the 3 types of treatment.

North Carolina Memorial Hospital
University of North Carolina School of Medicine
Chapel Hill, N. C.

1538 Nielsen, Moller, I., W., Lassen, N., Holm, T., & Petersen, P. V. Central depressant activity of some thiaxanthene derivatives. Acta Pharmacologica et Toxicologica, 1962, 19, 87-100.

The neuroleptic activity of 66 thiaxanthene derivatives was investigated and compared with that exhibited by several phenothiazines. Acute i. v. toxicity was determined in mice; LD_{50} (mg/kg) was measured by the method of Miller and Tainter. Spontaneous motor activity was determined by the dose (mg/kg i. p.) that reduced motility to 50% of control mouse activity, as determined by the method of Kopf et al. Potentiation of hexobarbital anesthesia was determined by administering the test compound (2.5 and 25 mg/kg i. p.) 30 minutes before i. v. injection of 50 mg/kg hexobarbital. The potentiating factor was recorded as the ratio of test animal sleeping time to control sleeping time. Like the phenothiazines, the thiaxanthenes were very potent central depressant drugs with fairly parallel potencies. The following 3 criteria seemed important for maximal central depressant activity: a double bond between carbon 9 and the side chain, substitution at carbon 2 and trans configuration at the double bond.

Department of Pharmacology
Research Laboratories
H. Lundbeck & Co.
Ottilavej 7, Copenhagen Valby
Denmark

1539 Bellville, J. Weldon, Aguto Escarraga, Lourdes, Wallenstein, Stanley L., Wang, Kuo Chen, Howland, William S., & Houde, Raymond W. Antagonism by caffeine of the respiratory effects of codeine and morphine. Journal of Pharmacology and Experimental Therapeutics, 1962, 136, 38-42.

The respiratory effects of caffeine (and sodium benzoate), codeine sulfate, and morphine sulfate alone and in xanthine-narcotic combinations were determined by a double-blind factorial study in 10 healthy volunteers. Ten (2 ml) solutions containing normal saline; caffeine 62.5, 125, and 250 mg; morphine sulfate 10 mg; codeine sulfate 60 mg; and narcotic combinations with the 2 lower dosages of caffeine were administered i.m. to 4 subjects, while the remaining 6 received an identical dosage schedule except for the administration of caffeine alone. According to the alveolar ventilation-alveolar P_{CO_2} response curve, caffeine alone did not cause a significant stimulation of respiration, perhaps due to low doses or insensitive techniques. Morphine (10 mg) produced a significantly greater degree of respiratory depression than codeine (60 mg). The simultaneous administration of caffeine with codeine or morphine produced a statistically significant decrease in respiratory depression caused by the narcotics. The dose-effect relationship is the greater the amount of caffeine, the greater the decrease in respiratory depression. The results, which suggest that the greater the respiratory depressant effects of the narcotic, the more effective caffeine may be in its antagonism, are in agreement with the findings of Stroud et al. (1955), who observed that aminophylline prevented meperidine-induced respiratory depression.

Department of Anesthesiology
Memorial Hospital
New York, N.Y.

1540 Mattila, M. The effects of morphine and nalorphine on the small intestine of normal and morphine-tolerant rat and guinea-pig. Acta pharmacologica et toxicologica, 1962, 19, 47-52.

Morphine and nalorphine receptor mechanisms were studied in rat intestine. Tests were conducted in vitro on pieces of small intestine from fasting male rats, stimulated at 6-minute intervals. Among drugs tested for degree of inhibition were nicotine (15-150 μg), pilocarpine (3-15 μg), barium chloride (250-750 μg) and 5HT (0.2-0.5 μg), Morphine (10-500 μg) and nalorphine (100-300 μg) were added 30 seconds before stimulation. Intestine from morphine-tolerant rats, and normal and morphine-tolerant guinea pigs, was also studied. Morphine proved to be an effective inhibitor of nicotine induced contractions and a poor inhibitor of those caused by 5HT and pilocarpine in rat intestine; all these contractions were prevented more readily by nalorphine. No morphine-nalorphine antagonism occurred in rat intestine. Intestine from some addicted rats was extremely sensitive to nalorphine; this was not observed in the intestine of tolerant guinea pigs, which showed a marked morphine tolerance.

Department of Pharmacology
University of Helsinki
Helsinki, Finland

1541 Chilton, J., & Stenlake, J.B. Dissociation constants of some compounds related to lysergic acid. Journal of Pharmacy and Pharmacology, 1962, 14, 367-370.

Dissociation constants were determined for ergometrine, ergometrinine, LSD, isolysergic acid and a number of alkanolamides of 3-dimethylaminopropionic acid, 1-methylhexahydronicotinic acid and arecaidine. The similarity of pK (amide) values for the alkanolamides to that for ergometrine offered evidence that such values might be taken as an indication of amino-carboxyl distances. The dissociation constants were determined by the method of Chilton and Stenlake in an aqueous medium containing carbonate-free potassium hydroxide; LSD and isolysergic acid required a small amount of carbonate to facilitate solubility (they were back-titrated immediately with dilute acid).

Department of Pharmacy
The Royal College of Science and Technology
Glasgow, Great Britain

1542 Supek, Z., Uroić, B., Gjuriš, V., & Marijan, N. The effect of adrenergic blocking agents and of chlorpromazine on blood pressure increase by vasopressin and angiotensin. Journal of Pharmacy and Pharmacology, 1962, 14, 284-287.

The i. v. influence of chlorpromazine (2-5 mg/kg), hydergine (0.3-0.9 mg/kg), dibenamine (25 mg/kg) and tolazoline (20-40 mg/kg) on the mean arterial response to i. v. vasopressin (0.1 I. U./kg), angiotensin (0.07 mg/kg) and barium chloride (0.5-1.0 mg/kg) was investigated in anesthetized mongrel dogs. The adrenergic blocking agents potentiated the pressor response to vasopressin but did not affect responses to angiotensin or barium chloride. Chlorpromazine potentiated the response to both vasopressin and angiotensin; this potentiation was not due to a decrease in blood pressure produced by adrenergic blocking or by chlorpromazine.

Department of Pharmacology
University of Zagreb
Zagreb, Yugoslavia

1543 Sloan, Jewell W., Brooks, J. W., Eisenman, Anna J., & Martin, W. R. Comparison of the effects of single doses of morphine and thebaine on body temperature, activity, and brain and heart levels of catecholamines and serotonin. Psychopharmacologia, 1962, 3, 291-301.

Single doses of morphine (15-60 mg/kg i. p.) were given to equal numbers of randomized Wistar rats, which were sacrificed 4 hours after treatment. Brains and hearts were analyzed for catecholamines; brains were also analyzed for serotonin. Animals were observed for changes in activity and body temperature. There were no significant changes in heart catecholamines, brain serotonin or catecholamines 4 hours after morphine. Brain catecholamines increased 2 hours after injection of morphine (60 mg/kg). Doses of 15-30 mg/kg resulted in an initial depression of activity followed by increased activity and body temperature, 60 mg/kg produced profound depression of activity and body temperature, which was maximal at 2 hours. Respiratory depression also occurred in these animals, with cyanosis in half of the cases. None

showed cyanosis with 15 mg/kg and very few with 30 mg/kg. In a comparative study, 20 mg/kg of thebaine produced a moderate decrease in brain and heart catecholamines, but no significant changes in brain serotonin within 30-60 minutes after drug administration. Fifteen of the 26 animals had convulsions, 7 had major seizures and 4 died. Animals appeared sedated inbetween seizures. No hyperthermia was observed.

Addiction Research Center
NIMH, USPHS
Lexington, Ky.

1544 Azima, H., Arthurs, Dorothy, & Silver, A. The effects of chlordiazepoxide (Librium) in anxiety states. A multiblind study. Canadian Psychiatric Association Journal, 1962, 7, 44-50.

The antianxiety properties of chlordiazepoxide (Librium) were evaluated in a multi-blind study on 2 randomly selected groups of 92 patients each (75 neurotics and 17 psychotics); 1 group receiving p. o. an average daily dose of 70 mg for an average of 3 weeks, the other (controls) receiving placebo; and a 3rd group of 15 neurotics receiving placebo and drug sequentially. Chi² analysis of data revealed that chlordiazepoxide had a highly significant effect ($P<0.001$) in neurotic states, but not in psychotics, while analysis of subgroup data in neurotics showed a statistically significant improvement rate in anxiety states and mixed states ($0.01>P>0.001$), but not in obsessive and depressive states. The most common side effects were headache, dizziness, hand tremors, drowsiness, nausea and vomiting. The efficacy of chlordiazepoxide as an adequate antianxiety and antitension drug may be limited to anxiety reactions and mixed neurotic states.

Allan Memorial Institute
McGill University
Montreal, Quebec
Canada

1545 Horovitz, Zola P., & Chow May-I. Effects of centrally acting drugs on the correlation of electrocortical activity and

wakefulness of cats. Journal of
Pharmacology and Experimental
Therapeutics, 1962, 137, 127-132.

Cats with chronically implanted electrodes
were used in the study of atropine, tetra-
hydroaminacrin (THA), N-ethylpiperidyl,
ethotrimeprazine, physostigmine salicylate,
chlorpromazine, triflupromazine
and imipramine, all injected i.p. Responses
i.e., behavior, and electrocortical recordings were used as test parameters.
Atropine and ethotrimeprazine produced
dissociation with the latter being about
10 times as potent. Physostigmine and
THA caused the opposite type of
dissociation with normal or low levels
of behavior being associated with a fast
low voltage electrocorticogram. Imipramine
did not produce any dissociation or stimulation but did depress the animal's behavior,
as did chlorpromazine and triflupromazine.

Squibb Institute for Medical Research
New Brunswick, N.J.

1546 Gabourel, John D., & Comstock,
John P. Effect of diacetylmonoxime on
the action of convulsant and sedative-
hypnotic barbiturates. Journal of
Pharmacology and Experimental
Therapeutics, 1962, 137, 122-126.

Male Swiss-Webster mice and male
Wistar rats were employed in the assessment of diacetylmonoxime (DAM). Also
rabbit microsomes were used for in vitro
metabolic studies according to Gillette et
al. (1957). Hexobarbital was assayed
photometrically and C^{14}-labeled pentobarbital by its radioactivity. Mice and
rats pretreated with DAM lose their
righting reflex when given injections of
25-35 mg/kg 3,5-dimethylbutylethyl
barbiturate (DMBEB). Although these
doses of DMBEB cause motor convulsions
and death in saline-injected controls,
DAM-treated animals do not exhibit motor
convulsions nor do they die. DAM-
pretreatment was also shown to prolong
barbiturate-induced loss of righting reflex
in mice, rats and rabbits, but it failed to
inhibit the metabolism of either hexobarbital
or DMBEB by liver microsomes. When
mice or rats were injected with DAM on

awaking from barbiturate sleep, they
again lost their righting reflex and studies
in mice with C^{14}-labeled pentobarbital
showed that here DAM did not elevate the
brain barbiturate level and therefore
prolongation of the righting reflex is
brought about either by a direct central
action of DAM or by barbiturate potentiation
of the weak neuromuscular blocking action
of this oxime.

Department of Pharmacology
Stanford University School of Medicine
Palo Alto, Calif.

1547 Maynert, E.W., & Kaji, Hideko, K.
On the relationship of brain γ-aminobutyric
acid to convulsions. Journal of Pharmacology
and Experimental Therapeutics, 1962, 137,
114-121.

Clonic seizures were electrically-induced
in Swiss mice and Sprague-Dawley rats.
Brain GABA was estimated chromatographically after sacrifice. Mice injected
i.p. with thiosemicarbazide showed a
significantly smaller decrease in brain
GABA than that found in animals similarly
treated with semicarbazide, acetone
semicarbazone, thiocarbohydrazide, iso-
nicotinic acid hydrazide or 3-deoxypyridoxine
phosphate (all at 2.67 μM/g i.p.). Compared
with the hydrazides, methylhydrazine and
1-phenyl-2-hydrazinopropane caused little
change in GABA while a convulsive dose of
hydrazine caused an increase in brain GABA.
Large doses of succinitrile (500 μg/g)
and diphenylhydantion (200 μg/g) were
almost as effective as hydrazides in lowering GABA. Metrazol, picrotoxin and
insulin caused smaller decreases and
reserpine had no effect. Brain GABA in
mice and rats was only elevated in level
by hydrazine and hydroxylamine, hydrazine
being more effective and less toxic. Neither
or these compounds altered the incidence
or duration of the electrically-induced clonic
seizures or modified the pattern of a maximal
seizure. Mice could not be protected against
pentylenetetrazol seizures by hydrazine
and hydrazine-treated mice injected with
semicarbazide exhibited maximal seizures
at supernormal concentrations of brain
GABA. Hydrazide-induced convulsions may
possibly cause a supernormal utilization

of GABA for energy-yielding reactions
in the brain.

Johns Hopkins University School of
    Medicine
Baltimore, Md.

1548   Davis, W.M. Day-night periodicity
in pentobarbital response of mice and
the influence of socio-psychological
conditions. Experientia, 1962, 18,
235-237.

Mice were given the customary 60 mg/kg
dose of pentobarbital i. p. and the
illumination in their environment automatically controlled. Twelve hours of
darkness alternating with 12 hours of
light were provided which corresponded
approximately to the natural daily cycle.
The anesthetic effect was marked during
the day and weak at night; this was true
for both experiments run at 26°C and at
36°C. The periodicity of analgesic effect
disappeared when the mice were kept under
continuous illumination and the degree of
periodicity diminished when mice were
kept isolated instead of grouped.

University of Oklahoma College of
    Pharmacy
Norman, Okla.

1549   Kraupp, O., Bernheimer, H.,
Heistracher, P., Papistas, D., &
Schiefthaler, Th. Die Wirkung von
Iproniazid sowie i. p. Zufuhr von
Katecholaminen und ihrer O-Methyl-
derivate auf die renale Ausscheidung von
Metanephrin und Normetanephrin an der
Ratte. [Effect of iproniazid and i. p.
administration of catecholamines and their
o-methyl derivatives on the renal excretion
of metanephrine and normetanephrine in
rats.] Archiv für Experimentelle Pathologie
und Pharmakologie, 1962, 243, 459-467.

Treatment of rats with iproniazid
(50 mg/kg/day i. p. for 3 days) increased
the urinary excretion of normetanephrine
from negligible values to 46 µg/kg/24 hours;
the recovery of metanephrine from the
urine after i. p. administration of 400 µg/kg
epinephrine or 800 µg/kg metanephrine

that of urethane. Control experiments showed that the effect of X-ray was not due to decreased food consumption, and administration of glucose had no effect. The prolongation of the hypnotic effect is probably due to interference with drug catabolism.

Medizinische Forschungsanstalt
Max Planck Gesellschaft
Göttingen, Germany

1552 Holck, Harald G.O., Demaree, Gale E., & Kaji, Hideko Katayama. Effects of β-diethylaminoethyl diphenylpropylacetate hydrochloride on three convulsants and on propallylonal. Journal of Pharmaceutical Sciences, 1962, 5 1, 739-742.

The effects of β-diethylaminoethyl diphenylpropylacetate (SKF 525-A) on 3 convulsants and propallylonal was studied in Swiss mice and Holtzman rats at various doses. The LD_{50}'s of nikethamide, pentylenetetrazol and picrotoxin were increased by pretreatment of mice 1 hour before drug injection with SKF 525-A. SKF 525-A markedly prolonged the hypnotic effect of propallylonal without increasing the number of delayed deaths in rats. The maximal picrotoxin action in mice pretreated with SKF 525-A s.c. developed in about 4 hours, was still marked at 8 hours, and was lost by 16 hours. SKF 525-A induced maximal effects when given i.p. immediately prior to picrotoxin; it also markedly facilitated the potency of picrotoxin in normal rats and in those receiving barbital, by a multiple injection technique. Using this same technique, barbital greatly increased LD_{50}'s of pentylenetetrazol and picrotoxin in rats. SKF 525-A did not influence the toxicity of pentylenetetrazol in normal rats or in those receiving barbital by the multiple injection method.

Department of Pharmacology
College of Pharmacy
University of Nebraska
Lincoln, Neb.

1553 Kapila, Kanti, & Arora, R.B. Anticonvulsant activity of procaine and its five congeners against experimentally

induced convulsions. Journal of Pharmacy and Pharmacology, 1962, 14, 253-254.

Procainamide, procaine and its 4 congeners were studied for anticonvulsant activity and compared with phenytoin against maximal electroshock and leptazol-induced seizures in rats. Neurotoxicity and acute toxicity were determined; ED_{50}, TD_{50}, LD_{50}, therapeutic indices and protective indices of the drugs were calculated. These compounds were effective only against maximal electroshock seizures, they were effective within 10 minutes and remained so for 2-3 hours, while the effect of phenytoin lasted much longer. Clonic convulsions preceded death during acute toxicity studies. Procaine, and to a greater degree, its methyl substituted congeners, had higher protective and therapeutic indices than did phenytoin, while these indices were lowest for procainamide.

Department of Pharmacology
All-India Institute of Medical Sciences
New Delhi 16, India

1554 Werdinius, Bengt. Effect of temperature on the action of reserpine. Acta Pharmacologica et Toxicologica, 1962, 19, 43-46.

An attempt was made to reproduce the results reported by previous authors on the effects of temperature on reserpine action. Male rats were exposed to various temperatures (-10°, 4° and 37°C) for various periods up to 16 hours, then given reserpine (1.0-2.5 mg/kg i.p.). After 4 additional hours in the same environment the animals were sacrificed and their brains analyzed for 5HT content (by a slight modification of Bertler's method). Controls were run in parallel, because of considerable normal variation in brain 5HT. All animals treated with reserpine were sedated, with ptosis and characteristic hunched posture, irrespective of thermal environment, 5HT content was comparably lowered by reserpine under all temperature conditions.

Department of Pharmacology
University of Göteborg
Göteborg, Sweden

1555   Feldman, Shaul, & Wagman, Irving
H.   Hypothalamic effects on spinal reflexes
and their alteration by pentobarbital.
Experimental Neurology, 1962, 5, 250-268.

Alterations in hypothalamic effects on
spinal reflexes were studied at various
levels of pentobarbital anesthesia in 15
intact cats.   Potentials evoked in the
hypothalamus upon peripheral stimulation
were studied concurrently.   In immobilized
and lightly anesthetized animals, high-
frequency hypothalamic stimulation usually
potentiated monosynaptic and depressed
polysynaptic reflexes.   Moderate pentobarbital anesthesia produced a diminution
of hypothalamic effects of spinal cord
reflexes with disappearance of the peripherally evoked hypothalamic potentials.
Deepening of anesthesia abolished hypothalamic facilitation of the spinal monosynaptic reflex.   Hypothalamic stimulation
had little or no effect on persistent
polysynaptic response.   High-voltage,
secondary, long-latency potentials were
evoked in the hypothalamus by peripheral
nerve stimulation at this stage of deep
anesthesia.   The effects noted were due
primarily to the actions of pentobarbital
in the hypothalamus and only partly to the
effect of anesthesia on the spinal mechanisms.
In the lightly anesthetized or immobilized
intact animal the facilitatory brainstem regions have a predominant effect on
spinal cord reflexes, and anesthesia (or
decerebration) attenuates this facilitatory
effect, thus allowing the inhibitory effect of
the bulbar reticular formation on the spinal
cord to be shown.

Department of Neurology
Mount Sinai Hospital
New York, N. Y.

1556   Essig, Carl F.   Convulsive and sham
rage behaviors in decorticate dogs during
barbiturate withdrawal.   Archives of
Neurology, 1962, 7, 471-475.

Three decorticate dogs, 27 to 37 days after
surgery, and intact controls received
increasing amounts of p.o. barbital until
final daily dose levels of 118 to 178 mg/kg
were attained (in periods varying from 202
to 372 days).   Following abrupt withdrawal,

A., Pieri, L., & Valzelli, L. Effect of
imipramine, amitriptyline and their
monomethyl derivatives on reserpine
activity. Journal of Pharmacy and
Pharmacology, 1962, 14, 509-514.

The effects of imipramine, amitriptyline
and their N-monomethyl derivatives (all
7.5-30 mg/kg i.p.), on reserpine
(2.5-5.0 mg/kg i.v. or i.p.) activity was
studied in female Sprague-Dawley rats,
Swiss mice and the zebra fish (Brachydanius
rerius). Demethylimipramine and
demethylamitriptyline reduced the reserpine-
induced hypothermia in rats more readily
than did the parent compounds, imipramine
and demethylimipramine decreased the
severity of gastric ulcers induced by
reserpine in restrained rats more so than
did amitriptyline or its desmethyl
derivative; desmethylimipramine did not
prevent the decrease in brain amine level
induced by reserpine. Imipramine, but
not demethylimipramine, antagonized
leptazol (0.5%) convulsions, failed to
potentiate the central effects of 5HTP and
5HT, and did not prevent the hypothermia
induced by 5HT, α-methyl dopa (500 mg/kg
i.p.) or chlorpromazine (10 mg/kg i.p.).

Department of Pharmacology
Medical School
University of Milan
Milan, Italy

1559 Hartry, Arlene L. The effects of
reserpine on the psychogenic production
of gastric ulcers in rats. Journal of
Comparative and Physiological Psychology,
1962, 55, 719-721.

The effects of low dosages of reserpine
(0.1 mg/kg i.m.) on the psychogenesis of
gastric ulcers was studied in 28 male
Wistar rats, with restraint stress used to
induce ulceration (Bonfils et al. 1957).
Four experimental conditions were
investigated: immobilization (plus hunger
and thirst) accompanied by injection of
reserpine, immobilization (plus hunger and
thirst) alone, reserpine alone and hunger
and thirst alone. Ulcers occurred primarily
in the immobilization-reserpine group and
secondly in the immobilization-no reserpine
group. Titration revealed less stomach

acidity in ulcerated rats. No relationship
was observed between weight loss and
frequency of ulceration. Titration values
indicated that ulceration was accompanied
by increased gastric motility or decreased
gastric secretion. Restraint stress may
provoke the physiological reactions of
anger rather than anxiety.

[No address]

1560 Malone, Marvin H., & Roth, Robert
H., Jr. Yohimbine potentiation of
reserpine blepharoptosis. Journal of
Pharmaceutical Sciences, 1962, 51, 345-348.

The mouse ptosis assay developed by
Rubin et al. was randomly employed in
216 mice to determine the effects of
yohimbine (2-16 mg) on potentiation of
reserpine (2-8 mg/kg). The oral LD_{50}
was 36.5 mg/kg for yohimbine and
150 mg/kg for reserpine. Various
reserpine-yohimbine mixtures were assayed
against reserpine alone in 4 balanced log
dose-response assays. Maximal mean
ptotic effects following reserpine
administration occurred within 10 hours.
Yohimbine produced detectable ptosis at
doses of 16 mg/kg but not at 8 mg/kg.
Statistical treatment involved analysis
of variance, factorial analysis, and
calculation of potency and confidence limits
according to the method of Bliss. Peak
potentiation occurred at 3 hours for 1:1
and 1:2 reserpine-yohimbine mixtures,
while peak effects were achieved at 10
hours with the 1:4 mixture, indicating
considerable distortion by yohimbine of
any ptotic assay documenting only reserpine
activity. Yohimbine, in a 1:1 ratio with
reserpine, potentiated ptosis for about
5 hours, ceased to be effective within 10
hours and may have aided reversal of
residual ptosis by 24 hours. With a 1:2
ratio, ptosis was unaffected at 24 hours.
Complete potentiation was obtained with
yohimbine in a 1:4 ratio at all times.
Males were considerably more susceptible to
reserpine-induced ptosis than females.
Yohimbine lacked true ptotic activity but
potentiated reserpine-induced blepharoptosis without altering slope or dose-
response relationships, thus indicating
that the mechanism of reserpine action may

be dependent upon depletion of levarterenol rather than upon release of serotonin.

Division of Pharmacology
University of Connecticut
Storrs, Conn.

1561 Schumann, E. L. , Paquette, L. A. , Heinzelman, R. V. , Wallach, D. P. , Vanzo, J. P. , & Greig, M. E. The synthesis and γ-aminobutyric acid transaminase inhibition of aminooxy acids and related compounds. Journal of Medicinal and Pharmaceutical Chemistry, 1962, 5, 464-477.

A series of 36 GABA analogues failed to inhibit GABA-α-keto glutaric acid (AKG) transaminase in vitro and in vivo. These compounds were also unable to raise GABA brain levels. Several of the 46 aminooxy derivatives synthesized were fairly active inhibitors of GABA-AKG transaminase in vitro and in vivo. All compounds were tested for their protective activity against thiosemicarbazide-induced convulsions (8 rats or mice received 10, 25 or 50% of the LD_{50} 1 hour before receiving thiosemicarbazide, 20mg/kg i. p.), and the resultant degree of protection paralleled the in vivo GABA transaminase inhibition. A significant degree of in vivo activity was limited to several α-amino-oxyacids or their easily hydrolyzed derivatives. No compound showed activity superior to that of aminooxyacetic acid. Most compounds were prepared by alkylation of a hydroxylamine derivative in the presence of base, followed by hydrolysis of the protecting group. Relevant data on all compounds is presented in tabular form.

Upjohn Company Research Laboratories
Kalamazoo, Mich.

1562 Remmer, H. , Siegert, M. , Nitze, H. R. , & Kirsten, I. Die Gewöhnung an langwirkende Barbiturate. [Tolerance to long-acting barbiturates.] Archiv für Experimentelle Pathologie und Pharmakologie, 1962, 243, 468-478.

Administration of phenobarbital (110 mg/kg) or barbital (150 mg/kg) s. c. to rats 3 times a week for 4 weeks produced no decrease in the duration of anesthesia following a test i. p. dose, compared to controls, although 5 out of 28 male rats and 17 out of 27 females died. Thus there seems to be chronic poisoning in females, with sufficient accumulation to produce tolerance. Daily administration of phenobarbital (50 mg/kg b. i. d. , s. c.) or barbital (200 mg/kg/day s. c.) did produce tolerance in rats, as measured by an increase in the concentration measured in the blood when the animals awoke. In dogs, which eliminate pheno-barbital more slowly, daily p. o. administration of increasing doses (2-30 mg/kg) also produced tolerance, as measured by the disappearance of ataxia at increasingly high blood levels. This tolerance was no longer demonstrable after 11 days without treatment when practically all of the phenobarbital had been eliminated. This type of tolerance is to be distinguished from the tolerance to short-acting oxidizable barbiturates due to an increase in their catabolic rate.

Pharmakologisches Institut
Freie Universität
Berlin, Germany

1563 Sammalisto, Lasse. Effect of glutamine on intoxication caused by ethyl alcohol. Nature, 1962, 185, 185.

A total of 57 fasting rats were divided into 7 groups of 6-10 animals which were tested for ethyl alcohol intoxication by placing each rat on an inclined plane with a rough surface; at a given angle of inclination the rat slid down the plane. Intoxicated rats slid down at lower angles than normal ones. The performance while intoxicated was expressed as a percentage of the value obtained while sober. Animals received the alcohol (3. 0-4. 5 mg/kg intragastrically) as a 30% v/v solution, glutamine [dose not stated] was administered in the alcoholic solution. Glutamine did not effect the blood alcohol level. However, it did offer variable degrees of protection against intoxication, which were contingent upon genetic and environmental conditions. Glutamine effects depended upon the role played by this compound in brain metabolism during alcohol intoxication.

Research Laboratories of the State
  Alcohol Monopoly (Alko)
Helsinki, Finland

1564 Callingham, B.A., & Cass, Rosemary. The effects of bretylium and cocaine on noradrenaline depletion. Journal of Pharmacy and Pharmacology, 1962, 14, 385-389.

Rats were used to study the effects of bretylium (30 mg/kg s.c.) and cocaine (10-50 mg/kg s.c.) on levarterenol depletion. Reserpine was administered s.c. at 0.1-1.0 mg/kg and guanethidine at 10 mg/kg to see if bretylium or cocaine might reduce their ability to deplete rat heart and spleen levarterenol levels; this reduction did not occur. Rats were sacrificed 6-18 hours after drug injection and catecholamine content (epinephrine and levarterenol) of heart and spleen assayed (method of Cass and Spriggs 1961) and expressed in terms of levarterenol. In additional experiments, 50 mg/kg cocaine failed to reduce the pressor action of physostigmine (20 μg ı.v.) in anesthetized rats; in fact it slightly potentiated the response. Bretylium probably acts by preventing levarterenol release, while cocaine prevents releasing agents from reaching levarterenol depots.

Department of Pharmacology
School of Pharmacy
University of London
29-39 Brunswick Square
London W.C.1, Great Britain

1565 Schmidt, G., & Meisse, P. Zentrale Wirkungen von Cocainhomologen und ihre Beeinflussbarkeit durch Reserpin oder Adrenolytica. [Central effects of cocaine homologs and the effect of reserpine or adrenolytic agents.] Archiv für Experimentelle Pathologie und Pharmakologie, 1962, 243, 148-161.

Pretreatment of guinea pigs with reserpine (5 mg/kg s.c.) abolished or markedly decreased the specific central sympathetic response to l-n-cocaine (increased motility, increased body temperature and hyperglycemia) and depressed the convulsive action, but had no effect on the toxic effects of d-4-cocaine. Similarly the ptosis due to reserpine was temporarily abolished by l-n-cocaine but not by d-4-cocaine. Pretreatment with iproniazid (100 mg/kg) potentiated the effects of l-n-cocaine but had no effect on the response to d-4-cocaine. The adrenolytic agents yohimbine (5 mg/kg s.c.) and phentolamine (0.05 mg/kg intracisternally) counteracted the pyrogenic effect of l-n-cocaine, but s.c. phentolamine was ineffective. In mice analgesic properties were shown by l-n-cocaine but not by d-4-cocaine. The psychopharmacological effects of l-n-cocaine are assumed to be mediated by an increased sensitivity to catecholamines in the CNS.

Pharmakologisches Institut
Universität Göttingen
Göttingen, Germany

1566 Friebel, H., & Kuhn, H.F. Uber husten- und atemdepressorische Wirkung. [Depressant effects on coughing and respiration.] Archiv für Experimentelle Pathologie und Pharmakologie, 1962, 243, 162-173.

In an attempt to differentiate pharmacologically between the regulatory systems for coughing and respiration, experiments were carried out on male guinea pigs forced to cough by inhalation of SO_2. Drugs were administered s.c. 30 minutes before SO_2. In other experiments, respiratory rate and minute volume were recorded kymographically. The ED_{50} for cough suppression was smallest with 1-phenethyl-4-(propin-2-yl)-4-propionoxypiperidine (1.6 mg/kg) and highest for hexobarbital (77.0 mg/kg). Codeine, pipazethate and 2-aminoindane all had ED_{50} values of 14.5-15.5, while pentoxyverin was 50.0 mg/kg. Respiration was markedly depressed by hexobarbital, even at 50 mg/kg, and moderately by codeine, but stimulated by 2-aminoindane; the other 3 drugs had little effect on respiration. Isoprenaline (0.01 mg/kg s.c.) did not alleviate the depression produced by hexobarbital, but had some effect on that produced by codeine. When given after

hexobarbital (50 mg/kg), 4 of the other
antitussives seemed to potentiate the
depressant effect on respiration while
2-aminoindane again stimulated respiration.
The results suggest that the central mechanism of the cough reflex is to a considerable
extent independent of the central mechanism
of the respiration.

Pharmakologisches Institut
Universität Bonn
Bonn 53, Germany

1567 Klärner, Paul. Über den Einfluss
von Barbituraten, Thiobarbituraten und
Barbitursäure auf celluläre Potentiale und
Kontraktionen des Meerschweinchenvorhofes.
[The effect of barbiturates, thiobarbiturates
and barbituric acid on cellular potentials
and contractions of the guinea pig auricle.]
Archiv für Experimentelle Pathologie und
Pharmakologie, 1962, 243, 269-278.

Comparative studies of hexobarbital,
pentobarbital, thiopental, methitural and
barbituric acid in the electrically stimulated
guinea pig auricle showed that low concentrations of all these drugs first prolonged the
90% repolarization time, while high
concentrations produced increasing shortening of the 20%, 50% and 90% repolarization
time. Very high concentrations decreased
the resting potential. Only thiobarbiturates
affected the rhythm of auricular contraction,
and they were more effective than barbiturates
in increasing the latent period. Thus, at
clinical dosage, barbiturates are less cardio-
toxic than thiobarbiturates. Barbituric acid
itself prolonged all phases of repolarization
only at high concentrations. These drugs
apparently act by changing ionic permeability.

Pharmakologisches Institut
Universität Mainz
Mainz, Germany

1568 Klinger, W., & Kersten, L. Die
analeptische Wirkung von Vanillinsäure-
diäthylamid. [The analeptic effect of
vanillic acid diethylamide.] Acta Biologica
et Medica Germanica, 1962, 9, 67-78.

Comparative studies of vanillic acid
diethylamide, metrazol and nikethamide in

1570 Carson, Richard P., & Domino,
Edward F. Synergistic and antagonistic
effects of premedication on general
anesthetics in mice. Anesthesiology,
1962, 23, 187-192.

The effects of preanesthetic medication
on the anesthetic and lethal concentrations
of general anesthetics were studied in
untreated, saline-control and drug-treated
mice. Premedication (all drugs given i. p.)
with subanesthetic doses of pentobarbital
(20-30 mg/kg) and phenobarbital (65 mg/kg)
had a synergistic effect on the anesthetic
concentration of diethyl ether, halothane,
and chloroform but no significant effect
on their lethal concentration. Atropine or
scopolamine premedication (1 mg/kg) had
no synergistic or antagonistic effect on the
anesthetic or lethal actions of diethyl
ether, halothane or chloroform. Morphine
premedication (5 mg/kg) did not affect
time to anesthesia with diethyl ether and
halothane but prolonged time to death.
Chlorpromazine and promethazine produced
variable results with doses of 5 mg/kg but
at 15 mg/kg, chlorpromazine reduced time
to anesthesia and prolonged the time for
death for diethyl ether and halothane but
not chloroform. In equal doses, promethe-
azine was less effective. Pentobarbital
and phenobarbital appear to have a
selective effect of increasing the anesthetic
but not the lethal potency of diethyl ether,
chloroform and halothane. Pentobarbital
premedication should therefore improve
the therapeutic index of these agents. The
variable results found with the phenothiazine
derivatives, particularly with smaller
doses, rules out definitive conclusions on
their utility.

Department of Pharmacology
University of Michigan
Ann Arbor, Mich.

1571 Kier, Lemont B., Fox, Lauretta E.,
Dhawan, D., & Waters, I. W. A new class
of central nervous system stimulants.
Nature, 1962, 195, 817-818.

An N-alkyl sydnone called compound I:

[N-isobutylsydnone]:

was studied pharmacologically. In male
brown mice (C57B x 1101 hybrids), the
s. c. LD_{50} is ca. 135 mg/kg and the convulsive dose ca. 117 mg/kg. Pentetrazole
under the same conditions had an LD_{50} of
ca. 75 mg/kg. Convulsions began less than
1 minute after administration, and caused
ticking in the facial musculature and fore-
limbs. This was followed by clonic
movements which frequently developed an
extensor component and almost all animals
died in tonic convulsions. A spinal cat,
transected at C-1, did not convulse at
100 mg/kg; 2 decerebrate cats showed
definite convulsive patterns at 200 mg/kg.
When 41 mg/kg of either compound I or
pentetrazole was administered i. v.
to a dog(given sufficient pentobarbital i. v.
to cause apnea) the more favorable response
and rise in blood pressure was obtained
with compound I. Respiratory stimulation
appeared to be predominantly central as
there was little decrease of activity after
vagotomy or carotid sinus denervation.
Compound I did not potentiate acetylcholine
and produced no acetylcholine esterase
inhibition. There was no antispasmodic
activity against acetylcholine or histamine
in guinea pig ileum. No spasmodic
activity was noted in isolated tissue although
a positive Straub test was observed in
Compound I-treated mice.

College of Pharmacy
University of Florida
Gainesville, Fla.

1572 Drain, D. J., Horlington, M.,
Lazare, R., & Poulter, G. A. The effect
of α-methyl DOPA and some other decarboxylase inhibitors on brain 5-hydroxy-
tryptamine. Life Sciences, 1962, 3, 93-97.

The effects of α-methyl DOPA, 3-hydroxy-
benzyloxyamine (NSD 1024) and N-(3-
hydroxybenzyl)-N-methylhydrazine (NSD

1034) on 5HTP decarboxylase were studied
in vivo and in vitro. In the first experiments, the minimum effective doses
necessary to prevent the characteristic
tremors following administration of 5HTP
(75 mg/kg) were determined in mice pretreated 2 hours before with the MAO
inhibitor N-(1-methyl-2-phenoxyethyl) -
hydrazine (5 mg/kg i. p.). In later
experiments, the 5HTP decarboxylase
activity of mouse brain homogenates was
compared in treated animals and untreated
controls; again, the amounts necessary to
produce 50% and 80% inhibition of decarboxylase activity were determined. All
3 drugs were found to be powerful inhibitors
of 5HTP decarboxylase in vivo and in vitro.
As previously reported, α-methyl DOPA
(400 mg/kg s.c.) also produces a marked
decrease in the mouse brain 5HT level. In
the case of NSD 1024, however, doses up
to 64 mg/kg) produced only a transitory
decrease in 5HT, the level returning to
normal long before the decarboxylase
activity. It is therefore unlikely that the
effect of α-methyl DOPA on cerebral 5HT
is mediated wholly via inhibition of 5HTP
decarboxylase.

Smith and Nephew Research Ltd.
Hunsdon Laboratories
Ware, Hertfordshire,
Great Britain

1573 Izquierdo, Juan A., Coussio, Jorge
D., & Kaumann, Alberto J. Effect of
imipramine on the pressor responses to the
afferent vagal stimulation in reserpinized
dogs. Archives Internationales de Pharmacodynamie et de Thérapie, 1962, 135, 303-
310.

The effect of levarterenol (0.5-2.0 μ g/kg),
epinephrine (1-2 μ g/kg) and imipramine
(3-10 mg/kg) injected into the external
iliac vein on the pressor response to
afferent vagal stimulation was studied in
anesthetized dogs (pentobarbital, 35 mg/kg)
given reserpine (250 mg/kg) 1-48 hours
earlier. Imipramine was found to oppose
reserpine-induced hypotension, antagonizing
the depressor response to vagal stimulation
and, 1 hour but not 48 hours after reserpine,
transforming it into a pressor response.
Imipramine accentuated the magnitude and

in mice and the prevention of convulsions due to i. v. strychnine. There was no potentiation, however, of either hexobarbital anesthesia or morphine analgesia. Other pig cerebral extracts not containing substance P (as shown by tests on isolated, atropinized, guinea pig ileum) also had central nervous system depressant properties.

Pharmacological Research Department
N. V. Organon Oss
The Netherlands

1576 Femmer, K. Antitremorin-Wirkung von quaternären Phenothiazinbasen. [Antitremorine activity of quaternary phenothiazine bases.] Arzneimittel-Forschung, 1962, 12, 706-707.

Comparative studies in mice and cats showed that both Wu 2505 (N-2-dimethylethylammonium-2-methylethylphenothiazine ethosulfate) and Wu 2506 (N-2-dimethylethyl.ammonium-1-methylethylphenothiazine ethosulfate) in doses of 5 mg/kg i. p. had a powerful and long-lasting anti-tremorine effect, as shown by the rotating-rod test and the hot-plate analgesia test in mice and tremorine-rage in cats; the effect of ethopropazine (5 mg/kg i. p.) was much more transitory. Both Wu 2505 and Wu 2506 also had significant anticholinergic activity on the isolated guinea pig ileum. This indicates that the anti-tremorine activity must be central in nature.

Forschungsabteilung I
VEB Arzneimittelwerk
Dresden, Germany

1577 Stock, K., & Westermann, E. Untersuchungen über den Mechanismus der narkoseverkürzenden Wirkung von Monoaminoxydase-Hemmstoffen. [Studies on the mechanism of the analeptic effect of monoamineoxidase inhibitors.] Archiv für Experimentelle Pathologie und Pharmakologie, 1962, 243, 44-64.

Measurements of the duration of hexobarbital (100 mg/kg i. p.) narcosis and of the cerebral catecholamine levels and MAO activity in male mice pretreated with

various MAO inhibitors and sedatives showed that the hydrazine MAO inhibitors iproniazid (100 mg/kg s. c.), nialamide (20 mg/kg s. c.) and JB 807 (benzylisopropylisopropylhydrazine; 20 mg/kg s. c.) prolonged hexobarbital anesthesia when given 1-6 hours earlier, but shortened it when given 20-48 hours before. The non-hydrazine MAO inhibitors pargyline (20 mg/kg s. c.) and tranylcypromine (10 mg/kg s. c.) shortened hexobarbital anesthesia when given 1-6 hours before, as did chlorpromazine (5 mg/kg s. c.) and SKF 525 A (diethylaminoethyl-diphenyl-propylacetate; 50 mg/kg s. c.) given 20-48 hours earlier. The cerebral serotonin level was increased by all MAO inhibitors, but the shortening of anesthesia 20-24 hours after iproniazid or nialamide still persisted when the increase in brain serotonin was prevented by harmaline (30 mg/kg s. c.). Hexobarbital catabolism by liver microsomes was strongly inhibited 1-6 hours after the hydrazine derivatives, but activated 48 hours after treatment. Neither the nonhydrazine MAO inhibitors nor chlorpromazine or SKF 525 A had any significant effect, but phenobarbital (100 mg/kg s. c.) also shortened the duration of hexobarbital anesthesia and stimulated its catabolism. Iproniazid, SKF 525 A or phenobarbital also decreased the hexobarbital concentration found in the brain after injection. Thus the shortening of hexobarbital sleeping time by various agents is due to different mechanisms of action.

Pharmakologisches Institut
Universität Frankfurt a. M.
Frankfurt, Germany

1578 Fink, Gregory B., & Swinyard, Ewart A. Comparison of anticonvulsant and psychopharmacologic drugs. Journal of Pharmaceutical Sciences, 1962, 51, 548-551.

Four anticonvulsant drugs and 7 tranquilizers were tested in male CF1 mice for their ability to increase hexobarbital sleeping time, abolish CAR's and reduce amphetamine toxicity in mice aggregated 3 per cage (more severe test) and 10 per cage (less severe test). All drugs were used at equitoxic doses, e.g., phenobarbital 70 mg/kg. Except for the 3 phenothiazine derivatives, all the drugs were ineffective in nontoxic doses in the 3 mice per cage test, while only phenobarbital, trimethadione, meprobamate and phenaglycodol were ineffective as measured by the 10 mice per cage test. Chlorpromazine, promazine and triflupromazine effectively reduced amphetamine toxicity in both situations. The phenothiazines, reserpine and hydroxyzine were active in the 10 per cage test; diphenylhydantoin and phenacemide were also effective which suggests that they have some tranquilizing properties. All drugs increased hexobarbital sleeping time. Chlorpromazine, promazine, triflupromazine, reserpine and hydroxyzine blocked CAR's and/or secondary conditioned responses. Meprobamate, phenaglycodol and the anticonvulsant drugs (diphenylhydantoin, phenacemide, phenobarbital and trimethadione) had little effect on CAR's in nontoxic doses.

Department of Pharmacology
University of Utah
Salt Lake City, Utah

1579 Noach, E.L., Bunk, J. Joosting, & Wijling, A. Influence of electroshock and phenobarbital on nucleic acid content of rat braing cortex. Acta Physiologica et Pharmacologica Neerlandica, 1962, 11, 54-69.

Studies were made in female rats to determine whether maximal electroshock evokes a decrease in brain nucleic acid, as reported for other species, and whether this decrease can be prevented with barbiturates in nonanesthetic, anticonvulsant doses. In addition, animals were housed either individually or in groups. Nucleic acids were estimated chemically (chromatography and spectrophotometry) in cerebral cortex slices from untreated controls, rats sacrificed 30-75 seconds after maximal electroshock, rats sacrificed 75 minutes after 15 mg phenobarbital, and rats sacrificed 30-75 seconds following maximal electroshock 75 minutes after 15 mg phenobarbital. No significant changes were observed in either amount or composition of DNA or RNA base composition. However, total RNA varied in 2 ways: in animals housed

together, the average cortical RNA level was lower than in animals kept in individual cages. In those housed separately a significant drop in RNA concentration was caused by maximal electroshock in phenobarbital-pretreated animals resulting in a suggestive increase in total RNA, as compared to unshocked, barbiturate-pretreated animals. Assuming a very rapid RNA turnover in the brain cortex, a rapid decrease (caused by maximal electroshock in unmedicated animals) may be due to an inhibition of RNA-biosynthesis or to an enhancement of its catabolism or decrease might be explained by an increase in both formation and breakdown of RNA with a slight predominance in breakdown. Also, electroshock after phenobarbital gives rise to an increase in RNA-turnover, synthesis being slightly predominant under these circumstances. This indicates that phenobarbital pretreatment inhibits RNA-breakdown in electrically shocked animals.

Department of Pharmacology
University of Leiden
Leiden, The Netherlands

1580 Griesemer, Ernest C., Gasner, Linda T., Clark, William G. Antagonism of reserpine hypothermia in mice by 3,4-dihydroxyphenylalanine (DOPA). Proceedings of the Western Pharmacology Society, 1962, 5, 7-8.

Reserpine (7 mg/kg i.p.) administered to mice produced a continuous prolonged decline in rectal temperature which remained consistently reduced for over 7 hours and was unaltered by administration of iproniazid 1 hour after reserpine. DOPA produced a temperature rise in normal and reserpinized mice which was markedly potentiated by iproniazid. Pargyline produced an equivalent potentiation of this response. Adrenergic blocking agents blocked the temperature rise. Two ergot derivatives, dichlorisoproterenol and atropine failed to block the rise, but it was potentiated by cocaine. The increase in temperature is apparently precipitated by conversion of DOPA to catecholamines. This effect may be mediated in the central temperature regulating mechanism and may be correlated with increased activity in the brain arousal centers.

VA Hospital
Sepulveda, Calif.

1581 Smith, Con L., & Robinson, Willaim A.
The effect of diphenhydantoin sodium on liver
restitution in the rat following hepatectomy.
Proceedings of the Western Pharmacology
Society, 1962, 5, 9-12.

Rats received diphenylhydantoin (10 mg/day
i.p. for 10 days before and 5 days after
hepatectomy or 10 mg/day i.p. for 5 days
after hepatectomy), 0.1 cc of commercial
diluent or nothing. Animals were sacrificed
0-5 days postoperatively and their livers
examined histologically. The amount of liver
tissue restitution in diphenylhydantoin-
treated animals was significantly greater in
all groups from days 2-5. The drug exerted
no significant proliferative effect upon the
liver before hepatectomy. Animals receiving only diluent showed no significant difference from controls at the end of a 5-day
period of restitution, nor did those who received diphenylhydantoin only after hepatectomy. Animals pretreated with diphenylhydantoin prior to hepatectomy exhibited
significant increases in hepatic parenchy-
mal tissue.

Department of Pharmacology
University of Colorado School of Medicine
Denver, Colo.

1582 Mackay, Frances, & Cooper, Jack R.
Hypnotic activity of chloral hydrate.
Anesthesiology, 1962, 23, 155.

In an attempt to correlate the degree of
neurological depression with the levels of
chloral hydrate and trichloroethanol in the
brain, mice were given 0.4 mg/g chloral
hydrate i.p. The animals were sacrificed
at different time intervals and the brains
analyzed for chloral hydrate and trichloroethanol. The injections caused the loss of
the righting reflex in 7-32 seconds. At this
time the chloral hydrate concentration was
283 μg/g brain and the trichloroethanol concentration only 31.1 μg/g brain. Another
group of mice was given 0.04 mg/g trichloroethanol i.v. and sacrificed 10 seconds later.
Although these mice showed no signs of
sedation, the average concentration of tri-

chloroethanol was 86.3 μg/g brain. Therefore the hypnosis observed in the mice
given chloral hydrate i.v. must have been
produced by the chloral hydrate itself rather
than by trichloroethanol.

Section of Anesthesiology
Yale University School of Medicine
New Haven, Conn.

1583 Sudak, Frederick N., Essman,
Walter B., & Hamburgh, Max. Anticonvulsive effects of 2, 4- dichlorophenoxyacetic
acid in mice susceptible to audiogenic seizures. Experimental Neurology, 1962, 6, 30-
35.

The anticonvulsive effects of 2, 4- dichlorophenoxyacetic acid were investigated in Swiss
mice predisposed to audiogenic seizures.
In 1 experiment 2, 4-dichlorophenoxyacetic
acid was given i.p., 25-150 mg/kg, to 56
animals, while 11 controls received saline;
all were then tested for seizures 30 minutes
postinjection. The ED_{100} was 100 mg/kg and
the ED_{50} was 75 mg/kg, well below the LD_{50}
of 375 mg/kg reported by Hill and Carlisle
(1947). The duration of protection was
investigated in a 2nd experiment with 38 mice
tested 24-72 hours after receiving 2, 4-di-
chlorophenoxyacetic acid. In a 3rd experiment, the time of onset of the protective
effect of 2, 4-dichlorophenoxyacetic acid,
100 mg/kg i.p., was determined. Animals
were protected against audiogenic seizures
by 100-150 mg/kg of 2, 4-dichlorophenoxy-
acetic acid; an increase in latency period
occurred in mice treated with 50-75 mg/kg.
The onset of protection by 100 mg/kg
occurred after 5 minutes, with complete
protection ensuing within 15 minutes; protection lasted for 24, but not 48 hours.

Department of Physiology
Albert Einstein College of Medicine
New York, N.Y.

1584 Kugita, Hiroshi., Saito, Seichi., &
May, Everette L. Structures related to
morphine. XXII. A benzomorphan congener
of meperidine. Journal of Medicinal and
Pharmaceutical Chemistry, 1962, 5, 357-
361.

The synthesis and chemistry of 5-carbethoxy-2-methyl-6,7-benzomorphan, essentially a hybrid of benzomorphan and meperidine, was described. Its s.c. analgesic activity (ED_{50} 10.0 mg/kg) was determined by the proceedure of Eddy and Leimbach and found to be comparable to meperidine ($ED50$ 9.9 mg/kg). The amide was about half as potent (ED_{50} 18.1 mg/kg) and the amine quite inactive.

Laboratory of Chemistry
NIH
Bethesda, 14, Md.

1585 Gaines, Thomas B. Poisoning by organic phosphorus pesticides potentiated by phenothiazine derivatives. Science, 1962, 138, 1260-1261.

Sherman rats received parathion (5 ml/kg intragastrically) followed by promazine and chlorpromazine (0.8 ml/kg intragastrically or i.p.) after which LD_{50} values were calculated by the method of Hitchfield and Wilcoxon. Groups of male rats received 1 oral dose of parathion (3-15 mg/kg) followed by oral doses of promazine or chlorpromazine (both 3 mg/kg). Treatment with promazine increased the toxicity of parathion by a factor of 2 and chlorpromazine increased it to a lesser degree. Administration of these drugs to parathion-poisoned rats altered neither the time of onset of symptoms nor the time of death. Male rats treated with promazine (up to 160 mg/kg) or chlorpromazine alone exhibited marked depression but recovered overnight upon drug withdrawal. Promazine (15 mg/kg) potentiated the toxicity of parathion (2.5 mg/kg) when administered to groups of 10 female rats within 30 minutes before or up to 1 hour after parathion. Minimal effects ensued with promazine given 4 hours after parathion. Groups of 10 female rats received promazine (50 mg/kg p.o.) 30 minutes before, at the same time, and at 2 intervals after a 13 mg/kg dose of Phosdrin. Promazine had no effect upon Phosdrin, all rats exhibiting typical symptoms of Phosdrin poisoning. In treating parathion or Phosdrin poisoning, phenothiazine derivatives should be avoided or utilized with extreme caution.

Toxicology Section
CDC
Atlanta 22, Ga.

1586 Shapiro, Seymour L., Parrino, Vincent A., Isaacs, Elaine S., & Freedman Louis. Indanols. IV. Indanoxypropanolamines. Journal of Medical and Pharmaceutical Chemistry, 1962, 5, 69-76.

A series of indanoxypropanolamines were evaluated as CNS depressants, and related compounds were evaluated as analgesics, hypnotics, anticonvulsants and muscle relaxants. The Muscle Relaxant Test and Audiogenic Seizure Test were used, as well as determinations of the lethal dose, analgesic and antitremorine effects and effect on spontaneous motility. The best muscle relaxant activity was obtained in $ROCH_2CHOHCH_2A$ compounds wherein R is 4-indanyl and A is a relatively weakly basic secondary amino group.

Research Laboratories
U.S. Vitamin & Pharmaceutical Corporation
Yonkers, N.Y.

1587 Polis, David B. Increase in acceleration tolerance of the rat by 2-dimethyl-aminoethyl P-chlorophenosyacetate (Lucidril). Aerospace Medicine, 1962, 33, 930-934.

Previous studies on centrophenoxine (Lucidril) which suggested involvement of the pituitary adrenal axis as well as the hypothalamic area of the brain led to this investigation of its effect on acceleration tolerance. Male Sprague Dawley rats, were given i.p. 5% Lucidril. A control group was given physiological saline. Tolerance to acceleration stress was evaluated using a small animal centrifuge and end point for acceleration tolerance determined by following the ECG (Sipple and Polis 1961). Tolerance to acceleration was significantly enhanced at 20 gravities. Median survival time of treated animals increased to 33.3 minutes compared to control survival time of 12.5 minutes. The effectiveness of the drug persisted for 4 hours after injection. Prior to apparent enhanced tolerance, a latent period of 3-4 days of drug treatment was necessary. Activity was dose-dependent. No significant changes in acceleration tolerance were found with a total injection of 50 mg, significant increments in tolerance were obtained with 75 mg and much larger increases in tolerance to acceleration followed administration of 100 mg. Centrophenoxine is probably mediated via the hypothalamic area, possibly by interplay with the biogenic amines. Its structural relationship to acetylcholine suggests additional areas for investigation of the mechanism of its action and also for the investigation of the role of this hormone in acceleration stress tolerance. As it has low toxicity and has already been used by humans in high doses, centrophenoxine may be effective in increasing human tolerance to acceleration.

Aviation Medical Acceleration Laboratory
U.S. Naval Air Development Center
Johnsville, Pa.

1588 Locker, A., & Ellegast, H. Librium als Strahlenschutzsubstanz für Mäuse. [Librium as a radioprotective agen in mice.] Experientia, 1962, 18, 363-364.

Male mice were subjected to total body X-ray dosages of 800 r (at the rate of 40 r/minute), 15 minutes after the injection of varying doses of chlordiazepoxide (Librium). The effective range for chlordiazepoxide was found to be very narrow, between 7.5 and 12.5 mg/kg. The chi-square test shows that the increase in survival rate in this range is statistically significant at the 0.05 probability level.

Institut für Biologie und Landwirtschaft
Reaktorzentrum Seibersdorf-Wien
Vienna, Austria

1589 Zbinden, Gerhard. Beeinflussung der experimentellen, durch Isoproterenol hervorgerufenen Myocardnekrose durch Aminoxydasehemmer, gefasserweiternde und tranquilisierende Arzneimittel. [Influence of amineoxidase inhibitors, vasodilators and tranquilizers on isoproterenol-induced myocardial necroses.] Arzneimittel-Forschung, 1962, 12, 635-638.

Isoproterenol (0.2-80.0 mg/kg s.c.) was injected into 597 rats and the influence of pretreatment with a number of drugs on the resulting infarct-like myocardial necroses was measured. Coronary dilators like sodium nitrite, aminophyllin, and dipyridamol, sedatives like reserpine, chlordiazepoxide, chlorpromazine, meprobamate, and adrenolytics like azapetine, did not affect the myocardial necroses. Aminoxidase inhibitors like iproniazid, isocarboxazid, and pivalylbenzylhydrazine significantly inhibited the isoproterenol necroses. Aminoguanidine and tranylcypromine were also ineffective. Calculation of significance levels was performed by the Fisher-Yates method.

Hoffmann-LaRoche, Inc.
Department of Biological Research
Nutley, N.J.

1590 Wulfsohn, N.L., & Politzer, W.M. 5-Hydroxytryptamine in anaesthesia. Anaesthesia, 1962, 17, 64-68.

Mice were anesthetized with ether, chloroform or halothane to the point of narcosis. The drugs administered i.p. were: a/ 2.5 mg/kg 5HT, b/ drugs which increase 5HT level-100 mg/kg iproniazid, 5 mg/kg reserpine and 5 mg/kg tetrabenazine and c/ 5HT blocking agents- 5 mg/kg methysergide, 0.1 mg/kg lysergide and 0.3 mg/kg hydergine. The duration of sleep was taken as the time required for the mice to right themselves. Sleeping time following general anesthesia is generally prolonged by 5HT and MAO inhibitors, while not necessarily shortened by 5HT blocking drugs. 5-Hydroxytryptamine causes an increase of respiratory rate which can be reduced by methysergide. 5-Hydroxy-indole acetic acid is not increased following anesthesia. The possibility of prolonging sleeping time in psychiatric patients receiving MAO inhibitors when administering general anesthetics should be accounted for.

South African Institute for Medical Research
Johannesburg, Union of South Africa

1591 Haeger-Aronsen, Birgitta. Porphyria induced in the rabbit by diethyl-1, 4-dihydro-2, 4, 6-trimethylpyridine-3, 5-dicarboxylate. II. Catalase activity and concentration of green porphyrins in the liver and a comparison with apronal-induced porphyria. Acta Pharmacologica et Toxicologica, 1962, 19, 156-164.

Hepatic porphyria was induced in 56 rabbits by administering p.o. 200 mg/kg of diethyl-1, 4-dihydro-2, 4, 6-trimethyl-pyridine-3, 5-dicarboxylate to 15 rabbits and the results were compared to those obtained in 9 rabbits with apronalide (apronal; 100-400 mg/kg p.o.). Four rabbits received only 10 ml of 96% ethanol (the vehicle). Urine and feces were analyzed during the period of drug treatment; animals were then sacrificed. Both drugs gave similar results; a substantial reduction in liver catalase and increase in green porphyrins, increased urinary excretion of 5-aminolevulic acid, porphobilinogen, uroporphyrin and coproporphyrin and increased fecal coproporphyrin and protoporphyrin. The metabolic block induced is assumed to be the same in these 2 types of porphyria.

Department of Clinical Chemistry
University of Lund
Malmo, Sweden

1592 Funcke, A. B. H., De Jonge, M. C., Tersteege, H. M., Mulder, D., Harms, A. F., & Nauta, W. Th. Preliminary communication; Pharmacological properties of 3-(10, 11-dihydro-5H-dibenzo [a,d] cyclohepten-5-yloxy)-tropane citrate (BS 6987, dibenzheptropine citrate). Acta Physiologica et Pharmacologica Neerlandica, 1962, 11, 104-112.

Dibenzheptropine citrate (BS 6987) was tested for: acute toxicity (mice, rats and dogs); chronic and subacute toxicity (rats); local tissue irritation (rabbits); antihistamine activity (guinea pig intestine, narcotized cat, guinea pigs); antiserotonin activity (isolated rat uterus, narcotized cat, rat hind paw, guinea pigs); cholinolytic action (isolated guinea pig intestine, narcotized cat, guinea pigs); spasmolytic action (isolated guinea pig intestine); adrenolytic action; antisecretory activity (alcohol-stimulated gastric juice secretion in dogs, histamine-induced secretion in the cat, gastric ulcers in the starved and cold-stressed rat, salivary flow in rabbits); mydriatic action (mice and dogs); CNS action (mouse, guinea pig, rat). BS 6987 was found to be decidedly active against experimental bronchospasms, both after parenteral and oral administration. Its strong peripheral histoaminolytic and cholinolytic activities play a part in this effect. In contrast to its marked peripheral actions, central effects were of minor importance, which makes it likely that it would be therapeutically active in patients suffering from asthmatic diseases, chronic bronchitis, rhinitis, etc.

Research Department N. V. Koninklijke
    Pharmaceutische Fabrieken
v/h Brocades Stheeman en Pharmacia
Amsterdam, The Netherlands

1593 Zarrow, M.S., Pawlowski, A.A, & Denenberg, V.H. Electroshock convulsion threshold and organ weights in rats after alcohol consumption. American Journal of Physiology, 1962, 203, 197-200.

The effect of ethyl alcohol (5-10% as the only drinking fluid for 141-157 days) was compared with that of stress (daily i.p. injection of 0.1cc 1.5% aqueous formaldehyde) in 137 Wistar rats. Thresholds for both the minimal and maximal seizure were determined. In the minimal seizure experiment, values were 21.4 ma for the control group and 25.7 for 10% alcohol-treated rats; in maximal seizure groups, the average threshold was 34.3 ma for the control group, 48.2 ma for the 10% alcohol-treated group, 39.5 ma for the 5% alcohol-treated group and 29.8 ma for the formaldehyde-stressed group. In both instances the threshold elevation was statistically significant at the 1% level. Postmortem examination revealed no significant changes in the liver or endocrine system, and it was concluded that the increased electroshock convulsion threshold after chronic alcohol consumption is probably due to a CNS depressant action of alcohol.

Department of Biological Science
Purdue University
Lafayette, Ind.

1594 Wolf, Harold H., Swinyard, Ewart
A., & Goodman, Louis S. Anticonvulsant
properties of some N-substituted hydantoins.
Journal of Pharmaceutical Sciences, 1962,
51, 74-76.

The anticonvulsant potencies (ED_{50}'s) of
3 N-substituted hydantoins, 1-methyl-5, 5-
phenylethylhydantoin (compound I), 1, 3-
dimethyl-5, 5-phenylethylhydantoin (II),
and 3-ethyl-5, 5-phenylethylhydantoin (III),
and of phenantoin and diphenylhydantoin
were determined in mice by the following
3 tests: maximal electroshock seizure
pattern (MES) test, low-frequency electroshock seizure threshold (1. f. EST) test,
and pentylenetetrazol seizure threshold
(s. c. Met.) test. In addition, neurotoxicity
(TD_{50}'s) was determined and the protective
index ($P. I. = TD_{50}/ED_{50}$) was calculated.
The TD_{50}'s for the 3 experimental drugs
were significantly higher than those for
phenantoin and diphenylhydantoin. The N-
substituted compounds showed activity in
all 3 tests; however, except for diphenylhydantoin by the s. c. Met. test and (II)
by the 1. f. EST test, they were less potent
than the 2 clinically employed agents.
(I) was more effective in elevating the
seizure threshold than in modifying the
maximal seizure pattern, whereas
diphenylhydantoin was more effective in
modifying the maximal seizure pattern.
(II), (III), and phenantoin showed no
striking selectivity of action. On the basis
of P. I.'s, (I) appears to be the most
promising of the 3 experimental drugs.
Structure-activity studies indicated that
mono-methyl substitution on a nitrogen of
the hydantoin ring exerted a more favorable
influence on anticonvulsant activity than
either di-methyl or mono-ethyl substitution
and that optimal activity was obtained when
the methyl substitution was on the nitrogen
in position 3 of the hydantoin ring.

College of Pharmacy and College of Medicine
University of Utah
Salt Lake City, Utah

1595 Courville, Jacques, Walsh, John, &
Cordeau, J. Pierre. Functional organization of the brain stem reticular formation
and sensory input. Science, 1962, 138,
973-975.

Small quantities of epinephrine, acetylcholine or procaine were injected slowly,
directly into the brain stem reticular
formation of unanesthetized encéphale
'isolé cats, of cats immobilized with
gallamine, and single-shock, square-wave
pulses were delivered to the optic chiasma
at a frequency of 1 pulse every 3 seconds;
the evoked potential, recorded from the
visual cortex of the posterolateral gyrus,
was displayed on a cathode-ray oscillograph.
Injection of $20\mu g$ epinephrine was followed
by a transient increase in the amplitude
of the cortical-evoked response while
injections of the same amount of acetylcholine produced a transient decrease.
Injection of procaine into the medial region
of the rostral pontine reticular formation
was followed by a long-lasting increase
in the amplitude of these evoked responses,
while the same injections at mesencephalic
levels produced a marked decrease. The
reticular formation must contain 2
antagonistic ascending systems: 1 adrenergic,
the other cholinergic, whose tonic activity
originates in the mesencephalic tegmentum
in 1 case and the caudal regions of the brain
stem in the other.

Department of Physiology
University of Montreal
Montreal, Quebec
Canada

1596 Sidhu, G. S., Sattur, P. B., &
Jaleel, Salma. Synthesis and anticonvulsant
activity of some N-phenethylacetamides.
Journal of Pharmacy and Pharmacology,
1962, 14, 125.

Two out of 5 chloroacetamides synthesized
had anticonvulsant activity. Rats were
given maximal electroshock seizures from
corneal electrodes. a-Chloro-N-
phenethylacetamide (I) was the most active
and its anticonvulsant activity was compared
to phenobarbital, phenytoin and troxidone.
The ED_{50} of these compounds administered
orally was 5 mg/kg for (I), phenobarbital

and phenytoin, and 100 mg/kg for troxidone.
The percentage of protection by oral doses
of 5, 10 and 15 mg/kg of the acetamide
was 64, 80 and 96, while corresponding
figures for phenobarbital were 48, 76 and
96;;for phenytoin 52, 64 and 76; for
troxidone 52, 64 and 72. The Peak Effect
was found at 4, 3, 4 and 2 hours respectively. Another compound, α-chloro-N-m-
chlorophenethylacetamide was about two-
thirds as potent as (I). The 3 other
compounds synthesized showed no significant
anticonvulsant activity and none of the
compounds protected against leptazol-
induced seizures.

Regional Research Laboratory
Hyderabad 9, India

1597 Von Euler, U.S., & Lishajko, F.
Release and uptake of catecholamines in
nerve storage granules in relation to
adrenergic neuro-transmission. Archives
Internationales de Pharmacodynamie et
de Thérapie, 1962, 139, 276-280.

Studies with sedimented bovine splenic
nerve granules showed that the liberation
of levarterenol into isotonic phosphate
buffer could be prevented by addition of
levarterenol to the medium at concentrations of 10 μg/ml. Previously depleted
granules took up added levarterenol
from the medium at a rapid rate, and
added epinephrine was taken up even without prior depletion. Some conclusions are
drawn with regard to the process of
transmitter release in vivo.

Department of Physiology
Faculty of Medicine
Karolinska Institute
Stockholm, Sweden

1598 Herz, Albert. Wirkungen des
Arecolins auf das Zentralnervensystem.
[Effects of arecoline on the central nervous
system.] Archiv für Experimentelle
Pathologie und Pharmakologie, 1962, 242,
414-429.

In rats, s.c. injections of arecoline
increased motor restlessness and had a
marked analgesic effect in doses (1-2 mg/kg)

1600 Pletscher, A. Basic aspects of psychotropic drug action. American Journal of Mental Deficiency, 1962, 67, 238-244.

With respect to the mechanism of action of psychotropic drugs affecting cerebral monoamines, rauwolfia alkaloids and benzoquinolizine derivatives with sedative action, reserpine and tetrabenazine, respectively, cause a marked decrease in cerebral 5HT, levarterenol and dopamine with concomitant increase in their urinary metabolites. Monoamine synthesis is blocked by the administration of α-methyl dopa or α-methyl 5HTP which cause a decrease of 5HT, levarterenol or dopamine in brain tissue due to decarboxylase inhibition. Repeated administration of inhibitors results in sedation. These drugs also release endogenous monoamines either by displacement or by impairing the storage capacity of brain tissue. MAO inhibitors (irreversible effects: hydrazine derivatives such as iproniazid, pheniprazine, phenelzine, etc.; reversible effects: harmane derivatives such as harmine or harmaline) produce rapid or sustained increases in endogenous monoamines in brain tissue due to drug-induced inhibition of monoamine degradation of 5HTP, dopa, etc., which produce marked CNS stimulation due to inhibition of MAO with accumulation of monoamines. Certain phenothiazines and thioxanthenes may inhibit penetration of monoamine through biological membranes. Chlorpromazine and chlorprothixene decrease the permeability of stored monoamine particles (stored in biologically inactive form), thus diminishing the degree of monoamine release by reserpine. A reduction in storage preceeds metabolic inactivation of newly formed monoamines. Hypothetically, psychostimulating effects from thymoleptic drugs like imipramine and amitriptyline may be derived from enhancement of the sensitivity of cerebral synapses for monoamines. Numerous experiments are mentioned which corroborate the above mechanisms as causative factors for the pharmacodynamic and clinical effects of psychotropic drugs.

Medical Research Department
F. Hoffmann-La Roche and Co., Ltd.
Basel, Switzerland

1601 Ayala, G. F. Un metodo per l'iniezione di farmaci in aree limitate del cervello del coniglio. [A method for the injection of drugs into a limited area of the rabbit brain.] Bollettino della Società Italiana di Biologia Sperimentale, 1962, 38, 157-160.

A surgical technique for localizing drugs to the cerebral circulation following injection into the subclavian artery, involving ligation of the basilar, external carotid, thyrocervical trunk and internal mammary arteries, insertion of a by-pass into the common carotid, and temporary clamping of the subclavian artery following injection so that the drug ascends the vertebral artery, is described in detail. The effectiveness of the technique was tested by injection of Monastral-blue, and it was confirmed that ligation of the basilar artery at the level of the pons per se and the injection of saline had no significant effect on the EEG.

Reparto Neurochirurgico
Ospedale Civico e Benfratelli
Palermo, Italy

1602 Pletscher, A., Besendorf, H., Steiner, F. A. & Gey, K. F. The effect of 2-hydroxy-benzoquinolizines on cerebral 5-hydroxytryptamine, spontaneous locomotor activity, and ethanol hypnosis in mice. Medicina Experimentalis, 1962, 7, 15-20

Mice received injections of 7 newly synthesized 2-hydroxy-hexahydro-benzo [a] quinolizines (5-50 mg/kg i. p. or s. c.) after which the following measurements were made: 5HT in total brain by spectrophotofluorometry, spontaneous locomotor activity by a modified photographic method and ethanol potentiation (drug treated mice received ethanol (4 g/kg i. p.) prior to measurement of sleeping time]. No strict correlation could be established between diminution of cerebral 5HT and reduction of spontaneous locomotor activity or ethanol potentiation. All 7 derivatives decreased motor activity and potentiated the effect of subhypnotic doses of ethanol, but only 4 compounds decreased brain 5HT. Pretreatment with iproniazid reversed the sedative action of 5HT lowering derivatives. Two different mechanisms may account for depression of locomotor activity, 1unrelated to mono-amine metabolism, the other predicated upon monoamine release. It appears un-likely that 5HT release is a major factor in producing ethanol potentiation. The action of these compounds on brain amines apart from 5HT remains to be established. Preliminary results indicate that levar-terenol behaves qualitatively like 5HT.

Medical Research Department
F. Hoffmann-La Roche & Co., Ltd.
Basel, Switzerland

1603 Bisson, Gabriele M.,) Muscholl, E. Die Wirkung von Guanethidin und Hexamethonium auf die Aufnahme zirkulierenden Noradrenalins in das Herz. [Effect of guanethidine and hexamethonium on the uptake of circulating levarterenol by the heart.] Naturwissenschaften, 1962, 49, 110.

Studies in spinal rats showed that the up-take of levarterenol (noradrenalin) by the heart following i.v. injection of $20 \mu g$ was prevented by guanethidine (15 mg/kg i.v.) but not by hexamethonium (20 mg/kg i.v.) Guanethidine alone had little immediate effect on the levarterenol content of the heart, but depleted it almost completely in 20 hours.

Pharmakologisches Institut
Universität Mainz
Mainz, Germany

1604 Zábojniková, M., & Kovalčik, V. Analgetické účinky inhibitorov MAO. [Analgetic effects of MAO inhibitors.] Ceskoslovenska Fysiologie, 1962, 11, 537. [Abstract]

Studies in mice using the method of Siegmund et al. showed that trans-2-phenylcyclopropylamine (SKF 385B) had a marked analgesic effect (ED_{50} 2.6mg/kg s.c. compared to 33 mg/kg for amidopyrine when given in combination. Thus, the ED_{50} of morphine was increased from 0.94 to 1.5 mg/kg s.c. by pretreatment with 1 mg/kg of SKF 385B, and that of amidopyrine was increased from 26 to 35 mg/kg s.c. No ED_{50} within the limits of toxicity could be determined for SKF 385B, however, by the method of D'amour Smith.

Charles University Medical School
Bratislava, Czechoslovakia

1605 Hapke, H. J. Die Wirkungen von Narkotika, Analeptika, Secale-Preparaten une Phenothiazin-Derivaten auf vagale Atem- und Kreislaufreflexe bei Ratten und Meerschweichen. [Effects of narcotics, analeptics, ergot alkaloids and pheno-thiazine derivatives on vagal respiratory and circulatory reflexes in rats and guinea pigs.] Medicina Experimentalis, 1962, 7, 77-84.

The response of the respiratory rate and carotid blood pressure to electrical stimulation of the vagus following admin-istration of various drugs was studied in 49 rats and 53 guinea pigs under urethane (chloralose urethane or pentobarbital anesthesia). Barbiturates (5-10 mg/kg) and morphine (2 mg/kg) produced slight respiratory depression themselves and usually intensified the effect of vagal stimulation, resulting in respiratory arrest; there was little effect on blood pressure from the barbiturates, but morphine or methadone (0.5 mg/kg) potentiated the hypotensive effect of vagal stimulation. Pentetrazol (5-10 mg/kg) and bemegride (2-5 mg/kg) counteracted the respiratory effects of vagal stimula-tion, while ergot alkaloids had little effect. The effects of chlorpromazine (0.05-2.0 mg/kg) on the respiratory re-sponse to vagal stimulation were quite variable, while promethazine and pro-pionylpromazine had no significant effect at 0.5-2.0 mg/kg; all 3 phenothiazines, however, as well as the ergot alkaloids, blocked the circulatory responses to vagal stimulation.

Pharmakologisches Institut der
Tierärztlichen Hochschule
Hannover, Germany

1606 Scocchera, Licia Fides. Un nuovo derivato fenotiazinico: la dixirazina. [A new phenothiazine derivative:

dixirazine.] Clinica Terapeutica, 1962, 23, 375-382.

After reviewing the structures of the phenothiazine and diphenylmethane derivatives and the initial attempts to combine their properties by synthesizing new compounds, the author reports extensive studies comparing the pharmacological properties of dixirazine, a new phenothiazine derivative containing the piperazine functional group of hydroxyzine, with those of promazine and chlorpromazine. The 3 drugs were found to be quite similar with respect to the potentiation of hexobarbitone narcosis in rats, the induction of hypotonic and catatonic states, the effects on behavior, motility, conditioned reflexes and amphetamine psychosis, and the antiapomorphine and antihistaminic properties, but dixirazine is less toxic. It was therefore tried clinically at doses of 20-75 mg/day with good preliminary results in gastrointestinal and cardiovascular conditions of neurotic origin, fever, pyloric spasm, vomiting, ulcerative colitis, asthma, insomnia, anxious depression and psychoneurosis.

No Address

1607 Delga, Jean, Laboure, Jacques & Olive, Georges. Etude de l'élimination et de quelques propriétés pharmacologiques du méprobamate et de trois de ses homologues. [A study of the elimination and some pharmacological properties of meprobamate and three of its homologues.] Annales Pharmaceutiques Françaises, 1962, 20, 121-126.

The effects and urinary excretion of meprobamate and the dicarbamates of ethylbutyl-, butylisopropyl- and butyl-isobutyl-propandiol-1,3 were compared in mice and rats. The water solubility and toxicity (LD_{50} i.p.) of the 4 compounds, as well as the hypnotic activity in mice (rotating rod test and potentiation of hexobarbital narcosis) , were found to decrease in the order listed. Studies of the urinary excretion following administration of 200 mg/kg i.p. to rats showed that the rapidity of elimination also decreased in the same order, 80% of the meprobamate

and only 9-27% of the other drugs being excreted in 48 hours. Permeability factors or rate of diffusion thus seem to play a primary role.

Laboratoire de Chimie
Val-de-Grâce
Paris, France

1608 Floris, V., Morocutti, G. & Ayala, G. F. Azione della nicotina sulla attività bioelettrica della corteccia del talamo e dell'ippocampo nel coniglio. Sus azione di "arousal" e convulsivante primitiva sulle strutture ippocampo-talamiche. [Effect of nicotine on the bioelectric activity of the thalamic and hippocampal cortex in the rabbit. Its "arousal" and primary convulsant effects on the hippocampal-thalamic structures.] Bollettino della Società Italiana di Biologia Sperimentale, 1962, 38, 407-410,

The site of action of nicotine on the CNS was studied by recording the EEG in 15 rabbits, including 4 in which the brain was isolated by section of the cerebral trunk and 4 in which the cortex was deprived of afferent innervation. In the intact rabbit or the isolated rabbit brain, 1-2 mg/kg i.v. produced general activation of the EEG, while 2-6 mg/kg produced generalized convulsions; these seemed to originate in the hippocampus. In the isolated cortex nicotine had no effect, although caridazol still produced the typical convulsive phenomena. Nicotine thus seems to act preferentially on the cholinergic portion of the ascending meso-diencephalic activating system.

Clinica delle Malattie Nervose e Mentali
Università di Cagliari
Cagliari, Italy

1609 Quevauviller, André, Blanpin, Odette & Garet-Pottier, Janine. Pharmacodynamie de la raugalline, nouvel alcaloide isole du Rauwolfia serpentina Benth. Apocynacées. [Pharmacodynamics of raugalline, a new alkaloid isolated from Rauwolfia serpentina Benth.(Apocynaceae).] Annales Pharmaceutiques Françaises, 1962, 20, 19-21.

Studies of the acute i. v. toxicity in mice
(LD_{50} - 33 mg/kg) , the effect on smooth
muscle (rat duodenum and guinea pig
ileum) and isolated rabbit heart, and the
hypotensive, antinicotinic and peristaltic
effects in dogs indicated that raugalline
may be indicated in cases of intestinal
atonia in view of its mild parasympatholyt-
ic and sympatholytic properties.

Faculté de Pharmacie
Université de Paris
Paris, France

1610 Lecoq, Raoul, Chauchard, Paul &
Mazoue, Henriette. Recherches chron-
aximétriques sur l'action qu'exercent
quelques psycholeptiques et psychotoniques
sur les effets nerveux de l'alcool éthylique.
Conclusions pratiques. [Chronaximetric
studies on the action of some psychotropic
and psychotonic drugs on the neurological
effects of ethyl alcohol. Practical conclusions.] Annales Pharmaceutiques
Françaises, 1962, 20, 607-622.

Measurements of chronaxy in the flexor
and extensor nerves of the toes in rats
following i. p. injection of 37 different
sedatives, tranquilizers, neuroleptics,
energizers and psychotomimetics, along
with experiments on the effect of these
drugs on the metachronoses due to ocular
compression, sharp noises or the injection
of anterior pituitary extract, showed that
these drugs can be classified into 3 groups:
the specific depressants of the basal regulatory centers, such as chlorpromazine;
the common hypnotics and general depressants, including reserpine; and agents such
as meprobamate which uncouple the
cerebral cortex from the periphery. The
authors then studied the effect of these
drugs on the response to i. p. ethyl alcohol,
which usually has a diphasic effect consisting of diminution and then increase in
neurochronaxy; this effect was suppressed
by most of the drugs tested, but was
accentuated by meprobamate, benactyzine,
methylpentynol carbamate and reserpine.
These results were confirmed by experiments with chronic administration of
alcohol (1 ml/day for 5 days) . Finally,
when the psychotropic drugs were combined
with disulfiram (0. 5 ml 1% dispersion i. p.)

some of those previously showing protective effects no longer did so (vinylbarbital,
isoamylethylmalonylurea, phenylbutazoline
chlordiazepoxide, methylpentynol carbamate, azacyclonol, prothipendyl,
thioridazine, nialamide, imipramine,
LSD and psilocybin) .

Laboratoire du Centre Hospitalier
Saint-Germain-en-Laye, France

1611 Sicuteri, F., Michelacci, S. &
Franchi, G. Contributo alla carat-
terizzazione della farmacologia della
reserpina sul sistema nervoso centrale.
Antagonismo di un bloccante adrenergico
sul fenomeno della eccitazione paradossa
da reserpina nel topo. [Contribution to
the characterization of the pharmacological
effect of reserpine on the central nervous
system. Antagonistic effect of an
adrenergic blocking agent on the paradoxical excitation due to reserpine in the
mouse.] Bollettino della Società Italiana
di Biologia Sperimentale, 1962, 38, 381-
384.

Studies on the spontaneous motor activity
of white mice showed that the usual motor
excitation produced by reserpine (10mg/kg)
following pretreatment with iproniazid
(200 mg/kg/day for 3 days) was completely prevented by the adrenergic blocking
agent phentolamine (1 mg/kg) , but was
unaffected by the antiserotonin drug
UML-491 (2 mg/kg) . Iproniazid or
UML-491 alone had no significant effect
on behavior, while phentolamine produced
slight depression and reserpine produced
a catatonic state. These results suggest
that the paradoxical excitation produced
by reserpine is due to catecholamines
and not to 5-HT.

Clinica Medica Generale
Università di Firenze
Florence, Italy

1612 Fadiga, E., Gessi, T. & Segata, L.
Modificazioni delle risposte del lembo
corticocerebellare per effetto di farmaci
provvisti di azione sinaptica. [Changes
in the response of the corticocerebellar
tract under the influence of drugs with

synaptic action.] Bollettino della Società Italiana di Biologia Sperimentale, 1962, 38, 440-442.

Studies of the response to electrical stimulation in the isolated cerebellar cortex of the cat following administration of various drugs (either applied directly to the cortex or injected i.a.) showed that only acetylcholine had the theoretically expected effect of a chemical mediator of nerve transmission (initial excitation followed by depression), making it unlikely that histamine (producing general excitation) or ATP (not producing any significant changes) play this role. The general excitation produced by strychnine and tubocurarine and the depressant effect of GABA confirm the hypothesis that they block the inhibitory synapses of the cortex.

Istituto di Fisiologia Umana
Università di Bologna
Bologna, Italy

1613 Heine, W., & Kirchmair, H. Tierexperimentelly Untersuchungen zur Frage der teratogenetischen Wirkung des Contergans. [Animal tests of the teratogenetic effects of thalidomide (Contergan).] Wochenschrift für die gesamte Medizin, 1962, 17, 1429-1431.

Thalidomide was administered to 3 groups of 12 gravid female rats at dosage levels of 2, 4, and 8 mg/kg/day, beginning 1-3 days after fertilization. The animals were killed on the 20th day and the fetus removed and examined. At 2mg/kg, 7 were gravid, with nearly normal numbers of fetuses, one uterus showing a number of placental fragments without fetuses. In the middle group, 4 were gravid and 3 bled from the vagina during the latter days of pregnancy. Of these, 1 had no fetuses. In the third group 5 were gravid, and of these 3 had placental fragments without fetuses. Among the living fetuses, particularly at 8 mg/kg, there was a marked tendency to dwarfism, and in some cases there was hydrocephalus.

Universitäts Kinderklinik
Rostock, Germany

1614 Böhmer, Dieter & Rügheimer, Erich. Die Folgen der intraarteriellen Injektion von Barbituraten und deren Therapie. [Consequences of intraarterial injection of barbiturates and their treatment.] Anaesthesist, 1962, 11, 112-113.

Hexobarbital and thiopental (50-350 mg) were injected into the femoral artery of 60 dogs in the form of 2.5, 5.0 and 10% solutions. Higher dosages were always fatal. Depending on the dosage, the effects varied from mild perivascular edema and muscular discoloration to swelling of the walls of the small arteries, vacuolar degeneration and necrosis. Hexobarbital was less toxic. In 2.5% solution, 300 mg of thiopental led only to slight discoloration, but at 5% there was vacuolar degeneration, well-defined edema, a washed-out appearance of the tissues, and swelling of the small arteries. A 10% solution intensified the damage. Spasms of the blood vessels occurred in all animals with both drugs, lasting for 4 minutes, but were not the cause of the later damage. The effects of intraarterial injection can be treated with hydergin, methylprednisolone, calcium and vitamin C. Some ways of avoiding intraarterial injections are suggested.

Chirurgische Universitäts Klinik
Erlangen, Germany

1615 Bräunlich, H. & Hofmann, H. Pharmakologische Studien über N-Allylnormorphinan. [Pharmacological studies on N-allylnormorphinan.] Arzneimittel-Forschung, 1962, 12, 174-178.

Measurements of respiration and blood pressure in rats showed that the effects of lethal doses of morphine (50 mg/kg) and codeine (150 mg/kg) could be counteracted by either prophylactic or subsequent administration of N-allylnormorphinan (1 mg/kg). With both drugs, respiration either reached or approached normality after repeated therapeutic doses, but the hypotensive effects of morphine could not be fully overcome. Prophylactic treatment was less effective and generally merely modified the response. The shorter the interval between morphine and N-allylnormorphinan injections, the more clearly were the depressant effects of the former expressed. The effects of codeine were generally more readily counteracted, but the antagonist was unable to overcome respiratory depression due to codeine if the respiratory volume was permitted to fall to values as low as 30% of the initial. At 1 mg/kg, N-allylnormorphinan also counteracted the analgesic effect of morphine (15 mg/kg) in mice. When administered by itself, however, the antagonist had an analgesic effect at doses of 50-100 mg/kg and showed depressive effects on respiration and blood pressure similar to those of morphine and codeine.

Institut für Pharmakologie
Friedrich Schiller Universität
Jena, Germany

See also 1381, 1523, 1639, 1640, 1646, 1616, 1627, 1630.

1616 Protiva, M., Rajsner, M., Seidlová, V., Adlerová, E., & Vejdelek, Z.J. Derivate des 6, 11-dihydrodibenz (b,e) thiepins, eine neue Gruppe von psychotropen Substanzen. [Derivatives of 6, 11-dihydrobenz (b,e) thiepins, a new group of psychoactive substances.] Experientia, 1962, 7, 326-328.

The chemical synthesis of a number of heterocyclic compounds from phthalide, 6-chlorophthalide and thiophenol is described and the melting points of the resulting derivatives are listed. Preliminary experiments showed that some of these compounds, particularly prothiaden, have ataractic activity in animals (rotating rod test, potentiation of thiopental narcosis) and an imipramine-like effect in man.

Research Institute for Pharmacy and
    Biochemistry
Prague, Czechoslovakia

1617 Milthers, Kirsten. The N-demethylation of morphine in rats. Quantitative determination of normorphine and morphine in the urine and faeces of rats given subcutaneous morphine. Acta Pharmacologica et Toxicologica, 1962, 19, 149-155.

Urinary and fecal excretion of normorphine and morphine was studied in male rats after s.c. treatment with morphine in increasing doses (10-50 mg/kg). A modification of the method of Milthers was used for the analyses. Morphine recovery was 40-50% in the urine and 7-10% in the feces; relative urinary excretion increased with increasing doses of morphine. Six or 7% normorphine was found in urine and 2-3% in feces, independently of the dose of morphine. It was concluded that 12-13% of the morphine administered was transformed to normorphine in rats.

Department of Pharmacology
University of Copenhagen
Copenhagen, Denmark

1618 Svendsen, A. Baerheim, & Brochmann-Hanssen, E. Gas chromatography of barbiturates. II. Application to the study of their metabolism and excretion in humans. Journal of Pharmaceutical Sciences, 1962, 51, 494-495.

A single p.o. dose of barbiturate (200 mg metharbital, 300 mg barbital, 200 mg phenobarbital, 150 mg mephobarbital and 150 aprobarbital) was administered to normal humans. Urine samples were collected at intervals from 9 to 48 hours after drug ingestion and analyzed by gas chromatography for unchanged compounds and metabolites. The demethylation of N-methyl substituted barbiturates could be followed, p-hydroxy phenobarbital was detected after ingestion of phenobarbital and mephobarbital. Only barbital was quantitatively excreted unchanged (for a period of up to 16 days).

School of Pharmacy
University of California
Medical Center
San Francisco, Calif.

1619 Kato, R., Chiesara, E., & Vassanelli. The in vitro inhibition of pentobarbital metabolism by chlorpromazine. Experientia, 1962, 18, 269-270.

Metabolized pentobarbital in liver slices from male Sprague-Dawley rats was estimated manometrically. The addition of 2×10^{-4} M chlorpromazine inhibited pentobarbital metabolism by 44% and 8×10^{-4} M chlorpromazine inhibited this activity by 81%. The inhibition of pentobarbital metabolism by chlorpromazine may not be due to a competitive requirement for TPNH, because the addition of TPN, glucose-6-phosphate and nicotinamide did not reverse the inhibition.

Istituto di Farmacologia e di Terapia
Università di Milano
Milan, Italy

1620 Garrett, Edward R. Characterization and mode of degradation of the neurophysiologically important transaminase inhibitors, the α-aminooxyalkanoic acids. Journal of Pharmaceutical Sciences, 1962, 51, 572-576.

The titrimetric characterization, stability

and possible modes of degradation of 2 representative compounds, aminooxyacetic acid and β-aminooxypropionic acid, were studied in order to obtain data to elucidate the differences observed in in vivo activity. The former compound showed good inhibition of enzymatic transamination of GABA-α-ketoglutaric acid to glutamate-succinic-semialdehyde; the latter acid was of low potency in this respect. The biological activity of aminooxyacetic acid may be due to the absence of basicity of the aminooxy group in aqueous solution perhaps due to a tendency to form a 5-membered ring, thus imparting to the molecule the ability to cross cellular membranes more readily. These α-aminooxyalkanoic acids may carry and release hydroxylamine (a transaminase inhibitor) at the physiological site, while hydroxylamine itself may not be readily transportable or metabolized. It is even possible that the intact acids may act as primary agents.

Research Division
Upjohn Company
Kalamazoo, Mich.

1621 Portmann, Glenn A., & Harris, Loyd E. Barbiturate glucosides. Journal of Pharmaceutical Sciences, 1962, 51, 780-782.

Nitrogen glucosides of barbital, phenobarbital, amobarbital, secobarbital and pentothal were prepared. Proof of the nitrogen glucosidic linkage was obtained by direct condensation of sym-di-(tetra-O-acetyl-β-D-glucopyranosyl)-urea with diethylmalonyldichloride. The syntheses and chemistry of these new compounds are described in some detail. A comparison is made between the barbiturates (40-200 mg/kg) and their glucosides (500-2000 mg/kg) for hypnotic activity in rats. Both the enolic tetraacetate and nitrogen type glucosides were inactive, even at 6-25 times the hypnotic dose of the corresponding barbiturate salt. No biological details were presented.

Research Department
White Laboratories, Inc.
Kenilworth, N. J.

1622 Ganrot, P.O., Rosengren, E., & Gottfries, C.G. Effect of iproniazid on monoamines and monoamine oxidase in human brain. Experientia, 1962, 18, 260-261.

Sixteen terminal cancer patients were investigated at autopsy; 5 received iproniazid and 11 served as controls. Bodies were sent to the mortuary within 2 hours after death and autopsied within 3-70 hours. Slices were taken from the parietal region of the cortex, head of the caudate nucleus unilaterally, the mesencephalon and the liver for estimations of MAO activity. The mean MAO activity found in the cortex according to the manometric method of Creasey (1956) in the 11 controls was 9 μM/g/hour. Activity in the caudate nucleus and mesencephalon was about 16 μM/g/hour; somewhat greater variation was observed in liver MAO activity, 50-100 μM/g/hour with a mean of 68 μM/g/hour. In the 5 cases treated with iproniazid the values found were much lower than those observed in controls, thus in 3 cases treated 1-3 weeks before death with 75-125 mg daily, the MAO activity was less than 5% of the mean control value, with an increase in cerebral catecholamines and 5HT. Conventional iproniazid treatment has an inhibitory effect on brain and liver MAO activity and increases the concentration of monoamines.

Department of Pharmacology
University of Lund
Lund, Sweden

1623 Popelak, A., & Lettenbauer, G. Rauwolfia Alkaloide IX. Über die Veräatherung der Yohimban-Alkaloide mit Diazomethan. [Rauwolfia alkaloids IX. Synthesis of the ethers of yohimbane alkaloids using diazomethane. Archiv der Pharmazie, 1962, 295, 427-430.

The methylation of alcoholic hydroxyl groups is discussed and chemical and chromatographic experiments with derivatives of yohimbine, α-yohimbine, methylreserpate and methyldeserpidate are reported briefly. Synthetic techniques and R_f values are given.

Forschungslaboratorium
Firma C. F. Boehringer u. Söhne G. m. b. H.
Mannheim-Waldhof, Germany

1624 Syner, Frank N. , & Shaw, Charles R.
Effect of schizophrenic serum on in vitro
synthesis of glutamine and gamma-amino-
butyric acid. Comprehensive Psychiatry,
1962, 3, 309-313.

A comparative study was carried out on the
effects of serum from 10 adult schizophrenic males, 9 adult males with personality disorders, 9 male schizophrenic children and 8 male children with other disorders
on the in vitro synthesis of glutamine and
GABA by rat brain acetone powder, using
glutamate as the substrate. Glutamine
production was markedly decreased by addition of either schizophrenic or control
serum, while GABA formation was unaffected by both. Thus, if there is an abnormal substance in schizophrenic serum,
it does not interfere directly with glutamine
or GABA synthesis. The selective inhibition
of glutamine synthesis by normal serum is
still unexplained.

Hawthorn Center
Northville, Mich.

1625 Amemori, T. Effect of dibenzyline
on serum cholesterol in rabbits. Experientia, 1962, 18, 331-332.

Levarterenol bitartrate was given i. m.,
0. 6 mg once a day for 2 days to 26 rabbits.
Twenty mg of 5HT were given i. m. to 12
animals as an aqueous solution of 5HT
creatinine sulfate once a day for 2 days.
Dibenzyline in doses of 2. 5 mg/kg was
injected into the ear vein of 17 animals
over a 20 minute period (1 rabbit died
and another showed serious symptoms of
adrenergic blockade, later recovering).
Blood was taken before and 24 hours after
injection and serum cholesterol was
eliminated. Cholesterol decreased slightly
(mean 3. 6%) after the administration of
levarterenol and the cholesterol change due
to serotonin treatment was insignificant.
However, 24 hours after single i. v.

injections of dibenzyline the cholesterol
level increased significantly (mean 13. 5%) .

Department of Anatomy
University of Saskatchewan
Saskatoon, Saskatchewan
Canada

1626 McDonald, Roger K. , & Weise,
Virginia K. The effect of certain psycho-
tropic drugs on the urinary excretion of
3-methoxy-4-hydroxy-mandelic acid in man.
Journal of Pharmacology and Experimental
Therapeutics, 1962, 136, 26-30.

The effect of single doses of reserpine
(2. 5 mg i. m.) , chlorpromazine (200 mg
p. o.), meprobamate (800 mg p. o.),
morphine sulfate (16 mg i. m.), pentobarbital
(200 mg p. o.) and d-amphetamine sulfate
(15 mg p. o.) on the urinary excretion of
3-methoxy-4-hydroxymandelic acid and
creatinine during the 24 hours following drug
administration was investigated in a placebo-
controlled study on 16 normal human subjects.
Only reserpine, morphine and chlorpromazine
had a significant effect. Whereas reserpine
increased 3-methoxy-4-hydroxymandelic
acid excretion and decreased that of
creatinine, morphine decreased both
significantly so that the ratio of the 2
compounds remained relatively constant,
and chlorpromazine decreased 3-methoxy-
4-hydroxymandelic acid excretion while that
of creatinine was unchanged. The increased
excretion of 3-methoxy-4-hydroxymandelic
acid following reserpine is thought to be
due to depletion of tissue catecholamines and
not to increased renal clearance; similarly,
the decrease following chlorpromazine can be
attributed to a direct effect on catecholamine
metabolism. The effect of morphine, however, was accompanied by a decrease in
urine volume and is attributed, at least in
part, to effects on renal function. Studies
of tryptamine excretion indicated that
amphetamine also had no significant effect
on MAO activity in these experiments.

Laboratory of Clinical Science
National Institute of Mental Health
NIH
Bethesda, Md.

1627 Doepfner, W. Biochemical observations on LSD-25 and Deseril. Experientia, 1962, 18, 256-257.

Extraction and fluorimetric estimation of LSD and methysergide (Deseril) were carried out on the brains of female rats 20 minutes after i. v. injection of the following doses of LSD: 1, 3 and 10 mg/kg and methysergide: 1, 3, 10 and 30 mg/kg. Almost instantaneously after the injection of LSD, as low as 1 mg/kg, the animals showed hyperactivity with convulsive movements and at higher doses generalized body tremors. After methysergide no behavioral changes were observed except slight hypersensitivity to noise and handling. Additionally lung, muscle and blood were assayed. The levels of LSD compounds in blood and muscle are about the same but definitely lower than those in the lungs. In the case of LSD the brain values closely resembled those found in muscle and blood, but much lower levels of methysergide were detected in this tissue. This difference in brain concentration is probably due to differential penetration across the blood-brain barrier. Only about 13% of methysergide reaches the brain.

Medizinisch-Biologische Forschungsabteilung
    der Sandoz A. G.
Basel, Switzerland

1628 Goldstein, M., & Contrera, J. F. The effect of pH on enzymatic formation and inhibition of norepinephrine synthesis. Experientia, 1962, 18, 332-333.

The effect of pH on the conversion rate of dopamine to levarterenol (norepinephrine) and epinine to epinephrine by phenolamine-β-hydroxylase was studied and the pH effect on the inhibition of the dopamine to levarterenol conversion by various inhibitors was examined. Maximal enzymic activity was established at pH 5.5. The formation of levarterenol and epinephrine was diminished in an incubation mixture with phosphate buffer compared to an incubation mixture containing acetate buffer; EDTA also inhibited levarterenol formation. The effects of pH may be due to ionization of enzymatically active sites or cofactors and may also affect the stability of the substrate-

Various benzyl derivatives of diphenylacetic acid were synthesized; their syntheses and chemistry are summarized. Lack of aqueous solubility limited pharmacologic testing. No toxicity was noted at 1.0 g/kg p.o., but antispasmodic activity similar in potency to that elicited by atropine was indicated for N-benzyl-N-methyl-2-chloro- and the N-benzyl-2-hydroxy-diphenyl-acetamides, as they inhibited the passage of a charcoal meal. No cardiovascular or respiratory effects were noted i.v. N-benzyl-2-hydroxy and N-benzyl-2-acetoxy diphenylacetamides (40 mg/kg) showed antipentamethylene tetrazol (100 mg/kg s.c.) activity i.p.; the former (at 100 mg/kg) also abolished the convulsive actions of electric shock. No sedative or tranquilizer activity was noted in the "wild" hamster (hungry or incited to anger) at 40 mg/kg.

Research Laboratory of Bilhuber-Knoll Corp. Orange, N.J.

1631 Yard, Allen S., & McKennis, Herbert, Jr. Aspects of the metabolism of iso-niazid and acetylisoniazid in the human and the dog. Journal of Medicinal and Pharmaceutical Chemistry, 1962, 5, 196-203.

The metabolism of isoniazid (100-150 mg/kg i.v. in dogs) and acetylisoniazid (265 mg i.v. in dogs and 500 mg p.o. in normal males) was studied in normal males and dogs. The urine was analyzed for drug metabolites, using extraction procedures, chromatography and ion exchange techniques. Administration of 1-acetyl-2-isoniazid yielded 1,2-diacetylhydrazine in human urine and acetylhydrazine in dog urine. Since the dog could not form 1,2-diacetylhydrazine from hydrazine or acetylhydrazine, it was concluded that the metabolism of isoniazid in man and certain other species (i.e., rabbit) involves the following route: isoniazid——→ 1-acetyl-2-isoniazid——→ acetylhydrazine——→ 1,2-diacetylhydrazine.

Department of Pharmacology
Medical College of Virginia
Richmond, Va.

1632 Ullmann, Elsa & Kassalitzky, Horst. Nachweis und Bestimmung von Reserpin in

Anwesenheit von Lösungsvermittlern. [Identification and determination of reserpine in the presence of surface-active agents.] Archiv der Pharmazie, 1962, 295, 37-40.

The ways in which solubilizing agents interfere with the classical analytical techniques for reserpine and rescinnamine are reviewed and experiments on the chromatographic separation of these alkaloids from Tween-20 on formamide-treated silica-gel plates are reported. The solvent system consisted of n-heptane and methylethylketone. After separation, reserpine was determined spectrophotometrically.

Institut für Pharmazie und Lebensmittel-
chemie
Universität München
Munich, Germany

1633 Balzer, H., & Palm, D. Über den Mechanismus der Wirkung des Reserpins auf den Glykogengehalt der Organe. [Mechanism of the effect of reserpine on the glycogen level in organs.] Archiv für Experimentelle Pathologie und Pharmakologie, 1962, 243, 65-84.

Administration of reserpine (5 mg/kg s.c.) to female mice increased the glycogen content of the brain, liver, heart and skeletal muscle, the increase being due entirely to free (trichloroacetic acid extractable) glycogen. Epinephrine (500 μg/kg i.m.) and levarterenol (500 μg/kg i.m.) produced transitory decreases in liver and muscle glycogen, but had no effect on the cerebral glycogen level. ACTH and hydrocortisone increased liver and muscle glycogen appreciably, but had little effect in the brain. Experiments with C^{14}-alanine showed that reserpine increased gluconeogenesis and glycogen turnover, with increased specific activity in both free and bound fractions. Experiments with C^{14}-γ-aminoisobutyric acid showed that reserpine increased the influx of amino acids into the liver but decreased their influx into the brain. Iproniazid (100 mg/kg i.m.), however, increased this influx into the brain.

Pharmakologisches Institut
Universität Frankfurt a. M.
Frankfurt, Germany

1634 Gunne, Lars-M. Catecholamine metabolism in morphine withdrawal in the dog. Nature, 1962, 195, 815-816.

Increasing doses of morphine (3-100 mg/kg/day) were administered to 10 dogs for 2 months, and 24 hours after 5 of the dogs served as controls and 5 received 2 doses of nalorphine (10 mg/kg) at 2 hour intervals animals were sacrificed, and their brains analyzed for catecholamine content. Previously collected urine eluates and adrenals were also analyzed for catecholamines. Nalorphine increased epinephrine excretion markedly. Morphine at minimal doses increased urinary excretion of epinephrine and levarterenol initially, but levels returned to the normal range within 10 days. After animals were sensitized to morphine (90 mg/kg/day), 1 injection of nalorphine resulted in a marked increase in epinephrine for 1 day, with a persistent concomitant increase of urinary levarterenol which continued for several days. Withdrawal of morphine was accompanied by a sharp rise in epinephrine excretion followed by a moderate increase in levarterenol. Morphine sensitized animals with nalorphine induced abstinence showed a significant decrease in brain and organ catecholamine content, and a particularly pronounced decrease was observed in animals which exhibited the severest abstinence symptoms.

Department of Physiology
Karolinska Institute
Stockholm, 60, Sweden

1635 Put, T.R., & Hogenhuis, L.A.H. Brain serotonin and thyroid function. Acta Physiologica et Pharmacologica Neerlandica, 1962, 10, 343-352.

Determinations of the cerebral 5HT levels at autopsy in rats treated for 2 weeks with either thyroxine (25 or 50 μg/100 g/day s.c.) on propylthiouracil (0.075% solution ad libitum) showed that both agents produced hypothyroidism and a significant increase in cerebral 5HT. Thyroidectomy, however, did not increase the cerebral 5HT level. Rats treated with propylthiouracil also showed adrenal hypertrophy, probably secondary to the increased blood levels of 5HT.

Pharmaceutical Sciences, 1962, 51, 393.

This brief communication reports the
separation and identification of micro-
quantities of sympathomimetic amines
by gas-liquid chromatography, at
temperatures ranging from 104° for
nonphenolic to 135° for phenolic amines.
A typical sample constituted 1.0 μl of
a solution containing 0.5-1.0% of each
amine. The substances mentioned include
amphetamine, methamphetamine, mephentermine, phenylpropanolamine, epinephrine
and pseudoepinephrine.

School of Pharmacy
University of California
San Francisco 22, Calif.

1639 Kato, Laszlo, Gozsy, Bela., Lehmann,
H.E., & Ban, T.A. Attempt to classify
psychotropic drugs, based on their affinity
to mucopolysaccharides in vivo. Journal of
Clinical and Experimental Psychopathology
and Quarterly Review of Psychiatry and
Neurology, 1962, 23, 75-90.

An attempt was made to classify many
different psychotropic drugs, used at
various dosages, based on their in vivo
i.v. effect in Sprague-Dawley rats on
the dextran (0.7-25 mg/0.5 ml) reactive
sites, one responsible for formation of
edema and the other for its inhibition. The
drugs were dissolved and diluted in dextran
solutions, then administered i.v. Evaluation
was based on a standard dose, the amount
of dextran evoking 100% intensity within
15 minutes in rats; the critical dose, the
amount that did not quite provoke increased
capillary permeability and visible edema;
and the degree (in percentage) of edema
compared to the maximum possible. Drugs
with established antipsychotic properties
reacted with both reactive sites of
dextran. CNS stimulants and antidepressants,
except MAO inhibitors, reacted exclusively
with the edema-inhibiting site. An attempt
was made to correlate these effects with
clinical behavioral effects. The method
is proposed as valuable for rapid drug
screening.

Institute of Microbiology and Hygiene
University of Montreal
Montreal, Quebec
Canada

1640 Fikrat, Hikmat T., & Oneto, J.F.
Derivatives of thiazolo[5,4-d]thiazole.
Journal of Pharmaceutical Sciences,
1962, 51, 527-529.

The chemistry, synthesis and biological
activity of a series of bis-2,5-substituted
thiazolo [5,4-d] thiazoles was described
in full. Rat blood cholesterol levels were
increased 20% by oral administration of
bis-(4-aminophenyl)-thiazolothiazole
(5 mg/day) for 7 days. The 1,1-dimethyl-
ā-cyanopropyl derivative induced normal
sleep in various animals at 2-200 mg/kg,
had an acute mouse LD50 of 1250 mg/kg
s.c., intensified the effect of pentobarbital
at 25-200 mg/kg i.p., showed only minor
protection against pentylenetetrazol
convulsions, had no autonomic or cardiovascular effects in anesthetized dogs
at 50 mg/kg (a dose tolerated by unanesthetized dogs) and no analgesic effect,
strychnine antagonism or protection
against apomorphine emesis. Unlike the
tranquilizers, it neither altered autonomic
function nor exhibited central stimulation.

School of Pharmacy
University of California Medical Center
San Francisco 22, Calif.

1641 Shapiro, Seymour L., Bazga,
Theodore, & Freedman, Louis, Indanols,
V. Indanoxyacetic acid derivatives.
Journal of Pharmaceutical Sciences, 1962,
51, 582-584.

A number of indanoxyacetic acid derivatives
were prepared, their chemical properties
were tabulated and their syntheses summarized. The hypocholesteremic effect
of α-(indan-4-oxy) butyric acid was observed
Other compounds from this group showed
adrenergic blocking and potentiating effects,
tranquilizing activity and antiinflammatory
action. No methodological details were
given for bioassay procedures.

Research Laboratories
U.S. Vitamin and Pharmaceutical Corp.
26 Vark Street
Yonkers 1, N.Y.

1642 Schieser, David W., & Tuck, Dallas L. Free radical studies by electron-spin resonance of some derivatives of phenothiazine. Journal of Pharmaceutical Sciences, 1962, 51, 694-695.

Prochlorperazine, chlorpromazine, triflupromazine and perphenazine were oxidized so that electron-spin resonance spectra of their free radicals could be determined. This technique demonstrated the existence of stable free-radical semiquinoid intermediates in the oxidation of these compounds. The spectra of the intermediates differed from those of the parent compounds in the lack of hyperfine structures. Relevant chemical details were presented briefly.

School of Pharmacy
University of California
San Francisco 22, Calif.

1643 Lange, Winthrop E., Candon, Basil H., & Chessin, Max. Metal chelates of oxazolidinones as central nervous system stimulants. Journal of Pharmaceutical Sciences, 1962, 51, 477-480.

A series of metal chelates was prepared of 2-imino-5-phenyl-4-oxazolidinone (pemoline), 2-imino-5,5-diphenyl-4-oxazolidinone and 2-imino-5-p-biphenyl-4-oxazolidinone, using cupric, nickel, magnesium and ferric ions. Their chemistry is described. The effects of chelation upon CNS stimulating activity were studied in mice. The compounds were usually tested at 100-500 mg/kg p.o. The magnesium chelate of pemoline exhibited the selective CNS stimulating characteristics of the parent compound, as well as an earlier onset of action and a relatively shorter span of activity. Substitution at position 5 inhibited the activity of these compounds.

Massachusetts College of Pharmacy
Boston, Mass.

1644 Nitze, H.R., & Remmer, H. Der Einfluss von Barbituraten auf die Förderung der Glucuronsäureausscheidung. [The effect of barbiturates on the stimulation of glucuronic acid excretion.] Archiv für Experimentelle Pathologie und Pharmakologie, 1962, 242, 555-563.

Administration of various barbiturates (80-200 mg/kg/day s.c.) to rats produced a significant increase in urinary excretion of glucuronic acid, but had no effect on glucuronide excretion, following administration of salicylamide or sodium salicylate. Glucuronide and glucuronic acid excretion was not affected by diethylaminoethylphenyl diallylacetate, which inhibits microsomal oxidative enzymes, so that stimulation of glucuronic acid excretion by barbiturates is a more unspecific process.

Pharmakologisches Institut
Freie Universität Berlin
Berlin, Germany

1645 Johannesson, Torkell. Morphine as an inhibitor of brain cholinesterases in morphine-tolerant and non-tolerant rats. Acta Pharmacologica et Toxicologica, 1962, 19, 23-25.

Large doses (600-780 mg/kg i.p.) of morphine were given to morphine-tolerant and nontolerant male rats. The nontolerant rats died 20-60 minutes after drug injection; tolerant rats were sacrificed at the same time. The cerebral morphine contents from both groups of rats was 20-40 μg/g, as determined by the polarographic method of Milthers. Brain cholinesterase activity was determined with and without added morphine by the method of Jensen-Holm et al. Using acetylcholine iodide (6.3×10^{-6} M) as the substrate, cholinesterase activity was found to be the same in both groups of rats; this activity was reduced 30-60% in either group by morphine. CNS cholinesterase inhibition following large doses of morphine was postulated as the cause of the excitation in both tolerant and nontolerant rats.

Department of Pharmacology
University of Copenhagen
Copenhagen, Denmark

Institut für Pharmazie und Lebensmittel-
chemie
Universität München
Munich, Germany

1646 Ebert, Andrew Gabriel. Barbital
C^{14} distribution and metabolism in
tolerant and non-tolerant rats. Ann
Arbor: University Microfilms Inc. No.
62-3447. Pp. 61.

Barbital tolerance was induced in male
Holtzman rats over a 2-week period through
administration of increasing i. p. doses.
Seventy-two hours after the last pretreatment dose, control and pretreated animals
were given 200 mg/kg barbital i. p. Lag
times between the 2 groups did not differ
but sleep times were 13-56% shorter in
the pretreated animals. Barbital C^{14}
was administered i. v. to tolerant and nontolerant groups. At 10-360 minutes after
drug administration the animals were
sacrificed. Brain, plasma and urine
samples were assayed for radioactivity.
No difference in brain, plasma or urine
barbital levels was observed between
tolerant and nontolerant rats, which
indicates that barbital tolerance cannot
be ascribed to decreased blood-brain
barrier permeability, decreased drug
absorption or increased drug excretion
in the tolerant animal; Monoethyl
barbituric acid and barbital were identified
chromatographically in the urine.

The Squibb Institute for Medical Research
New Brunswick, N. J.

1647 Thies, H. , & Özbilici, Z. Die
spektralen Eigenschaften der Sympatho-
mimetica und Weckamine. [The spectral
properties of sympathomimetics and
amphetamines.] Archiv der Pharmazie,
1962, 295, 194-196.

Typical UV-absorption spectra for
representatives of the phenylalkyl- and
phenylalkanolamines, p-hydroxyphenylalkyl-
amines, p-hydroxyphenylalkanolamines,
m-hydroxyphenylalkanolamines, 3, 4-
dihydroxyphenylalkanolamines and diphenol-
keto-bases are shown and described. The
spectral properties were found to be
correlated with chemical structure.

1648 Machata, G. & Kisser, W. Nachweis von Hydantoinderivaten in der
gerichtschemischen Praxis. [Determina-
tion of hydantoin derivatives in toxicologi-
cal practice.] Archiv für Toxikologie,
1962, 19, 327-338.

Since barbiturates and hydantoin derivatives
are usually prescribed together and
cannot be determined quantitatively in
tissue fluids and organs without previous
isolation, techniques for their separation
by sublimation or film chromatography
are discussed. Melting point data,
crystal forms, R_f values and ultraviolet
or infrared absorption spectra are
presented for the principal compounds, the
latter being most useful in the final
determination of relatively pure samples.
Finally, analytical data are presented
on tissue specimens from 4 fatal cases
of drug intoxication.

Institut für gerichtliche Medizin
Universität Wien
Vienna, Austria

1649 Lindfors, Raimo & Ruohonen, Aira.
Gerichtstoxikologische Identifiqierung
von Bromisoval, Karbromal and ihren
Entbromungsprodukten unter Verwendung
von Infrarotspektroskopie und Dünnschich-
tchromatographie. [Toxicological
identification of bromisoval, carbromal
and their debrominated derivatives using
infrared spectroscopy and film chromatography.] Archiv für Toxikologie, 1962,
19, 402-407.

R_f values for the chromatographic separation of bromisoval, 3-methylbutyrylcar-
bamide, carbromal, 2-ethylbutyrylcarbamide
and meprobamate are given and the isolation of these compounds from tissue
samples, urine and specimens of gastric
contents is discussed. Infrared spectroscopy is recommended for the final
quantitative determination. Finally,
analytical experience with 23 fatal cases

of bromisoval and/or carbromal
intoxication is reviewed briefly and the
analytical procedures carried out in 2
cases of intoxication due to meprobamate
and brominated sedative are presented
in detail.

Institute for Legal Medicine
University of Helsinki
Helsinki, Finland

1650 Pittman, J. A., & Brown, R. W.
Antithyroid activity of amphenidone.
Clinical Endocrinology and Metabolism,
1962, 22, 100-102. [Letter]

Two groups of female Sprague-Dawley
rats on I_2 enriched diets received
amphenidone (0.6-1.0 mg/g intragastrically
b. i. d.) for 7 days before sacrifice; 1 group
received a low I_2 diet 12 days before
amphenidone administration and a 0.2μc
dose of I^{131} i. p. on the 7th day of drug
administration; a 4th group received
amphenidone as a dietary constituent
(0.6% and 1% by weight) in a low I_2 diet
initiated on the day of drug administration.
An amphenone [dosage unspecified]
(administered s.c., b. i. d.) treated group
provided comparison. A dose of 0.6 mg/g
was moderately goitrogenic, and 1.0 mg/g
was markedly goitrogenic. The last 2
experiments confirmed the goitrogenicity
of amphenidone and demonstrated inhibition
of the thyroidal 24-hour uptake of I^{131}. All
thyroid changes were significant, except in
the 1st experiment ($p > 0.1$). Long term
studies by other investigators showed that
a slight increase in thyroid weight usually
occurred. On the basis of the above
information, it appears unlikely that·
clinical dosages currently advocated will
be associated with any overt thyroid
dysfunction.

Radioisotope Service
Birmingham VA Hospital
Birmingham, Ala.

1651 Zelnicek, Eman. Urinary excretion
of α-keto acids in phenylketonuria. Clinica
Chimica Acta, 1962, 7, 592-593.

Urine from 2 brothers aged 6 and 13 years

compound may be positively identified by using 2 gas chromatographic columns.

Lipid Research Center
Baylor University College of Medicine
Houston, Tex.

1653 Berry, Helen K., Scheel, Carolyn, & Marks, Joy. Microbiological test for leucine, valine, and isoleucine using urine sample dried on filter paper. Clinical Chemistry, 1962, 8, 242-245.

A microbiological assay with Lactobacillus arabinosus 17-5 was used to detect valine, leucine and isoleucine in urine specimens dried on filter paper obtained from 700 mentally retarded children under 6 years of age with maple sugar disease, Hartnup disease, etc. All 3 amino acids were detected in 3 specimens, 5 were positive for valine, 4 for leucine and 12 for isoleucine. Two of the 3 specimens that gave positive results in the microbiological assay were eluted for paper chromatographic testing, and showed a generalized amino-aciduria including, cystine, tyrosine, phenylalanine, glycine, alanine and glutamine in addition to valine, leucine and isoleucine. The 3rd specimen yielded valine and leucine/isoleucine upon chromatographic examination. The microbiological test is preferable to chromatographic evaluation to detect valine, leucine or isoleucine in the urine since it involves simple laboratory procedures and is an inexpensive and effective means of screening young children for metabolic disorders such as maple sugar disease.

Children's Hospital Research
    Foundation.
Cincinnati 29, Ohio

1654 Ernsting, M.J.E., Kafoe, W.F., Nauta, W.Th., Oosterhuis, H.K., & Roukema, P.A. Investigation into the effect of orphenadrine hydrochloride (Disipal) on the monoamine oxidase in the brain and liver of rats and guinea pigs. Medicina Experimentalis, 1962, 7, 119-124.

Orphenadrine (60 mg/kg) was administered orally to rats 1 hour prior to sacrifice,

after which MAO activity was determined in the brain and liver tissue. The serotonin content of rat brain was determined spectrofluorometrically 1 and 2 hours after oral administration of orphenadrine (100 mg/kg) and 1 hour after an injection of reserpine (1 mg/kg i.v.) preceded by oral administration of orphenadrine (100 mg/kg) 1 hour previously. In vitro experiments with orphenadrine (2.5×10^{-3}M-5×10^{-4}M) and diphenhydramine (5×10^{-4}M) as inhibitors and tyramine (0.01 M) as substrate were performed on rat brain and liver homogenates with and without KCN. With orphenadrine (5×10^{-4}M), harmine (5×10^{-4}M-1.4×10^{-6}M) and iproniazid (5×10^{-4}M) as inhibitors and tyramine (0.01 M) as substrate, MAO inhibition was determined in guinea pig brain and liver mitochondrial preparations. With 5HT (0.001 M) as substrate, and orphenadrine (5×10^{-4}M) and harmine (5×10^{-4}M) as inhibitors, MAO inhibition was determined in a mitochondrial suspension of rat liver and brain tissue. With respect to in vitro testing, Hope and Smith's method yields 60% MAO inhibition in brain and liver homogenates at a concentration of 2.5×10^{-3}M. KCN inhibits endogenous oxidation, but makes MAO more sensitive to inhibitors. The effect of orphenadrine is comparable to that of diphenhydramine. Orphenadrine shows hardly any effect on MAO with Gey and Pletscher's method, but harmine and iproniazid correspond to values obtained from the literature. Measurement of 5HT consumption revealed that orphenadrine failed to affect MAO. In vivo administration of orphenadrine to rats also failed to affect MAO activity or influence the 5HT content of rat brain. Reserpine-induced depletion of 5HT was not counteracted by orphenadrine.

N.V. Koninklijke Pharmaceutische
    Fabrieken
v/h Brocades-Stheeman & Pharmacia
Amsterdam, The Netherlands

1655 Madsen, Ole Drachmann. Colorimetric determination of meprobamate in blood. Clinica Chimica Acta, 1962, 7, 481-487.

Ten ml amounts of plasma or serum

(specimen), standard meprobamate
solution (10 mg/l) and a water blank are
placed in 40 ml tubes. Two drops of
ammonium hydroxide, 2 drops of saturated
potassium chloride and 25 ml of carbon
tetrachloride-chloroform are added. The
mixture is then centrifuged and the solvent
layer containing meprobamate removed
and filtered. A red-violet color is then
developed by the addition of 2 ml of a
saturated solution of antimony trichloride
in glacial acetic acid and 2 ml p-dimethyl-
aminobenzaldehyde reagent. Specimens
are then read colorimetrically at 550 mμ.
The method has an accuracy of $\pm5\%$, and is
suitable for clinical purposes. It has been
used to measure the dosage of meprobamate
during the treatment of tetanus, and in the
diagnosis of poisoning. The maximum
concentration in blood apears 2 hours after
administration of meprobamate. Poisoning
cases have shown a maximum of 120 mg/l
and therapeutic dosage a range of 1-33 mg/l.

Central County Hospital
Department of Clinical Chemistry
Nykoebing F., Denmark

1656 Van Pilsum, John F., & Halberg,
Franz. A method for the determination of
argininosuccinic acid in human urine.
American Journal of Mental Deficiency,
1962, <u>67</u>, 82-89.

A screening method for the determination
of argininosuccinic acid (in amounts above
approximately 300-500 mg/day) is
described which was used on 192 mentally
retarded patients, with no cases of
argininosuccinic aciduria found. As
argininosuccinic acid (anhydride form)
reacts with ortho-nitrobenzaldehyde in the
presence of alkali, the presumably oxidized
argininosuccinic acid derivative is converted
to arginine by heating the neutralized
solution. Creatinine, which reacts with
ortho-nitrobenzaldehyde in the presence of
alkali to yield oxalyl methylguanidine, is
converted to methylguanidine by heating
the neutralized solution. Treatment of
the solution containing methylguanidine and
arginine with $Ba(OH)_2$ and $ZnSO_4$ will
remove the arginine and allow the methylguanidine to remain in solution. Any
differences in the color intensities as

pigs receiving 300 mg/kg/day of ascorbic acid. The decrease became more marked with time and increasing dosage. Problems in the colorimetric determination of urinary vitamin C are discussed.

Instituto de Farmacología Experimental
Madrid, Spain

1659 Correale, P. Azione della reserpina e dell'iproniazide sulle nuove sostanze imidazoliche del cervello di rana. [Effect of reserpine and iproniazid on the new imidazol derivatives in frog brain.] Bollettino della Societa Medico-Chirurgica de Cremona, 1962, 38, 281-282.

Chromatographic determination of 2 imidazol derivatives (acid and amino acid) in acetone extracts of frog brain 24 hours after the end of 5 days' treatment with either reserpine (5 mg/kg/day) or iproniazid (100 mg/kg/day) showed that neither drug produced any significant change in the level of these imidazol derivates.

Istituto di Farmacologia
Università di Parma
Parma, Italy

1660 Hoffmann, Charles, Frossard, Jacques, Mai-Xuan, Kiem, & Karadavidoff, Isac. Hydrazines N_1N_2 disubstituées et monoamino oxydase. [N,N_2-disubstituted hydrazines and monoaminoxidase.] Annales Pharmaceutiques Françaises, 1962, 20, 539-544.

The authors discuss the synthesis and physical properties of 15 N, N-disubstituted hydrazines, especially derivatives of isopropylhydrazine, and report briefly that several of these are considerably more active against MAO in vivo than iproniazid, even though lacking in vitro activity (techniques not described). For reasons which remain obscure, dialkylhydrazines seem to attack liver MAO preferentially while those with aromatic substituents are more effective against cerebral MAO activity.

Laboratoires Allard
19 Quai du Port
Nogent-sur-Marne, France

1661 Opitz, Klaus, & Loeser, Arnold. Abschwächung der blutzuckersenkenden Wirkung antidiabetischer Substanzen durch Neuroleptika. [Abolition of the hypo-glycemic effect of antidiabetic substances by neuroleptics.] Deutsche Medizinische Wochenschrift, 1962, 87, 105-106.

Determinations of the blood sugar in rats following administration of either dimethyl-biguanide alone (300 mg/kg p.o.), dimethylbiguanide plus chlorpromazine (10 mg/kg i.p.), dimethylbiguanide plus chlorprothixene(10 mg/kg i.p.), tolbutamide alone (100 mg/kg p.o.), tolbutamide plus chlorpromazine, tolbutamide plus chlor-prothixene, insulin alone (2.0 IU/kg s.c. or 0.2 IU/kg i.v.), insulin plus chlor-promazine or insulin plus chlorprothixene showed that both neuroleptics had a marked hyperglycemic effect which completely abolished the hypoglycemic effects of the other drugs. Experiments with n-butylbiguanide (250 mg/kg p.o.) were inconclusive due to variability of the results. The neuroleptics probably act by inhibiting peripheral glucose catabolism.

Pharmakologisches Institut der
    Universität Münster
Münster/Westphalia, Germany

See also 1377, 1408, 1410, 1415, 1490, 1501, 1504, 1533, 1607.

PUBLICATIONS SCANNED BY PSYCHOPHARMACOLOGY ABSTRACTS

This list of publications is in 2 parts: the "core publications" are those containing a relatively large number of psychopharmacology articles. The "other publications" are scanned for the occasional psychopharmacological article they may contain.

CORE PUBLICATIONS

* ACTA NEUROLOGICA ET PSYCHIATRICA BELGICA

* ACTA NEUROPSIQUIATRICA ARGENTINA

* ACTA PHARMACOLOGICA ET TOXICOLOGICA

* ACTA PHYSIOLOGICA ACADEMIAE SCIENTIARUM HUNGARICAE

* ACTA PHYSIOLOGICA ET PHARMACOLOGICA NEERLANDICA

* ACTA PSYCHIATRICA ET NEUROLOGICA SCANDINAVICA

* ACTAS LUSO-ESPANOLAS DE NEUROLOGIA Y PSIQUIATRIA

* AGRESSOLOGIE

* AMERICAN JOURNAL OF MENTAL DEFICIENCY

* AMERICAN JOURNAL OF PSYCHIATRY

* ANIMAL BEHAVIOR

* ANNALES MEDICO-PSYCHOLOGIQUES

* ANNALS OF THE NEW YORK ACADEMY OF SCIENCES

* ARCHIVES INTERNATIONALES DE PHARMACODYNAMIE ET DE THERAPIE

* ARCHIVES OF GENERAL PSYCHIATRY

* ARZNEIMITTEL-FORSCHUNG

* BIOCHEMICAL PHARMACOLOGY

* BOLLETTINO DELLA SOCIETA ITALIANA DE BIOLOGIA SPERIMENTALE

* BRITISH JOURNAL OF MEDICAL PSYCHOLOGY

* BRITISH JOURNAL OF PSYCHIATRY

* BRITISH MEDICAL JOURNAL

* BULLETIN OF EXPERIMENTAL BIOLOGY AND MEDICINE /TRANSLATION
* BYULLETEN EKSPERIMENTAL NOI BIOLOGII I MEDITSINY

* CANADIAN MEDICAL ASSOCIATION JOURNAL

* CLINICAL MEDICINE

* CLINICAL PHARMACOLOGY AND THERAPEUTICS

* COMPREHENSIVE PSYCHIATRY

610

*COMPTES RENDUS DES SEANCES DE LA SOCIETE DE BIOLOGIE ET DE SES FILIALES/PARIS/

*CURRENT THERAPEUTIC RESEARCH, CLINICAL AND EXPERIMENTAL

*DEUTSCHE MEDIZINISCHE WOCHENSCHRIFT

*DIA MEDICO

*DISEASES OF THE NERVOUS SYSTEM

*ELECTROENCEPHALOGRAPHY AND CLINICAL NEUROPHYSIOLOGY

*ENCEPHALE

*EXPERIMENTAL NEUROLOGY

*FARMAKOLOGIYA I TOKSIKOLOGIYA

*FEDERATION PROCEEDINGS

*GAZZETTA MEDICA ITALIANA

*HOSPITAL /RIO DE JANEIRO/

*JOURNAL OF THE AMERICAN GERIATRICS SOCIETY

*JOURNAL OF THE AMERICAN MEDICAL ASSOCIATION

*JOURNAL OF CLINICAL AND EXPERIMENTAL PSYCHOPATHOLOGY AND QUARTERLY
                        REVIEW OF PSYCHIATRY AND NEUROLOGY

*JOURNAL OF COMPARATIVE AND PHYSIOLOGICAL PSYCHOLOGY

*JOURNAL OF MEDICINAL AND PHARMACEUTICAL CHEMISTRY

*JOURNAL OF NERVOUS AND MENTAL DISEASE

*JOURNAL OF NEUROCHEMISTRY

*JOURNAL OF NEUROPSYCHIATRY

*JOURNAL OF PHARMACEUTICAL SCIENCES

*JOURNAL OF PHARMACOLOGY AND EXPERIMENTAL THERAPEUTICS

*LANCET

*MEDIZINISCHE KLINIK

*MEDIZINISCHE WELT

*MODERN DRUGS

*NATURE

* NAUNYN-SCHMIEDEBERGS ARCHIV FUR EXPERIMENTELLE PATHOLOGIE UND PHARMAKOLOGIE
* NEUROLOGIA, NEUROCHIRURGIA I PSYCHIATRIA POLSKA
* NEURO-PSYCHOPHARMACOLOGY
* NEW ENGLAND JOURNAL OF MEDICINE
* NEW YORK STATE JOURNAL OF MEDICINE
* NORDISK MEDICIN
* ORVOSI HETILAP
* PAVLOV JOURNAL OF HIGHER NERVOUS ACTIVITY /TRANSLATION OF ZHURNAL VYSSHEI
                              NERVNOI DEYATELNOSTI IMENI I.P. PAVLOVA
* PHARMACOLOGICAL REVIEWS
* PHARMACOLOGIST
* PHARMACOLOGY AND TOXICOLOGY /TRANSLATION OF FARMAKOLOGIYA I TOKSIKOLOGIYA
* PRAXIS
* PRESSE MEDICALE
* PROCEEDINGS OF THE SOCIETY FOR EXPERIMENTAL BIOLOGY AND MEDICINE
* PROGRESS IN DRUG RESEARCH
* PSYCHIATRIA ET NEUROLOGIA
* PSYCHIATRIC QUARTERLY
* PSYCHOPHARMACOLOGIA
* PSYCHOSOMATICS
* RASSEGNA DI STUDI PSICHIATRICI
* RECENT ADVANCES IN BIOLOGICAL PSYCHIATRY
* REVUE CANADIENNE DE BIOLOGIE
* SCHWEIZER ARCHIV FUR NEUROLOGIE, NEUROCHIRURGIE UND PSYCHIATRIE
* SCIENCE
* SEMAINE DES HOPITAUX DE PARIS
* SEMANA MEDICA
* SVENSKA LAKARTIDNINGEN

KRFIT FOR LAEGER

STED DRUGS

ER MEDIZINISCHE WOCHENSCHRIFT

NAL NEVROPATOLOGII I PSIKHIATRII IMENI S.S. KORSAKOVA

NAL VYSSHEI NERVNOI DEYATELNOSTI IMENI I.P. PAVLOVA

OTHER PUBLICATIONS

ISITIONS MEDICALES RECENTES

BIOCHIMICA POLONICA

ALLERGOLOGICA

ANAESTHESIOLOGICA

ANAESTHESIOLOGICA SCANDINAVICA

ANATOMICA

BIOLOGICA ET MEDICA GERMANICA

CARDIOLOGICA

CHEMICA SCANDINAVICA

DERMATO-VENEREOLOGICA

ENDOCRINOLOGICA

HAEMATOLOGICA

MEDICA ACADEMIAE SCIENTIARUM HUNGARICAE

MEDICA ITALICA DI MALATTIE INFETTIVE E PARASSITARIE

MEDICA IUGOSLAVICA

MEDICA ORIENTALIA

MEDICA SCANDINAVICA

MEDICINAE OKAYAMA

NEUROLOGICA LATINO-AMERICANA

NEUROVEGETATIVA

PAEDIATRICA

PAEDIATRICA BELGICA

PAEDOPSYCHIATRICA

ACTA PHYSIOLOGICA LATINO-AMERICANA

ACTA PHYSIOLOGICA POLONICA

ACTA PHYSIOLOGICA SCANDINAVICA

ACTA PSYCHOSOMATICA □AMERICAN EDITION□

ACTA PSYCHOTHERAPEUTICA ET PSYCHOSOMATICA

ACTA SOCIETATIS OPHTHALMOLOGIAE JAPONICAE

ACTA TUBERCULOSEA SCANDINAVICA

ACTA UNIO INTERNATIONALIS CONTRA CANCRUM

ACTA UNIVERSITATIS CAROLINAE, MEDICA

ACTUALITES NEUROPHYSIOLOGIQUES

ACTUALITES PHARMACOLOGIQUES

ADVANCES IN PHARMACOLOGY

ALGERIE MEDICALE

AMERICAN HEART JOURNAL

AMERICAN JOURNAL OF CARDIOLOGY

AMERICAN JOURNAL OF CLINICAL PATHOLOGY

AMERICAN JOURNAL OF DIGESTIVE DISEASES

AMERICAN JOURNAL OF DISEASES OF CHILDREN

AMERICAN JOURNAL OF GASTROENTEROLOGY

AMERICAN JOURNAL OF HOSPITAL PHARMACY

AMERICAN JOURNAL OF THE MEDICAL SCIENCES

AMERICAN JOURNAL OF MEDICINE

AMERICAN JOURNAL OF NURSING

AMERICAN JOURNAL OF OBSTETRICS AND GYNECOLOGY

AMERICAN JOURNAL OF OCCUPATIONAL THERAPY

AMERICAN JOURNAL OF OPHTHALMOLOGY

AMERICAN JOURNAL OF ORTHOPSYCHIATRY

AMERICAN JOURNAL OF PHARMACY

MERICAN JOURNAL OF PHYSICAL MEDICINE

MERICAN JOURNAL OF PHYSIOLOGY

MERICAN JOURNAL OF PSYCHOLOGY

MERICAN JOURNAL OF PSYCHOTHERAPY

MERICAN JOURNAL OF PUBLIC HEALTH

MERICAN JOURNAL OF PUBLIC HEALTH AND THE NATIONS HEALTH

MERICAN PRACTITIONER AND DIGEST OF TREATMENT

MERICAN PROFESSIONAL PHARMACIST

MERICAN PSYCHOLOGIST

MERICAN REVIEW OF TUBERCULOSIS AND PULMONARY DISEASES

NAESTHESIA

NAIS PORTUGUESES DE PSIQUIATRICOS

NALES NEUROPSIQUIATRICOS

NALES DE LA REAL ACADEMIA DE FARMACIA

NALYST

NALYTICAL BIOCHEMISTRY

NALYTICAL CHEMISTRY

NATOMICAL RECORD

NESTHESIA AND ANALGESIA. CURRENT RESEARCHES

NESTHESIE, ANALGESIE, REANIMATION

NESTHESIOLOGY

NGIOLOGY

NNALES D'ENDOCRINOLOGIE

NNALES DE L'INSTITUT PASTEUR ¤PARIS¤

NNALES MEDICINAE EXPERIMENTALIS ET BIOLOGIAE FENNIAE

NNALES MEDICINAE INTERNAE FENNIAE

NNALES PHARMACEUTIQUES FRANCAISES

NNALI DI NEVROLOGIA

ANNALS OF ALLERGY

ANNALS OF INTERNAL MEDICINE

ANNALS OF SURGERY

ANNEE ENDOCRINOLOGIQUE

ANNEE PSYCHOLOGIQUE

ANNUAL OF CZECHOSLOVAK MEDICAL LITERATURE

ANNUAL REVIEW OF MEDICINE

ANNUAL REVIEW OF PHARMACOLOGY

ANNUAL REVIEW OF PSYCHOLOGY

ANTIBIOTIC MEDICINE AND CLINICAL THERAPY

ANTIBIOTICA ET CHEMOTHERAPIA

ARCHIV DER PHARMAZIE

ARCHIV FOR PHARMACI OG CHEMI

ARCHIV FUR PSYCHIATRIE UND NERVENKRANKHEITEN VEREINIGT MIT ZEITSCHRIFT
                              FUR DIE GESAMTE NEUROLOGIE UND PSYCHIATRIE

ARCHIV FUR TOXIKOLOGIE FUEHNER-WIELANDS

ARCHIVES OF BIOCHEMISTRY AND BIOPHYSICS

ARCHIVES OF DERMATOLOGY

ARCHIVES OF ENVIRONMENTAL HEALTH

ARCHIVES FRANCAISES DE PEDIATRIE

ARCHIVES OF INDUSTRIAL HYGIENE AND OCCUPATIONAL MEDICINE

ARCHIVES OF INTERNAL MEDICINE

ARCHIVES INTERNATIONALES DE PHYSIOLOGIE ET DE BIOCHEMIE

ARCHIVES DES MALADIES DE LAPPAREIL DIGESTIF ET DES MALADIES DE LA NUTRITION

ARCHIVES OF NEUROLOGY

ARCHIVES DOPHTHALMOLOGIE

ARCHIVES OF PATHOLOGY

ARCHIVES OF PEDIATRICS

ARCHIVES OF PHYSICAL MEDICINE AND REHABILITATION

ARCHIVES DES SCIENCES PHYSIOLOGIQUES

ARCHIVES OF SURGERY

ARCHIVIO E MARAGLIANO DI PATOLOGIA E CLINICA

ARCHIVIO ITALIANO DI SCIENZE FARMACOLOGICHE

ARCHIVIO DI PSICOLOGIA, NEUROLOGIA E PSICHIATRIA

ARCHIVIO PER LE SCIENZE MEDICHE

ARCHIVOS DEL INSTITUTO DE FARMACOLOGIA EXPERIMENTAL

ARCHIVOS MEDICOS DE CUBA

ARCHIVOS DE NEUROLOGIA Y PSIQUIATRIA

ARCHIWUM MEDYCYNY SADOWEJ, PSYCHIATRII SADOWEJ, I KRYMINALISTYKI

ARIZONA MEDICINE

ARMED FORCES MEDICAL JOURNAL —INDIA

ATTI DELLA SOCIETA ITALIANA DI CARDIOLOGIA

ATTI DELLA SOCIETA LOMBARDA DI SCIENZE MEDICHE F BIOLOGICHE

ATTI DELLA SOCIETA MEDICO—CHIRURGICA DI PADOVA E DELLA FACOLTA DI MEDICINA
                          E CHIRURGIA DELLA UNIVERSITA DI PADOVA

AUSTRALIAN ANNALS OF MEDICINE

AUSTRALIAN JOURNAL OF CHEMISTRY

AUSTRALIAN JOURNAL OF EXPERIMENTAL BIOLOGY AND MEDICAL SCIENCE

AUSTRALIAN SCIENCE INDEX

BEHAVIORAL SCIENCE

BEHAVIOUR

BELGISCH TIJDSCHRIFT VOOR GENEESKUNDE

BIBLIOTHECA PSYCHIATRICA ET NEUROLOGICA

BIOCHEMICAL AND BIOPHYSICAL RESEARCH COMMUNICATIONS

BIOCHEMICAL JOURNAL

BIOCHEMISTRY/ TRANSLATION OF BIOKHIMIYA/

BIOCHIMICA ET BIOPHYSICA ACTA

BIOKHIMIYA

BIOLOGIE MEDICALE

BIOLOGY AND MEDICAL SCIENCE

BOLETIN DEL CENTRO DE DOCUMENTACION CIENTIFICA Y TECNICA DE MEXICO SECCION ·4A

BOLETIN DEL INSTITUTO DE PATOLOGIA MEDICA, HOSPITAL GENERAL /MADRID/

BOLLETTINO CHIMICO FARMACEUTICO

BOLLETTINO DELLA SOCIETA MEDICO-CHIRURGICA DE DREMONA

BRAIN

BRAIN AND NERVE

BRITISH JOURNAL OF ADDICTION

BRITISH JOURNAL OF ANAESTHESIA

BRITISH JOURNAL OF CLINICAL PRACTICE

BRITISH JOURNAL OF PHARMACOLOGY AND CHEMOTHERAPY

BRITISH JOURNAL OF PSYCHOLOGY

BRITISH MEDICAL BULLETIN

BRUXELLES-MEDICAL

BULLETIN DE LACADEMIE NATIONALE DE MEDECINE

BULLETIN DE LACADEMIE POLONAISE DES SCIENCES

BULLETIN DE LACADEMIE ROYALE DE MEDECINE DE BELGIQUE

BULLETIN DE LASSOCIATION DES DIPLOMES DE MICROBIOLOGIE DE LA FACULTE DE

PHARMACIE DE NANCY

BULLETIN OF THE CHEMICAL SOCIETY OF JAPAN

BULLETIN DE LINSTITUT PASTEUR /PARIS/

BULLETIN OF THE MENNINGER CLINIC

BULLETIN ON NARCOTICS

BULLETIN OF THE NEW YORK ACADEMY OF MEDICINE

, UNIVERSITY OF MARYLAND

MIE DER MEDIZINISCHEN WISSENSCHAFTEN

CAL CENTER

IZATION

E MEDICALE DES HOPITAUX DE PARIS

AU STRASBOURG MEDICAL

RNAL

ND PHYSIOLOGY

DICINE AND VETERINARY SCIENCE

ES

ON E MEDICAL SCIENCES

OURNAL

CHEMISTRY AND INDUSTRY

CHEMOTHERAPIA

CHEMOTHERAPY REVIEW

CHINESE MEDICAL JOURNAL

CIBA SYMPOSIUM

CIRCULATION

CIRCULATION RESEARCH

CLINICA CHIMICA ACTA

CLINICA TERAPEUTICA

CLINICAL CHEMISTRY

CLINICAL RESEARCH

CLINICAL SCIENCE

CONCOURS MEDICAL

CONFINIA NEUROLOGICA

CONFINIA PSYCHIATRICA

CONNECTICUT MEDICINE

CONNECTICUT STATE MEDICAL JOURNAL

CONTEMPORARY PSYCHOLOGY

CURRENT MEDICAL DIGEST

CURRENT MEDICAL PRACTICE

CURRENT MEDICINE AND DRUGS

CURRENT THERAPY

DALLAS MEDICAL JOURNAL

DANISH MEDICAL BULLETIN

DANSK TIDSSKRIFT FOR FARMACI

DELAWARE MEDICAL JOURNAL

DENTAL SURVEY

DERMATOLOGICA

OGISCHE WOCHENSCHRIFT

 APOTHEKER-ZEITUNG

S GESUNDHEITSWESEN

S MEDIZINISCHES JOURNAL

F NEUROLOGY AND PSYCHIATRY

 OF THE CHEST

TION ABSTRACTS

NOARDS

 CHOICE

OLOGY

OLOGIE

GIA ACTA BIOCATALYTICA

A

N PSYCHIATRIQUE

 MEDICA SECTION XX GERONTOLOGY

 MEDICA SECTION VI INTERNAL MEDICINE

 MEDICA SECTION VIII NEUROLOGY

 MEDICA SECTION VII PEDIATRICS

 MEDICA SECTION II PHYSIOLOGY

 MEDICA SECTION XIX REHABILITATION

TIA

NTAL CELL RESEARCH

NTAL MEDICINE AND SURGERY

, NOSE AND THROAT MONTHLY

EDIZIONE PRATICA

EDIZIONE SCIENTIFICA

FIZIOLOGICHESKII ZHURNAL SSSR IMENI I M SECHENOVA

FIZIOLOGICHNYI ZHURNAL

FOLIA MEDICA /NAPLES/

FOLIA PHARMACOLOGICA JAPONICA

FOLIA PSYCHIATRICA

FOLIA PSYCHIATRICA ET NEUROLOGICA JAPONICA

FOLIA PSYCHIATRICA, NEUROLOGICA ET NEUROCHIRURGICA NEERLANDICA

FORTSCHRITTE DER MEDIZIN

FORTSCHRITTE DER NEUROLOGIE, PSYCHIATRIE UND IHRER GRENZGEBIETE

FORTSCHRITTE DER PSYCHOSOMATISCHEN MEDIZIN

FRANCE MEDICALE

FRIULI MEDICO

GASTROENTEROLOGIA

GASTROENTEROLOGY

GAZETA MEDICA PORTUGUESA

GAZETTE DES HOPITAUX CIVILS ET MILITAIRES

GAZETTE MEDICALE DE FRANCE

GAZZETTA INTERNAZIONALE DI MEDICINA E CHIRURGIA

GEBURTSHILFE UND FRAUENHEILKUNDE

GENEESKUNDIGE GIDS

GEORGETOWN MEDICAL BULLETIN

GERIATRICS

GERMAN MEDICAL MONTHLY

GERONTOLOGY

GINEKOLOGIA POLSKA

GIORNALE DI GERONTOLOGIA

GIORNALE DI PSICHIATRIA E DI NEUROPATOLOGIA

GP /KANSAS CITY, MO./

WTH

AECOLOGIA

EFUAH

LEM HOSPITAL BULLETIN

AII MEDICAL JOURNAL AND INTER-ISLAND NURSES BULLETIN

REW MEDICAL JOURNAL

TE ZUR UMFALLHEILKUNDE

VETICA CHIMICA ACTA

VETICA MEDICA ACTA

VETICA PHYSIOLOGICA ET PHARMACOLOGICA ACTA

RY FORD HOSPITAL BULLETIN

POKRATES

PITAL PROGRESS

GGYOGYASZATI SZEMLE

INOIS MEDICAL JOURNAL

EX MEDICUS

IAN JOURNAL OF EXPERIMENTAL BIOLOGY

IAN JOURNAL OF MEDICAL RESEARCH

IAN JOURNAL OF MEDICAL SCIENCES

IAN JOURNAL OF PHYSIOLOGY AND PHARMACOLOGY

IAN JOURNAL OF PSYCHIATRY

IAN MEDICAL RECORD

IAN PRACTITIONER

USTRIAL MEDICINE AND SURGERY

ERNATIONAL ARCHIVES OF ALLERGY AND APPLIED IMMUNOLOGY

ERNATIONAL JOURNAL ON ALCOHOL AND ALCOHOLISM

ERNATIONAL JOURNAL OF GROUP PSYCHOTHERAPY

ERNATIONAL JOURNAL OF NEUROLOGY

INTERNATIONAL RECORD OF MEDICINE

INTERNATIONAL REVIEW OF NEUROBIOLOGY

INTERNIST

IRISH JOURNAL OF MEDICAL SCIENCE

ISRAEL MEDICAL JOURNAL

ITALIAN JOURNAL OF BIOCHEMISTRY

JAPANESE JOURNAL OF PHARMACOLOGY

JAPANESE JOURNAL OF PHYSIOLOGY

JORNAL BRASILEIRO NEUROLOGIA

JORNAL BRASILEIRO PSIQUIATRIA

JORNAL DA SOCIEDADE DAS CIENCIAS MEDICAS DE LISBOA

JOURNAL OF ABNORMAL AND SOCIAL PSYCHOLOGY

JOURNAL OF THE ALBERT EINSTEIN MEDICAL CENTER

JOURNAL OF ALLERGY

JOURNAL OF THE AMERICAN CHEMICAL SOCIETY

JOURNAL OF THE AMERICAN MEDICAL WOMENS ASSOCIATION

JOURNAL OF THE AMERICAN OSTEOPATHIC ASSOCIATION

JOURNAL OF THE AMERICAN PHARMACEUTICAL ASSOCIATION / SCIENTIFIC EDITION

JOURNAL OF THE AMERICAN VETERINARY MEDICAL ASSOCIATION

JOURNAL OF APPLIED PHYSIOLOGY

JOURNAL OF THE ARKANSAS MEDICAL SOCIETY

JOURNAL OF BIOCHEMISTRY

JOURNAL OF BIOLOGICAL CHEMISTRY

JOURNAL OF CHILD PSYCHIATRY

JOURNAL OF CHRONIC DISEASES

JOURNAL OF CLINICAL ENDOCRINOLOGY AND METABOLISM

JOURNAL OF CLINICAL INVESTIGATION

JOURNAL OF CLINICAL PATHOLOGY

RNAL OF CLINICAL PSYCHOLOGY

RNAL OF COMPARATIVE NEUROLOGY

RNAL OF CONSULTING PSYCHOLOGY

RNAL OF THE EGYPTIAN MEDICAL ASSOCIATION

RNAL OF ENDOCRINOLOGY

RNAL OF THE EXPERIMENTAL ANALYSIS OF BEHAVIOR

RNAL OF EXPERIMENTAL PSYCHOLOGY

RNAL OF THE FLORIDA MEDICAL ASSOCIATION

RNAL OF GENERAL PHYSIOLOGY

RNAL OF GENERAL PSYCHOLOGY

RNAL OF GERONTOLOGY

RNAL OF THE HILLSIDE HOSPITAL

RNAL OF THE INDIAN MEDICAL ASSOCIATION

RNAL OF THE INDIANA STATE MEDICAL ASSOCIATION

RNAL OF THE INTERNATIONAL COLLEGE OF SURGEONS

RNAL OF INVESTIGATIVE DERMATOLOGY

RNAL OF THE IOWA STATE MEDICAL SOCIETY

RNAL OF THE IRISH MEDICAL ASSOCIATION

RNAL OF THE KANSAS MEDICAL SOCIETY

RNAL OF THE KENTUCKY STATE MEDICAL ASSOCIATION

RNAL OF LABORATORY AND CLINICAL MEDICINE

RNAL-LANCET

RNAL OF THE LOUISIANA STATE MEDICAL SOCIETY

RNAL DE MEDECINE DE BORDEAUX ET DU SUD-OUEST

RNAL DE MEDECINE DE LYON

RNAL OF THE MEDICAL ASSOCIATION OF GEORGIA

RNAL OF THE MEDICAL ASSOCIATION OF THE STATE OF ALABAMA

RNAL OF THE MEDICAL SOCIETY OF NEW JERSEY

JOURNAL OF MENTAL DEFICIENCY RESEARCH

JOURNAL OF MICHIGAN STATE MEDICAL SOCIETY

JOURNAL MONDIAL DE PHARMACIE

JOURNAL OF THE MOUNT SINAI HOSPITAL /NEW YORK/

JOURNAL OF THE NATIONAL MEDICAL ASSOCIATION

JOURNAL OF NEUROLOGY, NEUROSURGERY AND PSYCHIATRY

JOURNAL OF NEUROPHYSIOLOGY

JOURNAL OF OCCUPATIONAL MEDICINE

JOURNAL OF ORGANIC CHEMISTRY

JOURNAL OF PEDIATRICS

JOURNAL OF PERSONALITY

JOURNAL DE PHARMACIE DE BELGIQUE

JOURNAL OF PHARMACY AND PHARMACOLOGY

JOURNAL OF THE PHILIPPINE MEDICAL ASSOCIATION

JOURNAL OF PHYSIOLOGY

JOURNAL OF PSYCHIATRIC RESEARCH

JOURNAL OF PSYCHOLOGICAL STUDIES

JOURNAL DE PSYCHOLOGIE NORMALE ET PATHOLOGIQUE

JOURNAL OF PSYCHOLOGY

JOURNAL OF PSYCHOSOMATIC RESEARCH

JOURNAL OF REHABILITATION

JOURNAL OF THE SOUTH CAROLINA MEDICAL ASSOCIATION

JOURNAL OF SPEECH AND HEARING DISORDERS

JOURNAL OF SURGICAL RESEARCH

JOURNAL OF THE TENNESSEE STATE MEDICAL ASSOCIATION

JOURNAL OF THE WADSWORTH GENERAL HOSPITAL

KISERLETES ORVOSTUDOMANY

KLINICHESKAYA MEDITSINA

CHIRURGIE VEREINIGT MIT DEUTSCHE

SCHRIFT FUR CHIRURGIE

OLOGIAI ES ORVOSI TUDOMANYOK OSZTALYANAK

EMENYEI

RNING OG SOCIAL MEDICIN

COLUMBIA

627

MEDICAL TIMES /MANHASSET, N.Y./

MEDICAL WORLD /LONDON/

MEDICAL WORLD /NEW YORK/

MEDICAMENTA

MEDICAMENTA. FARMACEUTICA

MEDICAMUNDI

MEDICINA /PARMA/

MEDICINA EXPERIMENTALIS

MEDICINA INTERNA

MEDICINA DEL LAVORO

MEDICINA PSICOSOMATICA

MEDICINE ILLUSTRATED

MEDICINSKI ARHIV

MEDICINSKI PREGLED

MEDICO /PORTO/

MEDIZINISCHE MONATSSCHRIFT

MENTAL HOSPITALS

MENTAL HYGIENE

METHODS OF BIOCHEMICAL ANALYSIS

METHODS IN MEDICAL RESEARCH

MICHIGAN DEPARTMENT OF MENTAL HEALTH, RESEARCH SECTION REPORT

MILITARY MEDICINE

MIND

MINERVA ANESTESIOLOGICA

MINERVA FARMACEUTICA

MINERVA GASTROENTEROLOGICA

MINERVA GINECOLOGICA

MINERVA MEDICA

RVA MEDICOLEGALE

RVA PEDIATRICA

ESOTA MEDICINE

ISSIPPI DOCTOR

ISSIPPI VALLEY MEDICAL JOURNAL

OURI MEDICINE

RN MEDICINE

TSSCHRIFT FUR KINDERHEILKUNDE

TOR DE LA FARMACIA Y DE LA TERAPEUTICA

GOMERY COUNTY /MARYLAND/ MEDICAL SOCIETY MEDICAL BULLETIN

PELLIER MEDICAL

HENER MEDIZINISCHE WOCHENSCHRIFT

YA MEDICAL JOURNAL

RWISSENSCHAFTEN

ASKA STATE MEDICAL JOURNAL

RLANDS MILITAIR GENEESKUNDIG TIJDSCHRIFT

RLANDSCH TIJDSCHRIFT VOOR GENEESKUNDE

ENARZT

OBIOLOGIA

OLOGIA, PSIHIATRIA, SI NEUROCHIRURGIA

OLOGIE, PSIHIATRIE, NEUROCHIRURGIE

OLOGIE A PSYCHIATRIE CESKOSLOVENSKA

OLOGIYA I PSIKHIATRIYA

OLOGY /BOMBAY/

OLOGY /MINNEAPOLIS/

ONE, PERIODICO DI NEUROLOGIA, PSICHIATRIA E SCIENZE AFFINI

OPSICHIATRIA

OPSIHIJATRIJA

NEUROPSYCHIATRY

NEVRASSE

NEW ZEALAND MEDICAL JOURNAL

NIPPON SEIRIGAKU ZASSHI

NORTH CAROLINA MEDICAL JOURNAL

NORTHWEST MEDICINE

NOTE E RIVISTA DI PSICHIATRIA

NUTRITION REVIEWS

OBSTETRICS AND GYNECOLOGY

OHIO STATE MEDICAL JOURNAL

OKAYAMA IGAKKAI ZASSHI

OPHTHALMOLOGICA

ORAL SURGERY, ORAL MEDICINE AND ORAL PATHOLOGY

OSPEDALE PSICHIATRICO

PANMINERVA MEDICA

PATOLOGICHESKAYA FIZIOLOGIYA I EKSPERIMENTAL'NAYA TERAPIYA

PEDIATRIA /BARCELONA/

PEDIATRIA /BUCURESTI/

PEDIATRIA /NAPOLI/

PEDIATRIA /SANTIAGO/

PEDIATRIA POLSKA

PEDIATRIC CLINICS OF NORTH AMERICA

PEDIATRICS

PEDIATRIE

PEDIATRIYA

PENNSYLVANIA MEDICAL JOURNAL

PERCEPTUAL AND MOTOR SKILLS

PHARMACEUTICA ACTA HELVETIAE

ACEUTICAL JOURNAL

ACEUTISCH WEEKBLAD

AZEUTISCHE ZENTRALHALLE FUR DEUTSCHLAND

AZIE

  INDEX

OLOGIA BOHEMOSLOVENICA

OLOGIST

LINICO. SEZIONE PRATICA

I TYGODNIK LEKARSKI

PY HIGIENY I MEDYCYNY DOSWIADCZALNEJ

PY NEUROLOGII, NEUROCHIRURGII I PSYCHIATRII

RADUATE MEDICAL JOURNAL

IT.IONER

ISCHE PSYCHIATRIE

A MEDICA ARGENTINA

EME DE TERAPEUTICA

EMY ENDOKRINOLOGII I GORMONOTERAPII

EDINGS OF THE AMERICAN PSYCHOPATHOLOGICAL ASSOCIATION

EDINGS OF THE JAPAN ACADEMY

EDINGS OF THE ROYAL SOCIETY OF MEDICINE

EDINGS OF THE STAFF MEETINGS OF THE MAYO CLINIC

EDINGS OF THE UNIVERSITY OF OTAGO MEDICAL SCHOOL

EDINGS OF THE WESTERN PHARMACOLOGY SOCIETY

ITS PHARMACEUTIQUES

ES MEDICAL

ESOS DE PEDIATRIA Y PUERICULTURA

PROGRESOS DE TERAPEUTICA CLINICA

PROGRESSO MEDICO

PROGRESS IN NEUROBIOLOGY

PROGRESS IN NEUROLOGY AND PSYCHIATRY

PSYCHE /PARIS/

PSYCHE /STUTTGART/

PSYCHIATRIA, NEUROLOGIA, NEUROCHIRURGIA

PSYCHIATRIC BULLETIN

PSYCHIATRIC COMMUNICATIONS

PSYCHIATRIC RESEARCH REPORTS /AMERICAN PSYCHIATRIC ASSOCIATION/

PSYCHIATRIE DE L'ENFANT

PSYCHIATRIE, NEUROLOGIE UND MEDIZINISCHE PSYCHOLOGIE

PSYCHIATRISCH-JURIDISCH GEZELSCHAP

PSYCHIATRY

PSYCHOLOGICAL ABSTRACTS

PSYCHOLOGICAL BULLETIN

PSYCHOLOGICAL NEWSLETTER

PSYCHOLOGICAL REPORTS

PSYCHOLOGISCHE PRAXIS

PSYCHOLOGISCHE FORSCHUNG

PSYCHOSOMATIC MEDICINE

PUBLIC HEALTH MONOGRAPHS

PUBLIC HEALTH REPORTS

QUARTERLY JOURNAL OF EXPERIMENTAL PHYSIOLOGY AND COGNATE MEDICAL SCIENCES

QUARTERLY JOURNAL OF EXPERIMENTAL PSYCHOLOGY

QUARTERLY JOURNAL OF STUDIES ON ALCOHOL

RASSEGNA CLINICO-SCIENTIFICA DELL ISTITUTO BIOCHIMICO ITALIANO

RASSEGNA INTERNAZIONALE DI CLINICA E TERAPIA

MEDICA SARDA

DI NEUROPSICHIATRIA

I ISTITUTO SUPERIORE DI SANITA

F THE GROUP FOR THE ADVANCEMENT OF PSYCHIATRY

F THE U.S. AIR FORCE SCHOOL OF AVIATION MEDICINE

F THE U.S. ARMY MEDICAL RESEARCH LABORATORY

PUBLICATIONS /ASSOCIATION FOR RESEARCH IN NERVOUS AND MENTAL DISEASE/

E LA ASOCIACION MEDICA ARGENTINA

RASILEIRA DE GASTROENTEROLOGIA

LINICA ESPANOLA

ONFEDERACION MEDICA

SPANOLA DE OTO-NEURO-OFTALMOLOGIA Y NEUROCIRUGIA

SPANOLA DE PEDIATRIA

E LA FACULTAD DE MEDICINA

EDICA DE CHILE

EDICA CUBANA

E NEURO-PSIQUIATRIA

E PSIQUIATRIA Y PSICOLOGIA MEDICA DE EUROPA Y AMERICA LATINAS

ICALE DE NANCY

ICALE DE LA SUISSE ROMANDE

ROLOGIQUE

O-NEURO-OPHTALMOLOGIE

PRATICIEN

PSYCHOLOGIE APPLIQUEE

 SCIENCES MEDICALES

AND MEDICAL JOURNAL

VON VERGIFTUNGSFALLEN

SCANDINAVIAN JOURNAL OF CLINICAL AND LABORATORY INVESTIGATION

SCANDINAVIAN JOURNAL OF PSYCHOLOGY

SCHWEIZERISCHE MEDIZINISCHE WOCHENSCHRIFT

SCIENTIFIC AMERICAN

SCOTTISH MEDICAL JOURNAL

SEA VIEW HOSPITAL BULLETIN

SEIKAGAKU /JOURNAL OF JAPANESE BIOCHEMICAL SOCIETY/

SEISHIN SHINKEIGAKU ZASSHI

SEMAINE MEDICALE PROFESSIONNELLE ET MEDICO-SOCIALE

SEMAINE THERAPEUTIQUE

SETTIMANA MEDICA

SISTEMA NERVOSO

SOUTH AFRICAN MEDICAL JOURNAL

SOUTH DAKOTA JOURNAL OF MEDICINE AND PHARMACY

SOUTHERN MEDICAL JOURNAL

SOUTHWESTERN MEDICINE

SOVETSKAYA MEDITSINA

STRASBOURG MEDICAL

STUDII SI CERCETARI DE FIZIOLOGIE

STUDII SI CERCETARI DE MEDICINA

STUDII SI CERCETARI DE NEUROLOGIE

SUOMEN LAAKARILEHTI

SUVREMENNA MEDITSINA

SVENSK FARMACEUTISK TIDSKRIFT

TERAPIA

TEXAS REPORTS ON BIOLOGY AND MEDICINE

TEXAS STATE JOURNAL OF MEDICINE

THERAPEUTIC NOTES

THERAPEUTISCHE UMSCHAU UND MEDIZINISCHE BIBLIOGRAPHIE

THERAPIE

THERAPIE DER GEGENWART

THERAPIEWOCHE

TOHOKU JOURNAL OF EXPERIMENTAL MEDICINE

TOPICAL PROBLEMS OF PSYCHOTHERAPY

TOULOUSE MEDICAL

TOXICOLOGY AND APPLIED PHARMACOLOGY

TRANSACTIONS OF THE AMERICAN NEUROLOGICAL ASSOCIATION

TRIANGLE

TRI-STATE MEDICAL JOURNAL

TRUDY INSTITUTA FIZIOLOGII IMENI I.P. PAVLOVA

UNION MEDICALE DU CANADA

UNITED STATES ARMED FORCES MEDICAL JOURNAL

UNIVERSITY OF CALIFORNIA PUBLICATIONS IN PHARMACOLOGY

UNIVERSITY OF MICHIGAN MEDICAL BULLETIN

VENEFICUS. TIDSSKRIFT FOR FARMASI

VETERINARY MEDICINE

VIATA MEDICALA

VIE MEDICALE

VIRGINIA MEDICAL MONTHLY

VOPROSY KLINICHESKOY NEVROPATOLOGII I PSIKHIATRII

VOPROSY MEDITSINSKOY KHIMII

VOPROSY PSIKHIATRII I NEVROPATOLOGII SBORNIK TRUDOV

VOPROSY PSIKHIATRII SBORNIK NAUCHNYKH RABOT

VOPROSY SOTSIALNOY I KLINICHESKOY PSIKHONEVROLOGII

WESTERN JOURNAL OF SURGERY, OBSETETRICS AND GYNECOLOGY

WIENER ARCHIV FUR PSYCHOLOGIE, PSYCHIATRIE UND NEUROLOGIE

WIENER KLINISCHE WOCHENSCHRIFT

WIENER ZEITSCHRIFT FUR NERVENHEILKUNDE UND DEREN GRENZGEBIETE

WINNIPEG CLINIC QUARTERLY

WISCONSIN MEDICAL JOURNAL

WORLD HEALTH ORGANIZATION TECHNICAL REPORT SERIES

WORLD MEDICAL JOURNAL

WORLD MENTAL HEALTH

WORLD NEUROLOGY

YEAR BOOK OF NEUROLOGY, PSYCHIATRY AND NEUROSURGERY

ZEITSCHRIFT FOR ARZTLICHE FORTBILDUNG

ZEITSCHRIFT FUR DIE GESANTE EXPERIMENTELLE MEDIZIN

ZEITSCHRIFT FUR DIE GESAMTE INNERE MEDIZIN UND IHRE GRENZGEBIETE

ZEITSCHRIFT FUR HAUT- UND GESCHLECHTSKRANKHEITEN

ZEITSCHRIFT FUR KINDERPSYCHIATRIE

ZEITSCHRIFT FUR PSYCHO-SOMATISCHE MEDIZIN

ZENTRALBLATT FUR DIE GESAMTE NEUROLOGIE UND PSYCHIATRIE

Zuckerman's Affect Adjective Check List
adrenocorticotropic hormone
free choice
morning
American Medical Association
Article
adenosinetriphosphate

British antiLewisite
benzyl analogue of serotonin
twice a day
bromolysergic acid diethylamide
blood urea nitrogen

about
conditioned avoidance response
chronic brain syndrome
cubic centimeter
centimeter
square centimeter
cubic centimeter
Centre National de la Recherche Scientifique
central nervous system
catechol-o-methyl transferase
counts per second
conditioned reflex (response)
conditioned stimulus
Climbing Time Delay

dichlorodiphenyl trichloroethane
3, 4-dihydroxy-phenylalnine
diphosphopyridinenucleotide
reduced diphosphopyridine-nucleotide

electrocardiogram
editor
effective dose
ethylenediaminetetraacetic acid
electroencephalogram
for example
electroretinogram
and others
and so forth

free fatty acid

gram
γ-aminobutyric acid
γ-amino-β-hydroxybutyric acid

hypnotic dose
5-hydroxyindoleacetic acid
5-hydroxytryptamine

Abbreviation	Meaning
5HTP	5-hydroxytryptophane
i. a.	intraarterial
ibid.	in the same place
i. e.	that is
i. m.	intramuscular
IMPA	Lorr's Inpatient Multidimensional Psychiatric Scale
i. p.	intraperitoneal
IPAT	Cattell's Institute for Personality and Ability Testing Anxiety Scale
I. Q.	intelligence quotient
IU	international unit
i. v.	intravenous
kg	kilogram
K_i	Michaelis constant for an inhibitor
K_m	Michaelis constant for a substrate
lbs	pounds
LD	lethal dose
LSD	lysergic acid diethylamide
μ	micron
μc	microcurie
μg	microgram
μl	microliter
μM	micromolar
$m\mu$	millimicrons
M	molar
ma.	milliamperes
MACC	Motility Affect Cooperation Communication
MAO	monoamine oxidase
MAS	Taylor Manifest Anxiety Scale
meq	milliequivalents
ml	milliliter
mm_2	millimeter
mm	square millimeter
MMPI	Minnesota Multiphasic Personality Inventory
MSRLP	Multidimensional Scale for Rating Psychiatric Patients
N	normal
NEFA	nonesterified fatty acid
NIMH	National Institute of Mental Health
p	probability
PAH	para-aminohippuric acid
PBI	protein-bound iodine
pH	negative logarithm of the hydrogen ion concentration
P. M.	afternoon and evening
p. o.	by mouth

ppm	parts per million
PRP	Psychotic Reaction Profile
q. i. d.	four times a day
refs.	references
Rf	ratio of the distance of dissolved substance to solvent distance
RNA	ribonucleic acid
ru	rat unit
s. c.	subcutaneous
S. D.	standard deviation
SGOT	serum glutamic oxaloacetic transaminase
SGPT	serum glutamic pyruvic transaminase
sic	exactly as found
SOSAI	Springfield Outpatient Symptom and Adjustment Index
SRA	Science Research Associates
Suppl.	supplement
TH	thyroid hormone

t. i. d.	thrice a day
TPN	triphosphopyridinenucleotide
TPNH	reduced triphosphopyridine-nucleotide
TSH	thyroid-stimulating hormone
U	unit
UR	unconditioned response
US	unconditioned stimulus
USAF	United States Air Force
USDHEW	United States Department of Health, Education, and Welfare
USP	United States Pharmacopoeia
USPHS	United States Public Health Service
UV	ultraviolet
VA	Veterans Administration
viz.	namely
WAIS	Wechsler Adult Intelligence Sca
WPRS	Wechsler Psychiatric Rating Sc

DWYER BRIAN	1491	GREIG M E	1561	
EBERT ANDREW GABRIEL	1646	GRIESEMER ERNEST C	1580	
EISENMAN ANNA J	1543	GRUBER CHARLES M JR	1476	
ELLEGAST H	1588	GUNNE LARS-M	1634	
ERMER E	1657	GUNNER B W	1491	
ERNESTING M J E	1654	GUTMAN JEHUDA	1569	
ESSIG CARL F	1556	GUTZMANN HERMANN	1466	
ESSMAN WALTER B	1583	GWYNNE PETER H	1429	
FADIGA E	1612	GYLYS JONAS	1535	
FEINBLATT THEODORE M	1446	HAAHTI E O A	1652	
FELDMAN PAUL E	1413	HADDAD RAY	1432	
FELDMAN SHAUL	1555	HADLIK JOSEF	1461	
FEMMER K	1576	HAEGER-ARONSEN BIRGITTA	1591	
FERGUSON EDGAR A	1446	HALBERG FRANZ	1656	
FERRENO E	1471	HAMBURGH MAX	1583	
FFRENCH DEVITT R E	1509	HAMONEAU G	1469	
FIKRAT HIKMAT T	1640	HANKOFF LEON D	1445	
FINK GREGORY B	1578	HANNA CALVIN	1630	
FINK MAX	1468	HAPKE H-J	1605	
FINKE H	1467	HARGRAVE MICHAEL A	1407	
FLEMING H	1452	HARMS A F	1592	
FLORIS V	1608	HARRIS LOYD E	1621	
FOX LAURETTA E	1571	HART JOHN A	1535	
FOX RICHARD	1443	HARTRY ARLENE L	1559	
FRANCHI G	1611	HAVERBACK BERNARD J	1490	
FREEDMAN LOUIS	1586, 1641	HEARST ELIOT	1523	
FRIEBEL H	1566	HEATON-WARD W A	1453	
FRIEDMAN SAMUEL	1472	HECHT K	1531	
FROELICH ROBERT E	1525	HECKEL ROBERT V	1525	
FROSSARD JACQUES	1660	HEINE W	1613	
FUNCKE A B H	1592	HEINZELMAN R V	1561	
GABOUREL JOHN D	1546	HEISTRACHER P	1549	
GAINES THOMAS B	1585	HELLER BORIS	1445	
GALVIN JOHN W	1445	HERFORD MARY	1421	
GANDINI S	1435	HERZ ALBERT	1574, 1598	
GANROT P O	1622	HIMWICH HAROLD E	1399	
GARATTINI S	1558	HOAGLAND HUDSON	1415	
GARET-POTTIER JANINE	1609	HOFFER A	1457	
GARRETT EDWARD R	1620	HOFFMANN CHARLES	1660	
GARRISON HARVEY F JR	1489	HOFFMANN K	1410	
GASNER LINDA T	1580	HOFMANN H	1615	
GEIRNAERT G	1455	HOFMEISTER A	1425	
GELDER M G	1438	HOGENHUIS L A H	1635	
GESSI T	1612	HOHENSEE F	1575	
GEY K F	1602	HOLCK HARALD G O	1552	
GIACHETTI A	1558	HOLM T	1538	
GILBERT GORDON J	1372	HOLT N F	1441	
GJURIS V	1542	HORDERN ANTHONY	1441	
GOLDSTEIN M	1628	HORLINGTON M	1572	
GOMIRATO G	1435	HORNING E C	1652	
GOODMAN LOUIS S	1594	HOROVITZ ZOLA P	1545	
GORDON W F	1441	HOSAK LADISLAV	1461	
GOTTFRIES C G	1622	HOSBACH RICHARD E	1459	
GOZSY BELA	1639	HOUDE RAYMOND W	1539	
GRAHMANN HANS	1505	HOUGS W	1538	
GREEN CARL L	1475	HOWARD FRED J	1454	
GREENE BERNARD L	1500	HOWLAND WILLIAM S	1539	

HUNDZIAK MARCEL	1429	KRAUPP O	1549
HUNTER HARRY H	1447	KRAUSS STEPHEN	1380
HURST PAUL M	1524	KRONBERGER LEO	1465
IBE K	1504	KUGITA HIROSHI	1584
IM OBERSTEG J	1501	KUHN H F	1566
IMPASTATO DAVID J	1376	KURLAND ALBERT A	1431
IPPEN H	1405	KURLAND LEONARD T	1431
ISAACS ELAINE S	1586	LABORIT H	1369
ISRAELS M C G	1386	LABOURE JACQUES	1607
IZQUIERDO JUAN A	1573	LABURDETTE LEO	1436
JACOBS LIONEL A	1497	LAFORGE R A	1630
JACOBSON C R	1630	LAGAE J	1423
JACOBZINER HAROLD	1488, 1513	LAIR CHARLES V	1371
	1514	LANCET	1420
JALEEL SALMA	1596	LANG W	1599
JAROS MILOS	1461	LANGE WINTHROP E	1643
JOHANNESSON TORKELL	1645	LANGECKER H	1504
JOHNSEN U E	1630	LASAGNA LOUIS	1433
JONES CARROLL C	1451	LASSEN N	1538
JONES E B	1484	LATEUR J	1455
JONES THOMAS H	1448	LAURENCE D R	1396
JORI A	1558	LAZARE R	1572
JOURNAL OF IND MED ASSOC	1418, 1419	LEBENSOHN ZIGMOND M	1389
JOURNAL OF A M A	1422	LECHNER MICHAEL	1496
KAFOE W F	1654	LECOQ RAOUL	1610
KAJI HIDEKO K	1547	LEE HOWARD G	1447
KAJI HIDEKO KATAYAMA	1552	LEFEVER HARRY	1393
KAMBIN PARVIZ	1474	LEFTON MARK	1429
KAMINSKY DANIEL	1535	LEHMANN H E	1639
KAPILA KANTI	1553	LEITCH ALEXANDER	1440
KARADAVIDOFF ISAC	1660	LETTENBAUER G	1623
KASSALITZKY HORST	1632	LEWIS CHARLES E	1511
KATO LASZLO	1639	LIANG H S	1532
KATO R	1619	LIEBMAN S	1500
KATZ MARTIN M	1402	LINDFORS RAIMO	1649
KAUMANN ALBERTO J	1573	LISHAJKO F	1597
KAVTSCHITSCH JOSEPH	1429	LOCKER A	1588
KEATS SIDNEY	1474	LOESER ARNOLD	1661
KEBERLE H	1410	LOND M G	1515
KENNY SHEILA	1509	LONDON D R	1384
KERSTEN L	1568	LUKE ELIZABETH	1487
KESSEL M	1504	LUSTIG NOEL	1500
KHONCHAK M	1458	MACHATA G	1648
KIER LEMONT B	1571	MACKAY FRANCES	1582
KIESER JURGEN	1462	MADSEN OLE DRACHMANN	1655
KIRCHMAIR H	1613	MAERZ JOHN C	1447
KIRMAN BRIAN H	1518	MAI-XUAN KIEM	1660
KIRSTEN I	1562	MALITZ SIDNEY	1401
KISSER W	1648	MALONE MARVIN H	1560
KLARNER PAUL	1567	MANN DAVID E JR	1557
KLEIN DONALD F	1468	MARIJAN N	1542
KLINGER W	1568	MARKS JOY	1653
KLUTCHKO SYLVESTER R	1535	MARTIN W R	1543
KNIGHT DAVID A	1526	MASON ALAN	1520
KNOBLOGH HILDA	1411	MATIAR-VAHAR H	1502
KORNETSKY CONAN	1530	MATTHIES HANSJURGEN	1544
KOVALCIK V	1604	MATTILA M	1540

653

Psychopharmacology
ABSTRACTS

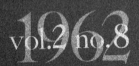

vol.2 no.8

U.S. DEPARTMENT OF HEALTH, EDUCATION, AND WELFARE
Public Health Service

PSYCHOPHARMACOLOGY ABSTRACTS is a publication of the
National Clearinghouse for Mental Health Information
of the National Institute of Mental Health. It is a
specialized information medium designed to assist the
Institute in meeting its obligation to foster and support
port laboratory and clinical research into the nature
and causes of mental disorders and methods of treatment and prevention. Specifically, this information
service is designed to meet the needs of investigators in the field of psychopharmacology for rapid and
comprehensive information about new developments and
research results.

PSYCHOPHARMACOLOGY ABSTRACTS is distributed gratis to
investigators doing research in psychopharmacology. It
is not available on a subscription basis. Requests
to receive the ABSTRACTS should be accompanied by a
brief statement of the research interests and scientific specialty of the investigator. Requests to receive the ABSTRACTS, address changes. and other communications should be addressed to:

Psychopharmacology Abstracts
National Clearinghouse for Mental
 Health Information
National Institute of Mental Health
Bethesda 14, Maryland

(The text of PSYCHOPHARMACOLOGY ABSTRACTS is prepared
under contract with the Literary Division of Biological and Medical Services, Philadelphia, Penna.)

U. S. DEPARTMENT OF HEALTH, EDUCATION AND WELFARE
Public Health Service
National Institutes of Health
National Institute of Mental Health
Bethesda 14, Maryland

PSYCHOPHARMACOLOGY ABSTRACTS

Volume 2, Number 8

vascular changes); trimethadıone
(hemopoietic disturbances, agranulocytosis,
increased grand mal attacks, dısturbances
of the central nervous system, damage to
sight, kidneys, liver, epidermis);
phenacemide (similar to above, also
personality changes). Percent frequencies
of the various side effects are given, as
reported in the literature. (127 refs.)

Pharmakologisches Institut der
    Universität Mainz
Mainz, Germany

1664 Arnold, Otto Heinrıch. Die Therapie
der malignen Hypertonie. [Treatment of
malignant hypertension.] Deutsches
Medizinisches Journal, 1962, 13, 502-507.

The author reviews the use of drugs for
the symptomatic treatment of hypertension.
These are classified according to the locale
of their action, i. e., the central sympathetic
nervous system (meprobamate, reserpine),
the sympathetic ganglia (ganglion-blockers),
the postganglionic adrenergic fibers
(sympathetic inhibitors), the sympathicolytics, and the saluretics. Indications,
and both relative and absolute contraindications for a variety of drugs falling
into the above classes are presented. In
malignant cases, when it is urgent to reduce blood pressure in the shortest possible
time, guanethidine may be used. In general,
and particularly in benign cases, even when
these occur in a severe form, the simplest
available hypotensive drug should be used,
in combination with saluretics together
with a salt-free diet (maximum intake,
5-8 g daily). The decision to use hypotensive drugs should be made only after
thorough examination of the patients'
general condition and family history.
(10 refs.)

Medizinische Klinik
Städtische Krankenanstalten
Essen, Germany

1665 Pougetoux, J., Campagnolle, A., &
Viader, A. Contribution à un essai
critique de classification des drogues
psychotropes. [Contribution to a critical
attempt to classify psychotropic drugs.]

Journal de Médecine de Lyon, 1962,
No. 1008, 648.

Brief mention is made of RP 1560, levomepromazine, thioproperazine, imipramine
and thioridazine in regard to classification
based on the evolution of neuromuscular
excitability curves, which parallel the
plasma sodium/erythrocytic potassium
ratio and plasma potassium. (No refs.)

[No address]

1666 Caffey, Eugene M. The use of
drugs in outpatient and inpatient psychiatric
practice. Virginia Medical Monthly, 1962,
89, 55-59.

Classification of the phenothiazine derivatives
based upon "low-dose" and "high-dose"
groups is discussed. Various side effects
are mentioned and the trend is toward
administration of "low-dose" drugs
because of relative freedom from undesirable
side effects. While drugs have been most
helpful, and the phenothiazines most effective
in the management of schizophrenic illnesses,
the trend should evolve from asking which
drug is most effective to whether or not a
drug is absolutely essential. Older somatic
therapies should not be denied consideration
and are frequently useful in combination
with drugs. With regard to antidepressants,
the side effects of imipramine and the MAO
inhibitors include rapid shifting into manic
states, marked vascular hypotension and
weight gain. Antidepressants can be used
with ECT and are also important in general
medical practice where they reduce the
incidence and severity of angina pectoris
and enhance psychomotor activity in
rheumatoid arthritis. Much additional study
of both the etiology of the disorders treated
and the action of the drugs used is necessary.
(No refs.)

VA Hospital
Perry Point, Md.

1667 Irvine, J.H. The differential
diagnosis of psychalgia and psychophysiologic
disease of the locomotor system. Intro-
ducing a new classification. Virginia
Medical Monthly, 1962, 89, 449-453.

Department of Psychiatry
Dalhousie University
Halifax, N.S.
Canada

1670 Ariens, E.J., & Simonis, A.M.
Drug-receptor interaction. Acta
Physiologica Pharmacologica Neerlandica,
1962, 11, 151-172.

A comprehensive review of drug-receptor
interaction encompasses 3 distinct part-
processes (overall metabolism, drug-
receptor interaction with drug stimulus,
and the relationship between the stimulus
induced and the effect obtained), affinity
and intrinsic activity (in terms of the
Michaelis-Menton equation), the processes
concerned with affinity and competition
(Van der Waals forces, Lineweaver-Burke
reciprocals, etc.), and irreversible and
noncompetitive blockade. Copious
experimental data illustrates the theories
mentioned above. Concentration-response
curves and Lineweaver-Burke reciprocals
are plotted in terms of competitive and
noncompetitive antagonism. Data
concerning the following types of compounds
is used to illustrate the basic principles
of drug-receptor interaction: carcinogens,
oxytocin derivatives, parasympathomimetics,
sympathomimetics, spasmogens and PABA
derivatives. Competitive antagonism,
noncompetitive antagonism and irreversible
drug blocking action are thoroughly
elucidated. (41 refs.)

Pharmacological Institute
R.C. University
Nijmegen, The Netherlands

1671 Knapman, William B. The basic
principles of psychosomatic disease.
British Journal of Clinical Practice, 1962,
16, 465-473.

Three aims are given relating to psychosomatic disease for the general practitioner:
a new classification of psychosomatic
disease; establishment of criteria for
the identification of psychological symptoms
in somatic disease, and elucidation of
general principles of treatment in the more
commonly recognized psychosomatic

diseases. The latter are classified under
4 major headings: the physical symptoms
in psychological disease which disappear
when the mental disease is cured; intermediate disease which includes both
mental and physical symptoms of unknown
etiology, e.g., anorexia nervosa, alcoholism,
epilepsy, migraine, etc; stress symptoms
which begin at a time of crisis but subside
when the stress is resolved, and finally
major psychosomatic disease, e.g.,
gastric ulcer or ulcerative colitis. A more
positive approach in treatment is needed,
hypnosis is often valuable, and in some
cases "simple" psychotherapy combined
with sedation such as amytal and phenobarbital is indicated; ECT is sometimes
necessary and leucotomy may be helpful
in chronic pain and occasionally in long-
standing "closed circuit" disease. The
general practitioner should assess the
patient since he probably knows the patient
best. The existence of free-floating anxiety
and hysteria concomitant with physical
disease and the physical side of psychosomatic disease must never be forgotten
or overlooked in psychiatric treatment.
(No refs.)

King George Hospital
Ilford, Great Britain

1672 Luby, Elliot D. Reply to the foregoing. American Journal of Psychiatry,
1962, 119, 591. [Letter]

The author of a paper entitled "Model
psychoses and schizophrenia" welcomes
the hypothesis postulated by a colleague
that the weird and terrifying body images
experienced by schizophrenics may have
their basis in defective screening of
afferent inflow, particularly from proprio-
ceptors. Dr. Jensen's comments are
particularly pertinent on the relationship
between psychopathology and the control
and switching of sensory input and attention.
Extensive testing of the above hypothesis
is anticipated. (No refs.)

Lafayette Clinic
Detroit, Mich.

1673 Burn, J. L. Treatment of addictions.

666

a depressant effect and LSD facilitating the arousal effects of sensory potentials. These drugs produce their effects by disturbing the relationship between specific and nonspecific afferent pathways in the brain. (15 refs.)

Department of Experimental Psychiatry
Medical School
Birmingham 15, Great Britain

1677 Jensen, S. E. Model psychoses and schizophrenia. American Journal of Psychiatry, 1962, 119, 590-591. [Letter]

The hypothesis of an aberrent proprioceptive feedback mechanism operant in both the phencyclidine induced state and chronic schizophrenia is promulgated. Corroboration is offered in the form of previous work on cats with implanted visual, auditory and subcortical electrodes. Responses to a flashing light recorded from the occipital cortex were almost abolished when the animal reduction was also observed in afferent leads from the optic tract and optic pathway, apparently due to a reduction in afferent inflow. Other experimental work indicates that reduction of inflow from one modality with concomitant augmentation of inflow through another modality is probably carried out at the lowest level in the afferent pathway. This evidence offers a new frame of reference from which various psychological anomalies such as sensory deprivation, model psychoses, schizophrenia, conversion hysteria and hypnosis (all conditions predicated upon abnormal input) may be evaluated. Further research on this hypothesis is contemplated with animals given LSD or phencyclidine and schizophrenics undergoing brain surgery. (No refs.)

[No address]

1678 Dundee, John W., & Barron, David W. The barbiturates. British Journal of Anaesthesiology, 1962, 34, 240-246.

Clinically efficacious barbiturates are derived from barbituric acid by alterations in the parent nucleus at the 1, 2 and 5, 5'

positions, and substitutions in the 5
position determine the degree and duration
of narcosis obtainable from the following
4 distinct chemical groups: barbiturates
(or oxybarbiturates), methylated oxybarbiturates, thiobarbiturates and methylated
thiobarbiturates. Classification is predicated
upon duration of drug action, i.e., ultra-
short, short, medium, intermediate and
long acting barbiturates. Replacement of
both H atoms on the 5-C by alkyl or aryl
groups confers hypnotic properties on the
barbiturates. Halogenation of the alkyl
substituents increases drug potency and
intensity of action. Long acting barbiturates
are typified by phenobarbital and barbital,
medium acting by amylobarbital, and rapidly
acting by thialbarbital, hexobarbital and
enallylpropymal. Sulphuration results in
a compound which has highly effective
soporific properties. 1-Methylation of a
barbiturate or thiobarbiturate confers
convulsive properties which are manifested
as anomalous skeletal muscle activity.
Certain side chains on the 5-C increase
the incidence of coughing and hiccoughing
for unknown reasons. Compounds of the
barbiturate group commonly used in
anesthesia are presented in tabular form
along with all relevant chemical data.
(7 refs.)

Department of Anaesthetics
The Queen's University of Belfast
Northern Ireland

1679 Schindel, L. E. Placebo in theory
and practice. Antibiotica et Chemotherapia,
Advances, 1962, 10, 398-430.

This general discussion of the placebo
starts with its historical origins and
theorizes that most medication up to and
including today is actually based on placebo
response. Pure and "impure" placebos are
differentiated in that impure is an active
substance administered under false premises
and/or in insufficient dosage. Other topics
covered are the placebo effect, magic,
suggestion, conditioning, the simple blind
test, the double-blind test, placebo reactors
and nonreactors. Studies in which placebos
are compared with tranquilizers and
energizers have often cast doubt upon the
drug's utility and conversely, placebos

existing medical or psychiatric institutions.
Group therapy, the establishment of
halfway houses designed to elevate the
derelict above the skid row environment,
teaching healthy attitudes toward alcohol
as a preventive measure, state programs
for rehabilitation, specialized treatment
centers in all major cities, and various
programs directed toward prevention
have all been instituted to curtail the
problem. The combined efficacy of such
a comprehensive plan of attack must be
thoroughly investigated before any
facsimile of the plan is adopted for Great
Britain. (12 refs.)

Maudsley Hospital
London, SE 5, Great Britain

1685 Macgregor, A. G., & Perry, W. L. M.
Detection of drug toxicity. Lancet, 1962,
No. 7244, 1406. [Letter]

A previous letter intimated that the antibiotics triacetyloleandomycin and
erythromycin have been withdrawn from
the British market due to hepatotoxicity.
These drugs have not been withdrawn.
However, the list of drugs which have
been banned due to unpredicted and undesirable toxicity includes thalidomide,
triparanol, zoxazolamine, furaltadone,
diathazanine and amphenidone. All of
these drugs have evidenced intolerable
toxicity. (No refs.)

University of Aberdeen
Aberdeen, Great Britain

1686 Macgregor, A. G., & Perry, W. L. M.
Detection of drug toxicity. Lancet, 1962,
No. 7241, 1233-1234. [Letter]

The thalidomide debacle precipitated an
acute awareness of drug teratogenicity
among members of the medical profession.
Stringent legislative controls should be
instituted to regulate the marketing of new
drugs. Toxic effects are divisible into
3 categories: those which have occurred
before that can be detected by a known test
in animals, those which are known but
for which no animal test has been devised

and those which have not occurred before.
Teratogenicity is detectable in rabbits
while agranulocytosis, aplastic anemia,
hepatotoxicity and carcinogenicity fall into
category 2, and future nebulous hazards
constitute category 3. Unpredicted and
undesirable toxicity has accounted for
withdrawal of the following drugs from the
market: thalidomide, triparanol, zoxazolamine, furaltadone, diathazanine and
amphenidone. Intolerable toxicity has also
been observed with triacetyloleandomycin
and erythromycin. Several proposals
have been suggested to formulate groups
designed to study various types of drug
toxicity. Bureaucratic inertia has precluded realization of these proposals. It
is imperative that adequate information
about the therapeutic efficacy of new drugs
be made available to physicians. A plea
is promulgated for the organized accumulation of information about drug toxicity and
efficacy, so control measures may be based
on knowledge rather than ignorant
supposition. (9 refs.)

University of Aberdeen
Aberdeen, Great Britain

1687 Merriman, B. Alcoholism. Lancet,
1962, No. 7241, 1238-1239.

The fact that England has 500,000 alcoholics
out of a population of 50 million people
indicates a crying need for some definitive
effective program of rehabilitation. The
public must be persuaded that alcoholism is
an urgent problem and a disease entity
rather than a condition of simple habitual
drunkenness. Alcoholism apparently
involves a chronic inability to abstain, so-
called "inveterate alcoholism", resulting
in CNS sensitization to a constant
relatively low blood alcohol concentration
called delta alcoholism, which fails to
produce acute intoxication but is progressively destructive to bodily functions and social
relationships. There is a current tendency
for the alpha alcoholic (purely psychological
dependence on alcohol or problem drinking
to relieve emotional tension) to progress
to delta alcoholism rather than the more
familiar gamma alcoholism. Public
opinion must be educated to accept
alcoholism as a disease entity in order to

cope with the problem on a national
scope. (No refs.)

[No address]

1688 Harris, E. L. Detection of drug
toxicity. Lancet, 1962, No. 7242, 1305.

A physician is aghast at the rather dogmatic
assertion of Macgregor and Perry that
drug teratogenicity will no longer endanger
mankind since the development and
application of testing procedures in rabbits
for detecting teratogenicity in new
pharmacological compounds. Such
optimism is apparently premature, and
extensive research in developing infallible
screening methods is indicated before we
can safely say that potential drug teratogenicity will invariably be detected before
a drug reaches the market. (No refs.)

Nicholas Research Institute Ltd.
Slough, Bucks
Great Britain

1689 Pliess, G. Thalidomide and congenital abnormalities. Lancet, 1962, No.
7239, 1128-1129. [Letter]

The Wiedmann syndrome (thalidomide
syndrome) consisting of characteristic
congenital anomalies resulted in 14
instances from thalidomide ingestion by
mothers during the 1st trimester of pregnancy. The teratogenic factor apparently
interferes with normal biochemical processes which govern the development of
mesodermal structures. Typical extremity
malformations probably originate during
the scleroblastemal stage. The precise
anomalies manifested should theoretically
correspond to the period of development
during which the noxious factor was administered. Coelomic malformations result
from interference with the critical determination phases of the mesenchymal derivatives, predominantly of the lateral and
intermediate mesoderm, rather than by
directly affecting the organ anlage.
Experiments with thalidomide administered
to pregnant rats have indicated that the
drug does not exert teratogenic effects in
rats. Malformations of exogenous origin

termination of pregnancy may be obtained
legally only if said pregnancy seriously
endangers the mental health of the mother.
Thalidomide was administered primarily
to women of nervous character who
required sedation, thus indicating a certain
degree of mental instability. The act of
abortion may be performed legally only
for the purpose of preserving the life or
mental or physical health of the woman in
question. (No refs.)

7 Adam Street
Adelphi
London W.C.2, Great Britain

1692 Busch, Harris, Adams, Helen, &
Muramatsu, Masami. Effects of alkylating
agents and thioacetamide on nuclear
metabolism. Federation Proceedings,
1962, No. 5323, 1093-1096.

A paper dealing primarily with the effects
of alkylating agents and thioacetamide on
nuclear and microsomal RNA content also
includes a brief discussion on phenothiazine
uptake in nuclear components. . The
implication of RNA as a vital information
agency in memory has suggested the
possibility that nucleolar phenothiazine
concentration may interfere with the
specific types of RNA which are essential
to the memory process. Purified
preparations of brain nucleoli will be
required for further investigation. (17
refs.)

Department of Pharmacology and
    Biochemistry
Baylor University College of Medicine
Houston, Tex.

1693 Spiers, Alexander L. Drug-induced
malformations in the fetus. American
Heart Journal, 1962, 5, 717-718.

A considerable body of information culled
primarily from the Continent has established
a definite correlation between ingestion of
thalidomide during the 1st trimester of
pregnancy and resultant fetal anomalies.
Characteristic thalidomide induced aberrations include gross limb defects, cardiac
malformations and gastrointestinal

abnormalities. Teratogenicity affects
tissues of mesenchymal origin, but
extensive research will be necessary to
determine the origin of deleterious effects
more precisely. The incidence of
thalidomide defects correlated rather
closely with the areas in which the drug
was freely obtainable. About 3,000
afflicted babies were born in West Germany
alone. The tragedy has precipitated a
widespread awareness of potential teratogenicity in new drugs, and testing procedures
will henceforth be required before a new
drug may be marketed. Drugs should be
used with the utmost caution in pregnancy
to prevent repetition of the thalidomide
disaster. (8 refs.)

Stirling Royal Infirmary
Stirling, Scotland

1694 Meyer, Joachim-Ernst. Prominent
trends in German psychiatry. South
African Medical Journal, 1962, 2, 150-152.

German psychiatry essentially originated
with the dictums of Kraepelin and progressed
to encompass the catholic concepts of
Sigmund Freud. Psychiatric research has
been based upon the concept of phenomenology
as introduced by Karl Jaspers which has
recently been enriched by the addition of
the concepts of gestalt psychology and
Jung's depth psychology. Existential
analysis added new depth and dimension to
psychiatry when promulgated by Martin
Heidegger. Genealogy has become obsolete
due to the political implications inherent
within its tenets. Biochemical research on
the endogenous psychoses flourishes in
present day Germany, along with concomitant
development of new drugs. Neurophysiology
provides a sound basis for a considerable
amount of significant research. Recent
events such as war neurosis, cerebral
atrophy from nutritional deficiency and
psychic trauma from concentration camp
sojourns have exerted a profound effect on
contemporary German psychiatry. Insulin
shock therapy, ECT, imipramine and the
MAO inhibitors, haloperidol and orphenadrine
are all important constituents in the modern
therapeutic armamentarium. (20 refs.)

Nervenklinik
University of Munich
Munich, Germany

Therapy for poisoning due to overdoses of
opium derivatives (morphine) and synthetic
analgesics such as meperidine, alpha-pro
deine and anileridine includes immediate
establishment of adequate pulmonary ventilation and circulatory support followed by
determination of the cause of coma, evaluation of the depth of depression and establishment of a tentative prognosis. Drug therapy
involves specific antagonists for opiate
poisoning such as nalorphine and levallorphan.
Deep coma responds to injections of pentetrazol, picrotoxin and methyl-ethyl-glutarimide,
and relatively mild narcotic depression may
by ameliorated by nikethamide, ephedrine,
caffeine and sodium benzoate. Apneic infants may benefit from administration of the
narcotic antagonists. Additional beneficial
therapy includes aspiration of stomach contents, catheterization, and tracheal aspiration with special emphasis on oral hygiene.
(No refs.)

School of Medicine
University of Pennsylvania
Philadelphia, Pa.

1699 Ryder, Henry W. Acute barbiturate
poisoning. In: Conn, Howard F. [Ed.]
Current Therapy. Philadelphia: W. B.
Saunders, 1962. Pp. 660-661.

Acute barbiturate poisoning is to be treated
as follows: remain with the patient until
consciousness is regained, keep the airway
open and gas exchange adequate, observe the
vital signs during adequate ventilation,
lavage the stomach, transfer the patient to
the recovery room if vital signs are normal,
administer phenylephrine and levarterenol
if the patient is in shock, review the mechanisms by which death is caused from barbiturate poisoning and maintain the patient's
general condition until definite signs of
recovery are observed. (No refs.)

Deaconess Hospital
Cincinnati, Ohio

1700 Hoffer, A., & Osmond, H. Adrenaline
and schizophrenia. Lancet, 1962, No. 7251
643-644.

Evidence is presented which suggests that 3
papers from NIMH which purportedly fail
to vindicate the adrenochrome-adrenolutin
theory of schizophrenia neither support nor
confute the hypothesis that schizophrenia is
characterized biochemically by increased
conversion of adrenochrome to adrenolutin,
a trihydroxy indole with toxicity which approx-
imates that of adrenochrome, which is
converted to 5:6 dihydroxy-N-methyl indole,
a nontoxic substance. Excess epinephrine is
metabolized to adrenochrome, an over-
abundance of which is present in schizophrenics. No direct correlation has been obtained experimentally, but the NIMH variables hardly lend themselves to a carefully
controlled study. It is unlikely that a typical
group of normal controls includes American
males who drink 1 cup of coffee per day and
smoke 1 1/2 cigarettes daily. La Brosse,
Mann, and Kety are also guilty of perpetrat-
ing the following misconceptions: the hypo--
thesis that dextro-epinephrine is probably
inert metabolically; the addition of ascorbic
acid, a known antioxidant, to every 100 ml
of epinephrine solution despite the fact
that it will undoubtedly hinder or prevent
the conversion of epinephrine to adrenochrome and the fact that epinephrine injections will probably reduce epinephrine
secretion from the adrenal medulla.
Esoteric techniques are required to isolate
adrenochrome or its metabolites from the
urine. Attschule (1961) found aminochromes
in schizophrenic urines, in experiments
which may prove crucial in ultimately
establishing the adrenochrome-adrenolutin
hypothesis. (10 refs.)

Department of Public Health
University Hospital
Saskatoon, Saskatchewan
Canada

1701 James, L. S. Apgar Scoring System.
Developmental Medicine and Child Neurology, 1962, 4, 444.

Critical comments by Dr. Crawford on the
Apgar Scoring System for neonates are
partially refuted, including the fact that
minimally depressed infants evince an absence of muscle tone. Rather, hypertonicity may be observed in the initial stages
of asphyxia, particularly with acute trachial

in moderate depression resulting from therapeutic doses of drugs including anesthetics. Analeptic drugs should never be utilized in these situations. In lieu of analeptics, good recovery room care including careful attention to airway management, maintenance of adequate ventilation, support of circulation and prevention of infection offers the highest rate of recovery with the lowest incidence of complications. Analeptics should never be used to supplement or substitute for good postoperative medical and nursing care. (No refs.)

Department of Anesthesiology
Columbia University College of Physicians
and Surgeons
New York, N. Y.

1704 Fouks, L., Laine, Mathis, Ferrant, Riou, & Boucher. Rapport sur l'essai clinique de la dixyrazine. [Report on the clinical trial of dixyrazine.] Annales Médico-Psychologiques, 1962, 1, 120, 636-637.

Dixyrazine, a methylated phenothiazine, is similar to levomepromazine in depressive and neurotic states because of its anxiolytic activity. It diminishes nervous tension and excitability. Its side effects are essentially those of piperazine-substituted phenothiazines (akinesia and psychomotor syndrome); these are minimal and easy to correct. The antihallucinatory and antipsychotic activity of dixyrazine is quite weak and it seems best used in cases of instability and character disorder. (No refs.)

[No address]

1705 Fouks, L., Lefèvre, Laine, Mathis, Ferrant, Riou, & Boucher. Essai clinique de la trifluopérazine. [Clinical trial of trifluoperazine.] Annales Médico-Psychologiques, 1962, 1, 120, 636.

Trifluoperazine is recommended as the best presently available neuroleptic, because of its antihallucinatory and antipsychotic properties and easily managed side effects. (No refs.)

[No address]

1706 Blaya, Marcelo. O uso de tranquilizadores na clinica. [The clinical use of tranquilizers.] Actas Luso-Españolas de Neurologia y Psiquiatría, 1962, 21, 153-158.

Tranquilizers are classified into 5 categories: Rauwolfia derivatives, phenothiazine derivatives, diphenylmethane (benactyzine) derivatives, propanodiolics and miscellany. A table of side effects (e.g., agitation, agranulocytosis) for 14 popular tranquilizers (e.g., chlordiazepoxide, reserpine, meprobamate) is also presented. Promazine is favored in psychotic syndromes, while in neurosis where anxiety is the main feature meprobamate is preferred. (7 refs.)

Av. João Pessoa, 925
Pôrto Alegre
Rio Grande do Sul
Brazil

1707 Linke, H. Kritik der Therapie: Nebenwirkungen and Gefahren der Anwendung psychotroper und schmerzstillender Pharmaka. [Critique of therapeutics: side effects and dangers of psychotropic and analgesic drugs.] Deutsches Gesundheitswesen, 1962, 17, 1095-1101, 1146-1156.

A classification of psychotropic and analgesic drugs based on their affinities for various parts of the nervous system is presented. Side effects are also discussed. The main classes are: neuroleptics; tranquilizers and ataractics; thymoleptics; psychotonics, and analgesics. The great dangers of misuse and addiction are pointed out, particularly in view of the pressures of modern living, the drive to increase individual living standards, the advertising by pharmaceutical houses, and the unwillingness of the overworked physician to deprive a suffering patient of the means of alleviating his pains or tensions. East Germany has gone far in the direction of passing laws for the provision of correct information on the properties of drugs, and for the control of their production. However, the physician owes it to his patient to understand his psychic needs and to treat these not only by drugs, but also by other means. (131 refs.)

Medizinische Klinik
Medizinische Akademie
Magdeburg, Germany

1708 Briggs, Michael H. Possible relations
of ascorbic acid, ceruloplasmin and toxic
aromatic metabolites in schizophrenia,
New Zealand Medicine Journal, 1962, 61,
229-236.

Numerous experimental studies have corroborated the fact that ceruloplasmin levels are higher in acute than in chronic
schizophrenia, while both groups evince
significantly higher plasma levels than
normal subjects. The increased concentration of ceruloplasmin in schizophrenics
catalyzes the oxidation of ascorbate to
dehydroascorbate, and the preferential
oxidation of ascorbate prevents oxidation
of circulating amines. Schizophrenics,
therefore, will exhibit lower blood ascorbate levels than normal persons, even when
an adequate dietary supply of the vitamin
is supplied. Schizophrenics tend toward
hypercupremia which in turn precipitates
a form of hypovitaminosis C. Since ascorbic acid activates the liver enzyme p-
hydroxyphenylpyruvic oxidase, the diminished ascorbate levels should result in a
corresponding decrease in the extent of
aromatic amino acid metabolism by the
phenylalanine oxidase system. With partial inhibition of this pathway, aromatic
amino acids are metabolized by an alternate pathway which favors increased
epinephrine synthesis. The major urinary
metabolite of epinephrine, 3-methoxy-4-
hydroxymandelic acid, is present in
significantly greater concentration in the
urine of schizophrenics than in normal
urine. It is conceivable that an abnormal
metabolite of epinephrine which structurally
resembles the psychotomimetic compounds
accumulates and exerts toxic activity. It
seems improbable that any drug therapy will
cure chronic schizophrenia since prolonged
action of these toxins on brain tissue has
probably induced the type of irreversible
cellular changes observed in experimental
animals maintained in a state of vitamin C
deficiency. Most major psychotherapeutic
drugs (chlorpromazine, reserpine, isocarboxazid, etc.) used to treat schizophrenia
are capable of altering brain amines related to epinephrine and serotonin and these
changes are compatible with the hypothesis
that toxic epinephrine metabolites induce
schizophrenic brain changes. (67 refs.)

Information on 86 deaths due to kidney damage caused by phenacetin is reviewed. The chief reasons for seeking medical aid on the part of phenacetin abusers are shortness of breath and fatigue. Anemia and renal insufficiency were often diagnosed clinically and commonly after 1-4 months the patients died in uremia. (No refs.)

[No address]

1712 Kasanen, A. Fenacetinproblemet i Finland. [The phenacetin problem in Finland.] Nordisk Medicin, 1962, 67, 755-756.

About 10% of factory workers, 34% of patients with kidney damage and 16% of others abuse sedatives in Finland. The incidence of papillitis necroticans has risen and about 60% of the cases are phenacetin users. Liver damage was also noted in some cases at autopsy, and changes are regularly seen in the EEG. (No refs.)

[No address]

1713 Björkman, Sven Erik. Njurskador genom fenacetinmissbruk. [Kidney damage due to phenacetin abuse.] Nordisk Medicin, 1962, 67, 755.

Prophylaxis against kidney damage caused by phenacetin is advocated, especially since the mechanism of this renal damage is unknown. (No refs.)

[No address]

1714 Naess, Knut. Barbitursyrefri hypnotica. [Barbiturate-free hypnotics.] Nordisk Medicin, 1962, 67, 734-735.

After discussing the disadvantages of barbiturates, the author remarks on glutethimide, methyprylon, ethinamate, chlorprothixene and thalidomide. The author warns against the injudicious introduction of new agents, as witnessed by the thalidomide tragedy. This is especially true since all of these agents are potential means of suicide. (No refs.)

[No address]

1715 Janssen, Paul. Zur Chemie morphinartiger Körper. [The chemistry of morphine-like substances.] Anaesthesist, 1962, 11, 1-7.

The structure of the piperidine derivatives is discussed, and a table presented in which the pharmacological properties of morphine, pethidine, phenoperidine, dextromoramide, pirinitramide, and diphenoxylate are compared. The important chemical features which are relevant to pharmacological properties are described for all known morphinelike analgesics. In view of their chemical similarity, these drugs are believed to act by "fitting" to a specific 3-dimensional receptor, probably located in the thalamus. (24 refs.)

Research Laboratory
Beerse, Belgium

1716 Quadbeck, G. Blut-Hirnschranke und Hirnernährung. [The blood-brain barrier and cerebral nutrition.] Medizinische Wochenschrift, 1962, 104, 24-26.

The concept of the blood-brain barrier as a functional rather than anatomic entity is discussed and the possibility of affecting cerebral transport mechanisms by means of pharmacological agents is pointed out. A decrease in barrier activity as can be produced by aminophyllin, nicotinic acid, reserpine, tetrabenazine, prothipendyl, chlorpromazine, chlorprothixene, triflupromazine and perphenazine permits the needs of the brain to be met by simple diffusion. However, as shown by experiments in mice, glucose uptake by the brain is not increased immediately by these agents, a period of metabolic adaptation being required. Thus 1 dose of aminophyllin (90 mg/kg) had no effect, but glucose uptake was increased significantly by 45 mg/kg/day for 8 days. (23 refs.)

Psychiatrische und Neurologische Klinik
Universität des Saarlandes
Homburg/Saar, Germany

1717 Lendle, L. Arzneimittelnebenwirkungen in der Kritik der Pharmakologie. [Drug side effects from the point of view of the pharmacologist.] Medizinische Wochenschrift, 1962, 104, 61-67.

In a general discussion of the causes, prediction and prevention of side effects due to
all types of natural and synthetic drugs,
including specifically the phenothiazines, the
author distinguishes between true dosage-
dependent side effects and allergic reactions,
and suggests that the risks of side effects
are often overrated. Particular attention
is paid to the pharmacological evaluation of
the risk of side effects by determination
of the spectrum of action, relative specificity, metabolism, biochemical effects and
immunological effects of drugs and their
combinations on a variety of animal species.
Even then final evaluation can only be made
on the basis of long clinical experience with
sick patients and accurate reporting. (6
refs.)

Pharmakologisches Institut
Uniersität Göttingen
Göttingen, Germany

1718 Sahli, M. Zur Analytik der
Rauwolfia-Alkaloide. [Quantitative determination of the Rauwolfia alkaloids.]
Arzneimittel-Forschung, 1962, 12, 55-61,
155-61.

Following a review of the chemical structure of the principal Rauwolfia alkaloids,
including the quaternary anhydronium bases
and the tertiary indol and indolin bases,
extraction methods used for their separation are briefly discussed. The spectrophotometric (UV and infrared), colorimetric and fluorometric determination of the
individual pure alkaloids, with particular
attention to reserpine and its degradation
products are reviewed; analytical results
on some of the commercial preparations
of reserpine are presented. Methods are
also described for the determination and
characterization of total Rauwolfia
alkaloids by means of countercurrent
distribution, chromatography on columns,
paper or films, and paper electrophoresis.
Finally the author's personal experience
with the paper chromatography of
serpentine, reserpine, reserpic acid,
rescinnamine, deserpidine and ajmalin is
reported. (138 refs.)

Laboratorium der Interkantonalen
   Kontrollstelle für Heilmittel
Bern, Switzerland

1719 Janz, Dieter. Gezielte Therapie der
Epilepsien. [Specific treatment in epilepsy.
Medizinische Welt, 1962, No. 12, 629-635.

After reviewing the etiology of epileptic
attacks and deploring the limited use of
anticonvulsive agents in practice, the
author points out that the type of treatment
should be determined by the type of attack
rather than by the etiology. The importance
of proper dosage is emphasized, and side
effects are grouped into 3 types; hypersensitivity reactions, effects on hematopoiesis,
and minor effects varying with the drug and
dosage used. Tables are presented listing
the chemical composition, dosage used, and
price of the anticonvulsive agents on the
German market. General suggestions for
the control of side effects and management
of treatment, the indications and contraindications for the most effective drugs in
the various types of epilepsy (on the
basis of 3350 cases), and the dosage and
side effects of 2 of the most important
barbiturates, hydantoins, succinimides
and oxazolidines are given. The sulfonamide derivative Ospolot, mentioned briefly,
does not seem to be effective in psychomotor epilepsy (61 cases). (10 refs.)

Nervenklinik der Universität Heidelberg
Heidelberg, Germany

1720 Lüth, Paul. Der praktische Arzt
und die neuen Medikamente. [The general
practitioner and the new drugs.] Münchener
Medizinische Wochenschrift, 1962, 104, 81-8
128-131.

In a general discussion of the requirements
for critical evaluation of new drugs in
general practice (animal experiments, toxicity studies in normal individuals, statistically evaluated placebo studies and pilot studie
to evaluate the dependability of patients),
presented at the Salzburg Congress of the
International Society for Applied Medicine in
1961, the author emphasizes that most of the
overwhelming numbers of new drugs are
directed at the hospitalized patient and that
the problems faced by the individual practitioner are quite different. The need for
complete information on the pharmacological
properties of new drugs is stressed, with

particular attention being drawn to the confusion in the field of psychopharmacology. (26 refs.)

Kaiserstrasse 8-3/10
Offenbach am Main, Germany

1721 Ulrich, J. Die konservative Therapie der Epilepsie. [Conservative treatment of epilepsy.] Praxis, 1962, 51, 62-67.

In addition to reviewing the psychological aspects of epilepsy and the general guide-lines for the management of this disease by proper living, the author classifies the currently used anticonvulsants into 2 groups: those which are effective in all cases except petit mal with 3/second spikes and waves (phenobarbital, diphenylhydantoin, meph-enytoin and primidone), and those which are effective only in this type (trimetha-done, trimethadione, acetazolamide and succinimide); dosages and side effects are listed, and the clinical characteristics of each of these classes of compounds are reviewed in detail. The lack of correlation between etiology and response to specific drugs is pointed out, and suggestions are made as to the best mode of treatment in particular situations. (30 refs.)

Medizinische Klinik des Kantonsspitals
St. Gallen, Switzerland

1722 Stucki, A. Angst, Hemmung, Minderwertigkeitsgefühl. [Anxiety, inhibi-tion and feelings of inferiority.] Praxis, 1962, 51, 148-154.

Following a general discussion of the nature, etiology and function of anxiety and its re-lationships to inhibition and feelings of inferiority, the author points out that psychotherapy is still the treatment of choice in such conditions. Various ways in which anxiety can be relieved are analyzed. Even though many psychotropic drugs, such as meprobamate, have a superficially beneficial effect on anxiety, they merely mask the underlying condition, destroying the body's alarm signal, often delaying causal therapy. Although tranquil-izers may be necessary temporarily in acute states, the dangers of addiction and

paradoxical effects are emphasized. The negative effects of meprobamate on per-sonality are illustrated by a personal experience. (23 refs.)

Bälliz 64,
Thun, Switzerland.

1723 Hartmann-von Monakow, K. Der heutige Stand der medikamentösen Therapie des Parkinsonsyndroms. [Present status of the drug therapy of the Parkinsonian syndrome.] Praxis, 1962, 51, 30-33.

The indications, clinical response and side effects of a large number of drugs are briefly reviewed. Agents used on the treat-ment of Parkinsonism are divided into alkaloids (tropeins, erthroidin, Rauwolfia), synthetics (aminoesters, phenothiazines, glycerol ethers, aminoethers, propanol derivatives and glutarimides), vitamins (B_6 and B_{12}), hydrazines (MAO inhibitors), and imipramine. Particular attention is devoted to cisternal therapy with Impletol (procaine and caffeine). All these agents, however, are purely symptomatic. (5 refs.)

Dufourstrasse 16
Zürich, Switzerland

1724 Merritt, H. Houston. The neurologi-cal and psychiatric implications of basic studies of the ultrastructure of the nervous system. Bulletin of the New York Academy of Medicine, 1962, 38, 813-816.

Despite the vast conglomeration of know-ledge which has been amassed about the CNS, the following information must be obtained to enable man to comprehend the more elusive aspects of mental and neuro-logical disease: the intimate structure and detailed biochemistry of the neurone, the means by which the cerebellum, brainstem nuclei and basal ganglia influence muscle tone and the mode of interaction between spinal cord, brainstem, thalamus and cerebral cortex. Only comprehensive knowledge of the chemical composition of the neurone and other CNS tissues accompanied by an understanding of the affiliated enzyme systems will explain the selective vulnerability which predis-poses certain cells to react selectively to

specific infections or toxins. Inherited
defects in the basal ganglia may lead to
greater vulnerability to certain exogenous
toxins, e. g., drug-induced parkinsonism.
Numerous degenerative diseases and
metabolic disorders await future elucidation
before they can be effectively ameliorated.
(No refs.)

Department of Neurology
Columbia University College of
    Physicians and Surgeons
New York, N. Y.

1725 Inglis, W. Drug company's
responsibility. New Zealand Medical
Journal, 1962, 61, 562. [Letter]

On behalf of the Geigy Chemical Co., the
medical director states that many years of
research and investigation preceded the
release of imipramine to the public.
Treatment of overdosages may be specified
only after sufficient data on the subject
has been accumulated. At present, the
dearth of available data means that treatment must be based solely upon knowledge
of the product especially with respect to
potential toxicity. Labels which extensively
proclaim possible deleterious drug effects
can only cause unnecessary consternation
on the part of the lay public. The drug
company should provide doctors with the
complete story of a drug, not an emphasis
on side effects. It is further suggested
that all potentially dangerous compounds
be packaged in the most unattractive form
possible. Parents should exercise extreme
caution in handling drugs where children
are concerned. (No refs.)

[No address]

1726 Cumming, A. Alcoholism. Medical
Services Journal (Canada), 1962, 18,
787-794.

Alcoholism, a personality disorder whose
chief symptom is chronic compulsive drinking, has roots which are deep in the unconscious. Signs which are suggestive of
alcoholism include: the morning drink,
severe and remorseful hangovers, sneaking
drinks, blackouts, loss of appetite, solitary
drinking, concealing liquor, decreased

efficiency, personal problems, lying about
alcohol consumption and characteristic
personality changes. Alcoholism exists in
people who require strong oral gratifica-
tion, and, while it cannot be cured, it can
be controlled. The Canadian army advo-
cates the following treatment regimen for
alcoholics suffering from acute withdrawal
symptoms: no alcohol, chlorpromazine
(50 mg t. i. d.), vitamin B complex (1 cc.
i. m. b. i. d.), crystalline insulin (5-10
units 30 minutes before meals) and sodium amytal (3 gr. at bedtime). Membership in Alcoholics Anonymous offers
the best opportunity for rehabilitation.
(No refs.)

[No address]

1727 Odegard, Ornulv. 3. internasjonale
kongress for psykofarmakologi i München
2. -5. IX. 1962. [Third International Congress
for Psychopharmacology in Munich, 2-5
Sept., 1962.] Nordisk Medicin, 1962, 68,
1457-1459.

The research departments of major drug
companies and the leading psychiatric
hospitals over the world were well
represented at the 3rd International
Congress for Psychopharmacology. About
350 delegates attended. The tone of this
congress was reserved compared to the
optimism exhibited in 1958. The debate
between the optimistic New York group
with Kline and the critical Maudsley
group with Shepherd was both useful and
entertaining. Placebo research appears
to be declining, and less interest was
expressed in the double-blind method as
the only method permitted in research.
In animal research the tendency is away
from Pavlovian methods to behavioral
research. Additionally a warning was
given against the promiscuous use of
minor tranquilizers. (No refs.)

[No address]

1728 Baeyerts, John D. The effect of
Librium. New Zealand Medical Journal,
1962, 61, 368-369. [Letter]

muscle can be obtained which render the
compounds valuable in the treatment of
extrapyramidal spasticity. (59 refs.)

Westendring 22
Dresden, Germany

1730 Voigt, R. Psychopharmaka. Chemie
und Wirkung pflanzlicher und synthetischer
psychotroper Verbindungen. [Psychotropic
drugs. The chemistry and pharmacology
of psychotropic substances, both synthetic
and those derived from plants.] Pharmazie,
1962, 17, 317-331.

In an extensive review of those agents with
a primary effect on the CNS, as distinguished
from alcohol, caffeine, morphine, etc.,
which have secondary psychotropic effects,
the author classifies psychotropic drugs
into 2 broad groups: psychotherapeutic
and psychotomimetic agents. The former
are subdivided into neuroleptics (Rauwolfia
derivatives, phenothiazines, azapheno-
thiazines, thiaxanthenes, diazepins),
ataractics (diphenylmethanes, aliphatic
alcohols, carbamates), psychotonics
(phenylethylamines, amphetamines) and
thymoleptics (hydrazines, dibenzoazepins).
Among the psychotomimetics, mescaline,
harmaline, tryptamine derivatives,
lysergic acid derivatives and psilocybin
are discussed, and some structure-activity
relationships are pointed out. (201 refs.)

Pharmazeutisches Institut
Humboldt Universität
Berlin, Germany

1731 Pfeifer, S. Zentrale Analgetica.
[Central analgesics.] Pharmazie, 1962,
17, 189-203.

This is an extensive review of the chemistry
and pharmacology of the principal types of
centrally acting analgesics, with particular
reference to structure-activity relationships.
A brief historical review of the development
of the semi-synthetic morphine derivatives
is followed by a detailed analysis of the
interrelationships in the morphinan,
pethidine, methadon and benzimidazol
groups. The principal structural components
in an analgesic include a central C or N atom

with decreased electron density, one or
more lipophilic aromatic rings, a cationic
group attached to the active center by a
C-C chain, and hydrophilic residues.
(178 refs.)

Pharmazeutisches Institut
Humboldt Universität
Berlin, Germany

1732 Dundee, John W., & Moore, James.
The phenothiazines. British Journal of
Anaesthesiology, 1962, 34, 247-250.

The phenothiazines, 7 with dimethyl amino
propyl side chains, 4 with piperazine side
chains and 2 with piperidine side chains
are classified in tabular form, replete
with information on proprietary names,
radicals, average clinical dosages, indications for common clinical usage and
frequently reported side effects. No
relationship has been observed between
analgesic activity and chemical grouping.
(46 refs.)

Department of Anaesthetics
The Queen's University of Belfast
Great Britain

1733 Kety, Seymour S. Regional neurochemistry and its application to brain
function. Bulletin of the New York Academy
of Medicine, 1962, 38, 799-812.

Esoteric experimental techniques have
enabled scientists to learn a considerable
amount about brain function, metabolism
and blood supply. The role of catecholamines
(such as levarterenol and serotonin) in
brain metabolism has been elucidated.
Psychoactive drugs like LSD, iproniazid
and reserpine have resulted from extensive
research. Neurochemistry provides the
key to unlock new thresholds of understanding
which will in turn provide the basis for
significant future achievement. (47 refs.)

Laboratory of Clinical Science
NIMH
Bethesda, Md.

1734 Amark, Curt. 5. Internationella

psykoterapikongressen i Wien, 21.-26.
VII.1961. [Fifth International Psychotherapy Congress in Vienna, 21-26 August,
1961.] Nordisk Medicin, 1962, 68,
1529-1533.

In the 5th International Psychotherapy
Congress in Vienna many talks centered
on the relationship between psychotherapy
and psychopharmacology. Drugs work
on mood but not individual experience.
Correct diagnosis is stressed in any event.
An ordinary drug can be used by a patient
as a defense so that he maintains his
neurotic symptom. Also complaints are
registered against the preponderance of
drug advertising. Finally, group therapy,
conjoint family therapy, etc., are mentioned.
(No refs.)

[No address]

1735 Shama Rau, T.H., & Mukerji, G.
Indigenous drug research. Probe, 1962,
1, 205-210.

A number of Indian plant species are
discussed, including Rauwolfia serpentina,
Nardostachys jatamansi (jatamansic acid
useful in the treatment of epilepsy,
hysteria and convulsions) and Echinops
echinatus (a nerve tonic; a crystalline
alkaloid which has been isolated and
found to be a smooth muscle relaxant).
Two works are cited: "Glossary of Indian
Medicinal Plants" by the Council of
Scientific and Industrial Research [India]
and the Indian Pharmaceutical Codex
published by the Central Drug Research
Institute, Lucknow, India. The latter
volume contains about 190 monographs on
Indian drugs. (No refs.)

Central Drug Research Institute
Lucknow, India

1736 Stephen, Elspeth. Carisoprodol.
Developmental Medicine and Child Neurology,
1962, 4, 80-83.

The value of carisoprodol in infantile
cerebral palsy and difficulties in evaluation
are discussed. In most cases there is no
way of determining the level of the lesion or

1739 Schou, Mogens. Klassificering af
nyere psykofarmaka. [Classification of
new psychopharmaca.] Nordisk Medicin,
1962, 68, 1431-1432. [Letter]

In a criticism of Lingjaerde (1962), the
writer took the view that his classification
was not new or different, and favored
Jacobsen's (1959) WHO report. (9 refs.)

[No address]

1740 McKay, D. N. The toxic substance
(thalidomide) prohibition notice, 1962.
New Zealand Medical Journal, 1962, 61,
474.

Thalidomide was prohibited in Wellington
on the 15th of August, 1962, by a proclama-
tion which decreed that the importation,
manufacture, sale, possession or use of
the toxic substance known as thalidomide
was henceforth prohibited by law for a
period of precisely 1 year. (No refs.)

Ministry of Health
Wellington, New Zealand

1741 Schmidt, Richard Penrose. Epilepsy
in adults. In: Conn, Howard F. [Ed.]
Current Therapy. Philadelphia: W. B.
Saunders, 1962. Pp. 508-511.

The following types of therapy are
advocated to ameliorate epilepsy in adults:
grand mal and focal cortical seizures
respond to diphenylhydantoin or primidone,
psychomotor attacks also respond to these
drugs, plus methsuximide where indicated.
Petit mal seizures may be alleviated with
trimethadione, phenobarbital, paramethadione or methsuximide while unclassified
seizures (myoclonic attacks, drop seizures,
minor seizures of uncertain origin) respond
more readily to primidone than to diphenylhydantoin. New compounds such as
ethosuximide are effective in petit mal
and psychomotor seizures. Severe
refractory epilepsy may respond to drugs
like methyl-phenyl-ethyl hydantoin,
phenacemide, mephobarbital or acetazolamide. Toxic effects are similar and
generally encompass excessive drowsiness,
unsteady gait, visual blurring with nystagmus
and, occasionally, granulocytopenia or

agranulocytosis. Surgical intervention
may sometimes be indicated. Status
epilepticus frequently responds to paraldehyde, amobarbital or tribromethanol.
Emotional rehabilitation is essential to
patient wellbeing. (No refs.)

[No address]

1742 Regan, Peter F. Psychoses: Delirium.
In: Conn, Howard F. [Ed.] Current
Therapy. Philadelphia: W. B. Saunders,
1962. Pp. 552-555.

Treatment of the initial phase of delirious
reactions involves diminution of all
excitatory external stimuli. During the
2nd phase, mounting anxiety and insecurity
necessitate precautions against suicide,
mandatory obviation of all excitatory stimuli
must be enforced, hypnotics may be used
to induce sleep and tranquilizers such as
chlorpromazine (25 mg q. i. d., i. m.) may
be found advantageous. The 3rd phase of
delusion is characterized by complete loss
of contact with reality, delusions, hallucinations and serious disorientation and the
patient must be prevented from committing
suicide. Agitation may be controlled by
administration of barbiturates or phenothiazines, particularly chlorpromazine,
with dosage regulated according to need.
The patient must receive adequate nourish-
ment with careful control of body processes.
Special treatment regimens are advocated
in instances of deliria occurring in drug
withdrawal, toxic and metabolic deliria,
deliria associated with drug administration,
postoperative deliria and deliria associated
with injury to the CNS. (No refs.)

University of Florida
Gainesville, Fla.

1743 Marks, John. Current views on
psychotropic drugs. New Zealand Medical
Journal, 1962, 61, 391-397.

Tranquilizers are classified primarily on
the basis of their pharmacological and
clinical properties rather than by their
chemical constituents. A 2nd method of
chemical classification divides the
compounds into 4 main groups : pheno-

psychological bolsters like Alcoholics
Anonymous in addition to familial
understanding and cooperation. (No refs.)

[No address]

1747 Payne, Charles E. The out-patient
treatment of depression. American
Practitioner, 1962, 13, 643-648.

Depression is manifested by early
awakening insomnia, anorexia, crying,
poor concentration, impaired thinking
ability, and a host of complaints which
often mimic somatic illness. Development
of the antidepressant drugs such as
imipramine and chlordiazepoxide have
enabled psychiatrists to treat depression
in ambulatory patients. Elucidation is
offered on the hazards of suicide, prognosis,
diagnosis and treatment of depression per
se. A hypothetical case is presented to
illustrate current modes of therapeutic
management. Emphasis is placed on
patient awareness of possible drug-induced
side effects, with precise instructions on
what to do in the event of an emergency.
Thorough explanation should precede any
therapy with psychoactive drugs. (1 ref.)

[No address]

1748 Regan, Peter F. Psychoses: Manic-
depressive reactions. In: Conn, Howard
F. [Ed.] Current Therapy. Philadelphia:
W. B. Saunders, 1962. Pp. 546-551.

The treatment of the depressive phase of
manic-depressive psychosis includes
protection of the patient by initially
determining suicide potential, followed by
stabilization by means of regular office
therapy, home or hospital treatment,
development of an activity program
encompassing patient mobilization,
occupational therapy, expansion of the
scope of interests and increasing satisfaction
obtained from daily pursuits, in conjunction
with a program of psychotherapy. Depression responds to meprobamate, ECT and
the antidepressant drugs (imipramine,
iproniazid and nialamide). Manic
excitement responds to similar therapy,
with considerable emphasis on protecting

the patient from bodily harm. Activity,
psychotherapy, ECT and the phenothiazines
are all efficacious in ameliorating mania.
Chlorpromazine, promazine, and trifluoperazine are particularly useful as adjunctive
therapy, despite the fairly serious side
effects which may be manifested. (No refs.)

University of Florida
Gainesville, Fla.

1749 Naess, Knut. Medikamenter og
blod-dyskrasier. [Drugs and blood
dyscrasias.] Nordisk Medicin, 1962, 67,
58-60.

In a general discussion centering largely
on the work done by the Study Group on
Blood Dyscrasias of the AMA Council on
Drugs, chlorpromazine-induced and
imipramine-induced blood dyscrasias
(leukopenia) are noted. (No refs.)

Sturegatan 16
Stockholm, Sweden

1750 Journal of the American Medical
Association. Glue-sniffing. Journal of
the American Medical Association, 1962,
184, 123. [Editorial]

Plastic cements and airplane glue are
currently inhaled by teenagers to induce
euphoria and exhilaration. Habitual
inhalation may lead to intoxication,
disorientation and coma. Detrimental
effects on the senses derived from vapors
of glue, paint thinners, lacquers, enamels
and marking pencils are apparently due to
the organic solvents within these products.
Glue-sniffing may also produce various
deleterious effects on different organ
systems. Apparently, glue-sniffing is
highly correlated with delinquency, and
frequently is the precipitating factor which
brings delinquents before the juvenile court.
In Denver alone, arrests for glue-sniffing
increased from 30 to 134 in 1 year. Further
investigations are contemplated on the
physical, social and emotional implications
of noxious vapor inhalation. (1 ref.)

Journal of the American Medical Association
535 N. Dearborn Street
Chicago 10, Ill.

conditions. Among the psychotropic drugs listed which produce thrombocytopenia are: apronalide, aminopyrine, chlorpromazine, imipramine, hydantoins and antihistamines which produce agranulocytosis, and phenacetin which may produce hemolytic anemia. (9 refs.).

[No address]

1754 Serra, Carlo. The enzymic activation of the electroencephalogram. Acta Neurologica Scandinavica, 1962, $\underline{38}$, 64-65.

Modifications of EEG recordings resulting from altered enzymatic activity in glucose metabolism include the following: i. v. cocarboxylase induces decreased electrocortical activity which migrates from temporal to anterior cortical regions, ATP administered i. v. to normal subjects produces photic driving patterns in response to intermittent photic stimulation which resemble patterns elicited from neurotics and interference with cytochrome systems produces EEG patterns which vary according to basic physiological conditions (e. g., congenital heart disease). Preliminary observations with malononitrile have corroborated the influence of cyanide on brain cytochrome systems, and consistent EEG changes observed as photic driving patterns have confirmed the importance of lipoic acid in the oxidative decarboxylation of pyruvic acid. These substances condition the complex physicochemical changes which are responsible at the cellular level for inducing continuous variations in electrical potential. (13 refs.).

Neurophysiological Department
Centro Traumatalogico Ortopedico, Inail
Naples, Italy

1755 Glatt, M. M. The abuse of barbiturates in the United Kingdom. Bulletin on Narcotics, 1962, $\underline{14}$, 19-37.

The historical background of the use of hypnotics in the United Kingdom, dating from the introduction of chloral hydrate in 1869, is reviewed with emphasis on the controversial aspects of use and abuse. Data is presented on barbiturate consumption, acute barbiturate poisoning (suicides and accidental deaths, and attempted suicides), barbiturate habituation, addiction and chronic intoxication, and information on alcohol. The need for education, psychotherapy and the development of less toxic drugs is stressed. The new nonbarbiturate hypnotics, while fairly satisfactory and probably less toxic and less habit forming, are not free from dangers and also seem slightly less effective than the barbiturates. (16 refs.)

[No address]

1756 Arlen, Monroe S. Emergency assessment and management of the potential suicidal patient. Clinical Medicine, 1962, $\underline{69}$, 1101-1118.

A comprehensive treatise on depression includes various analytically oriented definitions and theories of etiology, characteristics of depression, the relationship between grief and depression, and basic diagnostic categories (reactive depression, psychotic depressions, mania and involutional psychotic reactions). Suicide risk may be assessed on the basis of the following criteria: depth of depression, severity of despair, communication of suicidal intent, loss of contact with reality, previous suicidal attempts, suicide notes, traumatic anniversary reactions and various other indications. Indications and contraindications for hospitalization are presented, along with the need for a positive approach and avoidance of emotional blackmail. The physician should offer some support in making difficult but essential decisions. Elderly patients must be made to feel wanted. Several common misconceptions regarding suicide are dispelled in question and answer form. Drugs are of little value if results are mandatory in less than 12 hours. Anxiety, tension, irritability and restlessness may be ameliorated by meprobamate or chlordiazepoxide. Amphetamines may be helpful, and new antidepressants such as MAO inhibitors and imipramine may be efficacious over a period of several weeks. Sedatives and phenothiazines should be avoided, as they tend to deepen depression. (3 refs.).

Lawton, Okla.

1757 Córdova Castro, Armando. Aspectos psiquiátricos del asma bronquial. [The psychiatric aspects of bronchial asthma.] Revista Cubana de Medicina, 1962, 1, 33-38.

In a discussion of the psychogenic factors involved in asthma, the utility of chlorpromazine in small doses, meprobamate, reserpine, imipramine and methylphenidate, as well as Gorbadei's (1960) novocaine therapy are elucidated. (15 refs.).

Psiquiatra del Hospital Cmte. M. Fajardo
Havana, Cuba

1758 Liberson, W. T. Electroencephalography. American Journal of Psychiatry. 1962, 119, 607-611.

New developments on the use of electroencephalography in studying sleep, mental activity, evoked potentials, rheoencephalography (recording of intracerebral impedance contributing to the study of vascular lesions) and psychopharmacology. Comparison of the effect of chlorpromazine, imipramine and placebo suggests that EEG frequency analysis provides quantification of neurophysiological changes with psychotropic drugs for psychiatric research. Extensive studies were also performed with chlordiazepoxide. Considerable work has been done on determining abnormal EEG's in mental patients, free of any history of organic or epileptic disorder. Schizophrenic patients with abnormal EEG records showed a higher sensitivity to treatment, both from the clinical and EEG point of view.

V.A. Hospital
Hines, Ill.

1759 Ayd, Frank J. The impact of psychopharmaceuticals on psychiatric units in general hospitals. American Journal of Public Health, 1962, 52, 13-15.

Since 1955, the Franklin Square Hospital in Baltimore, a general hospital with no psychiatric division, has admitted over 1,000 psychiatric patients with acute brain syndrome, alcoholism, psychoneurotic disorders, schizophrenic reactions, manic-depressive reactions, etc.) on the medical service and treated them with psychotherapy, drug therapy, sleep therapy, ECT and psychosurgery, for an average hospital stay of 14 days. The current demand for psychiatric treatment in general hospitals far exceeds the facilities offered by the slightly more than 20% of our general hospitals which now accept the emotionally and mentally ill. Such facilities should multiply rapidly in the next few years due to greater improvement in psychoactive drugs and increased psychiatric acumen in utilizing these drugs, as well as increased coverage for psychiatric illnesses by commercial health insurance programs such as Blue Cross. Psychoactive drugs have reduced the number of institutionalized mental patients by more than 23,000 since 1955. The advent of the psychopharmaceuticals has enabled numerous general practitioners to successfully treat psychiatrically ill patients.

Franklin Square Hospital
Baltimore, Md.

1760 Arnold, O. H., Hift, St., & Hoff, H. The role of psychotropic drugs in current psychiatric therapy. Comprehensive Psychiatry, 1962, 3, 330-342.

Five groups of psychotropic drugs are discussed, particularly with regard to clinical effects. The following properties of neuroleptics (reserpine, harmaline, benzoquinolizines, phenothiazines, etc.) are reviewed including neurophysiologic-anatomic aspects, therapeutic applications and side effects. Tranquilizers mentioned included carbamate, bicyclic compounds and benzodiazepine, while antidepressants included imipramine, chlor-imipramine and amitriptyline. Stimulants included weckamine, oxazine derivatives, methylphenidates and hydrazides. Mescaline, LSD, psilocybin and dimethyltryptamine are noted as typical psychotomimetics. (35 refs.)

Psychiatrisch-Neurologische Klinik
Universität Wien
Vienna, Austria

diplegia, fructose intolerance, idiopathic
hypoglycemia (leucine-induced), sucrosuria,
gargoylism, Gaucher's disease, etc. Understanding of the pathogenesis of mental retardation is contingent upon the acquisition
of greater knowledge of the enzyme systems
involved and their biogenetics. (114 refs.)

Department of Pediatrics
University of Colorado Medical Center
Denver 20, Colo.

1763 Way, E. Leong, & Adler, T. K. The
biological disposition of morphine and its
surrogates. Geneva: World Health Organization, 1962, 1-117.

This study on the biology of morphine was
originally published in 4 installments in
the Bulletin of the World Health Organization (1961-1962). The first 3 parts, which
deal successively with morphine, the partially synthetic derivatives of morphine and
the wholly synthetic substances with morphine like action, are presented in the form
of individual monographs. The morphine and
morphinemimetic compounds, by class, are:
naturally occurring opium alkaloids, partially synthetic derivatives of morphine,
synthetic compounds - morphinans, methi-
dones, phenilpiperidines and miscellaneous
(ethoheptazine and phenazocine). The 4th
part is devoted to general considerations on
this group of drugs as a whole. Absorption,
distribution, biotransformation (N-demethylation, O-demethylation, conjugation and
hydrolysis) and the excretion of each compound, as well as techniques of evaluation
are detailed. (272 refs.).

Department of Pharmacology
University of California Medical Center
San Francisco, Calif.

1764 Bundock, J.B. Canada's new controls
of the barbiturates and the amphetamines.
Medical Services Journal, Canada, 1962,
18, 464-465. [Editorial]

New Canadian legislation has made trafficking in narcotics or possession for the purpose of trafficking a special offence with
appropriate penalties, as well as providing
for more effective legal control over the

importation, manufacture and distribution of these drugs in order to limit their legal use to exclusively medical purposes. The new act is administered by the Narcotic Control Division of the Department of National Health and Welfare, whose staff has considerable experience in enforcing laws pertaining to narcotics. Physicians should always be cognizant of potential misuse and addiction when prescribing controlled drugs. Only limited quantities of such drugs should be prescribed at a given time. The new law also endeavors to establish better control over "goofballs" and pep pills" now in circulation. (No refs.).

[No address]

1765 WHO Technical Report Series (1962), No. 229. World Health Organization Expert Committee on Addiction-producing Drugs: Twelfth report. Bulletin on Narcotics, 1962, 14, 42-43.

Discussion of the following topics comprised the 12th session of the Expert Committee on Addiction-producing Drugs of WHO: use and abuse of khat in East Africa and Arabia with full elucidation of the chemical and pharmacological properties of khat's active principles; the present disconcerting increase in the illicit production and traffic in heroin; an increase in codeine consumption resulting in all probability from the introduction of new proprietary analgesic preparations; the need for new legislation dealing with rehabilitation which aims at reducing the possibility of relapse, which must of course be preceded by successful drug withdrawal, the establishment of treatment and rehabilitation facilities to promote rehabilitation and the development of tests employing the dog and rat to detect addiction-liability. Research is currently being designed to encompass the basic mechanisms and epidemiology of addiction. (5 refs.).

WHO
Geneva, Switzerland

1766 Mol, W. Softenon en peromelie. [Softenon and peromelia.] Geneeskundige Gids, 1962, 40, 219-222.

Following a brief description, with X-ray photographs, of a 2.5 month-old child with multiple congenital obvious deformities, whose mother took thalidomide (Softenon) in early pregnancy, the influence of such deformities in the Netherlands is discussed. Brief abstracts of 17 articles taken from the literature (mostly British) are also presented. (17 refs.).

Groningen, The Netherlands

1767 Offenkrantz, William. Depression and suicide in general medical practice. American Practitioner, 1962, 13, 427-430.

Depression is predicated upon guilt, grief or shame, and a combination of psychotherapy coupled with mood-elevating drugs may result in significant amelioration of depressive symptoms in the hands of a competent physician. The etiology of depression is based primarily on somatic, psychic or a combination of somatic and psychic factors. Biochemically, serotonin and levarterenol may play significant roles in the complex regulation of affective states. Physical symptoms of depression include fatigue, insomnia, impotence, anorexia, constipation and true hypochondriasis. The omnipresent danger of suicide must always be considered in dealing with depressed patients, and restorative psychotherapy should always explore the patient's current life situation and psychological equilibrium with an eye to eliminating any such disastrous desire. (15 refs.)

University of Chicago School of
Medicine
Chicago, Ill.

1768 British Medical Journal. Powerful analgesics. British Medical Journal, 1962, No. 5325, 241-242. [Editorial]

The principal powerful analgesics fall into 3 chemical families typified by morphine, methadone and pethidine, all of which are antagonized by nalorphine, an analgesic structurally related to morphine. All of these have fundamentally similar modes of action and are readily able to cause addiction. Some nonaddictive analgesic derivatives are available, but their efficacy is limited to relieving mild or moderate pain. Optimal effects are obtained most readily by s.c. administration of morphine and its analogues. All of these analgesics depress respiration, but a combination of pethidine and levallorphan produces maximal analgesia with minimal respiratory depression. Several morphinelike drugs have become established antitussive agents. Decreased drowsiness may be obtained with levorphanol, methadone or pethidine rather than morphine. When analgesic efficacy is paramount, however, morphine is invariably the drug of choice. Chemistry, dosage, and other relevant information on various morphine analogues is presented in tabular form. (18 refs.)

British Medical Association
Tavistock Square
London W.C. 1, Great Britain

1769 Refshauge, W.D. Phenmetrazine and trifluoperazine. Medical Journal of Australia, 1962, No. 2, 58. [Letter]

Trifluoperazine, a pharmaceutical benefit, and phenmetrazine are contraindicated during pregnancy due to possible incipient teratogenicity. Trifluoperazine is not likely to be utilized by pregnant women to any extent, so it will not be removed from the list of drug benefits. Information which has been circulated to doctors in Canada by the Department of National Health and Welfare corroborates the extensive deleterious effects which may accrue from administration of trifluoperazine and phenmetrazine to pregnant women. Phenmetrazine produced extensive fetal diaphragmatic hernias, while trifluoperazine resulted in quadrilateral phocomelia and various other congenital deformities. (No refs.)

[No address]

1770 Winick, Charles. Maturing out of narcotic addiction. Bulletin on Narcotics, 1962, 14, 1-7.

Data for this study consists of the age and length of addiction of addicts in the files of the Federal Bureau of Narcotics who were originally reported during 1955 but not reported again by the end of 1960. There were 5,553 men and 1,681 women in this sample. Although the age range was from 18 to 76 years, a substantial concentration of addicts became inactive in their thirties. Various causes of drug discontinuance were speculated upon, e.g., whether the process is one of maturing out, as a reflection of the addict's life cycle, or as a reflection of the number of years that the addiction process per se continues. Further study of drug discontinuance should yield valuable information for the treatment and control of addiction. (12 refs.)

New York City Council
Narcotics Addiction Research Project
New York, N.Y.

1771 Endicott, Noble A. The problem of controls in the evaluation of psychotherapy. Comprehensive Psychiatry, 1962, 3, 37-46.

In evaluation of psychotherapy the problem of controls is one of the most troublesome. Several studies which demonstrate the necessity of including controls are reviewed as well as the methodologic difficulties which complicate the utilization of controls in psychotherapy outcome studies. Evaluation tests listed include: Thematic Apperception, Bell Adjustment Inventory, the Rorschach and Kent-Rosanoff Free Association. Psychotherapy given with and without a placebo has also been successfully used for assessment of results. Finally, a general discussion of probable solutions to the problem is presented. (42 refs.)

Albert Einstein College of Medicine
Jacobi Hospital
New York, N.Y.

1772 Barbeau, André. Etudes récentes sur les catécholamines. [Recent studies on catecholamines.] Union Médicale du Canada, 1962, 92, 42-51.

After reviewing various adrenal dysfunctions and catecholamine metabolism, the role of catecholamines in extrapyramidal disorders and mental conditions was elucidated. The advent of LSD, the mechanism of o-methylation, factors relating to epinephrine, adrenochrome, adrenolutin, taraxein, serotonin and ceruloplasmin, as well as the clinical use of phenothiazines, reserpine and antidepressants are noted. (119 refs.)

Section of Neurologie
Université de Montréal
Montréal, Quebec
Canada

1773 Taussig, Helen B. Thalidomide — a lesson in remote effects of drugs. American Journal of Diseases of Children, 1962, 104, 111-113. [Editorial]

Thalidomide ingested by 50 pregnant women between the 30th and 60th day after the last menstrual period invariably produced phocomelia in the infant. Accurate records from Lenz's study provide documentary proof that even a single dose of thalidomide can produce phocomelia. By August 1962, 3,500 thalidomide damaged infants will have been born in Germany and several hundred will also have been born in Great Britain. Definitive teratogenicity must be corroborated by extensive animal experimentation with thalidomide, but the welter of circumstantial evidence is damning. (No refs.)

Department of Pediatrics
Johns Hopkins Hospital
Baltimore, Md.

1774 Doshay, Lewis J., & Boshes, Louis D. Recent advances in the management of Parkinson patients. Current Medical Digest, 1962, 23, 53-62.

The aims of the National Parkinson Foundation and the Parkinson's Disease Foundation, in relation to the increasing incidence of Parkinson's disease are reviewed. Physical therapy, neurosurgery, etc. are detailed. The drugs of current utility are: trihexyphenidyl, cycrimine, procyclidine, benzatropine, orphenadrine, chlorphenoxamine, ethopropazine, diphenhydramine, scopolamine and dexamphetamine. (16 refs.)

935 Park Avenue
New York, N.Y.

1775 Kurland, Albert A. The clinical application of psychotherapeutic drugs. Bulletin of the School of Medicine of the University of Maryland, 1962, 47, 45-52.

Psychoactive drugs serve 4 major purposes in clinical psychiatry: therapeutic elimination or modification of psychopathological symptoms, transference of latent drug-induced mental phenomena into manifest phenomena by means of narcodiagnostic techniques, inducing psychotic states for experimental psychopathology and determining drug impact on the normal subject in order to interpret therapeutic effects. One clinical psychologist administered chlorpromazine, meprobamate, reserpine, iproniazid, phenobarbital, dexamphetamine and placebos to himself to determine his subjective interpretation of the resultant effects. Responses varied, even with repetition of the same drug. The major tranquilizers which produce antidelusional and antihallucinatory effects plus sedation include the phenothiazines (chlorpromazine, promazine, trifluoperazine and perphenazine) and the rauwolfia alkaloids (reserpine, rescinnamine, and deserpidine) Certain target symptoms are ameliorated by these drugs, but the underlying psychopathology remains unaltered. Treatment of minor emotional disorders accompanied by anxiety or apprehensive coloration entails use of the minor tranquilizers, such as meprobamate and chlordiazepoxide. Nonbarbiturate sedatives and hypnotics include glutethimide, ethchlorvynol and chlorpromazine. The antidepressant drugs are indicated whenever suicide is not immediately imminent, and drugs like imipramine, isocarboxazid and nialamide appear efficacious antidepres-

on chlordiazepoxide, prochlorperazine
and benactyzine have also been conspicuously
lacking in adequate controls. Depression
responds well to trifluoperazine. (10 refs.)

[No address]

1777 Ginsburg, Marshall. The treatment
of the problem drinker in an overseas
theatre by the general medical officer.
Military Medicine, 1962, 127, 416-422.

Alcoholism has always constituted a serious
problem for the military services, particularly in an overseas theatre with attendant
stressful conditions. The U.S. Armed
Forces have generally consigned treatment
of the problem drinker to the psychiatrist
and other specialized personnel. A
medical regimen is far more efficacious,
however, and is predicated upon treatment
of coexisting physical disorders frequently
associated with chronic alcoholism, as
well as vitamins, dietary regulation and
tranquilizers like chlordiazepoxide or
chlorpromazine. Disulfiram maintenance
therapy represents one of the most
significant advances in the medical treatment of the problem drinker, but should
only be utilized by a physician who is
thoroughly familiar with its indications and
contraindications. With respect to the
therapeutic aspects of the doctor-patient
relationship, the physician's acceptance of
the patient as a man with a problem
deserving medical attention, in place of
the moral condemnation he has come to
expect, greatly enhances the patient's
self esteem. Psychiatric consultations
should be obtained wherever possible.
Proper management of follow-up studies
are essential. The physician must respect
the patient's sensitive and exaggerated
pride, permitting him to use whatever
devices he requires to continue seeking
treatment, while simultaneously expecting
the patient to assume a considerable
degree of personal responsibility for his
participation in the treatment program with
absolute abstinence as his goal. (34 refs.)

Department of Psychiatry
Cincinnati General Hospital
Cincinnati 29, Ohio

1778 LaVerne, Albert A. [Editor]
Compendium of neuropsychopharmacology.
Psychotomimetic drugs. Journal of
Neuropsychiatry, 1962, 4, 63-67.

Perusal of numerous current references
has yielded considerable information
about psychotomimetic drugs like LSD,
mescaline, piperidyl benzilate and phencyclidine. These compounds have been
fully elucidated in chart form, offering
generic and trade-names, type and action,
indications for use, therapeutic rating,
side effects, contraindications and cautions,
recommended dosage and references under
the auspices of the compendium of neuropsychopharmacology. The format of the
compendium is also outlined. (22 refs.)

[No address]

1779 LaVerne, Albert A. [Editor]
Compendium of neuropsychopharmacology.
Preparations used in convulsive and other
biological therapies. Journal of Neuropsychiatry, 1962, 3, 399-409.

As a portion of the compendium of neuropsychopharmacology, the following
information is presented in tabular form
concerning psychopharmacological preparations utilized in convulsive and other biological
therapies: generic or trade name, type and
action, indications for use, therapeutic
rating (effectiveness and toxicity), side
effects, contraindications and cautions,
recommended dosage and references.
Compounds so elucidated include insulin,
glucagon, pentamethylentetrazol, succinylcholine, hexafluorodiethyl ether, tetramethyl-
succinimide and CO_2. Explanations for all
charts are provided. (49 refs.)

[No address]

1780 Evans, Wayne O. The synergism of
autonomic drugs on opiate or opiate-induced
analgesia: a discussion of its potential
utility. Military Medicine, 1962, 127,
1000-1003.

The autonomically active agents which
potentiate the analgetic activity of opiates
include parasympathomimetic agents

694

Department of Economic and Social Affairs
Division of Narcotic Drugs
United Nations
New York, N.Y.

1783 Shideman, Frederick E. The
pharmacology of hypnotics and sedatives.
I. South Dakota Journal of Medicine
and Pharmacy, 1962, 15, 438-441, & 445.

In general, serious CNS depression
results from administration of large doses
of barbiturates, but depressant effects
range from minimal sedation to anesthesia
and coma, depending upon the dosage level.
Sedative doses of these compounds are
capable of impairing the functional
capacity of the CNS. In hypnotic doses,
barbiturates depress respiration only
slightly, but more profound respiratory
impairment occurs with increased dosages,
due primarily to direct action on the
medullary respiratory center. The
barbiturates exert differential effects on
various autonomic functions, including
modification of the peripheral cardiac
action of the vagus. Different barbiturates
are bound in varying degrees to plasma
albumin and other cellular proteins;
pentobarbital and secobarbital are bound
to the greatest extent, phenobarbital to
a lesser degree and barbital the least.
Acute and chronic intoxication with
barbiturates has been widely recognized.
Chronic intoxication mimics the signs and
symptoms of chronic alcoholism, replete
with grand mal seizures and psychotic
behavior. (No refs.)

Department of Pharmacology and
      Toxicology
University of Wisconsin
Madison, Wisc.

1784 Hoch, Erna M. Psychotropic drugs
in the hands of the general practitioner.
Antiseptic, 1962, 59, 113-119.

There are 3 major types of psychotropic
drugs: tranquilizers (chlorpromazine),
ataractics and thymoleptics, all of which
are of value to general practitioners in
India in treating patients with psychotic,
neurotic or psychosomatic disorders.

Indications and contraindications for various drugs are briefly explained. (No refs.)

Nur-Manzil Psychiatric Centre
Lucknow, India

1785 Pagani, F. Allucinogeni e tranquillizzanti. [Hallucinogens and tranquilizers.] Gazzetta Medica Italiana, 1962, 121, 121-124.

The chemical structures and pharmacological details were given for some tranquilizers and psychotomimetics: lysergide, mescaline, the chlorpromazine group, the reserpine group, amphetamines, benactyzine, etc. The role of various amines, particularly 5HT, in mental processes is also noted. (8 refs.)

Istituto di Chimica Farmaceutica e
    Tossicologia
Università di Genova
Genoa, Italy

1786 Presse Médicale. Thalidomide et malformations congénitales. [Thalidomide and congenital malformations.] Presse Médicale, 1962, 70, 1241. [Editorial]

The worldwide spread of thalidomide syndrome is discussed with emphasis on the European situation. The laboratories which prepared thalidomide were among the 1st to suspect the possible role of thalidomide and they recalled it from the market in December, 1961. The necessity

Lancet, 1962, No. 7232, 725-726.

Parotid salivary cholinesterase was
measured in 29 psychiatric patients
(acute or affective schizophrenics) and 49
normal controls all with a median age of
24 years to detect diminutions in enzyme
concentration in psychopathological states.
In accordance with a modification of Ravin's
method, 8-10 ml of parotid saliva was
assayed in duplicate for titres of choline-
terase. Mean salivary cholinesterase in
the patient group was 58% of that in the
normal group, and salivary flow rate was
lower and less variable. Patients exhibited
either no measurable enzymic activity or
values approximating those of controls. No
enzyme was detectable in 7 patients. No
correlations were found among the cholin-
esterase-like substance, flow-rate,
Funkenstein test measures, physical
characteristics, or diagnostic category
for the entire group of patients. Enzyme
concentration increased in 9 patients
after i. m. injection of 10 mg methocholine.
The relation of the parotid enzyme to stress
was studied in a group of normal subjects
twice weekly for 3 months who were then
exposed to a variety of stressful experiences.
No subject showed a correlation between
enzyme concentration and parotid salivary
flow rate. Apparently, both enzyme concentration and flow rate were controlled
by the autonomic nervous system. Work
by other investigators was also cited.

Harvard School of Dental Medicine
Boston, Mass.

1790 Schlosberg, Arié. Treatment of
facial and head pain associated with
depression. Lancet, No. 7237, 1962,
1027. [Letter]

A 50-year-old-woman presenting with depression and excruciating residual facial
pain from trigeminal neuralgia unresponsive
to retro-gasserian neurotomy received
chlorpromazine (200 mg), methyl
phenidate (10 mg/day for 10 days) and
imipramine (200 mg/day for 10 days).
At discharge, her depression was alleviated,
she was more active, her weakness disappeared and her facial pain was no longer
intolerable. A maintenance dose of

imipramine (75 mg) for 6 months has almost completely obliterated the pain.

Shalvata Psychiatric Hospital
Magdiel, Israel

1791 Gahagan, L. H. , Intravenous atropine premedication before electroconvulsion therapy. Lancet, 1962, No. 7242, 1305.

A mixture of atropine (1,2 mg) and thiopental [dosage unspecified] is administered i. v. before ECT to prevent the undesirable cholinergic effects which are otherwise induced by ECT. Atropine premedication prevents cardiac arrhythmias of vagal origin and lessens internal secretion. Earlier experimental studies involved administration of double the above dosage, but the present amount suffices admirably. This premedication technique is a modification of the method of Hargreaves.

[No address]

1792 Beal, R. W. , & Blackburn, C. R. B. The effect of nialamide on endogenously elevated blood ammonia levels in patients with liver disease. Australasian Annals of Medicine, 1962, 11, 19-23.

Twelve studies were carried out on 9 patients with elevated blood ammonia levels due to liver disease (8 cases) or uremia (1). As well a second group of 8 patients, all with chronic liver disease, was treated. In the 1st group, venous blood ammonia levels were determined before and 60-120 minutes after i. v. nialamide (100 mg) and in each study blood ammonia levels were significantly reduced, the reduction ranging from 18-75%. For the 2nd group, 1 to 1 1/2 hours after a standard meal containing about 30 g protein, an i. v. infusion of ammonium chloride was begun after the resting blood ammonia level was determined. When a significant elevation of arterial blood ammonia concentration was obtained, 100 mg nialamide was administered i. v. Arterial blood ammonia levels in this group were also significantly lowered. With the exception of 2 patients, the clinical effects of nialamide did not correlate with the great improvement in circulating ammonia levels.

Thus further study is in progress to determine the manner in which nialamide lowers both endogenously and exogenously elevated blood ammonia levels.

Clinical Research Unit
Royal Prince Alfred Hospital
Sydney, Australia

1793 Evans, Raymond D. The successful management of a case of neonatal tetanus using paraldehyde and promazine hydrochloride (Sparine) for sedation. Archives of Pediatrics, 1962, 79, 299-301.

Paraldehyde (1 ml i. m. every 4 hours) and promazine (5-12.5 mg i. m.) administered to a 2 or 3 week old female with neonatal tetanus produced complete relaxation and cessation of tonic spasms within 30 minutes. Maintenance therapy was continued for 14 days. Penicillin and tetanus antitoxin were also administered to preclude spastic activity and intercurrent infection. Mortality rates in neonatal tetanus are still universally alarmingly high. Other investigators have curtailed spasms with barbiturates, phenothiazine derviatives, chlorpromazine and thiopentone.

Fairbanks Medical & Surgical Clinic
Box 1330
Fairbanks, Alaska

1794 Alcock, N. S. Clinical evaluation of 1-methyl-5, 5-phenylethyl-hydantoin in the treatment of epilepsy. Developmental Medicine & Child Neurology, 1962, 4, 465-466.

1-Methyl-5, 5-phenyl-ethyl-hydantoin (100 mg/day increased weekly by 50 mg increments to obtain control) was administered to 89 epileptics aged 2 to greater than 14 years for 6 or more months in an effort to control seizure activity. Seizures were completely controlled in 43 of the patients, 75% reduction in seizures occurred in 16, 50% reduction in 15, and no response in 15. Improvement was shown by 51 out of 59 with grand-mal seizures and 5 out of 10 with petit-mal seizures. Skin rashes developed in 4 patients 10 to 14 days after

was used in 82 neurosurgical operations
(excluding intracranial operations with
spontaneous respiration), and 33 angio-
grams and pneumoencephalograms. This
combination proved highly successful, the
patient being unconscious and areflexic
during surgery, but returning to normal
consciousness and reactivity levels within 2-5 minutes after discontinuation of
nitrous oxide administration. As a result,
the neurological course of the patient can
be followed with the assurance that postoperative changes in responsiveness are
due solely to changes in his neurological
condition, and not to any depression
caused by the anesthetic.

Department of Surgical Neurology
Western General Hospital
Edinburgh, Scotland
Great Britain

1797 De Castro, J., & Mundeleer, P.
Die Neuroleptanalgesie. (Auswahl der
Präparate, Bedeutung der Analgesie und
der Neurolepsie). [Neuroleptanalgesia.
(Drug selection, significance of analgesia
and neurolepsy.)]. Anaesthesist, 1962,
11, 10-17.

The authors tested 12 different analgetic
or neuroleptic drugs, employing 10 different treatment schemes, on about 8000
patients. The most effective combination
was found to be a balanced method employing haloperidol and phenoperidin in dosage
ranges of 2.2 - 5 mg and 2-15 mg, respectively, for adults. Succinylcholine (50 mg
i.v.) may be added when required for
muscle relaxation. Possible side effects
include bronchial spasm, bradycardia,
hypertension, tachycardia, etc. Reasons
for these side effects and their prophylaxis
and treatment are discussed. Nitrous oxide
and oxygen can be used for maintaining
anesthesia. Thiamine (0.5 - 1.0 g) has a
favorable effect on respiration. Neurolept-
analgesia is less dangerous and less toxic
than conventional general anesthesia.

Louis Caty Clinic
Baudour, Belgium

1798 Kapferer, J. M. Prinzipielle und
praktische Überlegungen zur "Neuroleptanalgesie". [Theoretical and practical
considerations concerning neuroleptanalge-
sia.] Anaesthesist, 1962, 11, 25-28.

The theoretical principle underlying neuro-
leptanalgesia is separation of the different
components, such as sleep, analgesia,
muscle relaxation, and inhibition of reflexes.
About 3100 patients were subjected to
neuroleptanalgesiá, using 50-300 mg thiopental for narcosis, which was maintained
with N_2O (50-80%). Analgesia was provided by dextromoramide (2900 cases) or
phenoperidine (200 cases), in doses of 1-1.5
mg/10 kg body weight. Muscle relaxation
was obtained with small doses of succinylcholine or curare. An antiemetic effect
was obtained with haloperidol (over 2900
cases) or methylperidol (over 200 cases)
in doses of 0.5-5.0 mg i.v. at the start of
narcosis. Side effects noted included dyspnea to apnea, which could be treated with
N-allylnormorphine. Bronchial spasms
can occur when phenoperidin is administered
too rapidly, and can be counteracted by
artificial respiration. Extrapyramidal
disturbances can occur at too high (over 5
mg) doses of haloperidol or methylperidol,
and can be controlled with barbiturates and
promethazine. Dextromoramide can lead
to addiction. The technique of neurolept-
analgesia is an improvement over older
methods and not expensive.

No. 6 Sennstrasse
Innsbruck, Austria

1799 Junkenitz, Karl Walter. Insidon in
der Allgemeinpraxis. [Insidon in general
practice.] Deutsches Medizinisches Journal,
1962, 13, 358-359.

The piperazinoiminostilbene derivative
iminostibene (Insidon) was tested in 153
patients over a 6-month period at a usual
dosage of 150-200 mg/day. Particularly
good results were obtained in anxiety or
insomnia due to emotional lability and lack
of self confidence (67 cases), essential (not
renal) hypertension (38 cases), climacteric
and post-climacteric syndromes (26 cases),
and migraine headache (22 cases). One
example of each group is reported in detail.

1801 Lindner, Wilhelm,& Spiegelberg, Hedwig. Klinische Erfahrungen mit Triflupromazin. [Clinical experiences with triflupromazine.] Medizinische Welt, 1962, No. 10, 546-549.

Triflupromazine (initially 40 mg i. m. 3-5 times a day, then 200-400 mg/day p. o. and finally 75-200 mg/day p. o.) was tried in 79 female hospitalized patients, including 63 manic-depressives (11 manic), 7 schizophrenics, 2 with CBS, 2 with exogenous psychoses and 5 neurotics, over a period of 7 months. Most of the patients also received glutethimide, and treatment was continued for an average of 2-4 months. Good to excellent results were obtained within 5-10 days in 49 cases, and 21 more responded after more prolonged treatment; these were mostly severe involutional psychoses characterized by paranoia and hallucinations; 8 patients failed to respond at all. Side effects were fairly common, including infiltrations at the site of injection, extrapyramidal reactions and convulsive symptoms, but were readily controlled with glutethimide. The drug thus has a definite tranquilizing effect, producing normalization of mood and initiative at doses considerably lower than those for chlorpromazine. Its action resembles that of chlorpromazine without all of the side effects.

Psychiatrische Abteilung
Allgemeines Krankenhaus Ochsenzoll
Hamburg-Langenhorn, Germany

1802 Stelzer, H. Erfahrungen mit Sedapon in Geburtshilfe und Gynäkologie. [Experiences with Sedapon in obstetrics and gynecology.] Medizinische Welt, 1962, No. 6, 321-322.

Sedapon, a psychoautonomic regulator containing 150 mg meprobamate, 2 mg yohimbine and 0.13 mg Belladonna alkaloids per tablet, was used in more than 400 obstetric and gynecologic patients over a period of 15 months. Among 54 patients suffering from nervous or autonomic complaints during pregnancy, 50 responded well to an initial dosage of 3-4 tablets/day, reduced 50% after 1-2 weeks and discontinued after 3-4 weeks. Hyperemesis gravidarum was controlled successfully in 24 of 32 patients

by 2-4 tablets/day and 6 more responded after addition of vitamins. Sedapon was also used before and during labor in 355 cases, with good effects on anxiety and agitation. The drug also shortened the first stage of dilatation, and had no effect on the fetus. Sedapon is also indicated in spastic or inflammatory pelvic disease, chronic constipation, menopausal syndromes (when hormones are contraindicated) and the premenstrual syndrome (good response in 24 of 29 patients at 3-4 tablets/day).

Frauenklinik Düsseldorf
Düsseldorf, Germany

1803 Roth, G. Elektrencephalographische Beobachtungen bei Anwendung von Thalidomid. [Electroencephalographic observations using thalidomide.] Nervenarzt, 1962, 33, 130-133.

Thalidomide (200 mg p. o. or rectally in adults, half that in children) was used for diagnostic purposes to provoke disturbances in the EEG in 60 patients with epilepsy (13 cases), cerebrovascular disease (14 cases), postencephalitic syndromes (4 cases), posttraumatic syndromes (6 cases), autonomic disturbances (9 cases), psychoses and neuroses (11 cases), Little's disease, multiple sclerosis and drug intoxication (1 case each). The 24 patients showing convulsive symptoms are tabulated in detail. Thalidomide had a marked activating effect in 6 of these 24, a moderate effect in 5, little or no effect in 12, and a normalizing effect on 1 case of paroxysmal dysrhythmia; the greatest effect was obtained on essentially normal EEG's. Several examples are given. The use of thalidomide is superior to other methods in that there is no β-activation and no clinical excitation.

II. Neurologische Abteilung
Nervenheilanstalt Wien-Rosenhügel
Vienna, Austria

1804 Anton, Alfred. Ergebnisse einer klinischen Prüfung des Neuroleptikums Ciatyl. [Results of a clinical trial of the neuroleptic drug Ciatyl.] Medizinische Welt, 1962, No. 12, 665-669.

Ciatyl, a chlorperphenthixene closely related to perphenazine, was tested in 115
hospitalized psychiatric patients suffering
from a variety of acute and chronic psychoses. Initial dosage was usually 150
mg/day i.m. (occasionally first 25 mg i.v.),
gradually reduced to 50 mg/day p.o. Four
illustrative cases are reported in detail.
The results indicate that Ciatyl is a highly
effective neuroleptic with a true antipsychotic action which far exceeds the sedative
effect of bromine and barbiturates. It is
particularly indicated in acute psychotic
agitation, anxiety and psychomotor excitation. The drug is less effective in defective
psychoses with loss of contact and initiative,
but even here it facilitates hospital care, and
can advantageously be combined with thymoleptics in cases of severe edogenous depression. Ciatyl is well tolerated, and the
occasional extrapyramidal reactions,
muscular dystonia and hypotension can
readily be controlled. Marked drowsiness
is common at the beginning of treatment.

Westfälisches Landeskrankenhaus
Münster, Germany

1805 Gómez-Reino y Filgueira, J., &
Fernández Vicente, L. Nuestras experi-
encias con el "Melleril" en la mania endo-
gena y en las esquizofrenias paranoides
cronicas. [Our experience with Melleril
in endogenous mania and in chronic schizophrenic paranoia.] Actas Luso-Españolas
de Neurologia y Psiquiatría, 1962, 21, 159-
164.

Thioridazine (Melleril), 200-400 mg/day,
was used in the treatment of 7 cases of
endogenous mania. Excellent results were
obtained in 5 cases and good results in 2.
Twenty-one schizophrenics were treated
for 2-6 months with 400-600 mg thioridazine
daily. Excellent improvement (remissions)
occurred in 15.7% of 19 paranoid schizophrenics, good results were obtained in 21%
and mediocre results in 5.2%; 1 case of
hebephrenic schizophrenia and another of
simple schizophrenia showed only mediocre
improvement. Target symptoms particularly susceptible to chemotherapy were
hyperexcitability, hallucinations, ideas of
reference (prejudicial, autoaccusatory, etc.),
anxiety and depression. Improvement for

all cases reported was 36.7%. No side
effects except slight drowsiness were
observed in any patients.

Sanatorio Psiquiátrico de Toen (P.A.N.A.
Orense, Spain

1806 Vintimilla Albornoz, Jaime. La
amitriptilina en el tratamiento de las
depresiones endogenas. [Amitriptyline
in the treatment of endogenous depressions
Antioquia Medica, 1962, 12, 494-501.

Fifty cases of endogenous depression, 30
hospitalized and 20 ambulatory, were
given amitriptyline, either 25 mg tablets
orally or 10 mg parenteral injections.
Usual dosage was 25 mg t.i.d., raised
to as much as 150 mg per day when
necessary. The treatment period ran
from 1-5 months. Thirteen cases had
concomitant ECT, 8 cases chlorpromazine
and 4 patients required psychotherapy.
The only side effect was 1 case of nausea.
In 14% the results were excellent, in 30%
good, in 30% fair, in 12% poor and in 14%
uncertain.

Hospital Mental de la Beneficencia de
Antioguia
Medellín, Colombia

1807 Merlis, Sidney, Turner, William J.,
& Halpern, Seymour. Chlordiazepoxide as
adjunctive therapy in convulsive disorders.
American Journal of Psychiatry, 1962,
119, 575-576.

Chlordiazepoxide (10-60 mg/day p.o.)
was administered to 86 epileptics aged 5-
66 years alone or in combination with
standard anticonvulsants for periods of up
to 16 months. Evaluation included serial
EEG's (in 30 patients) and clinical observation. Side-effects ensued in 43 cases:
17 evinced somnolence, 7 ataxia, 5 vertigo,
5 irritability, 2 restlessness, 2 fatigue
and 1 each headache, leucopenia, insomnia,
facial flushing and jaundice. Before treatment, 89% had fair or poor control of
seizures, whereas only 66% had fair or
poor seizure control after the introduction
of chlordiazepoxide. Chlordiazepoxide is
apparently efficacious as an adjunctive

fluphenazine for 2 months. Most manifested
psychosomatically influenced digestive or
cardiocirculatory disorders. Five patients
received 2 mg/day p. o. for the 1st month
and 1 mg/day for the following month. All
the rest received 1 mg/day, and 2 patients
received medication for 45 days. Improvement in 80% of the cases was considered
excellent. No toxicity was evidenced; this
was true even in a patient with auricular
fibrillation who was 84 years of age.
However, 1 patient showed drowsiness with
nausea and another drowsiness with depression during treatment for 45 days.

IPASE
Pôrto Alegre, Rio Grande do Sul
Brazil

1810 Mans, J.-P., & Cornil, J. Résultats
d'une année d'expérimentation d'un nouveau
neuroleptique, le chlorhydrate de prothipendyl, en psychiatrie. [The results of a year's
psychiatric experimentation with a new
neuroleptic: prothipendyl chlorhydrate.]
Annales Médico-Psychologiques, 1962, 1,
120, 637-638. [Abstract]

In the treatment of 39 cases, prothipendyl
[dosage unspecified] appeared to have good
sedative and neuroleptic action without the
production of side effects. Used initially in
agitated states the drug is not as potent as
chlorpromazine, but still useful. (No refs.)

[No address]

1811 Misrahi, R., Joubert, P., & Bernard-
Bouissières. Utilisation du niamide dans le
traitement des troubles digestifs psychoso-
matiques et plus particulièrement: la rec-
tocolite hémorragique. [The use of Niamide
in the treatment of psychosomatic digestive
disturbance, particularly, hemorrhagic
rectocolitis.] Annales Médico-Psychologiques,
1962, 1, 120, 630. [Abstract]

Three cases of hemorrhagic rectocolitis
improved in 3 months of treatment with
nialamide (Niamide) [dosage unspecified].

[No address]

1812 Fouks, L., Laine, Périvier,
Boucher, Mathis, Ferrant, & Riou.
Rapport sur l'essai clinique du S. 186
(Hexa-cyclonate de sodium). [Report on
a clinical trial of S. 186 (sodium hexa-
cyclonate).] Annales Médico-Psychologiques,
1962, 1, 120, 636. [Abstract]

Hexacyclonate, 25-150 mg/day, improved
the general and cardiovascular tone, as
well as alertness and mental efficiency of
patients. The drug is recommended for
use in arteriopathic senile states and
also in childhood oligophrenia, particularly
in cases of apathy. It is contraindicated
in the presence of convulsive tendencies.

[No address]

1813 Reichle, Claus W., Smith, Gene M.,
Gravenstein, Joachim S., Macris, Spyros
G., & Beecher, Henry K. Comparative
analgesic potency of heroin and morphine
in postoperative patients. Journal of
Pharmacology and Experimental Therapeutics,
1962, 136, 43-46.

The subjective reports of 522 patients with
steady incisional pain due to surgery were
used to compare the analgesic power of
heroin and morphine (double-blind basis).
Morphine, 10 mg/70 kg, was used as a
standard in an evaluation of pain relief
produced by 4 different dosages of heroin:
6, 4, 2, and 1 mg/70 kg. Heroin was
approximately 2-4 times as potent as
morphine in pain relief during the 1st
150 minutes after injection. At 45 minutes
equianalgesic doses of heroin, compared
to morphine, for moderate, severe and
very severe pain, were 3.2, 2.3 and 3.9 mg,
respectively. The corresponding values
90 minutes after medication were 4.0,
4.3 and 4.4 mg and those at 150 minutes
3.7, 5.2 and 4.8 mg.

Anesthesia Laboratory
Harvard Medical School
Massachusetts General Hospital
Boston, Mass.

1814 Walsh, P.J.F. Compulsive shouting
and Gilles de la Tourette's disease.
British Journal of Clinical Practice, 1962,

(Catran) in schizophrenia.] Nordisk
Medicin, 1962, <u>68</u>, 1165-1167.

One-hundred-and-ninety-five patients,
diagnosed as schizophrenic, were treated
with pheniprazine (β-phenylisopropyl-
hydrazine; 6-15 mg/day for 7 months).
After 2 weeks dosages were reduced to a
daily maximum of 12 mg. Phenothiazine
derivatives were administered concomitantly.
Fifty-eight percent of the cases improved.
The drug was especially effective against
depressive characteristics and secondary
hallucinations. In 6 cases treatment was
interrupted because of side effects:
jaundice in 1 and considerably increased
transaminase values in 5 cases.

Birgittas sjukhus
Vadstena, Sweden

1819 Kaartinen, Matti. Kliniska erfarenheter
av klorprothixen. [Clinical experiences
with chlorprothixene.] Nordisk Medicin,
1962, <u>68</u>, 1161-1164.

Two-hundred-and-eighty-two patients
(schizophrenia, mania, depression,
involutional psychosis, senile psychosis,
neurotic reactions, alcoholism, aggressive
oligophrenia and epilepsy) were treated;
172 with chlorprothixene only (15-600 mg
p.o. usually t.i.d.). The 110 other
patients received chlorprothixene and
insulin coma, ECT, reserpine and/or
imipramine. Overall results were
satisfactory; about 85% could be sent home
or were obviously improved. Psychomotor
agitation, restlessness, insomnia, anxiety,
apathy, withdrawal and hallucinations
showed the best improvement. The effect
on delusions, neurotic depressions and cases
of senile confusion was not as good. No
effect was observed in endogenous depression.
Side effects were: orthostatic vertigo and
collapse, tachycardia and allergic dermatosis.
Treatment had to be interrupted in 10 cases.
Also, an unsuccessful suicide attempt is
described where 2000 mg of chlorprothixene
was ingested.

Distriktssjukhuset
Halikko, Finland

1 820   Lapinsohn, L.I.   Anabolic steroids
in the treatment of psychiatric states.
(Effect of oxymetholone).   Diseases of
the Nervous System, 1962, 23, 226-230.

Following a detailed presentation of the
underlying concepts in the design of the
study and a review of the general indications
and contraindications for oxymetholone,
the results of a study of the adjuvant use
of this compound in 3 groups of psychiatric
patients are briefly reported.   The drug
was administered at a dosage of 2.5 mg
t.i.d., p.o. in 3 courses of 3 weeks each,
with 1-week intervals, in combination with
other types of treatment, to a total of
52 patients evaluated by 3 different
investigators.   Excellent results were
obtained in 10 of the 43 schizophrenics
and 1 case of posttraumatic encephalopathy.
Good results were obtained in 21 schizophrenics, 2 involutional psychoses, 1
phobic reaction and 1 postpartum psychosis.
Fair results were obtained in 11 other
schizophrenics, while 4 anxiety states and
1 schizophrenic showed no change.   Oxymetholone thus has considerable value as
an adjuvant in the treatment of certain
psychiatric conditions.

Psychiatry and Neurology Service
VA Hospital
Coral Gables, Fla.

1 821 Müllender, H.   Atarax in der
Geburtshilfe.   [Atarax in obstetrics.]
Praxis, 1962, 51, 475-476.

Hydroxyzine (Atarax; 100 mg i.m. at the
beginning of dilatation, repeated in 30
minutes) was tested in a double-blind study
on 90 parturient women, including 43
primiparas and 47 multiparas.   Hydroxyzine
produced good effects in 21 and moderate
effects in 19 out of 46 patients, and reduced
the consumption of pethidine 30%, while the
placebo produced good effects in 12 and
moderate effects in 7 out of 44 patients.
There were 4 surgical deliveries in each
group and no apparent effects on the fetus.

Frauenklinik des Kantonsspitals
St. Gallen, Switzerland

Schizophrenia is only slightly improved.

Heil- und Pflegeanstalt "Am Steinhof"
Vienna, Austria

1825 Flegel, Horst. Psyquil im Psychiatrischen Krankenhaus. [Psyquil in the
psychiatric hospital.] Medizinische
Welt, 1962, No. 2, 99-102.

A total of 70 female patients was treated
with triflupromazine (Psyquil) over a
1-year period at an oral dosage of 30-75 mg
per day initially, increasing to 150 mg/day,
if no improvement was evinced at the lower
doses. Of the 60 schizoform patients, 24
were discharged, but 6 of these relapsed
after 1-5 months. In addition, 7 others
improved sufficiently to be kept in open
wards, while 19 more, although restricted
to locked wards, could be assigned to
work therapy. Side effects, noted in 14
patients, consisted of stupor, pallor,
weakness, excessive perspiration, tachycardia, and a tendency to collapse.
Parkinsonian symptoms were displayed
by 29 patients. Triflupromazine is effective
in the treatment of schizophrenia of long
duration, and the side effects can be readily
controlled.

Rheinisches Landeskrankenhaus
Düsseldorf, Germany

1826 Flegel, Horst. Zur Dokumentation
und Auswertung psychiatrisch-klinischer
Verlaufsgegebenheiten für die Erprobung
von Psychopharmaka anlässlich Thioridazin-
medikation. [Documentation and evaluation
of data from the psychiatric clinic in the
testing of psychotropic drugs, with
particular reference to thioridazine.]
Nervenarzt, 1962, 33, 112-116.

A group of 80 women, including 55 schizophrenics and 12 depressives, was treated
with thioridazine over a 2-year period with
dosages of 75 mg and more per day. There
was no clear relationship between dosage
and percent discharged. Chronic schizophrenic patients could not be discharged
after treatment with the drug, but the
treatment proved effective in 10 out of 20
cyclic schizophrenics with a history of

previous acute attacks. Also, 4 depressives could be discharged. Relapses occurred in 2 cases. Of the remaining cases, 19 improved to the point where they could be assigned to work therapy. Side effects included lassitude, dizziness, tachycardia, gastric discomfort. One case of jaundice, in a patient previously treated with another phenothiazine derivative, was cured after withdrawal of the drug. Other symptoms were edema (in an edema-prone patient) and acne. Most symptoms disappeared after a 2-month period. Thioridazine is indicated for the treatment of more or less chronic psychoses. Severe agitation and acute psychotic syndromes require more powerful drugs. Psychopathic excitability is also controllable with thioridazine.

Rheinisches Landeskrankenhaus
Düsseldorf, Germany

1 827 Barron, David W. , & Dundee, John W. Clinical studies of induction agents. I: A comparison of the incidence of induction complications with nine barbiturates in electroconvulsive therapy. British Journal of Anaesthesiology, 1962, 34, 90-94.

Nine barbiturates: thialbarbital, thiamylal, Inactin, buthalital, methitural, hexobarbital, methohexital and B. 137 were administered to 1 0 1 0 patients (average age 39-45 years) as anesthesia for ECT 1 hour after atropine (0. 65-1. 3 mg) premedication and 1 minute before administration of suxamethonium. Resultant complications included excitatory phenomena (muscle tremor, twitchings and other involuntary muscle movement) and respiratory upset (coughing, hiccoughing and laryngospasm). Administration of anesthesia was assessed and graded according to the scheme designed by Dundee (1961). Hexobarbital, methohexital and B. 137 caused a significantly higher incidence of excitatory phenomena than thiopental. Although the incidence with Inactin was greater than that for thiopental at a 2% significance level, it was not different from that associated with thialbarbital, thiamylal, buthalital or methitural (p > 0. 05). Administration of buthalital and methitural was associated with a much higher incidence of respiratory upset than that which appeared with any of the other drugs. Seven of the above drugs were administered to 22 patients, and no respiratory aberrations were manifested, although hexobarbital and methohexital once again evinced excessive excitatory phenomena. An identical dose of thiopental and thiamylal was administered to 26 patients, and no complications ensued from either drug. Inactin (average dose 4. 07 mg/kg) and B. 137 (average dose 3. 71 mg/kg) were administered to 44 patients. Excitatory phenomena occurred in 6 patients with Inactin and in 13 with B. 137, but the difference between dosages failed to reach accepted levels of significance. Hexobarbital (average dose 4. 93 mg/kg) and thialbarbital (5. 79 mg/kg) were given to 32 patients. Excitatory symptoms occurred in 14 receiving hexobarbital and 1 given thialbarbital, with a highly significant difference (p < 0. 01). The thiobarbiturates produced a low incidence of side effects and a high incidence of respiratory upset, while the methylated barbiturates produced a high incidence of excitatory phenomena.

Department of Anaesthetics
The Queen's University of Belfast
Great Britain

1 828 Svendsen, B. Borup, Faurvye, A. , & Kristjansen, P. Sammenligning af thioridazin og klorpromazin over for kroniske skizofrene psykoser under anvendelse af placeboteknik. [Comparison of thioridazine and chlorpromazine in chronic schizophrenia using a placebo technique.] Nordisk Medicin, 1962, 67, 390.

In a double-blind crossover study 61 chronic schizophrenics received thioridazine or chlorpromazine for 12 weeks followed by 16 weeks of therapy with the alternate preparation. There were 9 dropouts. Thioridazine was similar in effectiveness to chlorpromazine. In cases where chlorpromazine produces extrapyramidal symptoms and/or a rash, then thioridazine is indicated. Some patients improved optimally on one drug, some on the other.

[No address]

agents, it produced a higher proportion of disturbed and turbulent children post-operatively than all other drug combinations except pentobarbital and atropine. Approximately 25% of the phencyclidine-treated patients observed preoperatively exhibited signs of emotional upset ranging from nausea and dizziness to agitation, extreme restlessness and delirium. About 50% of the children who appeared calm seemed completely detached and were quite phlegmatic about accepting an inhalational induction. Such serious side effects necessitated abandonment of phencyclidine as a premedicant.

The Royal Infirmary
Aberdeen
Great Britain

1832 Camilleri, Joe G. The use of phencyclidine (LI-395) in obstetric procedures. Anaesthesia, 1962, 17, 422-426.

Pethilorfan or pethilorfan combined with promethazine [dosage unspecified] was administered to 15 pregnant women within 4 hours before delivery, after which atropine (0.6 mg) and phencyclidine (10-15 mg) were given i.v. as premedication. Complete analgesia supervened within 3-6 minutes of injection, and lasted 30-45 minutes during which various obstetric procedures were performed without any discomfort to the patient. During the period of analgesia, the patient remained in a catatonic trance, staring fixedly into space. During obstetric procedures, the respiratory rate, pulse and blood pressure all rose slightly. No vomiting occurred before or after the procedure, and uterine contractions proceeded normally. Cyclopropane was used supplementally in 2 cases which required more extensive surgical procedures. No deleterious effects were observed in the babies thus delivered. Phencyclidine is highly recommended for use in obstetrics.

The Central Middlesex and Willesden
    General Hospitals
Middlesex
Great Britain

1 833 Joseph, Samuel R. Combined anti-depressant tranquilizer therapy in somatic and psychosomatic illnesses. Arizona Medicine, 1962, 19, 239-241.

Sixty-two ambulatory patients, aged 22-81 years, suffering from both anxiety and depressive symptoms were treated with a combination of trifluoperazine and tranylcy-promine for 3 months to 1 year. The usual dosage was 1-2 mg trifluoperazine b. i. d. and 10 mg tranylcypromine b. i. d. In 15 patients, the symptoms were associated with organic disease including arthritis, asthma, etc. Response was rated as excellent in 27%, good in 39%, fair in 13% and poor in 21%. No serious toxicity was encountered. Side effects in 19 included insomnia, dry mouth and drowsiness, which disappeared upon dosage reduction or cessation of the combination therapy. Distress was relieved in patients suffering from organic disease; all were better able to relate and gain insight.

2021 North Central Avenue
Phoenix, Ariz.

1 834 Kristensen, Keety Kjaerbye. Libriumbehandling af angstneuroser. [Librium therapy in neurotic anxiety reactions.] Nordisk Medicin, 1962, 67, 392-393.

Twenty-five patients, average age 37 years, were given 30-80 mg chlordiazepoxide daily (occasionally up to 150 mg/day), dosage was progressively increased to about 200 mg/day. One patient was cured spontaneously, 3 showed decided improvement, 12 some improvement, 7 remained unchanged, 1 worsened and 1 committed suicide. No toxicity was observed. Drowsiness was seen in about half the case load, disappearing on reduced dosage. One patient had fainting spells, 1 erythema and 3 euphoria. Chlordiazepoxide may be expected to compete with mepro-bamate in ameliorating mild neuroses.

[No address]

1 835 Kammerer, Th., Singer, L., Geissmann, P., & Wetta, J. -M. Utilisation d'un nouveau neuroleptique: la tétrabénazine Résultata cliniques, biologiques et électro-encéphalographiques. [The use of a new neuroleptic: tetrabenazine. Clinical, biological and electroencephalographic results.] Annales Médico-Psychologiques, 1962, 1, 120, 106- 115

Seventeen paranoid schizophrenics, (8 suffering delirium and 4 with chronic hallucinatory psychosis), aged 20-60 years, were treated for 3-7 weeks with tetrabenazine (average daily oral dose 90-135 mg). The doses were progressively augmented and usually given t. i. d. Tetra-benazine had a marked clinical action against hallucinations; in acute psychoses it had an immediate activity against anxiety, confusion and panic states in patients; in chronic psychoses delirium was diminished and patients adjusted better to reality. Encephalographically, disturbances were noted which contra-indicated the drug in cases of epilepsy or in subjects with a tendency towards epilepsy. Tolerance to tetrabenazine was highly variable and side effects notable, i. e., typical extrapyramidal syndrome. Untoward effects included moderate hypo-tension, dry mouth (in almost all patients), drooling, anorexia, constipation, daytime somnambulence (especially in the 1st week of treatment), fine tremor and agitation. Some of these effects were partially controlled by barbiturate administration.

[No address]

1 836 Mathisen, H. Storm. Hypertensjons-behandling med monoaminooxydase-hemmer og decarboxylasehemmer. [The treatment of hypertension with MAO and decarboxylase inhibitors.] Nordisk Medicine, 1962, 67, 459.

Thirty-seven hypertensive patients were treated with serine-N²-isopropylhydrazine (RO4 1038) and 10 with the decarboxylase inhibitor α-methyl-dopa. Also placebo effect was assayed as a control for the latter drug. α-Methyl-dopa was used for some days (0.5-2 g/day) without effect followed by RO4 1038 (usual dosage 15-20 mg/day). Both preparations lowered blood pressure (especially in the

free. Subsequently, 30 dysmenorrheic
patients of various ages have obtained either
ss, total or partial relief with administration of
chlordiazepoxide.

[No address]

1839 Lai, G., & de Penrot, E. Le Librium
dans le traitement du delirium tremens.
[Librium in the treatment of delirium
tremens.] Praxis, 1962, 9, 236-238.

Twenty-seven alcoholics suffering from
delirium tremens were treated with
chlordiazepoxide (Librium) and supportive
therapy. The dosage used was 100 mg,
repeated 3 times in the 1st 3 hours with a
maximal daily dose of 600 mg. The
preferred route of administration in severe
cases was i.v. and i.m. Injection was used
where agitation was somewhat attenuated.
This therapy usually lasted 4-5 days,
whereupon drug dosage was reduced
(75-150 mg/day) and maintained for 10-15
days. Agitation is quickly suppressed,
but therapy must be continued. No contraindications appeared. Excellent results
were obtained but true evaluation was
difficult because of lack of control in
relation to spontaneous cures.

Clinique Psychiatrique Universitaire
    de Lausanne
Lausanne, Switzerland

1840 Mall, G., Junnemann, H. J., Kruger,
H. J., & Schwartz, H. Contribution à la
thérapeutique clinique au moyen du librium.
[Contribution to clinical therapy, using
Librium.] Annales Médico-Psychologiques,
1962, 1, 120, 971.

Four-hundred-and-ten hospitalized psychiatric patients suffering from depression and/
or anxiety were given chlordiazepoxide (Librium); 30-70 mg at the beginning, reaching
up to 300 mg/day. Twenty percent of cases
showed improvement by the end of 10 days.
The least favorable effects, partially satisfactory, were obtained with other states of
depression (nonspecific, neurotic, obsessional and compulsive, depression accompanied by organic afflictions or senile
arteriosclerosis). In 55 cases, chlordiaze-

poxide was used in combination with
phenothiazine derivatives and in 23 cases
MAO inhibitors without untoward effects.

Clinique Neuro-psychiatrique de Landeck
Landeck, Austria

1 841 Grimaldi, Richard D. Propiomazine,
an adjuvant for obstetric analgesia. Anesthesia and Analgesia, 1962, 41, 487-496.

Propiomazine (15 mg i.m. to 249 patients
and 30 mg i.m. to 253) was administered
to 502 Negro and Puerto Rican women in
labor, in addition to meperidine (50 mg i.
m.) and scopolamine (0.04 mg i.m.). The
initial dose was repeated at 3-4 hour intervals depending upon patient response. Pain
relief was evaluated by the attending physician, and blood pressure, pulse, contractions, dilatation, descent and fetal heart
rate were charted before and after drug administration. Unless more frequent observations were necessitated, hourly recordings were obtained. Satisfactory analgesia was obtained by 80% on the lower
dosage schedule and 87% who received the
higher dosage. In general, those who received 30 mg propiomazine were quieter
and more cooperative. Among this group,
however, 1 case of coma occurred as did 1
case of hypotensive crisis. Results indicate that the lower dosage of propiomazine
should be administered to all initially and
dosage should be increased only on the
basis of individual requirements. From
this study, no conclusion could be drawn
as to whether propiomazine in combination with meperidine is less hazardous
than meperidine alone. A controlled
double-blind evaluation of meperidine
in combination with propiomazine, meperidine alone and morphine alone will be
undertaken.

Department of Obstetrics and Gynecology
New York Medical College
Metropolitan Medical Center
New York, N. Y.

1 842 Kammerer, Th., Geissmann, P.,
Wartel, R., & Lévy. Etude clinique,
biologique et électroencéphalographique
de l'action du KT 5 (Keithon) dans
certains syndromes psychiatriques.
[Clinical, biological and electroencephalographic study of the action of KT 5 (Keithon)
in some psychiatric syndromes.] Annales
Médico-Psychologiques, 1962, 1, 120, 119-130.

Thirty patients (8 psychotic, 7 psychoneurotic, 10 depressive neurosis with
asthenia and 5 behavioral disorder) were
treated with progressively increasing
doses of phenoethamine (KT 5; 50 up to
300 mg t.i.d.). Four out of 8 psychotics,
5 out of 7 psychoneurotics, 6 out of 10
cases of depression and 4 out of 5 cases
of behavioral disorder improved. Side
effects were highly variable. Drowsiness
and fine tremor (10-12 CPS) were
prominent. Extrapyramidal reactions
appeared during the 1st days of treatment
when encountered. EEG's taken on 21
patients showed some slowing in alpha
wave frequency with the appearance of
slow beta and delta waves. Phenoxethamine
is considered useful for its anxiolytic
properties.

[No address]

1 843 Pignataro, Frank P. Experience with
chemotherapy in refractory psychiatric
disorders. American Journal of Psychiatry,
1962, 119, 577-579.

Diazepam (10 mg b.i.d. or t.i.d. initially,
then 5-10 mg/day for maintenance) was
administered to 67 patients (16 schizophrenics, 9 with various psychoses and 42
psychoneurotics) with refractory illnesses
for 11 months, 14 of whom received isocarboxazid (5-10 mg/day) concomitantly to
combat severe depression. Laboratory
tests were performed on 32 patients. A
good to excellent response was obtained in
70% of all patients, 48% of psychotics and
83% of psychoneurotics, with extensive
amelioration of symptoms. Combination
therapy relieved all 14 depressed patients,
achieving good to excellent results in 12.
Good to excellent results were obtained in
7 out of 13 depressed patients treated only
with diazepam. Laboratory results were
well within normal limits. Side effects,
although infrequent, included drowsiness,

used as a further criterion in evaluation.
The 4 categories associated with tension-
anxiety which had the most patients were
422 dermatologic, 383 anxiety-tension and
neurosis, 198 cardiovascular and 124
menopausal. Seventy-nine percent of
patients experienced good to excellent
relief. Side effects in 6% were minimal
in all cases. Mild drowsiness occurred
in 55, dizziness in 17, fatigue in 11, and
gastrointestinal upset.

[No address]

1846 Wentzler, J. Donald. Triflupromazine
(Vesprin) as an adjunct to block anesthesia.
Contributory effects of single low-dosage
injections. Anesthesia and Analgesia, 1962,
41, 301-306.

Triflupromazine (Vesprin, 3-4 mg i.v.) was
administered to 84 patients, aged 19-70 /.
years, as an adjunct to block anesthesia
during 87 surgical and diagnostic procedures.
Premedication initiated 2 hours before surgery included: Morphine 1/6 grain, pentobarbital 1 1/2 to 2 grains, and scopolamine
1/150 grain. In 80% of the patients triflupromazine enhanced sedation and obviated
further narcotization or supplemental use
of general anesthesia. Sedation level was
excellent during 7 procedures, good during
64 and fair during 7. Degree of sedation
was poor in 9 operations. Patients were
readily placated with triflupromazine and
were more inclined to accept the block procedures. There were fewer complaints of
pain and awareness of the operative procedure. No untoward reactions of any consequence were encountered. One patient
had a fall in blood pressure of 20 mm of
mercury but no active intervention was
necessary and a normal level was reestablished. Thanks to the potent antiemetic
properties of triflupromazine, there were
no emetic reactions. Triflupromazine is
useful as a surgical premedicant in combination with traditional barbiturate-narcotic
preanesthetic agents since it greatly enhances sedation.

[No address]

1847 Sherline, D. M., & Roddick J. W. Jr.
A comparison of two narcotics, numporphan
and emerol, in obstetrics, by double-blind
technique. Quarterly Bulletin of Northwestern University Medical School, 1962,
36, 54-56.

In a double-blind study, 62 pregnant women
in labor received numorphan (0.75 mg
i. m.) and 62 received meperidine (100 mg
i. m.) in conjunction with scopolamine or
atropine (0.4 mg) to ascertain efficacy of
obstetrical analgesia. Patients were evaluated subjectively for relief of pain, and
infants were evaluated on 5 parameters of
the Apgar Rating. Results of maternal
analgesia indicated that 72% of the numorphan treated patients and 67% of the meperidine group experienced satisfactory analgesia. Decrease in fear and apprehension
without depression was difficult to assess,
but no patient was unduly depressed. No
significant statistical differences were observed for maternal analgesia ratings or
infant Apgar Ratings. No correlation was
observed between lower Apgar Ratings and
the time from medication to delivery with
either of the drugs used.

Department of Obstetrics and Gynecology
Northwestern University Medical School
Evanston, Ill.

1848 Hackstein, F.G. Die Behandlung
der enechetischen Wesensänderung mit
Chlorphenazine. [The treatment of
epileptic personality changes with chlorphenazine.] Medicina Experimentalis, 1962,
6, 265-273.

Fourteen patients with severe epileptic
character disturbances were treated with
chlorphenazine (8 mg b. i. d.). Nine showed
clear improvement in social behavior.
Symptoms such as irritability, self asser-
tiveness, awkwardness, etc. were favorably
affected, however neither the character disorder per se or individual symptoms peculiar to each case were remedied.
Rorschach and Behn-Rorschach tests were
used in evaluation.

Rheinisches Landeskrankenhaus Suchteln
Krefeld, Germany

1849 Baron, Seymour H., & Fishe,
Seymour. Use of psychotropic drug pre-
scriptions in a prepaid group practice plan.
Public Health Relations, 1962, 77, 871-881.

In 132 working days, nonpsychiatric physicians in the Group Health Association (GHA)
of Washington, D. C., wrote 1,072 prescriptions for psychotropic drugs, of which
3/4 were for psycholeptics and 1/4 was for
psychoanaleptic agents (antidepressants).
Tranquilizers accounted for 3% of all the
prescriptions written and filled at the GHA
pharmacy during the study period. Far
more psychotropic drugs, particularly the
amphetamines, were prescribed for females
than for males. Psychotropic agents were
prescribed infrequently for patients under
19 or over 70 years of age. Meprobamate
ranked 1st in the 40-69 age group, but
dropped in rank in the 40 and under category.
Psychotropic agents were frequently prescribed for the treatment of nonpsychologi-
cal symptoms. Median drug dosages appeared comparable to those prescribed else-
where by other nonpsychiatric physicians.
Commonly prescribed psycholeptics included
meprobamate, promethazine, prochlorperazine, reserpine and rescinnamine, etc.,
while psychoanaleptics included the amphetamines, methylphenidate and iproniazid.

Psychopharmacology Service Center
NIMH
Bethesda, Md.

1850 Lamphier, Timothy A. Evaluation of
chlormezanone as a clinical and postoperative
central relaxant and tranquilizer. Clinical
Medicine, 1962, 69, 109-111.

Eighty-three ambulatory patients, aged
13-72 years, with diversified musculoskeletal complaints received chlormezanone
(100-200 mg/day t. i. d. or q. i. d.). Response to therapy was excellent in 66%,
good in 20%, fair in 10% and poor in 4%.
Side effects occurred in 11 cases, consisting
of dizziness, nausea, weakness, rash and
flushing, all of which were alleviated by a
reduction in drug dosage. Therapy was
discontinued in only 1 patient due to
side effects. Chlormezanone safely and
effectively ameliorated a variety of
musculoskeletal conditions.

[No address]

1851 Beley, A., Girard, L., Leroy, C., &
Pinel, J.P. L'étude de l'action du N-benzyl-
beta-chloropropionamide dans les troubles
caractériels de l'enfant. [The study of N-
benzyl-β-chloropropionamide action in
behavioral disorders of children.] Annales
Médico-Psychologiques, 1962, 1, 120, 975.

Beclamide [dosage unspecified] was administered to children with behavioral problems.
On the whole the agent was efficacious in
controlling impulsiveness and instability
in nonepileptic subjects who had slightly
slow, dysrhythmic EEG's. Its best action
was related to the improvement of predominantly neurological instability. Clinical
improvement paralleled EEG improvement,
i.e., diminution of slow dysrhythmia

[No address]

1852 Mandell, Arnold J., Markham,
Charles H., Tallman, Frank F., &
Mandell, Mary P. Motivation and ability
to move. American Journal of Psychiatry,
1962, 119, 544-549; discussion, 549.

In a double-blind study the relationship
between akinetic and rigid neurological
features of Parkinson's disease, and mood
state was examined. Imipramine or placebo was administered to 42 patients with
Parkinson's disease. For the first week
100 mg/day was administered, followed by
150 mg in the second week and 200-250 mg
for the third week. They were given the
MMPI, Leary Interpersonal check list for
psychological evaluation, a physical therapy check list of 106 items (self-care, etc.)
and neurological examinations, as well as
psychiatric examinations for the assessment
of subjective mood. These patients appeared
more depressed than normal, and a relationship exists between the amount of apparent
subjective depression and the patient's ability to function neurologically. Tremor
tended to be characteristic of the least
debilitated patients, while akinesia and
rigidity were linked to the most depressed,
least mobile, poorly functioning group.
The latter group was most aided by imipramine; here 8 out of 9 patients showed

the highest degree of improvement. While
placebo effects paralleled that of the drug
generally, imipramine proved superior to
placebo, especially in relation to the suppression of neurological symptoms. In
the discussion L. B. Kalinowsky commented
favorably on the value of antidepressants in
atypical depression concerning the removal
of depression with concomitant improvement
in neurological function.

[No address]

1853 Ollendorff, R.H.V. A trial of
thioridazine (Melleril) in the maintenance
of chronic schizophrenics. British Journal
of Clinical Practice, 1962, 16, 183-186.

Thioridazine, 150 mg t.i.d., was administered to 49 chronic schizophrenics, most
in partial remission, as maintenance therapy.
They had been treated for the past year
with high dosage chlorpromazine. There
were 17 female and 32 male patients. Before thioridazine was substituted females
were generally maintained on a triad of
medicines - 100-200 mg chlorpromazine,
5-15 mg trifluoperazine and 50-100 mg
orphenadrine, all t.i.d. Two-and-one-half
to 3 months treatment was considered optimal. For evaluation, Baker and Thorpe's
interview method for deteriorated schizophrenics was employed. Marked improvement was observed in 2 patients, no change
in 16 and degrees of deterioration in 31.
Thioridazine was found less potent than the
original medications but its use is advocated, where possible, because of its lesser
side effects. Thioridazine should be tried
in chronic, catatonic and hebephrenic cases
with periodic remissions, particularly where
tension is marked.

St. Augustine's Hospital
Chartham Downs
Canterbury, Kent
Great Britain

1854 Brown, R. W. Barr, Hamilton-Hislop,
H. G., & Pritchard, J. G. A comparative
clinical trial in the elderly of Distaval.
British Journal of Clinical Practice, 1962,
16, 643-648.

Thalidomide (Distaval; 100 mg), glutethi-mide (Doriden; 500 mg) and Welldorm (chloral hydrate and phenazone; 1300 mg) were administered to 74 elderly patients, most 70-89 years of age, in order to determine which drug is the most useful in the management of insomnia. Observations were made on 36 nights; each drug administration was varied by means of a Latin square design in order to insure that all possible sequences were used. All drugs produced good sleep on most nights: 84.7% for thalidomide, 83.8% for Welldorm and 76.4% for glutethimide. No toxic or cumulative effects were noted, except that the incident of occasional hangover was greater for glutethimide.

Geriatric Unit
Queen's Hospital
Croydon, Surrey
Great Britain

1855 Gutiérrez Agramonte, E. El tratamiento preventivo de las depressiones con el Tofranil. [Preventive treatment of depression with Tofranil.] Revista Cubana de Medicina, 1962, 1, 110-112.

Eighteen depressed patients were given maintenance doses of 25-100 mg imipramine (Tofranil). Another group of 13 received 50-200 mg/day imipramine. Thirteen of the patients received 200-400 mg/day chlorpromazine concomitantly. The group receiving the higher dosage of imipramine were successfully maintained. This was also true for the 14 patients who received chlorpromazine-imipramine. The combined treatment is favored.

Psiquiatra Servicio
Hospital de Dementes
Havana, Cuba

1856 Gutiérrez Agramonte, Edmundo. Evolución histórica del tratamiento de la psicosis maniaco depresiva. [The historical development of treatment of manic depressive psychosis.] Revista Cubana de Medicina, 1962, 1, 78-84.

In a historical exposition of therapy for manic depression, the complementary roles of psychotherapy and chemotherapy are detailed. The high-dosage i.m. use of phenothiazine derivatives and/or ECT, as well as MAO inhibitors is advocated. Emphasis is placed on the value of imipramine. One-hundred-and-fifty depressed patients were treated with imipramine i.m. [dosage unspecified] or given 200 mg oral doses. In endogenous depression 68% recovered and in delusional melancholia 59%. Four additional cases of depression were completely cured.

Hospital Nacional de Dementes
Havana, Cuba

1857 Nussbaum, Harvey E. A new psychotherapeutic-anticholinergic combination for gastrointestinal disorders. American Journal of Gastroenterology, 1962, 38, 575-582.

Chlordiazepoxide combined with clidinium bromide (Librax) was studied for 12 months with 97 patients having symptoms referable to the gastrointestinal tract, and in whom anxiety was more or less prominent. Fifty were diagnosed as having gastrointestinal neurosis without evidence of organic disease, while the rest had somatic disorders, e.g., 8 with active duodenal ulcers. Several dosages were tried and the optimal dosage was concluded to be 1 capsule (5 mg chlordiazepoxide and 2.5 mg clidinium bromide) t.i.d. Other medications were also given, such as insulin in diabetic cases. In gastrointestinal neurosis improvement was marked in 30, moderate in 15, minimal in 3 and unchanged in 2; for the total caseload of 97 improvements were ibid., 56, 29, 5 and 7. For the target symptom anxiety present in all the patients, results were, ibid., 56, 29, 5, and 7. Nine patients complained of 1 or more side effects. These consisted of drowsiness in 3, dry mouth 7, forgetfulness 1, blurred vision 1, and hoarseness 1. Drowsiness in the 3 patients was sufficiently severe to necessitate discontinuation of the drug. Of 3 patients receiving placebo and active drug alternately

double-blind, improvement occurred
 the drug and symptoms returned
lacebo.

address]

See also 1726, 1728, 1752, 1759, 1948

1858 Schlake, Friedrich. Über den blutdrucksenkenden Effekt moderner Psychopharmaka und seine therapeutische Beeinflussbarkeit durch das Kreislaufmittel Novadral. [The hypotensive effect of modern psychotropic drugs and its management by means of the analeptic drug Novadral.] Münchener Medizinische Wochenschrift, 1962, 104, 555-557.

Studies of the blood pressure in 67 psychiatric patients under treatment with psychotropic drugs (phenothiazines and MAO inhibitors, not further specified) showed hypotensive effects in 36 cases, particularly in those with initial hypotension or given higher doses of the drugs. This side effect was successfully controlled by administration of m-hydroxyphenylethanolamine (Novadral) in doses varying from 15-40 drops t. i. d. p.o. with oral psychotropic drugs to 1 ampule b. i. d.–t. i. d. parenterally with parenteral psychotropic drugs or high oral doses. Two case reports are included, 1 of which showed that control of the hypotension may be accompanied by improvement in mood.

Nervenklinik Morija
Anstalt Bethel bei Bielefeld
Bielefeld, Germany

1859 Lenz, W., & Knapp, K. Thalidomide Embryopathy. Archives of Environmental Health, 1962, 5, 100-105.

One-hundred-and-twenty-nine reports of abnormal infants were collected in Hamburg and environs. In 90 cases there was convincing evidence of thalidomide intake in early pregnancy. An additional 203 cases were reported to the authors by letters from West Germany and abroad; parents or doctors usually wrote because the mothers had taken thalidomide. Types of malformations are discussed in an attempt to determine the critical period for embryopathy. Thalidomide intake between the 27th and 30th day after conception will affect the arms, and later intake damages the legs and to a lesser degree the arms.

Universitäts-Kinderklinik und Poliklinik
Martinistrasse 52,
Universitäts-Krankenhaus Eppendorf
Hamburg 20, Germany

1860 Grimlund, K. Fenacetinmissbruk i en svensk industri. [Phenacetin abuse in Swedish industry.] Nordisk Medicin, 1962, 67, 756.

One Swedish city, unspecified, had an incidence of phenacetin abuse 5-10 times higher than any other Swedish industrial town. Out of 200 phenacetin abusers, 34% had kidney damage while 700 nonusers showed an incidence of kidney damage of 2.5%. The number of deaths due to renal insufficiency has also shown a marked increase in the last 3 decades. Phenacetin had been ingested with the hope of increasing work capacity and not of suppressing pain.

[No address]

1861 Ringertz, N. Patologisk-anatomisk fynd i njurarna vid fenacetinmissbruk. [Pathological findings in the kidney in phenacetin abuse.] Nordisk Medicin, 1962, 67, 755.

At autopsy, a constant finding was chronic interstitial inflammation with atrophy of the kidney in persons habituated to phenacetin. Necrosis of the papillae without signs of myelitis is a common finding.

[No address]

1862 Ruikka, Ilmari, & Sourander, Leif B. Fenacetinmissbruk och njurfunktion i ett geriatriskt material. [Phenacetin abuse and kidney function in geriatrics.] Nordisk Medicin, 1962, 67, 756.

Two-hundred patients over 60 years of age (average age 75) had kidney dysfunction and pyelonephritis due to phenacetin abuse. Daily abuse was common and frequently of long standing. Pyelonephritis was more common in phenacetin users than in other patients. No significant differences could be found from normal in the plasma creatinine, the phenol red test and hemoglobin.

[No address]

and psychotherapy is detailed. She took
50 25/mg tablets of imipramine in a suicide attempt. She became confused,
drowsy and anxious. Intense headache,
nausea, loss of equilibrium, a tachycardia
of 97, mydriasis, lack of visual accommodation with visual blurring and diplopia,
dry mouth and skin, etc. were evident.
Treatment consisted of gastric lavage
with an aqueous suspension of charcoal
and then hypertonic magnesium sulfate was
administered every 6 hours. Additionally
6-methyl prednisolone was administered
every 12 hours. The patient recovered
uneventfully.

Hospital Psiquiátrico Provincial de Oviedo
Oviedo, Spain

1866 Hopkins, Paul, & Robertson, Duncan.
The effect of "Ancolan" and other drugs in
early pregnancy. Medical Journal of
Australia, 1962, No. 9, 329-330. [Letter]

Meclozine (Ancolan) and Ancoloxin (meclozine and pyridoxine) were administered
to 200 pregnant women prior to the 16th
week of pregnancy. Of the 200, 125 received meclozine and 75 received Ancoloxin; 187 had normal children, 8 babies were
stillborn and 5 evinced various fetal anomalies. The incidence of anomalies was
approximately normal, and, no correlation
could be detected with respect to the nature
of the defects. Apparently, meclozine and
Ancoloxin may be safely administered to
women during pregnancy.

Brisbane and Gordon Street
Mackay, Queensland
Australia

1867 Woodyatt, P. B. Thalidomide.
Lancet, 1962, No. 7232, 750. [Letter]

A 68-year-old-woman with an extensive
X-ray resistant mixed mesodermal
endometrioma received thalidomide (400
mg t. i. d.) for 8 days to investigate
potential anticarcinogenic drug effects.
The patient remained rather sleepy, and
the tumor apparently underwent a slight
increase in size. Therapy was maintained
for another week. Further trials to determine the cytotoxicity of thalidomide in

malignant disease are contemplated.

Hammersmith Hospital
London, W. 12, Great Britain

1868 Wigglesworth, Robert. Thalidomide-damaged infants. Lancet, 1962, No. 7251, 349. [Letter]

A 5 1/2-year-old girl afflicted with quadrilateral micromelia was readily accepted by her parents and family once the initial shock of her disability had been dissipated. Regular limb-fittings facilitated the development of grasping and walking skills at periods which were optimal psychologically. The child evidenced remarkable prowess in adjusting to and utilizing her prosthetic devices. Medical and financial support coupled with parental encouragement were important factors in contributing to this child's wellbeing and societal acceptance, including attendance in regular public schools rather than a school for the physically handicapped. Obviously, the initial step in dealing with thalidomide-damaged children who manifest similar disabilities involves the development of an understanding and cooperative parental attitude.

Kettering, Northamptonshire
Great Britain

1869 Taylor, S. W. Thalidomide in pregnancy. New Zealand Medical Journal, 1962, 61, 423.

A male child with typical congenital malformations was born to a woman who had ingested thalidomide, 100 mg/day, from the 4th to the 8th week of pregnancy. A direct correlation apparently exists between administration of thalidomide during gestation and resultant congenital anomalies.

[No address]

1870 Teitelbaum, I. Electrocardiographic changes associated with phenothiazine. Lancet, 1962, No. 7272, 115. [Letter]

In approximately 30% of the patients who had undergone [unspecified] phenothiazine therapy for varying periods of time, characteristic ECG changes were observed, including low voltage in the standard leads with widening QRS complexes and a flat or isoelectric T wave, especially in the AVL lead and an inverted T in the right precordial lead. Cessation of treatment resulted in restoration of normal ECG tracings. No underlying organic aberration could be detected.

Malben Hospital
Shaar-Menasch, Israel

1871 Wright, O. L. Thalidomide. New Zealand Medical Journal, 1962, 61, 56.

On the basis of reports from 2 overseas sources which associate thalidomide ingestion during early pregnancy with fetal defects, the Distillers Company Biochemicals Limited, has seen fit to withdraw all products containing thalidomide from the market pending further investigation.

[No address]

1872 Melvin, K. W. W. Tetanus-like reactions to the phenothiazine drugs "the grimacing syndrome." New Zealand Medical Journal. 1962, 61, 90-92.

A tentative diagnosis of tetanus was tendered for 10 patients with extensive intermittent muscle spasms involving the jaw, tongue, face, neck extensors and recti abdominis, 8 of whom had recently received prochlorperazine, 1 chlorpromazine and 1 perphenazine. Initial trismus precipitated facial muscle spasms which produced a typical risus sardonicus. Representative case histories included 4 women aged 20-72 with the above symptoms (which were really deleterious side effects from the respective phenothiazines, 25 mg/day i.m. to 25 mg t.i.d. p.o.) who experienced alleviation of spastic activity within 20 minutes to 4 hours following administration of pethidine, phenobarbital, amytal or amylobarbital. Symptoms appeared within 12-48 hours after phenothiazine injection, indicating an acute reaction. Symptoms which distinguish acute phenothiazine toxicity from tetanus include the painful, variable and intermittent nature of the masseter

A 28-year-old retarded woman overused
methylphenidate by giving herself i. v.
doses up to a level of 600 mg/day for about
5 months at which time she was admitted to
a state hospital. The patient showed paranoid symptoms after 14 days of methylphenidate abuse. In the week before admission she hallucinated. The patient recovered without withdrawal symptoms and
was released after 5 days. The symptoms
of methylphenidate psychosis are similar
to those of amphetamine psychosis.

[No address]

1875 Hangaard, Gunnar. Iproniazid som
arsak til hepatocellulaer icterus. [Hepa-
tocellular icterus caused by iproniazid.]
Nordisk Medicin, 1962, 68, 1071-1073.

A 38-year-old woman, treated for depression, ingested a total of 175 tablets of
iproniazid with a maximum daily dose of
150 mg. She suffered icterus, nausea and
pain, as well as pruritis. The clinical and
laboratory picture indicated hepatocellular
disease. While it has not been established
that iproniazid has caused such damage
care should be taken in the use of the drug.

Menighetssosterhjemmets Klinikk
Oslo, Norway

1876 Ahlberg, Ake. Decubitalsor efter
suicidalförsök. [Decubital ulcers following
suicide attempts]. Nordisk Medicin, 1962,
67, 376-377.

Case reports were presented for 6 cases
suffering from decubital ulcers following
recuperation from various suicide attempts.
In 1 case an unknown number of tablets of
meprobamate, prothipental, mebymal and
chlorpromazine had been ingested. The
patient was discovered unconscious and
it was impossible to discern the time factors involved. On admission he had sores
over the sacrum, heels and occipital
regions. These cases were treated with
plastic surgery.

Plastikkirurgiska Kliniken
Malmö, Sweden

1877 Hallwright, G.P. Agranulocytosis
with alpha methyl dopa. New Zealand
Medical Journal, 1962, 61, 470-472.
[Letter]

Agranulocytosis in a woman [age unspecified]
secondary to α-methyl-dopa (102 g)
administration over a period of 18 weeks
was ameliorated upon drug discontinuation.
Stabilization of the blood picture was
obtained with guanethidine (10 mg) combined
with hydrochlorothiazide. As a trial
measure, a specially purified preparation
of α-methyl-dopa (2.75 g) was subsequently
administered over a period of 16 days.
Blood counts were monitored constantly.
No untoward subjective reactions occurred,
other than hypotension when a single
750 mg dose was ingested rather than
the usual divided dose. Since no drug
hypersensitivity was observed, the previous
agranulocytosis could have been due to
the presence of trace amounts of an
impurity such as D-α-methyl-dopa or
ammonium chloride. To preclude the
possibility of an endogenous change in
reactivity, purified α-methyl-dopa (total
dose 6, 250 mg) plus hydrochlorothiazide
(25 mg/day) were administered for 12
days, after which a slight neutropenia was
observed which persisted for 2 weeks after
drug discontinuation. No true hypersensitivity was manifested, but the discomfort
and inconvenience attendant upon continual
blood studies precipitated a return to
guanethidine.

Hypertension Clinic
Wellington Hospital
Wellington, New Zealand

1878 Bargues, R., Planques, L., Cohadon,
S., & Loiseau, P. A propos d'une série
récente d'accidents nerveux dus aux
hydantoines. [On a series of recent nervous
accidents due to hydantoins.] Annales
Médico-Psychologiques,1962,1, 120, 968-969.

Twenty cases of intoxication caused by
N-3-methyl-5,5-diphenylhydantoin are
reported. However, the supposition is put
forth that the toxicity was due to impurities
accidently incorporated at manufacture.
Acute cerebello-labyrinth syndrome,
regressing several days after cessation of

Westminster Hospital
London, Ontario
Canada

1883 Weir, D.G., & Carson, J.F. A
further fatal case of Doriden intoxication.
Irish Journal of Medical Science, 1962,
No. 433, 20-22.

A 64-year-old chronically depressed woman
was admitted unconscious with pupils
dilated; corneal and gag reflexes were
absent and the fundi were normal; all
reflexes were very sluggish and no positive
Babinski sign, after apparently ingesting
25 g glutethimide (Doriden). In the 5
hours after admission respiration rate fell
but this was corrected by 2 ml 5% vanillic
acid diethylamide i.v. given hourly and then
5 ml i.m. 6-hourly. Standard gastric lavage
and prophylactic antibiotic therapy were
given. Some 21 hours later the blood
pressure had fallen to 80/40 and continued
to fall in spite of i.m. amphetamine. Some
6 hours later she died.

School of Medicine
Trinity College
Dublin, Ireland

1884 Pretto, John I. Observations on the
effects of a narcotic, including accidental
overdosage. Clinical Medicine, 1962, 69,
2011-2013.

An overdosage of piminodine (300 mg p.o.
within 2-4 hours) was taken by 2 men 52 and
66 years of age, who were members of a
group of 42 patients receiving the drug in
conjunction with x-ray therapy for cancer.
Both men rapidly developed tachycardia and
tachypnea, with diminution of peripheral
pain sensation but no disturbance of mental
alertness, intellect or consciousness.
Nausea and vomiting occurred in 1 patient.
Following ingestion of the standard dose of
piminodine (50 mg p.o. every 4 hours),
another patient showed allergic urticaria
which was promptly alleviated by parenteral
antihistamine. Piminodine seems able to
produce analgesia without causing euphoria
or narcosis.

Department of Radiology
College of Medicine
University of Illinois
Chicago, Ill.

1885 Benitz, K.-F., Moraski, R., Roepke,
R.R., & Wozniak, Lillian A. Toxicity
studies on mephenoxalone in rats and dogs.
Toxicology and Applied Pharmacology, 1962,
4, 220-237.

Toxicity data for mephenoxalone after oral
administration to beagle dogs (1-month and
6-month studies) and Sherman rats (1-month
study) are reported. In the dog, daily doses
of 480 and 600 mg/kg administered for 3-4
weeks produced toxic effects such as
anorexia, loss of body weight, ataxia, hemolytic anemia, etc. Slight hemolytic anemia
was detected in the dogs on 200 mg/kg for
1 month. No toxicity was observed with daily
doses as high as 120 mg/kg for a period of
6 months. Daily oral doses of approximately
1000 mg/kg for 30 days to rats produced
decreased food intake and body weight gain.
Slight decrease in body weight gain was
observed in the female rats receiving
280 mg/kg. Daily doses of 70 mg/kg for
1 month were well tolerated.

Lederle Laboratories Division
American Cyanamid Company
Pearl River, N.Y.

1886 Algeri, Elvera J., Katsas, George
G., & Luongo, Michael A. Determination
of ethchlorvynol in biologic mediums, and
report of two fatal cases. American Journal
of Clinical Pathology, 1962, 38, 125-130.

Two suicides (ingestion of unknown amounts
of ethchlorvynol) prompted the establishment
of a method for its determination, based
on the color reaction produced in compounds
with an allyl group on treatment with phloro-
glucinol and concentrated HCl. The procedure
was applied to 7 samples of whole blood and
liver. As well, blood samples from 2 healthy
adults were analyzed following ingestion of 2
500 mg capsules (ca. 12 mg/kg) of ethchlorvynol at 0.5 hour intervals for 2 hours, then
at 3, 4, 6 and 24 hours after ingestion. The
side effects produced (which disappeared 3
hours after ingestion) included: drowsiness,
slurring of speech, unsteady gait, double
vision and muscular incoordination. Analysis
was also made of concentrations of ethchlorvynol in blood, liver and kidneys of the 2
described cases of suicide. Attempts to
determine whether unchanged drug or
metabolites were extracted were unsuccessful.

and morphine ingested 10 100 mg tablets
of Tuinal (amobarbital and secobarbital)
and a large amount of whiskey the night
before she swallowed 215 25 mg tablets
of imipramine (5375 mg) in a suicidal
attempt. Within 3 1/2 hours she was apneic
and deeply comatose, with marked hypotension and absent corneal and plantar
reflexes. Gastric lavage, dextran and
metaraminol failed to control hypotension.
Tonic-clonic seizures were relieved by
amobarbital (0.25 g i. v.). Levarterenol
i. v. maintained blood pressure. Dialysis
on an artificial kidney for 5 1/2 hours was
initially complicated by generalized
convulsions and 2 episodes of cardiac
arrest. Administration of mannitol (50 g
i. v.) induced osmotic diuresis. The
temperature of the dialysis bath was lowered
to 95°F, to decrease the patients temperature from 107°F to 96°F. Levarterenol
and methoxamine controlled hypotension
after cessation of dialysis. Analysis of the
dialysis bath water revealed only 30 mg of
imipramine in 300 liters. Early recovery
was characterized by myoclonic jerking
and athetoid movements as well as auditory
and visual hallucinations. No neurological
damage was evidenced 3 months after the
above episode and the ECG was normal.

Massachusetts General Hospital
Boston, Mass.

1891 Alajem, N., & Albagli, Ch. Severe
imipramine poisoning in an infant. American
Journal of Diseases of Children, 1962, 103,
702-705.

A 1 1/2 year old girl accidental ingested
375-500 mg imipramine and became comatose with gross neurological disturbances
and severe myocardial damage with
corresponding EEG and ECG changes. She
was treated symptomatically with barbiturates
and made a complete clinical, electroencephalographic, and electrocardiographic
recovery.

"Asaf Harofe" Government Hospital
Zerifin, Israel

See also 1663, 1674, 1683, 1685, 1686,
1688, 1689, 1691, 1693, 1698, 1699, 1706
1707, 1711, 1712, 1713, 1725, 1749, 1753,
1761, 1773, 1827, 1906, 1908, 1909, 1914,
1915, 1917, 1931, 1933, 1938, 1968, 1969

1892 Ostfeld, Adrian M., & Aruguete, Alayne. Central nervous system effects of hyoscine in man. Journal of Pharmacology and Experimental Therapeutics, 1962, 137, 133-139.

A series of experiments was performed with 54 normal paid volunteers in order to assess hyoscine CNS effects (EEG and behavior). Subjects reported in the fasting state, their pupils were dilated with 10% phenylephrine and, after 10 minutes of rest, pulse rate and saliva volume were measured. A Clyde Mood Scale was completed, electrodes were applied and the room darkened for photic stimulation. EEG's were recorded during the 30 minute control period. Hyoscine hydrobromide 0.15-0.80 mg was then injected s.c. The test parameters were recorded thereafter at intervals of a half hour. A metronome tapping task (Wilker 1954) was employed as a simple measure of alertness; the Wechsler Memory Scale, the buzzer press test, the Stroop color naming test and the card-object recall test (Terman and Merrill 1937) were also employed. The Clyde Mood Scale was retaken at 1 hour and again at 4 hours after hyoscine. EEG and gross behavioral observations were continued for at least 5 hours. Hyoscine induced a moderate bradycardia and a marked decrease in salivation and in the duration of the EEG arousal response. These effects were maximal at 1-2 hours after administration, but no longer present at 4 hours. Consistent behavioral effects in EEG experiments were a decrease in spontaneous speech and movement and a significant decrease in the "Energetic" Scale of the Clyde Mood Scale. The spontaneous EEG exhibited a consistent shift toward lower amplitude of the 5-8 cycles per second activity. The alpha index significantly decreased. The depression of the EEG arousal response may be attributed to the action of hyoscine on the ascending reticular activating system which occurs independently of the action on the spontaneous EEG rhythm. The larger hyoscine dose was associated with a decrease in performance on behavioral tests. When arecoline and methacholine were employed, in doses which antagorized the peripheral effects of hyoscine, e.g., salivation, they did not antagonize hyoscine effects on behavior.

Department of Preventive Medicine
University of Illinois College of Medicine
Chicago, Ill.

1893 Collins, William E., & Poe, Robert H. Amphetamine, arousal, and human vestibular nystagmus. Journal of Pharmacology and Experimental Therapeutics, 1962, 138, 120-125.

Twelve mg racemic amphetamine or saline was administered s.c. to normal human subjects 20 minutes before trials in order to examine the effects of the clinical dose on the vestibular response under conditions of mental activity and reverie. A rotary turntable (Guedry and Kalter 1956), located in a light-proof room, was used and the subjects were seated at the center of the apparatus in a normal sitting position. A reference electrode on the forehead and an electrode taped at the outer canthus of each eye served to record horizontal components of eye movement. Two groups were used: a "naive" group which had no previous turntable or caloric stimulation experience and an "experienced" group that had been rotated many times previously under a variety of conditions. For the 1st 2 trials on each day, mental arithmetic problems (continuous division) were assigned; for the 3rd and 4th trial, the subjects were instructed to relax and daydream, keeping the eyes open. The drug produced significant increases in cardiovascular activity. However it did not affect significantly the total amount of slow-phase nystagmus induced by rotation when instructions influencing mental activity were employed. The mentally active state resulted in greater output and longer durations of nystagmus than did the relaxed state.

Civil Aeromedical Research Institute
FAA
Oklahoma City, Okla.

1894 Korman, Maurice, Knopf, Irwin J., & Leon, Robert L. Alcohol as a discriminative stimulus. A preliminary report. Texas Reports on Biology and Medicine, 1962 20, 61-63.

administration of pheniprazine to rats and dogs appears to be due to a depression of spinal synaptic pathways.

Department of Pharmacology
University of Pittsburgh School of Pharmacy
Pittsburgh, Pa.

1896 Gylys, J. A., Hart, J. J. D., & Warren, M. R. Chlorphentermine, a new anorectic agent. Journal of Pharmacology and Experimental Therapeutics, 1962, 137, 365-373.

Chlorphentermine reduced food intake in rats, dogs, mice and in gold thioglucose obese mice. The oral anorectic potencies of chlorphentermine and diethylpropion in rats were about 1/5 and in dogs 1/10 that of dexamphetamine. The acute oral toxicities of these drugs were respectively 1/8 and 1/15 that of dexamphetamine. The anorectic response of chlorphentermine in rats was prolonged and without any increase of motor activity while the effects of diethylpropion and dexamphetamine were shorter and accompanied by hyperactivity. All 3 compounds caused autonomic sympathomimetic side effects at anorectic doses which produced a prolonged anorectic response. At anorectic doses chlorphentermine and dexamphetamine increased the sensitivity of rats to quinine as reflected by an increased aversion to the drinking of quinine containing milk. The locomotor activity profile of chlorphentermine as shown with mice in rotating cages was different from that seen with dexamphetamine and diethylpropion; dexamphetamine was stimulating while diethylpropion had no consistent effect. Chlorphentermine did not antagonize chlorpromazine or reserpine depression, while diethylpropion and dexamphetamine induced reversal. Chlorphentermine had no effect on body temperature in rats in contrast to the pyrexic responses caused by dexamphetamine and diethylpropion to induce increased spontaneous activity, pyrexic responses or to reverse reserpine or chlorpromazine depression.

Department of Pharmacology
Warner-Lambert Research Institute
Morris Plains, N. J.

1897 Smith, Gene M., & Beecher, Henry K. Subjective effects of heroin and morphine in normal subjects. Journal of Pharmacology and Experimental Therapeutics, 1962, 136, 47-52.

Twenty-four healthy, nonaddicted college men between 21 and 30 years of age were used as subjects. Each was given 10 mg/70 kg morphine on one occasion, 4 mg/70 kg-heroin on another and placebo on still another. The drug order was counterbalanced so that each of the 6 possibilities of ordering the 3 medications were used with 4 subjects. Subcutaneous injections were made on a double-blind basis. The most definite subjective effects (90-item check-list of Smith and Beecker 1959) of both opiates were mental clouding, mental and physical "deactivation" and "somatic" effects such as dizziness, itching, sweating, numbness, nausea and visual difficulties. The effects on responses in the emotional areas were weaker than those aforementioned but were internally consistent. Although most subjects reported unpleasant emotional effects, 2 reported pleasant ones. The effects of the 2 opiates were similar; the main differences were that the heroin effects were stronger and reached peak degrees earlier than those of morphine. Undesirable side effects were more marked with heroin than with morphine.

Anesthesia Laboratory
Harvard Medical School
Massachusetts General Hospital
Boston, Mass.

1898 Smith, Gene M., Semke, Charles W., & Beecher, Henry K. Objective evidence of mental effects of heroin, morphine and placebo in normal subjects. Journal of Pharmacology and Experimental Therapeutics, 1962, 136, 53-58.

Forty-eight nonaddicted male students, 21-32 years of age received s.c. injections of morphine (10 mg/70 kg), heroin

ın simultaneous discrimination learning.
Six minutes before the start of the
training trials on the discrimination
problem (procedure similar to that of
Thompson and Bryant 1955), 16 were given
0.33 mg/kg strychnine i.p. and 16 given
saline. There was a significant difference
in the number of trials to criterion;
the mean for all strychnine-treated
animals was 30.5 and that for controls
81.5 The overall median of strychnine-
treated subjects was 13.0, while that of
controls,40.5. Females gave superior
performance, possibly either due to
their lighter weight or in response to
shock. Further, no significant difference
was noted between strains.

Department of Psychology
University of Oregon
Eugene, Ore.

1902 Hollister, Leo E „ & Hartman, Alan
M. Mescaline, lysergic acid diethylamide
and psilocybin: comparison of clinical
syndromes, effects on color perception
and biochemical measures. Comprehensive
Psychiatry, 1962, 3, 235-241.

Mescaline (5mg/kg), LSD (1 μg/kg) and
psilocybin (150 μg/kg) were randomly
administered p.o. to 20 subjects (18
received all 3 drugs), who were free from
overt psychopathology, in a single-blind
study. Evaluation included a questionnaire
of 43 items, completed by the subjects,
regarding signs and symptoms experienced
with each drug. Color perception was
measured by the Farnsworth-Munsell Hue
Discrimination test. Various biochemical
tests (total lipids, inorganic phosphate,
creatinine, etc.) were also performed.
Similar clinical syndromes resulted
from all 3 drugs, that from mescaline
being the most pronounced. Somatic
manifestations predominated and psychotomimetic symptoms were uncommon
except for visual hallucinations. Color
perception was altered significantly
only after inadequate stimuli, a fact which
tends to support the hypothesis that heightened and unusual perception of colors
following psychotomimetics may result
from the action of normally inadequate
stimuli. The urinary excretion of inorganic

9

phosphate usually decreased, total circulatory eosinophils decreased and plasma FFA
increased. Except for an increase in copper
oxidase activity after psilocybin, all other
biochemical measurements were not significantly changed. Many common mechanisms
of action apparently existed.

VA Hospital
Palo Alto, Calif.

1903 Frankenhaeuser, Marianne, Myrsten,
Anna-Lisa, & Järpe, Gundla. Effects of a
moderate dose of alcohol on intellectual
functions. Psychopharmacologia, 1962, 3,
344-351.

In a single-blind study, the performance of
8 healthy subjects, aged 20-27 years, was
examined in 4 tests of intelligence (verbal,
numerical, inductive and spatial) following
an oral dose of alcohol (0.8 g/kg). In order
to maintain the blood alcohol at a constant
level during psychological testing, a level
of about 0.1 g/kg/hour was maintained by
a 5% alcohol i.v. infusion. Two test sessions
a few days apart were given each subject
and the testing sequence rotated so that each
test was given 1st, 2nd, 3rd or 4th an equal
number of times. Comparison with placebo
results showed that numerical and spatial
test performance was significantly impaired,
wheras verbal and inductive test performance
was unaffected. Performance speed was less
affected than accuracy. As the affective
test is considered the most complex, results
do not confirm the belief that more complex
tasks are those affected by alcohol.

Psychological Laboratory
University of Stockholm
Stockholm, Sweden

1904 Posluns, Donald. An analysis of
chlorpromazine-induced suppression of the
avoidance response. Psychopharmacologia,
1962, 3, 361-373.

Male Long-Evans rats were used in a
conditioned avoidance experiment with or
without 3 mg/kg chlorpromazine given i.p.
before test phases. The avoidance response
required moving from 1 end of 1 compartment in a 2-compartment box (electrified

Peak effects of mescaline occurred 2.5 hours
and persisted longer than the effects of
either LSD or psilocin. With peak values
for pupillary dilatation, 1 μg/kg LSD was
equivalent to 45 μg/kg psilocin, and 1 μg/kg
psilocin was equivalent to 66 μg/kg mescaline. Nearly identical values were obtained
with the data for peak pupillary response,
total or peak number of answers on the
questionnaire and clinical grade.

NIMH Addiction Research Center
USPHS Hospital
Lexington, Ky.

1906 Somers, G. F. Thalidomide and
congenital abnormalities. Lancet, 1962,
No. 7775, 912-913. [Letter]

Eight New Zealand rabbits received thalidomide (150 mg/kg/day p.o.) from day 8
to 16 of pregnancy. Litters produced by 3
of the rabbits contained stillbirths and
young with deformities. The 4th yielded
evidence of fetal autolysis. Characteristic fetal defects were observed. In a 2nd
experiment involving 8 does, thalidomide
administered as above induced similar
malformations in the 1st 4 litters. Improved screening methods for new drugs
must be instituted. Detailed results of
similar experiments with mice, rats and
hens' eggs will soon be published.

Distillers Co. (Biochemicals) Ltd.
Speke, Liverpool
Great Britain

1907 Feldman, Shaul. Electrophysiological alterations in adrenalectomy. Changes
in brain stem conduction, excitability, and
sensitivity to anesthesia in adrenalectomized cats. Archives of Neurology, 1962, 7,
460-470.

Chronically adrenalectomized hydrocorti-
sone-supported cats were studied and compared with intact animals in order to study
possible neurophysiological disturbances in
hypoadrenalism. Blood level determinations for glucose, sodium, and chloride
were made for 7 adrenalectomized cats
prior to surgery. Concentric electrodes
were introduced stereotaxically into the
medial lemniscus, midbrain reticular
formation and ventromedian and the posterolateral hypothalamic regions. At the
end of surgery the cats were immobilized
with gallamine triethiodid (Flaxedil) and
maintained on artificial respiration.
Stimuli were delivered to the contralateral
sciatic nerve. The evoked potentials were
recorded monopolarly in the different brain
stem regions. Neuronal recovery in the
medial lemniscus, the midbrain reticular
formation and the hypothalamus was studied
by delivering paired shocks to the sciatic
nerve at varying intervals. The neuronal
recovery was determined by expressing
the amplitude of the response to the second

and a propylene glycol-water solution of
carisoprodol, 5.1 or 8.0 mg, labeled in
the carbonyl position with C^{14}, administered i.v. Urine was collected and 3 ml
volumes of blood were withdrawn through
the catheter at appropriate intervals. In
the dog, carisoprodol is largely metabolized to a compound tentatively identified as
hydroxycarisoprodol. Hydroxymeprobamate
and small quantities of meprobamate also
occur in the urine. Carisoprodol itself is
excreted unchanged in trace amounts.
After i.v. administration of carisoprodol
to dogs, the major circulating carbamate
is the unchanged drug. Hydroxycarisoprodol, hydroxymeprobamate and meprobamate
are also present in the blood.

Wallace Laboratories
Cranbury, N. J.

1911 Koechlin, Bernard A., Schwartz,
Morton A ., & Oberhaensli. Metabolism of
C^{14}-iproniazid and C^{14}-isocarboxazid in
man. Journal of Pharmacology and Experimental Therapeutics, 1962, 138, 11-20.

The metabolic fates of iproniazid labeled in
the isopropyl group at C_2 and isocarboxazid labeled in the benzyl moiety in human
subjects were investigated and compared
to previous results in rats. Both drugs
were rapidly absorbed after oral administration of therapeutic doses. C^{14}-Isocarbox-
azid was metabolized by oxidation of the
labeled isopropyl substituent resulting in
the elimination of 50-60% of the radioactive
dose as pulmonary carbon dioxide within
24 hours. The oxidation rates differed
markedly between individuals as did the
patterns of the radioactive urinary excretion products. C^{14}-Isocarboxazid was metabolized analogously by oxidation of the
labeled benzyl moiety to C^{14}-benzoic acid
which was excreted as urinary C^{14}-hippu-
rate and accounted for 56% of the dose in
24 hours. Comparison of the fate of the
2 drugs in man with that in rats revealed
identical major pathways of oxidative degradation but characteristic differences of the
degradation rates. Much higher doses of
both drugs are required in the rat than in
man to elicit measurable pharmacological
effects. In both species isocarboxazid
seemed to be oxidized faster than iproniazid

while faster rates of oxidation of both drugs in the rat than in man were indicated.

Department of Pharmacology
Hoffmann- La Roche Inc.
Nutley, N. J.

1912 Albaum, Harry G. The effect of central nervous system drugs on the enzyme activity of rat brain. Acta Neurologica Scandanavica, 1962, 38, 68.

The effect of 5 psychoactive drugs [concentrations unspecified] on 10 CNS enzyme systems were studied in rat brain tissue. Significant alterations of enzyme activity were observed with pentobarbital (malic dehydrogenase and hexokinase), meprobamate (hexokinase and lactic dehydrogenase) and reserpine (enolase and myokinase). None of the drugs affected aldolase, glutamic oxalacetic transaminase, glutamic pyruvic transaminase, phosphoglycerokinase or transaminase, phosphoglycerokinase or glyceraldehyde phosphate dehydrogenase. In view of the fact that both of the rate-limiting steps in glycolysis were unaffected by drugs, it seems highly unlikely that these drugs exert their metabolic effects on the glycolytic sequence.

Department of Biology
Brooklyn College
Brooklyn, New York, N. Y.

1913 Martin, W.R., &Eisenman, A.J. Interactions between nalorphine and morphine in the decerebrate cat. Journal of Pharmacology and Experimental Therapeutics, 1962, 138, 113-119.

Acute physical dependence can be produced by a single dose of morphine in the decerebrate cat and the acute abstinence syndrome of the acutely physically dependent cat consists of a sequence of changes in respiratory and cardiovascular functions that are similar to the changes observed in severely narcotized subjects treated with nalorphine. Morphine [11-20 mg/kg] decreased respiratory rate, respiratory minute volume, pulse rate and blood pressure, increased serum CO_2 concentration and decreased serum pH in the decerebrate cat. Nalorphine (5-10 mg/kg) in contrast produced a moderate increase in respiratory rate and minute volume, and a modest decrease in serum CO_2 and blood pressure. Nalorphine when administered to decerebrate cats severely depressed by morphine produced a transient and

of amphetamine. Within a temperature
range of 20 to 27.5°C each 2.5°C rise in
temperature produced a significant increase in amphetamine toxicity. A significant interaction occurred between degree
of aggregation and temperature. The size
of the cage in which the mice were confined
(degree of confinement) had little influence
on the toxicity of amphetamine in mice
grouped 10 per cage. A decrease in cage
size augmented amphetamine toxicity in
mouse groups of 5 per cage.

College of Pharmacy
Washington State University
Pullman, Wash.

1917 Clausen, Ebba. Fenacetins og
acetylsalicylsyres nefrotoksiske effekt
belyst ved dyreksperimentelle undersøgel-
ser. [The nephrotoxic effect of phenacetin
and acetylsalicylic acid in animal experiments.] Nordisk Medicin, 1962, 67, 755.

Ten rabbits were given phenacetin, 10
acetylsalicylic acid and 8 placebo. After
11 months of daily feeding [dosage unspec-
ified] 1/2 of the animals in each group were
injected i. v. with a coliform bacterium.
Histopathologically, both the phenacetin and
acetylsalicyclic acid groups showed dilatation of the tubules, interstitial hyperplasia
with round-cell infiltration and abcess
formation. Similar histopathologic changes
were observed in all animals which had not
been given a bacterial suspension. In the
placebo-bacteria and in the uninoculated
group some inflammation was noted in 1
out of 4 and 2 out of 4 animals, respectively.
Kidney damage may be due to direct drug
toxicity or to a lowering of resistance to
infection.

[No address]

1918 Chusid, Joseph G. , & Kopeloff, Lenore
M. Chlordiazepoxide as an anticonvulsant
in monkeys. Proceedings of the Society for
Experimental Biology and Medicine, 1962,
109, 546-548.

Chlordiazepoxide was tested in 11 rhesus
monkeys, 5 of which had been made chronically epileptic by the application of alumina

cream to the cerebral cortex. The drug was injected i. v. (0. 55-35 mg/kg) and followed 1/2 hour later by an i. m. injection of pentetrazol (24 mg/kg for epileptic and 64 mg/kg for normal monkeys). Intravenous chlordiazepoxide in large doses prevented clinical and EEG convulsant effects of the challenge pentetrazol doses in both epileptic and normal monkeys. The only toxicity noted was transient hematuria on 3 occasions in 2 monkeys at the highest dosage (35 mg/kg).

Department of Bacteriology
New York State Psychiatric Institute
New York City, N. Y.

1919 Greef, K., Kasperat, H., & Osswald, W. Paradoxe Wirkungen der elecktrschen Vagusreizung am isolierten Magen- und Herzvorhofpräparat des Meerschweinchens sowie deren Beeinflussung durch Ganglienblocker, Sympathicolytica, Reserpin und Cocain. [Paradoxical effects of electrical stimulation of the vagus in isolated guinea pig stomach- and atrium preparations, and the effects of ganglionic blocking agents, sympathicolytics, reserpine and cocaine.] Archiv für Experimentelle Pathologie und Pharmakologie, 1962, 6, 528-545.

Tests were performed on 28 isolated stomachs and over 70 isolated atria from guinea pigs, as well as on a few preparations of guinea pig and rabbit ileum, and cat and rabbit atria. Pretreatment of the isolated guinea pig stomach with atropine and histamine reverses the usual effect of electrical stimulation of the vagus or injection of dimethylphenylpiperazinium iodide, which produces paradoxical inhibition of gastric contraction. This paradoxical effect can be prevented by addition of hexamethonium (10 μg/ml), azamethonium (30 μg/ml), chlorisondamine (5 μg/ml), thymoxyalkylamine (10-20μg/ml), darethin (10-20 μg/ml) and cocaine (2. 5-5 μg/ml), but not by pretreatment of the animals with reserpine (1 mg/kg b. i. d. for 2 days). Similar effects were obtained in the isolated ileum. In the isolated atrium, atropine again reverses the usual inhibitory effects of vagal stimulation, resulting in a positive inotropic and chronotropic action. This paradoxical effect can be prevented by pretreatment with reserpine or by addition of hexametho-

nium, chlorisondamine or nicotine, but is potentiated by dibenzyline (10 μg/ml), phentolamine (5-10 μg/ml) and cocaine. Some of the interactions of reserpine, butyrylcholine, epinephrine, methamphetamine, tyramine and guanethidine on these preparations are also discussed.

Pharmakologisches Institut der Medizinisch Akademie
Düsseldorf, Germany

1920 Baruk, H., & Launay, J. Action du chlorhydrate de prothipendyl sur le comportement psychomoteur du singe. Comparaison avec l'action de la chlorpromazine. [The action of prothipendyl chlorhydrate on the psychomotor behavior of monkeys. A comparison with the action of chlorpromazine.] Annales Médico-Psychologiques, 1962, 1, 120, 638.

In monkeys, 5 mg/kg prothipendyl caused sedation with diminution in aggressiveness, drowsiness without the induction of deep sleep, and a general slowing of movements. At high doses (20 mg/kg) catalepsia was induced. However the catatonigenic qualities of prothipendyl are less than those of chlorpromazine.

[No address]

1921 Volle, Robert L. Enhancement of postganglionic responses to stimulating agents following repetitive preganglionic stimulation. Journal of Pharmacology and Experimental Therapeutics, 1962, 136, 68-74.

Experiments were conducted on the superior cervical ganglia of urethane-anesthetized cats. Acetylcholine, carbamylcholine, tetramethylammonium chloride (TMA), hexamethonium and procaine were administered, either by rapid injection or by infusion, into the common carotid artery before and after repetitive preganglionic stimulation. Postganglionic responses to acetylcholine, carbamylcholine and TMA were enhanced markedly following repetitive preganglionic volleys at frequencies ranging from 5-100 cps for durations of 10 seconds to 5 minutes. Both amplitudes and time

depression of the phasic component was
seen after doses of scopolamine which produce cholinergic blockade at peripheral
autonomic sites. The order of potency
of the agents in producing 50% depression
of the tonic reflex was: zoxazolamine,
mephenesin, carisoprodol, caramiphen,
pentobarbital, chlorpromazine, and
scopolamine. Scopolamine was approximately 20 times as potent as zoxazolamine.
For 75% depression of the tonic component
of the reflex the order of potency was:
zoxazolamine, carisoprodol, mephenesin,
caramiphen, scopolamine, pentobarbital
and chlorpromazine. Chlorpromazine was
almost 16 times as potent as zoxazolamine.

Department of Pharmacology
University of Illinois College of Medicine
Chicago, Ill.

1923 Mulé, S. J., & Woods, L. A. Distribution of N-C^{14}- methyl labeled morphine:
I. In central nervous system of nontolerant
and tolerant dogs. Journal of Pharmacology and Experimental Therapeutics. '962,
136, 232-241.

N-C^{14}-methyl labeled morphine was synthesized with a specific activity of about
0.4 mc/mM. Selected areas of the CNS
of dogs were separated into gray and white
matter where possible; recoveries of 15-
150 mμ/g and 150-1500 mμ/g of labeled
morphine from dog brain tissues were
approximately 90 and 95%, respectively,
and recoveries of 50-4000 mμ/g from suit-
ably diluted plasma and urine were ca. 95
and 99%, respectively. Total radioactivity
was determined in toluene extracts, employing descending paper chromatography
as an additional control procedure. Concentrations of free labeled morphine were
lower in the CNS of tolerant dogs in comparison to nontolerant dogs at various
intervals of time after a single 2 mg/kg s.c.
injection of labeled drug. The levels of
free morphine in the CNS of tolerant dogs
following consecutive 2 mg/kg s.c. injections as compared to consecutively injected
nontolerant dogs were higher at 35 minutes,
similar at 4 hours, and much lower at 8
hours. Generally the cerebral cortical
gray matter contained the highest concentrations of free morphine in both nontolerant.

and tolerant dogs. Predominantly cellular subcortical areas of the CNS occasionally contained levels of free morphine equal to cerebral gray matter values. Cerebral and cerebellar white matter levels of free morphine were lower than gray during the early time intervals and approximately the same as gray matter or higher at later time periods. Small quantities of conjugated morphine were observed in the temporal cortex of nontolerant and tolerant dogs. The rate of disappearance of free morphine from plasma and CSF was faster in tolerant than in nontolerant dogs following a single injection of labeled morphine. Egression of free morphine from plasma and CSF following consecutive labeled morphine injections were quite similar in nontolerant and tolerant dogs. Conjugated morphine levels in plasma were much lower in tolerant dogs as compared to corresponding values in nontolerant dogs after consecutive injections. The differences in the physiological disposition of free morphine between nontolerant and tolerant dogs do not appear to be of sufficient magnitude to account for tolerance development.

Department of Pharmacology
University of Michigan Medical School
Ann Arbor, Mich.

1924 Mulé, S. J., Woods, L. A., & Mellett, L. B. Distribution of N-C^{14}-methyl labeled morphine: II. Effect of nalorphine in the central nervous system of nontolerant dogs and observations on metabolism. Journal of Pharmacology and Experimental Therapeutics, 1962, 136, 242-249.

The effect of nonlabeled nalorphine on the distribution of labeled morphine in the CNS (nalorphine-morphine antagonism), and the chromatographic analysis of the CNS and urinary extracts of nontolerant and tolerant dogs following the administration of labeled morphine was studied. The s.c. administration of labeled morphine (2 mg/kg) before nonlabeled nalorphine (2 mg/kg), given s.c., resulted in a significant increase in the CNS levels of morphine in nontolerant dogs. Simultaneous injection of both drugs, or pretreatment with nalorphine resulted in an increase or no change in morphine levels in nontolerant dogs compared to morphine

control dog values. Effect of nalorphine on the plasma and CSF concentrations of free morphine was somewhat variable. Paper chromatographic studies provided no evidence for the presence of an N-C^{14}-methyl labeled metabolite of morphine in the CNS or urinary extracts of nontolerant and tolerant dogs.

Department of Pharmacology
University of Michigan Medical School
Ann Arbor, Mich.

1925 Anderson, E. G., Markowitz, S. D., & Bonnycastle, D. D. Brain 5-hydroxytryptamine and anticonvulsant activity. Journal of Pharmacology and Experimental Therapeutics, 1962, 136, 179-182.

Electroshock seizures were induced in male Sprague-Dawley rats. An animal was considered protected against the shock on failure to manifest a maximal extensor reflex (MER). Diphenylhydantoin (12.5 mg/kg), pheniprazine (4 mg/kg) and 5HTP (100 mg/kg) were administered i.p. The comparison of relative drug induced effects on the MER in response to electroshock and rise in brain 5HT showed a complete lack of correlation. 5-Hydroxytryptamine elevation alone may play no significant role in the production of the anticonvulsant effect; however, with a better knowledge of the factors relating to binding and release and precise localization in the CNS it is possible that such relationships can be reassessed.

Department of Pharmacology
Seton Hall College of Medicine and Dentistry
Jersey City, N. J.

1926 Green, Harry, Greenberg, Samuel M., Erickson, Robert W., Sawyer, John L., & Ellison, Theodore. Effect of dietary phenylalanine and tryptophan upon rat brain amine levels. Journal of Pharmacology and Experimental Therapeutics, 1962, 136, 174-178.

Female weanling Long-Evans rats were used in the study of dietary effects of phenylalanine and tryptophan on brain amine levels. The basal diet was modified with respect to these amino acids. Diets enriched

zamine, pretreatments known to affect the
sensitivity and/or levarterenol content of
this organ. No relationship was found between the sensitivity to levarterenol and the
levarterenol content. Hypersensitivity to
levarterenol appeared whenever, for a
period of 7-14 days, the nictitating membrane was deprived of the usual influence
of tonic impulses. This was observed after
chronic denervation, chronic decentraliza-
tion, or 7 days of pretreatment with reserpine, TM 10 or chlorisondamine. Brief
depletion, caused by pretreatment with a
single large dose of reserpine, did not
cause hypersensitivity. Hypersensitivity
to i.a. injections of acetylcholine paralleled that to levarterenol in these procedures.
Hyposensitivity to tyramine was observed
after any type of depletion of levarterenol
stores, whereas hypersensitivity to this
substance was found when the levarterenol
stores were normal or only slightly affected.
Thus tyramine acts by liberating endogenous
levarterenol,. Prolonged reserpine pretreatment does not increase the plasma half-life
of injected levarterenol.

Department of Pharmacology
Harvard Medical School
Cambridge, Mass.

1928 Smith, Cedric M., Budris, A. V., &
Paul, J. W. Quantification of phasic and
tonic stretch reflexes: effects of neuromuscular blocking agents. Journal of
Pharmacology and Experimental Therapeutics, 1962, 136, 267-275.

In order to determine if any curariform
agent produces selective blockade of the
mammalian intrafusal neuromuscular junc-
tion, experiments were performed on pentobarbital anesthetized cats suspended in a
stereotaxic apparatus. Transection of the
brain stem at the level of the colliculi was
accomplished by electrocoagulation, the
cauterized area corresponded to that area
encompassed by the following stereotaxic
coordinates: anterior 1 to posterior 1, right
lateral 6 to left lateral 6 and vertical -8 to
+ 4. Of 80 animals operated upon 45 died
within the 1st 24 hours and 40 of these died
within the 1st 12 hours (hemorrhage at the
site of the lesion). Rigidity appeared in the
survivors 6-8 hours after section with

recovery from the pentobarbital anesthesia. Results were obtained with 25 out of 35 cats which exhibited extensor tone. Reflex contractions of the gastrocnemius and soleus muscles to stretch were obtained and contractions of the contralateral muscles induced by tetanic sciatic nerve stimulation were recorded. The total tension developed upon stretching was characterized by initial peak contraction (phasic) with a decrement to a lower sustained tension (tonic). Muscle tension obtained after section of the sciatic nerve or after succinylcholine-induced neuromuscular blockade was taken as a measure. Cumulative dose-effect relationships for depression of the above responses were established for tubocurarine, decamethonium and 4 polymethylene bis-isoquinolinium derivatives. Tubocurarine produced depression of the sustained tetanic nerve-muscle response followed, in order of inhibition, by the initial tetanic response, the tonic reflex, the twitch, and finally, the phasic reflex. The sustained tetanic response was 8 to 9 times more sensitive than the phasic reflex or twitch response. The patterns of effects of the 4 bis-isoquinolinium derivatives were similar to those of tubocurarine. In contrast, given doses of decamethonium produced almost equal inhibition of all the responses assessed. The postulate that these agents act primarily at the neuromuscular junctions of extrafusal muscle fibers and that any depression of the fusimotor nerve-muscle transmission takes place with doses equal to or larger than those required to block extrafusal junctions appears true.

Department of Pharmacology
University of Illinois College of Medicine
Chicago, Ill.

1929 Chai, C.K., Roberts, Eugene, & Sidman, Richard L. Influence of aminoxy-acetic acid, a γ-aminobutyrate transaminase inhibitor, on hereditary spastic defect in the mouse. Proceedings of the Society for Experimental Biology and Medicine, 1962, 109, 491-495.

Homozygous spastic mice (spa/spa) were tested for righting time, tremor, flexibility of trunk movement and alertness. Diphenylhydantoin (50 μg per mouse),

trimethadione (a 100 μg dose) and aminoxyacetic acid (AOAA; 5-30 μg), were given i.p. Paper chromatography was conducted on brain extracts. When single doses of these drugs were administered only AOAA was effective in decreasing symptoms. Subcutaneously injected AOAA (5-15 μg/g) produced a marked improvement which was the same for 12-24 hours or more. In some animals which received continued injections of the drug there was a depression of motor activity, decreased alertness and loss of weight. Brain extracts showed no significant alteration in the distribution of ninhydrin-positive constituents in comparison to normal.

Roscoe B. Jackson Memorial Laboratory
Bar Harbor, Me.

1930 Green, Harry, Sawyer, John L., Erickson, Robert W., & Cook, Leonard. Effect of repeated oral administration of monoamine oxidase inhibitor on rat brain amines. Proceedings of the Society for Experimental Biology and Medicine, 1962, 109, 347-349.

Repeated daily oral administration of tranylcypromine (5 mg/kg b.i.d.) or iproniazid (50 and 100 mg/kg b.i.d.) to rats for 3-10 days resulted in cumulative increases in brain 5 HT concentration 2-4 times that produced by a single administration of the drug. Levarterenol concentration was not appreciably different from that following a single drug administration. The rats showed no overt pharmacologic responses. No significant or consistent effect upon the motor activity pattern of drug-treated rats compared to untreated rats was observed.

Research and Development Division
Smith Kline and French Labs.
Philadelphia, Pa.

1931 MacKenzie, Robert D., & McGrath, W. Robert. Absorption of thalidomide in the rat. Proceedings of the Society for Experimental Biology and Medicine, 1962, 109, 511-515.

1933 Eerola, Risto. The combined action
of morphine and atropine. Annales
Medicinae Experimentalis et Biologiae
Fenniae, 1962, 40, 83-90.

Male mice were injected s.c. with varying
amounts of morphine and/or atropine.
Twenty-four hour toxicity was studied,
i.e., lethality between 5 and 95% (LD5
and LD95). For atropine, mortality
fluctuated between 10 and 85% and the
LD50 was established at 400 mg/kg.
For morphine, mortality fluctuated
between 10 and 90% and the LD50 was
300 mg/kg. For the combination of drugs
mortality ranged from 15 to 100%.
Here the doses were presented in a rectang-
ular coordinated system according to
Gaddum (1959). The lethality areas of the
individual drugs were presented by thickened
segments of the coordinative axis. This
analysis revealed an additive synergism
between morphine and atropine.

Institute of Pharmacology
University of Helsinki
Helsinki, Finland

1934 Casier, H., & Merlevede, E. On the
mechanism of the disulfiramethanol
intoxication symptoms. Archives Internationales de Pharmacodynamie et de
Thérapie, 1962, 139, 165-177.

Arterial blood pressure, heart rate and
respiration were followed in morphinized,
chloralosed dogs. Disulfiram (0.05%) was
infused into the femoral vein at a rate of
4 ml/minute; no reactions were observed
after 25 mg/kg. In other experiments ethanol (133-960 mg/kg) and acetaldehyde
(3.3-5.0 mg/kg) were infused with and
without disulfiram. Administration of a
compound obtained by the chemical reaction
in vitro between disulfiram and ethanol
induces all the physical symptoms provoked
by the administration of disulfiram and
ethanol. Disulfiram, i.v., induced a marked
and prolonged output of carbon disulfide in
the expired air. Neither acetaldehyde nor
the metabolites of disulfiram, diethyldithio-
carbamate, diethylamine and carbon disulfide,
are responsible for the acute toxic effects
encountered. The positive compound
obtained in vitro is probably a quaternary

ammonium base.

J. F. Heymans Institute of Pharmacology
University of Ghent
Ghent, Belgium

1935 Drucker, William R., Kingsbury,
Bryant, Powers, Adie, & O'Reilley,
Mark. Metabolic changes in lethal
shock produced by norepinephrine.
Journal of Laboratory and Clinical
Medicine, 1962, 60, 871.

Variable amounts of l-levarterenol
(norepinephrine; 1.9-4.8 μg/kg/minute)
were given as a 4-hour constant i.v.
infusion to 10 well fed normovolemic
dogs. Serial analyses were made of
blood glucose and carbohydrate
intermediaries, arterial pH, blood volume,
hematocrit, and arterial pressure. All
animals manifested a similar rise in
blood pressure, blood glucose (20 to
90 mg%), pyruvic acid (1 to 2 mg%), and
inorganic phosphate (407 mg%). The
5 dogs in which the infusion of levarterenol
exceeded 2.6 μg/kg/minute died. Death
occurred from 1/2 to 30 hours following
discontinuation of the infusion and was
associated with a gradual decline in
blood pressure and pH with an accumulation of lactic acid (over 100 mg%). These
changes began during the infusion. By
contrast, there was neither a rise in
excess lactate nor a fall of pH in the survivors. Blood volume fell in 8 of 10 dogs
during the infusion and remained low for
several hours thereafter; the mean fall
was 11% for nonsurvivors and 16% for
survivors. Similar metabolic changes
are characteristic of the severe oligemic
and hypotensive phase of hemorrhagic
shock. Here these changes were produced
by the severe vasoconstriction caused by
levarterenol with minimal hypovolemia
and similar fatal consequences.

[No address]

1936 Winter, D., & Timar, Magda.
Experimentelle Untersuchungen über
das Wiedereinschlafen aus der Barbiturat-
narkose erwachter Tiere. [Experimental
studies on the rehypnosis of animals just
awakened from barbiturate anesthesia.]
Pharmazie, 1962, 17, 454-455.

The number of rats falling back to sleep
when a 2nd drug was given i.v. immediately
upon awakening from the anesthesia produced
by 100 mg/kg of sodium amobarbital i.p.
(lasting 71 ± 5 minutes) varied from 80-100%
for chlorpromazine (2 mg/kg), imipramine
(10 mg/kg), serotonin (1.25 mg/kg),
epinephrine (0.05 mg/kg) and acetylcholine (0.1 mg/kg) to 40-60% for imipramine (5 mg/kg), methocarbamol (125 mg/kg),
reserpine (5 mg/kg), methylcellulose
(125 mg/kg), heparin (250 U), histamine
(0.01 mg/kg) and diethylaminoethylbenzylate
(5 mg/kg) and to 0% for reserpine (1 mg/kg),
dimethylaminoethyl-p-acetamidobenzoate
(5 mg/kg), procaine (12.5 mg/kg) and
polyvinylpyrrolidone (175 mg/kg). A 2nd
dose of amobarbital produced rehypnosis
in 20% at 7 mg/kg and 100% at 15 mg/kg.
This technique is not adequate as a specific
test to distinguish narcosis-potentiating
agents from neurotropic drugs with
additive effects.

Pharmaceutical Division
Chemical-Pharmaceutical Research
   Institute
Bucharest, Romania

1937 Buchel, L., Levy, Jeanne, & Tanguy,
O. Rapport entre constitution chimique
et action pharmacologique. Influence de
la nature de l'amine sur les propriétés
pharmacologiques dan quelques amino-
esters X-CO$_2$(CH$_2$)$_2$-N< et quelques
amino-esters phenoliques Y-O(CH$_2$)$_2$-N< .
[Relationship between chemical constitution
and pharmacological activity. Effect of
the nature of the amine on the pharmacological properties in some amino-esters
X-CO$_2$(CH$_2$)$_2$-N< and some phenolic aminoethers Y-O(CH$_2$)$_2$-N< .] Archives des
Sciences Physiologiques, 1962, 16, 57-70.

A comparison of the diethylamino-,
piperidyl- and methyl-4-piperazinyl-
derivatives of either cyclohexyl-1-cyclohexane
carboxylic acid ethyl ester or cymene-
ethyl ether with respect to their acute
toxicity (LD$_{50}$ i.p.), hypothermic activity
and effect on exploratory behavior, chloral
hydrate and hexobarbital anesthesia, cylin-

diethylamino-> methyl-4-piperazinyl-,
while the order was generally piperazinyl-
> diethylamino- for the other properties of
the amino esters and consistently the
opposite for the amino ethers.

Laboratoire de Pharmacologie Chimique
Faculté de Médecine
Paris, France

See also 1716, 1822, 1885, 1897, 1946,
    1981

1938 Kaye, Sidney. Simple, reliable tests for some common poisons and drug overdosage. Clinical Medicine, 1962, 69, 1971-1975.

Germane to the need for simple reliable tests to detect various poisons and drugs, clinical procedures are delineated for determining the presence of barbiturates, CO, methanol, arsenic, mercury, antimony or bismuth, salicylates, sulfanilamide derivatives and phenothiazine compounds in the human body.

State Health Department
Commonwealth of Virginia
Richmond, Va.

1939 Long, R.F. Reversible inhibition of brain monoamine oxidase in vitro and in vivo. Acta Neurologica Scandinavica, 1962, 38, 27-28.

In vitro studies on the action of reversible inhibitors on human brain MAO required different substrates for each inhibitor concentration to reduce the rate of oxidation. With harmaline, 50% inhibition was produced by 10^{-3}M with tryptamine and 2×10^{-7}M with levarterenol or 5HT as the substrate, all substrates stabilized at a concentration of 2×10^{-3}M. Differences were observed, however, among enzyme preparations from the brains of different species both in the relative rates of oxidation of different amines and in their relative affinities as measured by the action of reversible inhibitors. Harmaline or α-methyltryptamine administered to mice in doses which caused marked rises in brain 5HT and levarterenol levels failed to raise the level of dopamine. Since irreversible MAO inhibition produces a rise in dopamine, 5HT and levarterenol levels, it appears probable that the differential increase observed was due to the selective inhibition of MAO by the reversible inhibitors utilized.

Research Department
Roche Products Ltd.
Welwyn Garden City, Great Britain

1940 Baxter, Claude F. Metabolism of γ-aminobutyric acid in vivo. Acta Neurologica Scandinavica, 1962, 38, 20.

A constant ratio is found in different areas of guinea pig brain between the level of endogenous GABA and the maximal potential activity of glutamic acid decarboxylase. An exception to this correlation is found in the olfactory lobes which contain a much higher GABA level per unit of decarboxylase activity. Large doses of GABA injected parenterally into rats elevate GABA levels in the olfactory lobes but not in other brain areas. The activity of GABA α-KG transaminase in normal animals appears unrelated to GABA levels found in different areas of the brain. The effect of pyridoxal phosphate antimetabolites and carbonyl trapping agents on α-KG transaminase, GABA transaminase and GABA in brain, and β-alanine in liver has been studied. Within the brain of the intact rat, amino-oxyacetic acid appears to inhibit GABA transaminase without affecting α-KG decarboxylase, while thiosemicarbazide inhibits this decarboxylase preferentially. Both enzymes are equally susceptible to inhibition by either of these compounds in vitro. Differences may be attributable to structural barriers in vivo.

Department of Biochemistry
Medical Research Institute
City of Hope Medical Center
Duarte, Calif.

1941 Van der Helm, H.J. Electrophoretic separation of enzymes in the central nervous system. Acta Neurologica Scandinavica, 1962, 38, 64-65. [Summary]

Lactic dehydrogenase isoenzymes from homogenates of human brain were compared with lactic dehydrogenase isoenzymes in CSF and serum. The diagnostic value of enzyme activity in the CSF will be enhanced by such chemical procedures since medicine is currently limited by a rather nebulous understanding of the role played by the CNS in these activities. This approach may also be advantageous in interpreting alterations in CSF enzyme activity. Agar electrophoresis of enzymes is discussed, along

chloroform (10:0-0:10), petroleum, cyclo-
hexane, CCl_4, benzene or chloroform on
formamide-treated paper. R_f values are
given and the separation of these 4 drugs
is discussed. The best separation of all
4 components could be achieved with
formamide/benzene. All 4 drugs could be
detected on the paper with short wavelength
UV light, while for aminopyrine and
phenazone, Dragendorff's reagent and
$K_3Fe(CN)_6$-$FeCl_3$ were also useful.

Laboratory for Toxicology and
    Legal Chemistry
Charles University
Prague, Czechoslovakia

1944 Dreyfus, Pierre M. Microchemical
enzyme studies of the rat nervous system
in experimental thiamine deficiency. Acta
Neurologica Scandinavica, 1962, 38, 69-70.

The distribution of thiamine-dependent
CNS enzymes was determined in normal
and thiamine-deficient rats in various
stages of thiamine deprivation to elucidate
the selective vulnerability of specific CNS
areas to thiamine deficiency. Quantitative
histochemical methods facilitated the use
of microgram quantities of tissue as well
as histological controls. Transketolase
activity was estimated by measuring
sedoheptulose-7-phosphate production
during the incubation of fresh frozen
tissue slices or homogenates in a buffered
medium containing ribose-5-phosphate as
substrate. Sedoheptulose-7-phosphate and
ribose-5-phosphate were determined by
microspectrophotometric methods. Histological controls, dry weight, fat free dry
weight or protein determinations were
obtained on all samples. The 1st hour of
incubation represented the activity of
transketolase, the rate-limiting enzyme,
which was manifested by linear Lineweaver-
Burke plots. Transketolase activity (μM
sedoheptulose-7-phosphate/g protein/minute)
was 2.3 in white matter and 1.5 in frontal
cortex and sciatic nerve. Enzyme activity
in normal rats paralleled total lipid content
of the samples. Transketolase activity
was considerably diminished in excessive
thiamine depletion. Results indicate that
the monophosphate shunt may play an
important role in developing and maintaining

the functional integrity of the medullated portions of the CNS.

McLean Hospital Research Laboratory
Waverly, Mass.

1945 Cremer, J. E. A study of amino acid metabolism in rat brain using $[C^{14}]$-glucose and inhibitors. Acta Neurologica Scandinavica, Supplement I, 1962, 38, 22-23.

An in vitro comparison of triethyl tin and triethyl lead with other known metabolic inhibitors of the oxidation of C^{14}-labeled substrates by slices of rat brain cortex revealed that the 2 compounds selectively inhibited glucose oxidation. Preliminary in vitro experiments with these 2 compounds and other known inhibitors on the levels of amino acid in brain tissue and their degree of labeling from C^{14}-labeled glucose have shown that for a given inhibitor there is a definite change in the amino acid pattern of brain slices incubated with labeled glucose. Thus, changes in GABA were not necessarily a reflection of changes in glutamic acid. Unlike glutamic acid, the concentration of GABA within a brain slice was not readily lowered in the presence of inhibitors but its specific activity was markedly reduced. Incorporation of C^{14}-labeled amino acids into the protein fraction of brain slices was particularly sensitive to the inhibitors tested.

Toxicology Research Unit
Woodmansterne Road
Carshalton, Surrey
Great Britain

1946 van Rees, H., & Noach, E. L. Reserpine-induced changes in insulin action in the rat. Acta Physiologica et Pharmacologica Neerlandica, 1962, 11, 264-265.

In intact rats, insulin hypoglycemia was unchanged by concomitant reserpine treatment, and decreased by reserpine pretreatment. In the latter experiment, reserpine was shown to have a long-lasting blood sugar elevating action of its own. The reserpine-induced impairment of insulin activity was proven not due to acute catecholamine release, as it was also present in adrenomedullectomized animals

and after dihydroergotamine pretreatment in such animals. An acute insulin-induced increase in corticosteroid levels could not be excluded by experiments in animals adrenalectomized 14 hours after reserpine pretreatment and 2 hours before insulin administration. Also the enhancing influence of in vitro insulin addition to glucose uptake by isolated rat hemidiaphragms was unmodified by in vivo reserpine pretreatment

Department of Pharmacology
University of Leyden
Leyden, The Netherlands

1947 Eggels, P.H., Hoekstra, M.H., & Rolkens, P.W.A. The chemical assay of norepinephrine and serotonin in the rat's brain. Acta Physiologica et Pharmacologica Neerlandica, 1962, 11, 300-302.

Spectrofluorophotometric estimation of levarterenol (norepinephrine) and serotonin in the whole brain of the rat yielded the following concentrations: levarterenol content, ca. 0.50 μg/g (tissue wet weight) and serotonin content, ca. 0.56 μg Recovery rates with levarterenol and serotonin added to the tissue ranged from 90-100%. Shore and Olin's (1958) acid purification method gave the same results for serotonin as did the alkaline purification method (Bogdanski), indicating a dearth of 5HT in rat brain. Results obtained with iproniazid and reserpine agreed with those found in the literature.

Department of Pharmacology
University of Utrecht
Utrecht, The Netherlands

1948 Gibbons, James L., & McHugh, Paul R. Plasma cortisol in depressive illness. Journal of Psychiatric Research, 1962, 1, 162-171.

Plasma cortisone (cortisol) was measured at weekly intervals in 17 depressed patient All except 1 case received small amounts of hypnotics (200-400 mg amylobarbital) because of insomnia. Later treatment consisted of ECT in 12 cases and imipram in 5, 2 of whom had ECT as well. The

phrenic and normal subjects. Journal of
Psychiatric Research, 1962, 1, 101-105.

Twelve schizophrenics and 11 volunteer
control subjects were given identical
diets for the experiment. Radioactive
l-histidine-C^{14} was administered orally
to these subjects and the radioactive
urinary metabolites were separated by
column chromatography and measured by
isotope dilution techniques. There was no
significant difference between the normal
and schizophrenic groups in the fraction
of radioactivity excreted, the amount of
C^{14} lost after urine concentration, the
urinary hydantoin-propionic acid-C^{14},
histidine-C^{14}, l-methylhistidine-C^{14} or
the combined value for free and conjugated
radioactive imidazoleacetic acid. No
evidence was found for the purpose of
qualitative differences in metabolites in
the schizophrenic group, nor did any
subject in either group lack any of the
known major histamine derivatives.

Laboratory of Clinical Science
NIH
Bethesda, Md.

1951 Mueller, Peter S. Plasma free fatty
acid concentrations (FFA) in chronic
schizophrenia before and after insulin
stimulation. Journal of Psychiatric
Research, 1962, 1, 106-115.

Two series of studies were undertaken
involving 12 male chronic schizophrenics
without somatic illness and 20 normal male
subjects. The same 12 schizophrenics
participated in both studies compared to 7
normal volunteers in the 1st and 13 in the
2nd, dealing respectively with plasma FFA
and blood glucose before and after 10/U
insulin i. m. Both studies were performed
after an overnight fast. In both studies
preinsulin FFA means of the normal and
schizophrenic patients were identical.
Mean fasting blood glucose concentrations
were significantly higher in the schizophrenic
group in the 2nd experiment. No other
significant difference was noted in blood
glucose. Both groups of subjects had
decreases in blood glucose of similar proportions. In both studies all normal subjects
had falls in FFA within a very narrow

range. Three patients in the 1st study and 4 in the 2nd had rises or no decreases in FFA after insulin. Eight schizophrenics in the 1st study and 5 in the 2nd had post-insulin FFA concentrations above the highest normal postinsulin FFA. Correlations showed a fair degree of consistency in both studies.

Laboratory of Clinical Science
NIMH
Bethesda, Md.

1952 McDonald, R.K., & Weise, V.K. The excretion of 3-methoxy-4-hydroxy-mandelic acid in normal and in chronic schizophrenic male subjects. Journal of Psychiatric Research, 1962, 1, 173-183.

Urinary vanilmandelic acid (VMA) was assayed by a modification of the tracer technique described by Weise (1961); urinary creatinine was determined by the alkaline picrate method. Seventeen healthy volunteers, 10 chronic and 3 acute schizophrenics, all male, were studied. Significant diurnal changes in VMA excretion rate occurred in both normal and chronic schizophrenic subjects. The VMA excretion rate was greater during the waking hours (8 a.m.-12 p.m.) than during the sleeping hours (12 p.m.-8 a.m.); this difference was not a function of the physical activity attending ordinary ambulatory activity. The chronic schizophrenic subjects tended to have a higher VMA excretion rate than the normal subjects, and the difference in excretion rates was significant when the subjects were kept on a 24-hour period of bed rest. The chronic schizophrenics excreted less creatinine than the normal subjects. This difference may be due to a difference in body composition between the 2 groups. Reserpine administration (2.5 mg i.m.) caused a similar increase in VMA excretion in both groups. Chlorpromazine administration (200 mg p.o.) caused a similar decrease in VMA excretion in both groups.

Laboratory of Clinical Science
NIMH
Bethesda, Md.

1953 Novák, I., Buzás, G., Tóth, L., & Simon, L. Beiträge zur vergleichenden Untersuchung des ungarischen und indischen Hanfes. [A comparative investigation of Hungarian and Indian hemp.] Pharmazie, 1962, 17, 95-98; 166-173.

In a 2-part article based on a contribution to a Hungarian symposium on medicinal plants, the authors first discuss the morphology and histology of hemp and then report the results of comparative studies of the ash, sand and moisture content and of the color reactions of approximately 20 varieties of Hungarian and Indian hemp using the alkaline Beam, acid Beam, Ghamrawy, Duquenois-Negm, modified British Pharmacopoea Codex, Rathenasinkam and Viehoever reactions. The results show that Hungarian hemp contains only traces of physiologically active alkaloids.

Institute of Pharmacognosy
Medical University
Szeged, Hungary

1954 Lewis, J.J., & Van Petten, Garry R. The effect of amphetamine and related compounds on the concentration of adenine nucleotides, inorganic phosphate and creatine phosphate in the rat brain. Journal of Pharmacology and Experimental Therapeutics, 1962, 136, 372-377.

Male Wistar rats were given i.p. injections of methamphetamine, amphetamine, dex-amphetamine, phenmetrazine (the bitartrate), phenmetrazine, l-phendimetrazine bitartrate and d-phendimetrazine bitartrate. After 1/2, 1 1/2, 3 or 4 hours, the rats were decapitated and the brain assayed for adenine nucleotides, inorganic phosphate and creatine phosphate, using a spectro-photometer. The order of treatment in each group was randomized, e.g., three 3 x 3 Latin squares. Four hours after treatment with methamphetamine, amphetamine, dexamphetamine, ephedrine, phenmetrazine and d-phendimetrazine there was an increase in the ATP/ADP ratio as a result of the increase of ATP level with concomitant decrease in ADP. The dose required to produce this effect appears to be correlated with the potency

is ca. 5 hours.

Wallace Laboratories
Cranbury, N. J.

1956 Irwin, Richard L., & Hein, Manfred
M. The inhibition of rat brain cholinesterase after administration of the dimethyl-
carbamates of deoxy-demethyl-lycoramine,
neostigmine or physostigmine. Journal of
Pharmacology and Experimental Therapeutics, 1962, 136, 20-25.

Male Osborne-Mendel rats were injected
i. p. with varying doses (0.084-1.14 mg/
kg) of the dimethyl-carbamate of deoxy-
demethyl-lycoramine methiodide (MCDL),
its tertiary analogue HCDL, neostigmine
bromide and physostigmine salicylate.
Each surviving animal was decapitated and
the entire brain removed (caudal part discarded) and used in the analysis of cholinesterase activity. After the administration
of ca. 20 doses (0.108 mg/kg) of MCDL the
activity of brain cholinesterase is essentially unchanged. When 1.39 mg/kg of MCDL,
the approximate LD 20 of HCDL, was given
to 9 rats pretreated with 2.0 mg/kg atropine, none survived. Two of the 5 animals
given 0.5 mg/kg atropine and 1.01 mg/kg
MCDL survived and had brain cholinesterase values within the normal range. In
contrast to MCDL the passage of neostigmine into the brain was detected in 1/3 of
the animals, occurring at both 0.069 mg/
kg and 0.835 mg/kg. The convulsions and
deaths observed after neostigmine or MCDL
occurred in 8-15 minutes. Using the tertiary
drugs physostigmine or HCDL these effects
were observed in 6-9 minutes. After physostigmine a rapid and marked inhibition of
brain cholinesterase occurred. Physostigmine was the only drug of the 4 tested
which reduced the level of cholinesterase
activity in the brain to less than 20%.

National Institute of Neurological Diseases
    and Blindness
NIH
Bethesda, Md.

1957 Guth, Paul S. Effect of phenothiazines
on neurohumor-containing particles from
mammalian brain. Federation Proceedings,
1962, 21, 1100-1102.

Isolated nerve endings from guinea pig brain tissue (0.4-2.0 g) containing synaptic vesicles were treated with varying concentrations of chlorpromazine ($5x10^{-5}$) under several releasing procedures to determine the efficacy of chlorpromazine in preventing acetylcholine release from vesicular membranes. Parallel work involved acetylcholine release in isolated guinea pig ileum by $100^{\circ}C$ at pH 4 followed by identification of the released neurohumor by destruction with acetylcholinesterase and alkaline blocking, atropine blocking and parallel assay procedures. With the isolated nerve ending preparations, chlorpromazine could not prevent release produced by incubation at $37^{\circ}C$ or dilution to 0.032M sucrose. Chlorpromazine inhibited release more at 4-fold dilution than at 5-fold, and still more at 6-fold dilution. Graphic illustration of results indicates a curvilinear relationship between drug concentration and inhibition. Addition of exogenous acetylcholine indicated that the particles rejected the neurohumor. However, application of massive concentrations forced a small fraction of acetylcholine into the nerve endings, which is termed input rather than uptake. Chlorpromazine inhibits input almost as effectively as it inhibits release. The brain apparently does not contain a membrane which is selectively permeable to chlorpromazine; rather, certain brain areas are believed to concentrate the drug to a considerable extent.

Department of Pharmacology
Tulane University School of Medicine
New Orleans, La.

1958 Phillips, Barrie M., & Miya, Tom S. Excretion of S^{35}-prochlorperazine to rats subjected to experimental stress. Proceedings of the Society for Experimental Biology and Medicine, 1962, 109, 576-577.

Male Holtzman rats stressed for 12 hours by the bilateral hind leg ligation method according to Dexter et al. (1953), received $10/\mu c$-175 g in an i.p. dose of 25 mg/kg prochlorperazine. They were placed in metabolism cages for 96 hours during which time urine and feces were collected. Rats subjected to experimental ligation excreted significantly smaller amounts of S^{35} in the urine following administration of S^{35}-prochlorperazine than did control animals. This

decreased excretion may be the result of diminished urine formation in stressed rats.

Department of Pharmacology
Purdue University
Lafayette, Ind.

1959 Gal, E. M., & Drewes, P. A. Studies on the metabolism of 5-hydroxytryptamine (serotonin). II. Effect of tryptophan deficiency in rats. Proceedings of the Society for Experimental Biology and Medicine, 1962, 110, 368-371.

Male Sprague-Dawley rats were divided into 4 groups; the 1st and 2nd groups were kept on tryptophan-sufficient diet with and without sulfasuxidine (10 g/kg), while the 3rd and 4th groups were on tryptophan-deficient diet with and without sulfasuxidine. The animals were fed these diets for a maximum of 6 weeks. Blood and weighed tissue samples were analyzed for 5HT content according to a modified method of Bogdanski et al. (1956). In some cases the animals were given a single i.p. injection of 1.86 mg/kg pheniprazine. Tryptophan-deficient rats showed significant decrease of 5HT in all their tissues analyzed. Feeding of sulfasuxidine, presumably through its antibacterial action, led to greater recovery of intestinal serotonin in tryptophan-deficient rats. Injection of pheniprazine resulted in a statistically significant increase of 5HT in the blood but not in the brain of deficient animals.

Department of Psychiatry
College of Medicine
State University of Iowa
Iowa City, Iowa

1960 Rosen, Lawrence, & Goodall, McC. Identification of vanillic acid as a catabolite of noradrenaline metabolism in the human. Proceedings of the Society for Experimental Biology and Medicine, 1962, 110, 767-769.

Four normal subjects were infused over a 1-hour period with 9.5 μc d,l-levarterenol-2-C^{14} (d,l-noradrenaline-2-C^{14}; specific activity 20 mc/mM). Vanillic acid was identified as a urinary catabolite of levarterenol in man through column chromatography and scintillometric measurement. The ultimate formation of a small amount of vanillic acid from levarterenol involved

In order to determine the rate of P^{32} incorporation into adenine nucleotides, the following fractions were isolated: inorganic phosphorus, hexose diphosphate, ADP and ATP. The inorganic phosphorus levels rose in each group during incubation. Hexose diphosphate levels decreased moderately in normal patients and nonpsychotics, but rose slightly in schizophrenics. Adenosinediphosphate levels decreased significantly ($p < 0.001$) in schizophrenics, but remained constant in other groups. Schizophrenics show a reduced requirement for high energy phosphate bonds over a period of time.

[No address]

1963 Gardner, Thomas S., Wenis, Edward, & Lee, John. Monoamine oxidase inhibitors. III. Structural variations in 1-alkyl and 1-aralkyl-1 (or 2) acyl-hydrazines. Journal of Medicinal and Pharmaceutical Chemistry, 1962, 5, 503-513.

Modifications were made in iproniazid for the purpose of achieving a more specific distribution of the drug in various tissues. A number of sugar acyl, 4-hydroxybutyryl and D-pantoyl derivatives of benzylhydrazine, 4-dimethylaminobenzylhyrazine, and α-methylphenethylhydrazine were prepared by reaction of the corresponding lactones with the substituted hydrazines. The reaction product of D-ribonolactone with benzylhydrazine was shown to be a N^1, N^2-hydrazine derivative. The most interesting compounds were 1-benzyl-2(D-ribonoyl) hydrazine, and 1-benzyl-2-(D-pantoyl) hydrazine. The variation of the structures of active MAO inhibitors, such as 1-isopropyl-2-isonicotinoylhydrazine, 1-benzyl-2-(5-methyl-3-isoxazolylcarbonyl)-hydrazine and 1-benzyl-2-picolinoylhydrazine, either eliminates or reduces MAO inhibitory activity. In one case, quaternization of 1-benzyl-2-picolinoylhydrazine with methyl iodide or methyl bromide increased response to 5HTP.

Hoffmann-La Roche Inc.
Nutley, N. J.

Biochemistry
Abstracts 1964-1967

1964 Anton, Aaron H., & Sayre, David F.
A study of the factors affecting the aluminum
oxide trihydroxyindole procedure for the
analysis of catecholamines. Journal of
Pharmacology and Experimental Therapeutics, 1962, 138, 360-375.

A reliable quantitative method for catecholamine estimation in diverse biological material, mainly urine, from various vertebrate species is presented. It involves the
selective adsorption of catecholamines onto
a constant amount of aluminum hydroxide,
elution with a constant volume of 0.05 N
perchloric acid and measurement by the
formation of fluorescent trihydroxyindole
derivatives in the presence of potassium
ferricyanide and 10 N alkali ascorbate.
The relative fluorescence for 25 analogues
of levarterenol are given.

Department of Psychiatry
University of Florida College of Medicine
Gainesville, Fla.

1965 Kopin, Irwin J., & Gordon, Edna K.
Metabolism of norepinephrine-H^3 released
by tyramine and reserpine. Journal of
Pharmacology and Experimental Therapeutics,
1962, 138, 351-359.

In order to study the fate of levarterenol-H^3
(norepinephrine-H^3) released from binding
sites by reserpine and tyramine, male
Sprague-Dawley rats were given d,l-levar-
terenol-7-H^3 (100/μc in 2 ml saline) i.v.
followed 10 hours later by either 4 i.v.
doses of 10 mg/kg tyramine at 15 minute
intervals or 2.5 mg/kg reserpine i.p.
Also levarterenol-H^3 (1.0/μc) or normetan-
ephrine-H^3 (1.0/μc) was slowly infused or
injected in divided doses over a 1-hour period with 2.5 mg/kg reserpine or with 10 mg/
kg tyramine in various schedules. As a result of tyramine administration, the bound
catecholamines are released directly into
the circulation; a small portion is metabolized in the tissue before release, predominantly by deamination; little levarterenol
is released in an active form.

Laboratory of Clinical Science
NIMH
Bethesda, Md.

1966 Resnick, Robert H., Gray, Seymour
J., Koch, James P., & Timberlake,
William H. Serotonin metabolism in
paralysis agitans. Proceedings of the
Society for Experimental Biology and
Medicine, 1962, 110, 77-79.

Metabolic observations in 10 cases of
paralysis agitans and 12 control patients
affected with other neurological diseases
were conducted. The cases collected were
free from liver dysfunction and azotemia,
and were not receiving psychoactive drugs.
In both groups endogenous 24-hour urinary
excretion of 5HT and its major metabolic
derivative 5HIAA were measured by standard techniques; these measurements were
repeated following i.v. administration of
0.66 mg/kg 5HTP. Determination of total
5-hydroxyindole excretion by a modification
of Udenfriend's procedure (1955) and paper
chromatography were also carried out on
urines collected following 5HTP infusion.
The metabolism of 5-hydroxyindolic compounds in paralysis agitans is similar to
that observed in other unselected neurological disorders. No clarification has yet
been made in relation to the possibility that
drug-induced extrapyramidal syndromes
may be caused by 5HT deficiency.

Department of Medicine
Harvard Medical School
Cambridge, Mass.

1967 Carver, Michael J. Effects of
sodium phenylpyruvate on brain amino
acids. Proceedings of the Society for
Experimental Biology and Medicine, 1962,
110, 171-173.

Brain slices from Sprague-Dawley rats
were incubated in air with 0.01 mM glucose
0.001 8mM sodium phenylpyruvate was adde
to the experimental Warburg flasks. The
free amino acids were isolated from the
tissue by the picric acid technique and
chromatography. Addition of phenylpyruvate resulted in an increase in brain phenylalanine with a decrease in aspartic and
glutamic acids, and glutamine. The concentration of other brain amino acids was
unaffected.

Blegdamshospitalet
Epidemisk afdeling
Blegdams, Denmark

1970 Eränkö, Olavi, Kokko, Aulikki, &
Söderholm, Ulla. Starch electrophoretic
separation of esterases in the adrenal
medulla, adrenal cortex and the brain of
the rat and the hamster. Annales Medicinae
Experimentalis et Biologiae Fenniae, 1962,
40, 146-161.

Extracts of rat and hamster brain, adrenal
medulla and cortex were subjected to
starch gel electrophoresis, according to
the method of Markert and Hunter (1959).
In all organs examined several reacting
esterase bands were observed using the
substrates α-naphthyl acetate, α-naphthyl
butyrate, acetylthiocholine and butyrylthiocholine, alone or with an inhibitor such as
eserine or 3 other compounds; inhibitor
concentrations were usually 10^{-5} M. The
bands differed from each other not only in
electrophoretic mobility but also in regard
to substrate and inhibitor characteristics.
Carbolic esterases appear to form a large
family of enzymes, all members of which
cannot be demonstrated with a single method.

Department of Anatomy
University of Helsinki
Helsinki, Finland

1971 Briggs, Michael H., Andrews, E.
David, Kitto, G. Barrie, Segal, Leah,
Graham, Venise, & Baillie, W. Jeavons. A
comparison of the metabolism of ascorbic
acid in schizophrenia, pregnancy and in
normal subjects. New Zealand Medical
Journal, 1962, 61, 555-558.

Urine samples collected from 15 male
schizophrenic patients (mean age 40 years,
mean duration of illness 12 years), 12 males
with various psychoses (i.e., manic-depressive, senile mania, etc., mean age 44 years,
mean duration of illness 7 years), 8 pregnant females (mean age 28 years), 9 normal females (mean age 31 years) and 16
normal males (mean age 29 years) were
analyzed to determine the concentrations of
ascorbate, dehydroascorbate and diketogu-
lonate by a differential 2,4-dinitrophenol

method. Results indicated an impairment in ascorbate metabolism in schizophrenics, based primarily upon continual partial inhibition of p-hydroxyphenylpyruvate oxidase, which interferes with phenylalanine oxidase and results in engorgement of tissues with excessive aromatic compounds. In all groups, the total percentage of free ascorbic acid correlated with total metabolites about 0.1%. In order to minimize variations in ascorbic acid intake, 24-hour-urine samples were obtained from 8 pregnant females and analyzed for the above metabolites to determine whether or not increases in ceruloplasmin and plasma copper were related to excessive breakdown of ascorbic acid. Low urinary ascorbate metabolite values were found for both pregnant females and schizophrenics. This evidence may support the findings of Adelstein et al (1956) and others that a sharp rise occurs in ceruloplasmin and plasma copper during late pregnancy.

Victoria University of Wellington
Wellington, New Zealand

1972 Novák, I., Háznagy, A., & Szendrei, K. Beiträge zur UV-spektrophotometrischen Untersuchung und zu den "Beam-Chlorwerten" des ungarischen und indischen Hanfes. [Contributions to the UV-spectrophotometry and the "Beam chlorine values" of Hungarian and Indian hemp.] Pharmazie, 1962, 17, 294-297.

The previously established fact that Hungarian hemp contains only traces of physiologically active substances was confirmed by the results of a semi-quantitative modification of the Beam reaction in petroleum-ether extracts and by UV absorption curves. The size of the secondary absorption maximum provides a quantitative indication of the content of physiologically active substances, while the Beam chlorine values are only suitable for a qualitative judgment.

Institute of Pharmacognosy
Medical University
Szeged, Hungary

1973 Vecerkova, J., Sulcova, M., & Kacl, K. Über den papierchromatographischen Nachweis der Antihistaminica und Atarac-

tica durch Umkehrphasenchromatographie im System Petroleum-Athanol/Wasser/ Ammoniak. [The paper-chromatographic determination of antihistamines and tranquilizers by reversed-phase chromatography in the system petroleum-ethanol/water/ ammonia.] Pharmazie, 1962, 17, 22-29.

Determination of the R_f-values of 24 antihistamines and tranquilizers (including 20 with a tertiary N and 4 with a quaternary N) in 5 solvent systems with a constant ammonia concentration (2%) and an ethanol concentration varying from 55 to 95% (descending chromatography at 12-15°C) showed that the mobility of compounds with a tertiary N increased with increasing ethanol concentration while that of quaternary compounds could be divided into 3 subgroups: 5 compounds in which there was a linear relationship between R_f-value and ethanol concentration, 9 compounds in which there was a more pronounced increase in R_f at lower ethanol concentrations, followed by leveling off, and 6 compounds which practically accompanied the solvent front. This system is therefore most useful for separating mixtures containing only 1 compound from each subgroup. A chart showing the color reactions of these compounds with H_2SO_4, HNO_3, $PdCl_2$, $FeCl_3$, $AuCl_3$, $Ce(SO_4)_2$ and Ehrlich's reagent is also presented.

Laboratory for Toxicology and Legal Chemistry
Charles University
Prague, Czechoslovakia

1974 Klöcking, H.-P., & Walter, H. Über eine modifizierte Murexidreaktion zum qualitativen Nachweis von Barbitursäure- und Thiobarbitursäurederivaten. [A modified murexide reaction for the qualitative detection of barbituric acid and thiobarbituric acid derivatives.] Pharmazie, 1962, 17, 277-280.

Two simplifications of Handorf murexide reaction were used for the identification of barbiturates and thiobarbiturates in either pure form or commercial mixed preparations. The sensitivity thresholds of the 2 methods are given for 20 barbiturates and

coprecipitation (incomplete precipitation of other alkaloids by molybdate). The method is therefore usable only for a limited range of concentrations of pure morphine.

Pharmazeutisches Institut
Humboldt - Universität
Berlin, Germany

1977 Gonnard, Pierre. Effect of hydrazides and hydrazones of pyridoxal-5-phos-
phate on the cerebral glutamic decarboxylase and pyridoxal phosphokinase. Acta
Neurologica Scandinavica, 1962, 38, 28-29.

Warburg manometric measurement of CO_2
output in cerebral glutamic acid decarboxylase of the rat, guinea pig and rabbit invariably demonstrates a deficiency of coenzyme
in reference to the apoenzyme. Addition of
pyridoxal phosphate greatly enhances CO_2
output. Pre-incubation of ATP pyridoxal
and rabbit cerebral pyridoxal phosphokinase
without preliminary incubation with glutamic
decarboxylase and its substrate prevents
phosphorylation of the pyridoxal. Although
the pyridoxal phosphate hydrazones can
function as coenzymes, the possibility of
hydrazone hydrolysis releasing the pyridoxal phosphate during incubation must be
discarded on the basis of evidence obtained
by paper chromatography, the kinetics of the
decarboxylation itself, and the lack of
hydrolysis undergone by the hydrazone in
pre-incubation studies. Therefore, the in
vivo and in vitro pyridoxal phosphate
deficiency induced by isoniazid cannot be
attributed to a blocking of the coenzyme,
for the above results confirm those formerly obtained with other pyridoxal enzymes.
Other results indicate that addition of a
small quantity of isoniazid to the pre-
incubation medium completely inhibits
pyridoxal phosphate formation without
enhancing subsequent decarboxylation. Addition of isoniazid, decarboxylase and substrate after pre-incubation in no way inhibits
decarboxylation.

Nouvelle Faculté de Médecine
45 Rue des Sts-Pères
Paris 6e, France

1978 Barron, Kevin D., Bernsohn,
Joseph, & Hess, Adeline R. Electrophoretic

analysis of human brain esterases. Acta Neurologica Scandinavica, 1962, 38, Suppl. 1, 61-62.

Postmortem human brain esterases were studied by vertical starch gel electrophoresis of saline homogenates followed by application of histochemical staining techniques to the gel (zymogram). Enzymic activities of grey and white matter from the frontal, temporal, parietal, occipital and limbic lobes, telencephalic and diencephalic nuclei, brain stem and cerebellum were studied employing various esters of α-naphthol and β-naphthol, thioesterase iodides, chlorides, N-benzoyl-DL-arginine-β-naphthylamide (BANA) etc. as substrates. Enzyme activities have been surveyed over a pH range of 5.0-8.0 with determinations of susceptibility to fixation, aging and heat. Sixteen bands of nonspecific esterolytic activity occur against α-naphthyl acetate in normal white matter, while several additional bands occur with propionate and butyrate esters. Thioesterase resolves into 3 major bands. At least 4 zones of enzymic activity occur against BANA. Multiple bands of cholinesterase activity are also demonstrable and, in caudate-putamen, acetylcholinesterase activity resolves into 3 distinct zones. Nonspecific esterase and thioesterase are largely inhibited by cupric salts (10^{-3}M). Cholinesterase activities are eliminated by eserine (10^{-5}M) E 600 (10^{-6}M) TEPP (10^{-6}M) and DFP (10^{-5}M). Quantitative estimations of enzyme activities were made by reflection densitometry. Differences in substrate optima and inhibitor sensitivity have supported the concept that the numerous bands of activity shown by the varied staining techniques are due to specific molecular species of enzymes.

Neuropsychiatric Research Laboratory
VA Hospital
Hines, Ill.

1979 Carlsson, Arvid, Falck, Bengt, Hillarp, Nils-Ake, & Torp, Alf. Histochemical localization at the cellular level of hypothalamic noradrenaline. Acta Physiologica Scandinavica, 1962, 54, 385-386.

Catecholamines of the freeze-dried hypothalamus (mouse, rat, rabbit) were condensed with formaldehyde to highly fluorescent isoquinoline derivatives; serial sections were examined in a fluorescence microscope and then stained with toluidine blue. A rather intense yellow-green fluorescence develops in 3 circumscript and bilaterally symmetrical areas within the hypothalamus: a large area in the preoptic region just ventrally and slightly dorsally to the anterior commisure with its largest extension in the lateral part; the supraoptic nuclei and the paraventricular nuclei. The fluorescent products are localized to very fine fibres running between and partially enclosing the nerve cells which themselves, like the glia cells, showed no fluorescence. The fibres, although finer, have the same characteristic appearance as the adrenergic nerve terminals in peripheral tissues, with small intensely fluorescent enlargments dispersed at irregular intervals. However they are not ordinary adrenergic nerves to blood vessels, as bilateral cervical sympathectomy does not cause them to disappear. The fibres probably represent synaptic terminals derived from brain neurons. The fluorescing substances are probably levarterenol(noradrenaline), dopamine and 5HT. Fluorescence disappears within 24 hours after the administration of 5 mg/kg reserpine s.c. to rats, and does not reappear for days. Administration of m-tyrosine in doses that deplete the hypothalamus of catecholamines but not 5HT also caused the fluorescence to disappear. Thus it appears that levarterenol in the hypothalamus is accumulated in what appears to be synaptic nerve terminals. Also there seems to be a local accumulation of levarterenol or possibly dopamine in the median eminence where the hypophysial porta system arises.

Department of Pharmacology
University of Göteborg
Göteborg, Sweden

1980 DeGiacomo, Piero. Histochemical research on some aspects of acetylcholinesterase and its inhibitors in the CNS. Acta Neurologica Scandinavica, 1962, 38, Suppl. 1, 55-56.

Gomori's method was used to determine the effect of certain reversible and irreversible inhibitors of cholinesterase on the CNS and

phosphatidylinositol uptake and no action on
phosphatidic acid. Lower concentrations
$(10^{-4}M)$ however stimulated phosphate
exchange in phosphatidic acid, had no effect
on other phospholipids. Addition of ATP
had no effect on chlorpromazine action.
If the ATP was added 20 minutes before
chlorpromazine, then the uptake into
phosphatidic acid and phosphatidylinositol
was partially restored to control levels
though uptake into phosphatidylcholine and
-ethanolamine was still completely inhibited.

Department of Experimental Neuropharma-
    cology
University of Birmingham Medical School
Birmingham 15, Great Britain

1982 Lagnado, J.R. Electrophoretic
separation of rat brain esterases in starch
gel medium. Acta Neurologica Scandinavica,
1962, <u>38</u>, 63-64.

Electrophoresis of particle-free extracts
of rat brain in starch gel medium resulted
in the separation of 9-10 esterase bands as
revealed by a technique similar to that of
Hunter & Markert (1957). α-Naphthylacetate
was used as a substrate. Cholinesterases
were distinguished from other esterases by
the use of neostigmine or eserine sulphate
$(10^{-5}M)$; acetylcholinesterases were
specifically inhibited by 62 C 47 $(10^{-5}M)$.
E 600 $(10^{-6}-10^{-5}M)$ and p-chloromercuri-
benzoate $(10^{-4}M)$ were employed to
differentiate between arylesterases,
carboxylesterases and C-esterases. Plani-
metry of the stained gel scans showed that
cholinesterases (both types) contributed
45-55% of the total amount of developer
deposited (naphthalene black 10 B); the
remainder was contributed by arylesterases
(ca. 35%), carboxylesterases (ca. 12%)
and C-esterases (ca. 8%). Esterase zymo-
grams obtained using extracts of newborn
rat brains differed from those from adults
in that carboxylesterase was virtually absent
and the two arylesterases migrated more
slowly.

Medical Research Council
Neuropsychiatric Research Unit
Carshalton, Surrey
Great Britain

See also 1680, 1690, 1692, 1715, 1718,
1754, 1762, 1808, 1886, 1910, 1911, 1912,
1930

α-KG	α-ketoglutarate	HD
AACL	Zuckerman's Affect Adjustive Check List	5HIAA
		5HT
ACTH	adrenocorticotropic hormone	5HTP
ad lib.	free choice	
ADP	adenosinediphosphate	i. a.
AM	morning	ibid.
AMA	American Medical Association	i. e.
Art.	Article	i. m.
ATP	adenosinetriphosphate	IMPS
BAL	British antiLewisite	i. p.
BAS	benzyl analogue of serotonin	IPAT
b. i. d.	twice a day	
BOL	bromolysergic acid diethylamide	IQ
BUN	blood urea nitrogen	IU
		i. v.
ca.	about	
CAR	conditioned avoidance response	kg
CBS	chronic brain syndrome	K_i
cc	cubic centimeter	K_m
CDC	Communicable Disease Center	
cm^2	square centimeter	lbs
cm^3	cubic centimeter	LD
C. N. R. S.	Centre National de la Recherche Scientifique	LSD
CNS	central nervous system	μ
COMT	catechol-o-methyl transferase	μc
cpm	counts per minute	μg
cps	counts per second	μl
CR	conditioned reflex(response)	μM
CS	conditioned stimulus	m
CTD	climbing time delay	M
		ma.
DDT	dichlorodiphenyl trichlorethane	MACC
DNA	deoxyribonucleic acid	
DOPA	3, 4-dihydroxy-phenylalanine	MAO
DPN	diphosphopyridinenucleotide	MAS
DPNH	reduced diphosphopyridine-nucleotide	meq
		ml
		mm
ECG	electrocardiogram	mM
Ed.	editor	mm^2
ED	effective dose	MMPI
EDTA	ethylenediaminetetraacetic acid	
EEG	electroencephalogram	MSRPP
e. g.	for example	
ERG	electroretinogram	
et al.	and others	N
etc.	and so forth	NEFA
		NIH
FFA	free fatty acid	NIMH
g	gram	p
GABA	γ-aminobutyric acid	PAH
GABOB	γ-amino-β-hydroxybutyric acid	PBI

negative logarithm of hydrogen
  ion concentration
afternoon and evening
by mouth
parts per million
Psychotic Reaction Profile

four times a day

references
ratio of the distance of dissolved
  substance to solvent distance
ribonucleic acid
rat unit

subcutaneous
standard deviation
serum glutamic oxaloacetic
  transaminase
serum glutamic pyruvic
  transaminase
exactly as found
Springfield Symptom and
  Adjustment Index
Science Research Associates
supplement

TD	toxic dose
TH	thyroid hormone
t. i. d.	three times a day
TPN	triphosphopyridinenucleotide
TPNH	reduced triphosphopyridine-nucleotide
TSH	thyroid-stimulating hormone
U	unit
UR	unconditioned response
US	unconditioned stimulus
USAF	United States Air Force
USDHEW	United States Department of Health, Education, and Welfare
USP	United States Pharmacopoeia
USPHS	United States Public Health Service
UV	ultraviolet
VA	Veterans Administration
viz.	namely
WAIA	Wechsler Adult Intelligence Scale
WHO	World Health Organization
WPRS	Wechsler Psychiatric Rating Scale

	HAMILTON-HISLOP H G, 1854
6, 1930	HANGAARD GUNNAR, 1875
	HARENKO A, 1879
	HARMANN-VON MANOKOW K, 1723
	HARRIS E L, 1688
	HART J J D, 1896
	HARTHORNE J W, 1890
	HARTMAN ALAN M, 1902
	HAYDU GEORGE G, 1808
1805	HAZNAGY A, 1972
812	HEARST ELIOT, 1901
	HECHT R A, 1845
	HEIN MANDRED M, 1956
	HESS ADELINE R, 1978
26	HIFT ST, 1760
	HIGHMAN B, 1909
	HIGHMAN BENJAMIN, 1915
812	HILLARP NILS-AKE, 1979
	HIRSCH SOLOMON, 1669
	HOBBS G E, 1882
E, 1903	HOCH ERNA M, 1784
	HOEKSTRA M H, 1947
95	HOFF H, 1760
	HOFFER A, 1700
	HOFMANN A, 1715
	HOFMANN VOLKER, 1815
	HOHMAN LESLIE B, 1702
	HOLLISTER LEO E, 1674, 1902
2	HOLMBERG GUNNAR, 1822
	HOPKINS PAUL, 1866
	HUBATA J A, 1845
	HUVANANDANA MALAI, 1751
	IISALO ESKO, 1830
	INGLIS W, 1725
	IRVINE J H, 1667
7	IRWIN J, 1894
	IRWIN RICHARD L, 1956
	ISBELL HARRIS, 1905
A, 1805	JAMES L S, 1701
	JANSSEN PAUL, 1715, 1737
	JANZ DIETER, 1719
	JARPE GUNDLA, 1903
	JENSEN S E, 1677
1813	JORGENSEN FINN, 1874
	JOSEPH SAMUEL R, 1833
	JOUBERT P, 1811
0	JOURNAL OF THE AMA, 1750
26	JUNKENITZ KARL WALTER, 1799
41	JUNNEMANN H J, 1840
	KAARTINEN MATTI, 1819
	KACL K, 1943, 1973
	KAMMERER TH, 1835, 1842
	KAPFERER J M, 1798
	KASANEN A, 1712
1855, 1856	KASPERAT H, 1919
	KATSAS GOERGE G, 1886
	KAYE M, 1890
	KAYE SIDNEY, 1938
	KETY SEYMOUR S, 1733
	KINGSBURY BRYANT, 1935

KINNARD WILLIAM J, 1895
KITTO G BARRIE, 1971
KLOCKING H-P, 1942, 1974, 1975
KNAPMAN WILLIAM B, 1671
KNAPP K, 1859
KOCH JAMES P, 1966
KOECHLIN BERNARD A, 1911
KOHLICEK J, 1943
KOKKO AULIKKI, 1970
KOPELOFF LENORE M, 1918
KOPIN IRWIN J, 1965
KORMAN MAURICE KNOPF, 1894
KRISTENSEN KEETY K, 1834
KRISTJANSEN P, 1828
KRONHOLM V, 1829
KRUGER H J, 1840
KURLAND ALBERT A, 1775
LAGNADO J R, 1982
LAI G, 1839
LAINE, 1704, 1705, 1812
LANCET, 1691
LAPINSHON L I, 1820
LARSON ROBERT E, 1916
LAUNAY J, 1920
LAVERNE ALBERT A, 1778, 1779
LEDOUX MICHEL, 1787
LEE JOHN, 1963
LEFEVRE, 1705
LENDLE L, 1717
LENZ W, 1859
LEON ROBERT L, 1894
LEREBOULLET JEAN, 1787
LEROY C, 1851
LEVY, 1842
LEVY JEANNE, 1938
LEWIS J J, 1954
LIBERSON W T, 1758
LINDER WILHELM, 1801
LINGJAERDE ODD, 1710, 1738
LINKE H, 1707, 1761
LISANTI VINCENT F, 1789
LOISEAU P, 1878
LONG R F, 1939
LUBY ELLIOT D, 1672
LUDWIG B J, 1910, 1955
LULLMANN H, 1663
LUONGO MICHAEL A, 1886
LUTH PAUL, 1720
MACGREGOR A G, 1685, 1686
MACKENZIE ROBERT D, 1931
MACRIS SPYROS G, 1813
MALING H M, 1909
MALING HARRIET M, 1915
MALL G, 1840
MANDELL ARNOLD J, 1852
MANDELL MARY P, 1852
MANN WARREN A, 1746
MANS J P, 1810
MARCUS A M, 1890

MARK LESTER C, 1703
MARKHAM CHARLES H, 1852
MARKOWITZ S D, 1925
MARKS JOHN, 1743
MARSHALL ARTHUR, 1822
MARSHALL E F, 1981
MARTIN W R, 1913
MASERA ALVARO, 1809
MATHIS, 1704, 1705, 1812
MATHISEN H STORM, 1836
MATTSSON EIRA, 1822
MATTSSON NILS, 1822
MAX PAUL, 1882
MCALLISTER DONALD, 1838
MCCLEERY W N C, 1887
MCDONALD, 1950
MCDONALD R K, 1952
MCGAUGH JAMES L, 1901
MCGRATH W ROBERT, 1931
MCHUGH PAUL R, 1948
MCKAY D N, 1740
MCLOUGHLIN GEORGE, 1887
MELLETT L B, 1924
MELVIN K W W, 1872
MENDELSON JOSEPH, 1903, 1905
MERLEVEDE E, 1934
MERLIS SIDNEY, 1807
MERRIMAN B, 1687
MERRITT H HOUSTON, 1696, 1724
MEYER JOACHIM-ERNST, 1694
MEYLER L, 1753
MINER E J, 1905
MISRAHI R, 1811
MIYA TOM S, 1958
MOL W, 1766
MONTANARI R, 1908
MOORE JAMES, 1732
MORASKI R, 1885
MOSHEIN PETER, 1904
MOYER K E, 1904
MUELLER PETER S, 1951
MUKERJI B, 1735
MULE S J, 1923, 1924
MULLENDER H, 1821
MUNDELEER P, 1797
MURAMATSU MASAMI, 1692
MYRSTEN ANNA-LISA, 1903
NAESS KNUT, 1714, 1749
NESSWETHA LIESELOTTE, 1864
NILSSON E, 1795
NOACH E L, 1946
NORDENFELT OLOF, 1711
NORREDAM KAI, 1969
NOVAK I, 1953, 1972
NUSSBAUM HARVEY E, 1857
OBERHAENSLI WILLIAM E, 1911
ODEGARD ORNULV, 1727
OFFENKRANTZ WILLIAM, 1767
OLLENDORFF R H V, 1853
OREILLEY MARK, 1935

WALSH P J F, 1814
WALTER H, 1942, 1974, 1974
WARREN M R, 1896
WARTEL R, 1842
WAY E LEONG, 1763
WEINER HERBERT, 1695
WEINER MYRON F, 1682
WEINER N, 1927
WEIR D G, 1883
WEISE V K, 1952
WENIS EDWARD, 1963
WENTZLER J DONALD, 1846
WETTA J M, 1835
WHALEN RICHARD E, 1901

WHO TECHNICAL REPORT, 1765
WICKSTROM LENNART, 1818
WIESER STEFAN, 1662
WIGGLESWORTH ROBERT, 1868
WINICK CHARLES, 1770
WINTER D, 1937
WOLBACH A B, 1905
WOODS L A, 1923, 1924
WOODYATT P B, 1867
WOZNIAK LILLIAN A, 1885
WRIGHT O L, 1871
WUNDERLICH H, 1729
ZIFFER HERMAN, 1961
ZIMMERMAN GEORGE B, 1914,

EX
bstracts
subject headings

N DOGS, 1934

TS, 1936

 1754

1907

1880
1741, 1753, 1775, 1877

N DOGS, 1934

684, 1746

ESERINE, 1980
ESTERASE
    ELECTROPHORETIC SEPARATION IN BRAIN AND ADRENALS IN VITRO, 1970
ETHCHLORVYNOL, 1775
    OVERDOSAGE, 1886
ETHOPROPAZINE
    IN PARKINSON DISEASE, 1696
    IN THE TREATMENT OF PARKINSONS DISEASE, 1774
EUPHORIA AS SIDE EFFECT, 1834, 1836, 1905
EXTRAPYRAMIDAL REACTIONS AS SIDE EFFECT, 1788, 1798, 1801, 1825, 1828,
                1831, 1834, 1835, 1842
    TREATMENT, 1723
FAINTING AS SIDE EFFECT, 1834
FARNSWORTH-MUNSELL HUE DISCRIMINATION TEST, 1901
FATAL POISONING, 1873
FATIGUE AS SIDE EFFECT, 1807, 1845
FATIGUE TREATMENT, 1767
FETAL DEVELOPMENT, 1866, 1869, 1871
FETAL MALFORMATION, 1686, 1689, 1693, 1766, 1769, 1781, 1866, 1869,
                1871, 1906
FLUPHENAZINE
    IN GERIATRICS, 1809
    SIDE EFFECTS, 1880
GASTROINTESTINAL DISORDER AS SIDE EFFECT, 1663
GASTROINTESTINAL DISORDER TREATMENT, 1857
GERMAN PSYCHIATRY
    TRENDS IN, 1694
GILLES DE LA TOURETTES DISEASE, 1814
GLUCAGON, 1779
GLUE SNIFFING
    DETRIMENTAL EFFECTS, 1750
GLUTETHIMIDE, 1714, 1714, 1775
    IN INSOMNIA, 1854
    IN TREATMENT OF NEUROLEPTIC SIDE EFFECTS, 1801, 1831
    INTOXICATION, 1883
GRIMACING AS SIDE EFFECT, 1872
GUANETHIDINE
    IN THE TREATMENT OF HYPERTENSION, 1664
GUINEA PIG, 1914, 1919, 1940, 1957, 1977
HABITUATION
    COCA, 1782
HALLUCINATIONS AS SIDE EFFECT, 1822
HALLUCINOGENS SEE PSYCHOTOMIMETICS
HALOPERIDOL, 1787, 1788, 1795, 1797
    SIDE EFFECTS, 1880
    SURGICAL ANESTHESIA, 1798
HAMSTER, 1970
HARMALINE, 1760
    EFFECT ON HUMAN BRAIN MAO IN VITRO, 1939
    EFFECT ON MOUSE BRAIN MAO IN VITRO, 1939
HARTNUP DISEASE, 1762
HEADACHE AS SIDE EFFECT, 1807, 1824, 1829, 1865
HEBEPHRENIA SEE SCHIZOPHRENIA HEBEPHRENIC TYPE
HEDONAL
    EFFECT ON CRS IN RATS, 1900
HEMODIALYSIS, 1889, 1890

HEMP HUNGARIAN, 1735
    ALKALOID CONTENT, 1953, 1972
    MORPHOLOGY, 1953
    SPECTROPHOTOMETRY, 1972
HEMP INDIAN, 1735
    ALKALOID CONTENT, 1953, 1972
    MORPHOLOGY, 1953
    SPECTROPHOTOMETRY, 1972
HEPATIC DAMAGE SEE LIVER DAMAGE
HEPATOTOXICITY SEE LIVER DAMAGE
HEROIN
    EFFECT ON MENTAL PERFORMANCE, 1898
    SUBJECTIVE EFFECTS, 1897
    SURGICAL ANALGESIA, 1813
HEXACYCLONATE
    ANALEPTIC EFFECTS, 1812
    IN CBS, 1812
    IN OLIGOPHRENIA, 1812
HEXAFLUORODIETHYL ETHER, 1779
HEXAMETHONIUM
    EFFECT ON ATRIUM TO VAGUS STIMULATION AFTER ATROPINE, 1919
    EFFECT ON STOMACH TO VAGUS STIMULATION AFTER ATROPINE, 1919
    POSTGANGLIONIC RESPONSE IN CATS, 1921
HICCOUGH AS SIDE EFFECT, 1827
HIDDEN FACES, 1898
HISTIDINE
    METABOLISM IN SCHIZOPHRENICS, 1950
HISTOCHEMISTRY, 1980
    CEREBRAL CATECHOLAMINES, 1979
HUNTINGTONS CHOREA, 1788
HYDANTOINS, 1878
    AGRANULOCYTOSIS AS SIDE EFFECT, 1753
    IN EPILEPSY, 1719
HYDERGINE, 1795
HYDRAZIDES, 1760
    EFFECT ON CEREBRAL GLUTAMIC DECARBOXYLASE, 1977
    EFFECT ON PYRIDOXAL PHOSPHOKINASE, 1977
HYDROXYAMPHETAMINE
    IN OBSTETRICS, 1821
HYDROXYMEBUTAMATE
    TOXICITY IN MICE, 1955
M-HYDROXYPHENYLETHANOLAMINE
    IN TREATMENT OF HYPOTENSION DUE TO PSYCHOTROPIC DRUGS, 1858
HYDROXYPETHIDINE
    IN MENOPAUSE, 1845
    IN NEUROSIS, 1845
HYDROXYTRYPTAMINE SEE DOPAMINE
5-HYDROXYTRYPTAMINE SEE SEROTONIN
HYDROXYZINE
    IN INSOMNIA, 1816

MECLOZINE
    EFFECT ON FETAL DEVELOPMENT, 1866
    WITH PYRIDOXINE EFFECT ON FETAL DEVELOPMENT, 1866
MEGACOLON AS SIDE EFFECT, 1914
MELANCHOLIA, 1856
    , 1802, 1845
MENTAL RETARDATION, 1762
    BIOGENETICS, 1762
MENTAL STRESS SEE STRESS
MEPERIDINE, 1841, 1847
    IN PORPHYRIA, 1887
MEPHENESIN
    EFFECT ON STRETCH REFLEX IN CATS, 1922
MEPHENOXALONE
    TOXICITY IN DOGS, 1885
    TOXICITY IN RAT, 1885
MEPHENYTOIN, 1663
MEPROBAMATE, 1775
    ADDICTION, 1882
    EFFECT ON CRS IN RATS, 1900
    EFFECT ON ENZYMATIC ACTIVITY, 1912
    EFFECT ON PERSONALITY, 1722
    IN ANXIETY, 1722
    IN ASTHMA, 1757
    IN DEPRESSION, 1756
    IN MANIC DEPRESSIVE REACTION DEPRESSED TYPE, 1748
    IN NEUROSIS, 1837
    IN THE TREATMENT OF HYPERTENSION, 1664
    WITH IMIPRAMINE IN ACUTE ALCOHOLISM, 1837
    WITH IMIPRAMINE IN AGITATION, 1837
    WITH IMIPRAMINE IN DEPRESSION, 1837
    WITH IMIPRAMINE IN MELANCHOLIA, 1837
    WITH PROTHIPENDYL AND CHLORPROMAZINE OVERDOSAGE, 1876
    WITH YOHIMBINE AND BELLADONNA IN HYPEREMESIS GRAVIDARUM, 1802
    WITH YOHIMBINE AND BELLADONNA IN MENOPAUSE, 1802
    WITH YOHIMBINE AND BELLADONNA IN OBSTETRICS, 1802
    WITH YOHIMBINE AND BELLADONNA IN PREMENSTRUAL TENSION, 1802
MERCAPTOTHIAZINYL, 1968
MESCALINE, 1760, 1778, 1785, 1901
METHAMINODIAZEPOXIDE SEE CHLORDIAZEPOXIDE
METHAMPHETAMINE, 1780
    EFFECT ON BRAIN ADENINE NUCLEOTIDES AND CREATINE PHOSPHATE, 1954
METHOCARBAMOL
    POTENTIATING EFFECT ON AMOBARBITAL IN RATS, 1936
1-METHYL-5,5-PHENYLETHYLHYDANTOIN
    IN EPILEPSY, 1794
A-METHYL-DOPA
    CAUSING AGRANULOCYTOSIS, 1877
    EFFECT ON MOUSE BRAIN MAO IN VITRO, 1939
    IN HYPERTENSION, 1836
N-METHYLATION
    ENZYMATIC, 1949
METHYLPENTYNOL CARBAMATE
    SURGICAL ANESTHESIA, 1798
METHYLPHENIDATE
    IN ASTHMA, 1757

METHYLPHENOBARBITAL, 1760
    ADDICTION, 1874
    ANALGESIC EFFECT ON TRIGEMINAL NEURALGIA, 1790
    IN DEPRESSION, 1703, 1790
A-METHYLTRYPTAMINE
    EFFECT ON HUMAN BRAIN MAO IN VITRO, 1939
METHYPRYLON, 1714
MINNESOTA MULTIPHASIC PERSONALITY INVENTORY, 1852
MIRROR DRAWING, 1822
MONKEY, 1918, 1920
    SQUIRREL, 1909, 1915
MONOAMINE OXIDASE INHIBITORS, 1800, 1963
    IN DEPRESSION, 1666, 1681, 1756
    IN MANIC DEPRESSIVE REACTION, 1856
    IN SCHIZOPHRENIA, 1666
    SIDE EFFECTS, 1666 , 1888
    WITH PHENOTHIAZINES SIDE EFFECTS, 1864
MORPHINE, 1780
    ABSORPTION, 1763
    ADDICTION, 1913
    BIOTRANSFORMATION, 1763
    CHEMISTRY AND PHARMACOL PROPERTIES, 1715
    CONJUGATION, 1763
    DISTRIBUTION, 1763
    DISTRIBUTION AND METABOLISM, 1924
    DISTRIBUTION IN CNS, 1923
    EFFECT ON MENTAL PERFORMANCE, 1898
    EFFECT ON SERUM TRANSAMINASE LEVELS, 1969
    EXCRETION, 1763
    HYDROLYSIS, 1763
    MECHANISM OF ACTION, 1737
    METABOLISM, 1763
    N-DEMETHYLATION, 1763
    O-DEMETHYLATION, 1763
    OVERDOSAGE TREATMENT, 1698
    PHARMACOLOGICAL EFFECTS, 1913
    QUANTITATIVE DETERMINATION, 1976
    SUBJECTIVE EFFECTS, 1897
    SURGICAL ANALGESIA, 1813
    TOLERANCE IN DOGS, 1923
    TOXICITY, 1933
    WITH ATROPINE TOXICITY, 1933
MORPHINE DERIVATIVES, 1768
MOUSE, 1716, 1780, 1895, 1896, 1916, 1929, 1932, 1933, 1937, 1939,
        1955, 1968
MUREXIDE REACTION, 1942, 1974
MUSCULAR INCOORDINATION AS SIDE EFFECT, 1886
MYDRIASIS AS SIDE EFFECT, 1865
NALORPHINE
    EFFECT ON DISTRIBUTION OF MORPHINE IN CNS, 1924
    EFFECT ON MORPHINE ADDICTION IN CATS, 1913
NAME-FACE TEST, 1898
NARCOTICS, 1770
NATIONAL PARKINSON FOUNDATION, 1774
NAUSEA AS SIDE EFFECT, 1775, 1806, 1809, 1823, 1824, 1831, 1865, 1875
NEOSTIGMINE, 1780
    EFFECT ON CEREBRAL CHOLINESTERASE IN RATS, 1956

51, 1952, 1962, 1971

22
SE, 1774
RUG EVALUATION

IN INSOMNIA, 1816

4

6
N RATS, 1936
7

1683, 1715, 1729, 1730, 1731,

1

834, 1865, 1876, 1886

1823, 1825, 1826, 1837, 1864,

```
 1930
 LEVELS, 1926
1926

TABOLISM IN RATS, 1945

TABOLISM IN RATS, 1945

9
R, 1716

E, 1814

 1833
ON, 1833

1846


RESSED TYPE, 1801, 1831

31


ISEASE, 1774

IN MICE, 1929


LS IN RATS, 1959
 LEVELS, 1926
MINES TO TRANYLCYPROMINE, 1926
1926



SM IN RATS, 1965




IN MAN, 1960

ICS, 1952

663, 1865

1726



785
```

If you do not wish to continue receiving this publication, please check here ☐ tear off this label and return it to the address shown above. Your name will then be removed from the mailing list.

PSYCHOPHARMACOLOGY ABSTRACTS is a publication of the
National Clearinghouse for Mental Health Information
of the National Institute of Mental Health. It is a
specialized information medium designed to assist the
Institute in meeting its obligation to foster and support laboratory and clinical research into the nature
and causes of mental disorders and methods of treatment and prevention. Specifically, this information
service is designed to meet the needs of investigators in the field of psychopharmacology for rapid and
comprehensive information about new developments and
research results.

PSYCHOPHARMACOLOGY ABSTRACTS is distributed gratis to
investigators doing research in psychopharmacology. It
is not available on a subscription basis. Requests
to receive the ABSTRACTS should be accompanied by a
brief statement of the research interests and scientific specialty of the investigator. Requests to receive the ABSTRACTS, address changes, and other communications should be addressed to:

>   Psychopharmacology Abstracts
>   National Clearinghouse for Mental
>   Health Information
>   National Institute of Mental Health
>   Bethesda 14, Maryland

(The text of PSYCHOPHARMACOLOGY ABSTRACTS is prepared
under contract with the Literary Division of Biological and Medical Services, Philadelphia, Penna.)

U. S. DEPARTMENT OF HEALTH, EDUCATION AND WELFARE
Public Health Service
National Institutes of Health
National Institute of Mental Health
Bethesda 14, Maryland

PSYCHOPHARMACOLOGY ABSTRACTS

Volume 2, Number 9

reserpine casts some doubt on this premise.
Possible mechanisms of action and the
possibilities of reciprocal relationships
are discussed. (83 refs.)

Department of Pharmacology
University of Washington Medical School
Seattle, Wash.

1986 Harney, Malachi L.   Current provisions and practices in the United States
of America relating to the commitment of
opiate addicts. Bulletin on Narcotics, 1962,
14, 11-24.

The history of narcotic addiction in the USA,
its characteristics, the necessity for added
control, the federal narcotic hospitals (Lexington, Ky. and Fort Worth, Tex.) and their
contributions, the series of opiate addiction
treatments, the New York, California, Michigan and Illinois programs, other programs,
arguments pro and con compulsory treatment, and particularly emphasis on the use
of nalorphine in the detection and attempted
control of addicts are reviewed. A small
dose of nalorphine (3 mg) will promptly
produce enlargements of the pupils in opiate
usage, the change depending to some extent
on the degree of dependence to the opiate.
Yet this dose is small enough so that severe
and disagreeable withdrawal symptoms are
not produced. Nalorphine programs have
substantially contributed toward reducing
the incidences of relapses to narcotics by
addicts and have enabled authorities to
detect very quickly those who do relapse
before serious addiction can be resumed.
(No refs.)

[No address]

1987 Bulletin on Narcotics.   Estimated
world requirements of narcotic drugs in
1962.   Bulletin on Narcotics, 1962, 14,
47-48. [Editorial]

The Drug Supervisory Body of the United
Nations publishes an annual statement of
estimated world requirements for 60 narcotic drugs which enabled the Permanent
Central Opium Board to calculate manufacture and import limits on these drugs
for 116 countries and 64 nonmetropolitan

territories for the forthcoming year. Consumption figures on the 60 narcotics are given for 1956-1962. (No refs.)

United Nations
New York, N.Y.

1988   Public Health Reports. Thalidomide. Public Health Reports, 1962, 77, 946. [Editorial]

A survey of 1,258 physicians in the USA interviewed by the FDA revealed that 20,771 patients received thalidomide, of which 3,879 were women of child-bearing age and 624 were pregnant. Most had not delivered and 9 cases of abnormality have been reported in offspring of patients who took thalidomide. Thalidomide was definitely not at fault in 1 instance, but 8 cases remain under investigation. Most of the physicians reported that they received admonitions from the manufacturer to discontinue thalidomide administration, but 85 stated that they were not warned of adverse drug reactions and 42 received no communication from the manufacturer. Thalidomide may still be found in medicine cabinets in the United States. (14 refs.)

Superintendent of Documents
Government Printing Office
Washington 25, D.C.

1989   Current Medical Digest. Emotional disorders of menopause. Current Medical Digest, 1962, 23, 139-142. [Editorial]

Caldwell (1961) administered thioridazine to 150 women with menopausal symptoms. Anxiety, tension and depression were markedly improved in all patients. Drowsiness, the only side effect, was rectified by decreasing drug dosage. Oral estrogens were required as adjunctive therapy in 30 patients to control hot flashes and night sweats. Another 40 found that thioridazine controlled these symptoms, while the remaining 20 required brief intermittent therapy with stilbestrol. Reassurance and a thorough explanation of menopausal symptoms does much toward restoring the confidence of these patients. (1 ref.)

PSYCHOPHARMACOLOGY ABSTRACTS

Volume 2, Number 9

reserpine casts some doubt on this premise.
Possible mechanisms of action and the
possibilities of reciprocal relationships
are discussed. (83 refs.)

Department of Pharmacology
University of Washington Medical School
Seattle, Wash.

1986 Harney, Malachi L. Current provisions and practices in the United States
of America relating to the commitment of
opiate addicts. Bulletin on Narcotics, 1962,
14, 11-24.

The history of narcotic addiction in the USA,
its characteristics, the necessity for added
control, the federal narcotic hospitals (Lexington, Ky. and Fort Worth, Tex.) and their
contributions, the series of opiate addiction
treatments, the New York, California, Michigan and Illinois programs, other programs,
arguments pro and con compulsory treatment, and particularly emphasis on the use
of nalorphine in the detection and attempted
control of addicts are reviewed. A small
dose of nalorphine (3 mg) will promptly
produce enlargements of the pupils in opiate
usage, the change depending to some extent
on the degree of dependence to the opiate.
Yet this dose is small enough so that severe
and disagreeable withdrawal symptoms are
not produced. Nalorphine programs have
substantially contributed toward reducing
the incidences of relapses to narcotics by
addicts and have enabled authorities to
detect very quickly those who do relapse
before serious addiction can be resumed.
(No refs.)

[No address]

1987 Bulletin on Narcotics. Estimated
world requirements of narcotic drugs in
1962. Bulletin on Narcotics, 1962, 14,
47-48. [Editorial]

The Drug Supervisory Body of the United
Nations publishes an annual statement of
estimated world requirements for 60 narcotic drugs which enabled the Permanent
Central Opium Board to calculate manufacture and import limits on these drugs
for 116 countries and 64 nonmetropolitan

territories for the forthcoming year. Consumption figures on the 60 narcotics are given for 1956-1962. (No refs.)

United Nations
New York, N.Y.

1988   Public Health Reports. Thalidomide.
Public Health Reports, 1962, 77, 946. [Editorial]

A survey of 1,258 physicians in the USA interviewed by the FDA revealed that 20,771 patients received thalidomide, of which 3,879 were women of child-bearing age and 624 were pregnant. Most had not delivered and 9 cases of abnormality have been reported in offspring of patients who took thalidomide. Thalidomide was definitely not at fault in 1 instance, but 8 cases remain under investigation. Most of the physicians reported that they received admonitions from the manufacturer to discontinue thalidomide administration, but 85 stated that they were not warned of adverse drug reactions and 42 received no communication from the manufacturer. Thalidomide may still be found in medicine cabinets in the United States. (14 refs.)

Superintendent of Documents
Government Printing Office
Washington 25, D.C.

1989   Current Medical Digest. Emotional disorders of menopause. Current Medical Digest, 1962, 23, 139-142. [Editorial]

Caldwell (1961) administered thioridazine to 150 women with menopausal symptoms. Anxiety, tension and depression were markedly improved in all patients. Drowsiness, the only side effect, was rectified by decreasing drug dosage. Oral estrogens were required as adjunctive therapy in 30 patients to control hot flashes and night sweats. Another 40 found that thioridazine controlled these symptoms, while the remaining 20 required brief intermittent therapy with stilbestrol. Reassurance and a thorough explanation of menopausal symptoms does much toward restoring the confidence of these patients. (1 ref.)

tor-patient relationship, assessment of the patient's allergic and toxic history of susceptibility to drugs and regular evaluation of biological state of the patient plus a thorough study of few drugs in clinical trials. The psychoactive drugs may be utilized to improve the doctor-patient relationship by providing symptomatic relief and reduction in the patient's anxiety-hostility responses.

Dallas Medical Journal
Dallas, Tex.

1995 Groh, Ch. Therapie der Epilepsie im Kindesalter. [The therapy of epilepsy in childhood.] Monatsschrift für Kinderheilkunde, 1962, 110, 96-103.

The development of the chemotherapy of epilepsy over the last 100 years is briefly reviewed; a table lists the predominant types of epilepsy, the drugs recommended and the daily oral dosage according to age groups. Treatment with anticonvulsants is still regarded as the main pillar of treatment. The psychopharmaca (the "nonspecific" drugs) which influence the general condition of the patient are also considered important, as are general hygienic and dietetic measures, and psychologic and pedagogic guidance of the patient in his environment. Therapy with ACTH and cortisone-derivatives, which was initiated in 1958, especially for "propulsive petit mal" in infants, has brought about a decisive change in management. Different types of side effects are discussed; side effects affecting the CNS often are signs of overdosage. This is true also for damage to the hematopoietic system, as well as damage to the liver or kidneys. The necessity of checking the EEG and blood count regularly is emphasized. The gradual reduction in the dosage of anticonvulsive drugs throughout at least 1.5-2 years is stressed, especially during puberty.

Universitäts-Kinderklinik
Vienna, Austria

See also 2057, 2105

1996   Wrede, Josef. Beitrag zur medikamentösen Behandlung von Angst- und
Zwangsvorstellungen. [Contribution to the
chemotherapy of anxiety and compulsive
obsessions.] Therapie der Gegenwart, 1961,
100, 568-570.

Thirty-seven patients were treated with
chlordiazepoxide (Librium). The maximal
dose was 10 mg t.i.d. The patients were
suffering from anxiety in varying degree,
compulsive obsessions, phobias and slight
depressions coupled with fear. No side
effects were noted during 2-3 months of
treatment except in 1 case. All patients
whose anxieties and phobias were not of
psychotic origin were greatly improved.
Far-reaching insight by the patient into
his own problem could often be achieved.

Krankenhaus für Nerven- und Gemütsleiden
Rottenmünster bei Rottweil
Rottweil, Germany

1997   Wieck, H.H., Brilmayer, H., & Picka,
N. Durchgangs-Syndrome infolge von Vergiftungen mit Barbituraten. [Temporary
degeneration syndromes following barbiturate intoxications.] Neurologie, Psychiatrie, Neurochirurgie, 1962, 30, 304-324.

The reversible psychic degeneration syndrome which occurs when overdosages of
barbiturates are taken was measured in
141 patients and related to barbiturate
blood concentrations. Measurements of the
severity of the syndrome were obtained by
calculating the Bücker test score, which
combines in a single figure the reaction
and resolution times and number of errors
made in the solution of a series of problems involving recognition, recall, color
differentiation, ordering ability, verbal reproduction and nonverbal contact recept-
ivity. The general time sequence pattern
in severe intoxications is (1) unconscious-
ness, (2) complete mental and physical
confusion, (3) severe degenerative syndrome, (4) moderate syndrome and (5) mild
syndrome. In the case history reported
here as typical of such conditions, the
duration of the above states was 2, 3, 2,
1, 1 and 7 days, corresponding to barbiturate concentrations in the patient's serum
which declined from a maximum of about

to achieve sleep threshold in this study
(6.0 mg/kg) was remarkably close to that
(6.1 mg/kg) determined in a study by
Shagass (1958).

Department of Psychiatry
University of California School of Medicine
San Francisco, Calif.

2001 Goldman, Douglas, & Rosenberg,
Brigitte. Electro-encephalographic observ-
ations in psychotic children. Comprehensive
Psychiatry, 1962, 3, 93-112.

Over a period of 1-10 years, social studies, physical and mental status examinations, various psychological tests and EEG
observations were performed on 132 hospitalized, psychotic children, aged 6-13
years, (35 CBS, 31 schizophrenic, 52 personality disorders, 7 mentally deficient
and 7 miscellaneous cases). A normal
EEG was rare among these mentally disturbed children. The effect of small, subanesthetic doses (25-75 mg i.v.) of pentothal during the EEG was studied, and a
correlation with the nature of the illness
was established (i.e., in schizophrenic functioning), but residual inconsistencies occurred chiefly in patients with personality
disorders. Prochlorperazine and Win-13,
645-5 [dosages unspecified] were used to
indicate a correlation between EEG and
clinical improvement.

Department of Psychiatry
Good Samaritan Hospital
Cincinnati, Ohio

2002 Boatman, Maleta, & Berlin, I..N.
Some implications of incidental experiences
with psychopharmacologic drugs in a children's psychotherapeutic program. Journal
of Child Psychiatry, 1962, 1, 431-442.

Eighteen children, aged 2 1/2-21 years,
exhibiting hyperactivity and aggressive behavior (1 phobic, 13 psychotic, primarily
schizophrenic, 3 epileptic and 1 with borderline intelligence) were treated with tranquilizers. Nine were analyzed in case
history form. They received psychotherapy
and various psychoactive drugs, including
reserpine (0.1-0.3 mg t.i.d.), chlorpro-

mazine (20 mg/day-200 mg q.i.d.), diphenylhydantoin, meprobamate (400 mg t.i.d. or
every 4 hours) and prochlorperazine (60 mg
per day). Medication was clearly helpful
to 6 and largely detrimental to 4 children.
The 6 clearly showed reduction of excited,
aggressive and destructive behavior. For
2 of these, however, onset of behavioral
alterations was too rapid to be credited
to drug action, and for the rest, the behavioral changes that occurred seemed
related to the psychological climate surrounding the prescription and administration of the drugs. For the same 6 children
similar changes in behavior were also
noted during psychotherapy without medication. In the other 12 out of 18 children,
no clear behavioral changes were noted.
There were psychological factors which
may have contributed to chemotherapeutic
failure. As the psychological circumstances
involved in the prescription and administration of psychopharmacological drugs may
be of importance in evaluating their efficacy, such data should more frequently be
included in reports on these drugs.

Children's Service
Langley Porter Neuropsychiatric Institute
San Francisco, Calif.

2003 Diethelm, Oskar, & Barr, Rosalie
M. Experimental study of amnestic periods in acute alcohol intoxication. Psychiatria et Neurologia, 1962, 144, 5-14.

Fifteen severe alcoholics, aged 22-48 years,
received ethanol (75-100 cc in 450-500 cc
of saline i.v.) infusions over an 18-22
minute time span, after and during which
all conversation was recorded on tape for
45 minutes in order to determine the occurrence of amnestic episodes. All patients
exhibited alcoholism related to an ill-
defined psychoneurotic illness or anxiety
reaction. The observer asked the patient
to describe all details which he could
remember 24 hours after the infusion.
When amnesia occurred, the patient was
permitted to listen to a recording of the
incidents in question. Amnestic episodes
were of short duration and contained psychologically meaningful material which would
have been unpleasant for the patient to
remember. Most patients felt intoxicated

2006   Fisher, G.W., Murray, F., Walley,
M.R., & Kiloh, L.G. A controlled trial of
imipramine in the treatment of nocturnal
enuresis in mentally subnormal patients.
American Journal of Mental Deficiency,
1962, 67, 536-538.

Thirty-four mentally subnormal or severely
subnormal epileptics with nocturnal enuresis, aged 7-67 years, were divided into
2 groups and given imipramine (25-50 mg
per day) or inert placebo alternated on a
double-blind basis for 8 weeks, preceded
by 4 weeks during which frequency of "wet
nights" was determined. Aside from the
epileptics, all patients exhibited a tendency
toward somewhat fewer episodes of enuresis with imipramine than with placebo.
These differences were not statistically
significant. Imipramine is apparently ineffective in controlling enuresis, at least
at the dosages employed.

Prudhoe and Monkton Hospital
Prudhoe-on-Tyne, Northumberland
Great Britain

2007   Vyas, K.J. Hydroxyzine hydrochloride in paediatrics. Antiseptic, 1962, 59,
877-878.

Hydroxyzine drops (2-7 drops b.i.d. or
t.i.d.) were administered to 60 children
aged 1-18 months (22 with evening colic,
10 with abdominal colic, 8 with acute
diarrhea and 20 with acute upper respiratory tract infections). Results were
excellent in 54 children and good in 6.
Effects were palliative, and the drug's
antihistaminic property was beneficial in
the respiratory tract infections. Crying
children were promptly pacified after drug
administration. The drops were given for
1.5-2.0 months to 2 infants who cried
persistently, and improvement was promptly sustained. No toxic effects were observed.

Children's Ward
General Hospital
Junagadh, India

2008   Chatterji, N.N. Psychopharmacology
of phenothiazine. Antiseptic, 1962, 59, 120-
124.

Chlorpromazine [dosage unspecified] was administered to 364 patients (112 schizophrenics, 25 paranoids with systematized delusions, 65 manic-depressives and 75 psychoneurotics). Trifluopromazine [dosage unspecified] was administered to 64 patients (40 schizophrenics and 24 manic-depressives). Prochlorperazine (75-125 mg per day) was given to 68 patients (40 chronic schizophrenics and 28 with acute manic states). Trifluoperazine [dosage unspecified] was given to 100 schizophrenics. Thioridazine (75-400 mg per day for 3-4 months) was administered to 30 schizophrenics. Chlorpromazine was particularly effective in catatonic schizophrenia, offering amelioration of symptoms like mutism, catatonic stupor and cerea flexibilitus. Results with trifluopromazine were optimal in the paranoid group, obliterating delusions and hallucinations. Prochlorperazine was most efficacious in chronic schizophrenia, particularly the paranoid variety, and was superior to chlorpromazine in allaying excitement. Trifluoperazine was very effective in paranoid schizophrenia and catatonic states but its action in other psychoses was most discouraging. Paranoid schizophrenics with prominent hallucinations responded best to thioridazine. The postulated mechanism of action for the phenothiazine tranquilizers involves direct action on the hypothalamic stores of bound levarterenol and serotonin which in turn precipitate alterations in the patient's psyche.

Lumbinipark Mental Hospital
Calcutta, India

2009 Lamphier, Timothy A., Chin, Stanley, Crooker, Lester, Arthurs, Alexander, & Goldberg, Ronald I. Chlordiazepoxide as a preoperative and postoperative medication. Clinical Medicine, 1962, 69, 2466-2469.

Chlordiazepoxide (30-80 mg/day p.o. or i.m.) was administered as presurgical adjunctive medication to 287 anxious patients, aged 9-78 years, from 1-4 days preoperatively and 50-80 mg i.m. q.i.d. was continued postoperatively. Inert placebo was administered to 56 patients who served as controls. To ascertain the feasibility of this study, 35 patients also received

Department of Anesthesia
Pascack Valley Hospital
Westwood, N.J.

2012 Krawiec, Jaime S., Desiderio, Vincent, Bodi, Tibor, & Gambescia, Joseph M. Effect of oxyphencyclimine-hydroxyzine on gastric acid. American Journal of Gastroenterology, 1962, 38, 460-469.

The effect on gastric acidity of the combination oxyphencyclimine-hydroxyzine was examined in a group of 50 patients, using multiple intragastric electrodes to follow focal gastric pH in 25, and aspiration and titration of gastric contents in the other 25. Typical diagnoses were: duodenal ulcer, benign gastric ulcer, etc. The usual choice was 10 mg oxyphencyclimine and 25 mg hydroxyzine; onset of action varied from 18 to 120 minutes with a duration of 1-4 hours. Oxyphencyclimine was somewhat effective as an anticholinergic and its action was potentiated by its combination with hydroxyzine. Twenty-five of the patients were evaluated clinically and the combination found effective in relieving symptoms of gastrointestinal origin, regardless of the fact that the mechanism of such symptoms is not understood.

Section of Gastroenterology
Department of Medicine
Hahnemann Medical College and Hospital
Philadelphia, Pa.

2013 Berthier, Ch. J., Bouvard, J., & Viret, G. A propos de deux psychoses puerpérales. Evolution clinique et thérapeutique. Intérêt des courbes d'excitabilité neuromusculaire. [On 2 cases of puerperal psychoses. Clinical and therapeutic course. The importance of the neuromuscular excitability curves.] Lyon Médical, 1962, No. 1008, 647-648. [Abstract]

Two cases of postpartum psychosis are described. One woman responded to neuroleptics [unspecified], perfusion and cortisone; the other, after the failure of the neuroleptics, recovered after 1 series of insulin shock therapy. Repeated studies of these patients using excitability curves guided proper therapy and confirmed the validity of the concepts of Laborit, Coirault, et al.

[No address]

2014 Stucki, D., & Gross, J. Etude clinique du "Librium" au cours de l'accouchement. [Clinical study of Librium used at delivery.] Praxis, 1962, No. 24, 624-633.

One-hundred women were given 50 mg i.m. injections of chlordiazepoxide (Librium), sometimes repeated, at childbirth. Fifty-five were primaparas. In 17 cases chlordiazepoxide was used with morphine, while in the remaining 83 it was used alone. Behavior was much improved in 40 and improved in 15. Control of pain was excellent in 25 instances and average in 15. Chlordiazepoxide is useful in obstetrics because of its psychorelaxant, myorelaxant and analgesic properties.

Hôpital de district de Porrentruy
Service de gynécologie et d'obstétrique
Porrentruy, Switzerland

2015 Bhaskaran, K., & Nand, D. Satya. Prochlorperazine in chronic schizophrenia. Journal of the Indian Medical Association, 1962, 39, 91-93.

Prochlorperazine (25 mg t.i.d. p.o. for 1 week, then 50 mg t.i.d. for 3 weeks, continued if necessary as maintenance therapy) was administered to 45 chronic schizophrenics (31 unclassified, 9 paranoid and 5 catatonic) aged 20-44 years (mean duration of illness 4.2 years) for 22-60 days. Routine laboratory tests were performed. Clinical response was assessed by 2 investigators. Of the 45 patients, 14 recovered, 3 improved markedly, 15 improved, 12 were unchanged and 1 was withdrawn from the study due to development of severe extrapyramidal symptoms. Comparatively severe extrapyramidal symptoms occurred in 3 other patients, but concurrent administration of promethazine effectively controlled these reactions. No other side effects were encountered. Overall, 32% of the patients recovered, 41% improved and 27% failed to improve.

i.v. injection of 50 mg acetylcholine; blood pressure levels were determined before and after 3, 5, 8, 10 and 20 minutes. Imipramine was better tolerated by patients with sympathicotonic or fast vagotonic responses. A major drop in arterial pressure without recovery at the final reading, characteristic for marked vagotonus, indicates a poor tolerance for imipramine.

[No address]

2020   van Leeuwen, D.P., & Scholl, F.S.K. Promazine hydrochloride (Prazine) tijdens de baring. [Promazine hydrochloride (Prazine) during delivery.] Geneeskundige Gids, 1962, 40, 161-164.

A mixture of promazine and pethidine (25 mg of each i.m., i.v. or both) was used during labor in 32 obstetric patients, including 20 primiparas. Analgesic and sedative effects were excellent, especially by the i.v. route, and there were no side effects in either the mother or the infant. The use of promazine significantly reduced the total amount of opiates and other narcotics required during labor. Figures for forceps deliveries and total duration of labor were within normal limits.

Gynaecologische-Verloskundige afdeeling Gemeenteziekenhuizen te Gravenhage Hague, The Netherlands

2021 Hanna, Calvin, Mazuzan, John E., Jr., & Abajian, John, Jr. An evaluation of dihydromorphinone in treating postoperative pain. Anesthesia and Analgesia, 1962, 41, 755-760.

Following major surgical procedures expected to produce moderate to severe pain, 76 patients, aged 21 to 67 years, in a double-blind study comparing the pain-relieving action of dihydromorphinone to morphine, meperidine and alphaprodine (all drugs in mg/70 kg i.m.), received dihydromorphinone (1-4 mg), morphine (7-10 mg), meperidine (75-100 mg) or alphaprodine (40 mg) with levallorphan (0.8 mg). Of the 76 patients, 39 received a 2nd injection in a crossover study. Drugs used in the crossover (mg/70 kg i.m.), received dihydromorphinone (1-4 mg), morphine (7-10 mg), meperidine (75-100 mg) or alphaprodine (40 mg) with levallorphan (0.8 mg). Of the 76 patients, 39 received a 2nd injection in a crossover study. Drugs used in the crossover (mg/70 kg i.m.) were: dihydromorphinone (1-2 mg), morphine (7-10 mg) and meperidine (75-100 mg). Within 3 hours , 10 mg of morphine was equivalent to ca. 1.5 mg of dihydromorphinone (ratio 1:7) with respect to onset, maximal activity and length of drug action. Meperidine at 75 mg or alphaprodine at 40 mg manifested similar onset of action and time of maximal activity but a decrease in duration of effect. Nausea and vomiting were not troublesome side effects with dihydromorphinone. Dihydromorphinone has several advantages over the newer narcotics, but additional evaluations are strongly recommended.

Department of Pharmacology
University of Arkansas Medical Center
Little Rock, Ark.

2022 Geissmann, P., & Sichel, C. A propos d'un nouveau cas d'hallucinose visuelle verbale chez un névrosé obsessionnel. Résultats favorables du traitement par l'imipramine. [On a new case of visual-verbal hallucinosis in an obsessional neurotic. Favorable results with imipramine treatment.] Annales Médico-Psychologiques, 1962, 120, 1, 403-404.

A second case of visual-verbal hallucinosis, analogous to that first reported by Kammerer, Israel and Geissmann (1959), in a 27-year-old man, is reported. He suffered from repeated depressive episodes with hallucinations. Treatment with high doses [unspecified] of imipramine suppressed hallucinations and depressive phases so that the subject could undergo psychotherapy.

[No address]

2023 Dunlop, Edwin. Inhibition of enzymic activity by intravenous drug therapy. Acta Neurologica Scandinavica, 1962, 38, 71-72.

Over 100 patients with diversified depressive conditions, who failed to respond to

version reaction, depressive reaction with anxiety, CBS, etc.), average duration of disease 2.7 years, received diazepam (5-10 mg t.i.d., with slight variations) as an adjunct to intesive psychotherapy given for an average of 14 weeks. In addition to diazepam, 2 patients received progesterone, 1 chlordiazepoxide and 5 ECT. A very satisfactory response was obtained in 66 patients, a moderate response in 24 and an unsatisfactory response in 18. Considerable improvement was shown, with diminution of tension, increased optimism and renewed interest in everyday events. Patients became more amenable to psychotherapy. Many elderly patients experienced significant improvement in mood, with resultant augmentation of insight. Side effects occurred in 33 patients (lassitude, ataxia, dizziness, gastrointestinal distress, etc.) and necessitated discontinuance of therapy in 9. Diazepam was by far the most effective chemotherapeutic agent for psychomotor depression, and involutional and postinvolutional psychotic reactions. It is less effective than chlordiazepoxide as an anxiolytic agent except in patients with concomitant depressive symptoms.

[No address]

2027 Royer, P., Poire, R., Rayel L., & Trouvenot, P. Action du Daranide dans l'epilepsie. Premiers essais cliniques. [The action of Daranide in epilepsy. Initial clinical trials.] Annales Médico-Psychologiques, 1962, 120, 1, 402.

Daranide [no details], in addition to the barbiturates, has a particularly favorable effect on the classic components of psychic epilepsy, having a tranquilizing action on ideomotor processes.

[No address]

2028 Bobon, J., Collard, J., & Demaret, A. L'imipramine (Tofranil) à faibles doses en gériatric mentale. [Imipramine (Tofranil) at low doses in psychiatric geriatrics.] Annales Médico-Psychologiques, 1962, 120 1, 424.

Imipramine (10-40 mg/day) was adminis-

tered to elderly mental patients. Global
therapeutic results were variable. The 2
symptoms most influenced were depression,
and social and locomotor inertia. In some
cases the side effect excitation necessitated
interruption of treatment. Imipramine has a
decidedly favorable effect in a significant
minority of cases.

[No address]

2029   Singer, L., Geissmann, P., Depoutot,
J. C., & Gutbub, Th. Resultats thérapeutiques du 2028 M.D. [Therapeutic results
with MD 2028 M.D.] Annales Médico-Psycholo-
logiques, 1962, 120, 1, 402.

Sixty-three cases of agitation were treated
with MD 2028 [dosage unspecified]. The
agent had excellent psychiatric activity, allowing a better therapeutic approach, especially in relation to the suppression of
psychomotor excitation. MD 2028 potentiates phenothiazine derivatives. Side effects
include parkinsonism, and cardiovascular
and respiratory reactions. The latter reactions necessitate strict medical surveillance. MD 2028 should not be used in combination with phenothiazine derivatives.

[No address]

2030   Schlemm, Walter. Erfahrungen mit
einem neuen Phenothiazin-Derivat in der
Gynäkologie und Geburtshilfe. [Results with
a new phenothiazine derivative in gynecology
and obstetrics.] Mediziniscle Monatsschrift
1962, 16, 33-34.

Six-hundred hospitalized female patients
received triflupromazine in doses of 10-20
mg i.m. The drug was very effectively used
in post-operative patients (vomiting was
controlled in 89.8%), and in patients with
hyperemesis gravidarum (vomiting was controlled in 78.7%). It also proved to be a very
efficient tranquilizing agent in cases of excessive agitation due to emotional factors
and cerebral sclerosis. In these cases 1 injection (20 mg i.m.) was administered, followed by 10 mg p.o. t.i.d. Triflupromazine
was very effective during delivery when
10 mg i.m. was given during cervical
dilatation.   Triflupromazine reduces the

the greatest diminution of lethargy, boredom and withdrawal were least likely to have an increase of overt anger and hostility. Side effects in 10 of the 32 cases included involuntary body movements characterized by stammering, difficulty in swallowing and involuntary twitching of the mouth and face, suggestive of myoclonic seizures. Reduction in drug dosage resulted in amelioration. The 4 young, bizarrely ruminative schizophrenic males, who were worse after imipramine was added to the regimen, became subjectively happier but more overtly psychotic with combined drug therapy.

Department of Experimental Psychiatry
Hillside Hospital
Glen Oaks, L. I., N. Y.

2035 Hsu, B., & Kin, K. C. Pharmacological study of tetrahydropalmatine and its analogs. A new type of central depressants. Archives internationales de Pharmacodynamie et de Thérapie, 1962, 139, 318-327.

A series of animal experiments and trials on hospital patients were designed to test the effects of tetrahydropalmatine (THP) and its analogues since 1955. In studies of THP analgesic effects and sedative-tranquilizing action, rabbits, hospital patients, mice, cats and monkeys were used in tests which included: prolongation of hexobarbital sleeping time, influence on spontaneous motor activity, action on amphetamine toxicity, influence on mescaline action, influence on avoidance conditioning, behavioral influence (in monkeys) and influence on cerebral electrical activity (in rabbits). Results indicate that THP, which has marked analgesic, sedative and hypnotic activity, may be a new type of CNS depressant. Its levorotatory isomer exerts inhibitory effects, while the dextrorotatory isomer does not, and sometimes even provokes transient excitation. THP exerts considerable effects on the cerebral cortex and subcortical structures. The main site of its action is probably located in the subcortical areas. Among the THP analogues, Corydalis L (which contains the aporphine nucleus) has marked analgesic potency with weak sedative and hypnotic activity, while the tetrahydroberberine exerts a stronger sedative-tranquilizing action with a slight analgesic effect. Study of the structure-activity relationships indicates that the integrity of the mother nucleus of THP and the saturation of the 3rd ring are essential for central depressant action. For tetrahydroberberine the methylenedioxy group is 1 of the active groups. A working hypothesis is proposed for further synthesis of new tranquilizing drugs.

Institute of Materia Medica
Academia Sinica
Shanghai, China

2036 Vidal, M. G., Vidal, B., & Valery, M. B. Essais cliniques de la trimeproprimine (7162 RP). [Clinical trials with trimeproprimine (RP 7162)]. Annales Médico-Psychologiques, 1962, 120, 1, 422.

Trimeproprimine (300 mg/day) was used in the treatment of 50 cases [depression]. Global improvement was 15 remissions, 13 markedly improved, 14 slightly improved and 8 were failures. Two patients suffered an epileptic fit during therapy. The antidepressive, sedative and anxiolytic actions of trimeproprimine make this drug a valuable antidepressant.

[No address]

2037 Kramer, John C. Single daily dose schedules of imipramine (Tofranil). Comprehensive Psychiatry. 1962, 3, 191-192.

Imipramine (75-300 mg/day, mean dosage 150 mg/day) was administered in a single daily dose (SDD) or as a multiple daily dose (MDD) to 14 voluntary hospitalized patients, aged 17-60 years, for 1-5 months. Behavioral alterations observed with SDD and MDD regimens included decreased depression, decreased apathy and withdrawal, diminished preoccupation with somatic symptoms or obsessions and increased activity. In 6 patients who received imipramine initially on a SDD basis, therapeutic response varied from minimal to good. Of 8 patients placed on the SDD regimen after previous MDD therapy, 4 showed additional behavioral improvement and 3 maintained the behavioral changes initiated during the MDD period. On SDD, 1 patient became increasingly hostile towards a new physician although

Promethazine was given as premedication
for endoscopy in 100 patients, the majority
of whom were bronchoscoped. Promethazine
was given i.m. 90 minutes before endoscopy;
65% of the patients were given 50 mg, and
the remaining 35% received 25 mg. Additionally, 15 patients received 100 mg promethazine on the night before endoscopy;
there was a tendency to give very anxious
subjects heavier premedication. Other drugs
used at conventional dosages were meperidine, morphine, codeine, scopolamine and
atropine. Suitable relaxation and appropriate responses were obtained from 80% of
the patients. Maximal drying effect was obtained from 80% of the patients. Maximal
drying effect was obtained from promethazine in conjunction with either atropine or
scopolamine, while the combination of promethazine with meperidine lessened apprehension. Promethazine materially aided in
predicting patient response.

Francis Delafield Hospital
New York, N. Y.

2042   Hussen, Jan-Hinnerk, & Scholz,
Werner. Psychopharmakotherapie mit Librium in der Tuberculose-Behandlung. [Psy-
chotherapeutic use of Librium (chlordiazepoxide) in the treatment of tuberculosis.]
Medizinische Monatsschrift, 1962, 16, 176-
178.

Fifty-six tubercular patients, 8 of whom
were female, from 25 to 29 years of age,
were treated with 10 mg chlordiazepoxide
usually t.i.d. with some variation. Psychically labile patients and those who were
troubled, querulous, or agitated or suffering
from anxiety, depression or insomnia, were
treated with satisfactory to excellent results
in 52 cases, and without success in 4 cases.
These 4 patients were extremely ill, suffering also from considerable reduction of the
breathing surface and dyspnea, and in 3 of
these cases side effects were noted, consisting of vomiting (1), increased depression
(1) and general malaise (1). Otherwise no
side effects were noted.

Städtisches Waldkrankenhaus
Berlin-Frohnau, Germany

2043   Hashkes, Henry R. Evaluation and

803

pattern response of a benzquinamide in 50 patients. Clinical Medicine, 1962, 69, 2239-2244

Fifty patients, aged 14-80 years, with acute, subacute, chronic or reactivated anxiety and tension, nausea and vomiting or muscular spasms received benzquinamide (25 mg p.o., q.i.d.) for an average of 2 weeks. Some patients with severe nausea, cardiac neurosis and palpitation received 50 mg t.i.d. or q.i.d., p.o. Initial response to the average dose fluctuated from a few hours to a few days, while those receiving the 50 mg dose schedule frequently responded within 1 hour. Of the 36 acute reactions, 23 had excellent responses, 8 good, 1 fair and 4 poor. Psychiatric referral was necessary for 2 individuals (schizoid and involutional reactions). Benzquinamide provided varying degrees of effective relief from anxiety (27 excellent, 10 good, 1 fair and 2 poor responses) and nausea (5 excellent and 1 good response) in the majority of patients, with an excellent or good response achieved by 86%. The drug was not valuable in alleviating muscle spasms (1 fair and 3 poor responses). No untoward side effects occurred in any of the patients. Concurrent therapy in 5 cases with an analgesic, vasodilator, or anticholinergic resulted in marked potentiation of drug effects.

[No address]

2044   Bram, G. Treatment of psychoneurotic conditions with long acting trifluoperazine (Stelazine), spansule capsules. British Journal of Clinical Practice. 1962, 16, 143-145.

Trifluoperazine sustained release capsules (supplemented when necessary by 1 mg tablets) were administered p.o. b.i.d. or t.i.d. for 2 months to 114 psychoneurotic patients suffering from tension, restlessness and panicky attacks. Individual adjustments in dosage produced marked improvement or complete relief from symptoms in 39 patients, marked improvement in 56, slight improvement in 6 and no demonstrable change in 13. Patients with endogenous depression and agitation failed to respond uniformly to the drug. No significant side effects were observed. Illustrative case histories of 4 patients, aged 34-62 years, are presented.

admission, their average hospital stay being 48 days. Of 145 readmissions, 93 (64%) were in remission and out of the hospital within 90 days. Of 62 patients returned from furlough with relatives, 30 (43%) were in remission and on furlough again within 90 days of their return. The proper ratio of convulsive and non-convulsive electrical stimulation in combination with trifluoperazine offers the fastest and most efficient means of relieving the psychotic symptoms in schizophrenia.

Wichita Falls State Hospital
Lake Wichita, Tex.

2049   Maletz, Leo. Use of a neuroleptic-antidepressant combination in office practice. Journal of Neuropsychiatry, 1962, 4, 35-38.

A combination tablet containing trifluoperazine (1 mg) and tranylcypromine (10 mg) was administered t.i.d. to 54 psychiatric patients, aged 23-72 years, most of whom had acute depressive reactions accompanied by mild to moderate anxiety, for 1-9 months. Dynamic psychotherapy was performed concomitantly. Close supervision minimized the danger of suicide. Criteria for improvement included overall symptomatic relief, ability to participate in psychotherapy, degree of insight attained and changes in capacity to function socially and vocationally. Results revealed that 24 patients (44%) were much improved, 18 (34%) were improved, and 12 (22%) remained unchanged or unimproved. Symptomatic improvement usually occurred within 5 days of treatment. Restoration of concupiscence heralded rapid overall improvement. During the course of the evaluation, treatment was discontinued in 11 patients who had experienced initial improvement, and treatment with other tranquilizers or antidepressants was substituted. While 3 continued to improve, 8 experienced a return of their symptoms within 1 week. Symptoms were again alleviated by the drug combination. Side effects occurred in 12 patients and included insomnia, headache, constipation, dizziness and restlessness.

80 Nahant Street
Lynn, Mass.

2050 Roper, Peter, Effect of multiple-shock electroconvulsive therapy on a para-noid delusional system. Journal of Neuro-psychiatry, 1962, 4, 28-30.

A 42-year-old man with a highly systema-tized paranoid delusional system received chlorpromazine (50 mg q.i.d.) and 9 ECT treatments within 12 days, after which he was less agitated. More intensive ECT was instituted on a daily basis for 4 consecutive days, whereupon the patient's delusional system disappeared completely. After 9 intensive ECT sessions, a program of 3 reg-ular ECT treatments per week was re-instituted. A total of 22 ECT treatments (9 Page-Russell intensive treatments) were administered over 1 month, and the pa-tient recovered sufficiently to be discharged from the hospital 6 weeks after admission.

Allan Memorial Institute
McGill University
Montreal, Quebec
Canada

2051 Papadopoulos, C. N., & Keats, Arthur S. Specific and nonspecific antagonism of morphine-induced respiratory depression. Anesthesiology, 1962, 23, 86-91.

To compare the efficacy of nalorphine to that of methylphenidate against a thera-peutic dose of morphine, 6 healthy men, aged 22-27 years, received morphine (10 mg/day) for 4 days in tests at intervals of 4-25 days. Placebo, 7 mg nalorphine and 10-30 mg methylphenidate were adminis-tered i.v. in randomized order. As well, 3 subjects were given 30 mg methylpheni-date i.v. without morphine in a separate study and effects were measured 1 and 3 hours later. Morphine effects were mea-sured 60-90 minutes following drug admin-istration and antagonist effects were deter-mined 120-150 minutes after morphine administration. Measurement of respira-tory depression was made in terms of the displacement of each subject's alveolar CO_2 tension-alveolar ventilation curve produced by the drug when compared to a control curve which was previously obtained. Alveo-lar air was continuously sampled and passed through an infrared CO_2 analyzer. Subjec-tive effects were estimated by questioning

2054 Monnerot, E., Chabert, G., & Barre,
R. L'éventail thérapeutique: un correcteur
des neuroleptiques, le R. 381-382 (Califon).
[Clinical note: an antineuroleptic, R 381-382
(Califon).] Annales Médico-Psychologiques,
1962, 120, 1, 419.

Eighteen cases of drug-induced extrapyramidal reaction were treated with phenmetrazine [(Califon; R 381-382) dosage un-
specified]. The drug was capable of suppressing neuroleptic side effects and inhibited weight gain caused by neuroleptics, No
side effects occurred with phenmetrazine.

[No address]

2055 Dornette, William H. L., Poe, Mary
F., Cavallaro, Richard J., & Sheffield,
William E. A double-blind study of Tacaryl
as a narcotic potentiator when used for preliminary medication. Anesthesia and Analgesia, 1962, 41, 32-36.

In a double-blind study methdilazine (Tacaryl) was used as a narcotic potentiator in
4 groups comprising 195 patients awaiting
surgery. This drug is classified as an
antihistaminic. One hour before anesthesia,
in addition to 0.43 mg atropine i.m., the
following schedules were followed: 31 patients received palcebo (0.5 cc), 55 50 mg
pethidine and 12.5 mg methdilazine, 51 100
mg pethidine and placebo, and 58 12.5 mg
methdilazine. No clearcut differences were
noted in any of the 3 drug groups, but the
combination gave a higher influence of respiratory minute volume depression than either drug used alone. Methdilazine potentiated pethidine so that the pethidine dosage
could be reduced by half.

Department of Anesthesiology
University of Tennessee College of Medicine
Memphis, Tenn.

2056 Ekbom, K. A. Treatment of migraine,
Horton's syndrome and restless legs with
Deseril (UML-491). Acta Neurologica Scan-
dinavica, 1962, 38, 313-318.

Methysergide (UML-491; 4-6 mg/day p.o.)
was administered to 64 patients (42 with
migraine, 4 with Horton's syndrome, 5 with

chronic headache and 16 with restless legs)
for several months to over a year. Side
effects, predominantly nausea and vomiting,
occurred in 25 patients, and were severe
enough to necessitate drug discontinuation
in 14 patients'. Migraine headaches were
ameliorated in 26 patients. In Horton's syndrome, some improvement was noted but
too few patients were treated to permit
definite conclusions. Methysergide produced
no improvement in chronic headache. While
8 patients with restless legs showed improvement, earlier studies in which placebos caused improvement in this syndrome
cast doubt on the validity of the improvement observed.

Akademiska Sjukhuset
Uppsala, Sweden

2057 Wright, Stanley W., Valente, Mario,
& Tarjan, George. Medical problems on a
ward of a hospital for the mentally retarded.
American Journal of Diseases of Children,
1962, 104, 111-113.

This report, intended as an aid for physicians in counseling parents before and after
institutionalization of the young, severely
mentally retarded child, gives a general description of the daily activities, medical
care and common illnesses of 76 children,
most from 2 to 10 years of age, hospitalized in the Pacific State Hospital. Chlorpromazine, prochlorperazine, trifluoperazine,
meprobamate and promazine [no dosage
schedules] are efficacious in controlling
serious behavior problems in these children; phenobarbital, often with diphenylhydantoin, is used in the control of seizures.
Facilities, personnel, and budgets are briefly reviewed. Information which should be
supplied to parents is cited. Pediatricians
should assume a leadership role in the improvement of such institutional programs.

Research Department
Pacific State Hospital
Pomona, Calif.

2058 Wrede, J. Erfahrungen mit Marsilid
bei Depressionen. [Results with Marsilid
in depressions.] Der Nervenarzt, 1962,
33, 30-32.

2061 Plotz, Milton. Oxanamide in anxiety
and tension states. Clinical Medicine, 1962,
69, 708-712.

In a single-blind 10 week study, 39 office
patients suffering mild anxiety and tension
were treated with either a vitamin fortified
400 mg oxanamide capsule, given q.i.d., or
a vitamin capsule alone on alternate weeks.
Most patients ultimately refused the vitamin
capsule due to ineffectiveness in comparison
to the drug. Improvement was noted in 70%
on the drug, while there was no real response
to the vitamins alone. Drug response was
best in mild neurosis and poorest in those
with more serious difficulties. Side effects,
most occurring within the 1st 2 weeks of
the study, included gastrointestinal upset
and drowsiness. Oxanamide administration
on alternate days is adequate for many patients with temporary or minor emotional
disturbances. Its use in agina pectoris
should be further investigated.

Brooklyn State Hospital
Brooklyn, N. Y.

2062 Hüter, K. A. Vergleichende Untersuchungen zur psychoprophylaktischen und
medikamentösen Geburtsleitung unter besonderer Berücksichtigung der Neugebor-
enenasphyxie [Comparative investigations
on the "psychoprophylactic" and drug-sup-
ported delivery, with special consideration
of the asphyxia of the newborn.] Geburtshilfe und Frauenheilkunde, 1962, 3, 279-
289.

Four-hundred-and thirty-six women were
thoroughly prepared for natural childbirth.
The aim was to shorten the duration of delivery, ease labor pains, avoid complications, keep the mother aware of the childbirth and avoid possible harm to the breathing center of the newborn. For evaluation,
the women were grouped in 4 groups. 85.6%,
groups I and II, were regarded as complete
success. In group I the duration of delivery
was normal, little pain was felt, the patient
was quiet and disciplined and no medication
was needed. Group II differed only in one
respect: antispasmodic medication or pethidine was administered. Groups III and IV,
a total of 14.4%, were regarded as "failures".
The patients were restless, complained of

severe labor pains and demanded medication. They received a lytic mixture, consisting of 50 mg chlorpromazine, 100 mg pethidine and 50 mg promethazine. The deliveries in these last 2 groups took twice as long as in Groups I and II. The quota of asphyxia of the babies, and therefore the danger of physical and mental damage to the baby, is directly proportional to the duration of the delivery, concerning frequency of incident as well as severeness.

Frauenklinik der Medizinischen Akademie
Düsseldorf, Germany

2063   Ramquist, Nils,& Jonsson, Carl-Otto. Insulin-glykosterabi vid schizofreni. [Insulin-glucose therapy in schizophrenia.] Nordisk Medicin, 1962, 67, 371-375.

The milder therapeutic effects of insulin-glucose therapy were compared to standard insulin coma therapy at conventional dosages in 109 schizophrenic females. In order to make the 2 groups of patients comparable they were matched according to the type of schizophrenic reaction, length of illness and age, etc. No serious side effects were seen with insulin-glucose therapy but some cases showed gastrointestinal symptoms resulting from heavy glucose intake. No definitive rate of improvement was stated because the standard, insulin coma therapy, has not been conclusively shown superior to placebo or barbiturate induced sleep. In cases where insulin coma therapy is considered, insulin-glucose therapy is advocated because it offers less risk.

Beckomberga Sjukhus
Bromma, Sweden

2064   Itil, T. Die Problematik der Schlafstörungen und deren Beeinflussung. [Problems of disturbances of sleep and their treatment.] Arzneimittel Forschung, 1962, 12, 399-407.

EEG methods were used to determine the effects on duration and depth of sleep of 11 patients following i.v. administration of a combination drug Itridal, (40 mg prothipendyl and 150 mg cyclobarbital in 2 ml Homburg-Solution B). The effects of the

consisting of 10 mg thiopropazate and 30, 15 and 25 mg respectively of KSW 788 (a bicyclical central stimulant). MF 11a and b are tablets, and 11d is in ampoule form. Doses varied from 3-8 tablets daily, and in acute psychoses to as much as 12 tablets daily. Ampoules were used parenterally only when tablets could not be administered. MF 11b was used at the end of the treatment period, which lasted 2-4 months. Tolerance was good. Side effects included psychomotor unrest, esophageal spasms, and parkinsonism, the latter being noted in patients who had similarly reacted to other drugs including perphenazine. MF 11 was administered with fair to excellent results to 40 patients, and with no effect or poor results in 33. The drug is effective in rigid, catatonic or hebephrenic schizophrenics, as well as in the majority of chronic schizophrenics.

Heil- und Pflegeanstalt
Lohr am Main, Germany

2068 Archer, Joel S., Smessaert, Andre A., & Hicks, Robert G. Phenothiazine tranquilizers in anesthesia. Review with report on fluphenazine. New York State Journal of Medicine, 1962, 62, 828-833.

In a double-blind study on over 200 women, aged 20-45 years, scheduled for dilatation and curettage, fluphenazine or placebo was administered postoperatively. A 5% incidence of retching and vomiting occurred with fluphenazine and a 14% incidence with placebo. With fluphenazine, recovery was more serene; there were no noticeable differences in blood pressure and pulse. Although hypotension and tachycardia are possible complications, judicious use of the newer phenothiazine derivatives with the piperazine nucleus poses no threat.

Department of Anesthesiology
St. Vincent's Hospital
New York, N. Y.

2069 Carpenter, Frederick A., Steinhaus, John E., Webb, Sam C., & Thompson, Raleigh. Evaluation of preanesthetic medication. Anesthesiology, 1962, 23, 141-142.

Skin resistance and the psychogalvanic reflex (PGR) were used as criteria in a
double-blind study of apprehension following
administration of surgical preanesthetic a-
gents (all on a weight basis, 3.0 ml/150
pounds i.m.). Immediately before surgery,
50 patients (10 in each group), 15-60 years
of age, received pentobarbital (90 mg/150
pounds), meperidine (75 mg/150 pounds),
promethazine (37.5 mg.150 pounds), hydroxyzine (150 mg/150 pounds) or placebo.
A 15-minute control period before drug
administration was used to determine
changes in skin resistance caused by the
PGR (stimulated by standardized light flashes.). Drug administration was followed by
a test period of 1 hour divided into 4
15-minute periods during which the light
flash occurred 3 times at random intervals.
The resultant skin resistance changes were
read directly from the recorder. Although
the group slope of meperidine showed considerable difference from placebo, a scattergraph of meperidine indicated wide variability in individual response. Promethazine's group slope differed least from placebo, but a scattergraph showed consistent
action. Differences between the scores of
each drug and placebo were highly significant. To test correlation of rating scales
and the PGR, an additional study was undertaken with 5 patients using the same drugs
and placebo at 3 dose levels. Each patient
was simultaneously evaluated by PGR
changes and 7-point rating scales by 2 independent observers. The correlation was
highly significant at the 0.5% level of confidence. The PGR may merely mirror changes
in peripheral autonomic reactions due to the
drugs tested. Further studies will attempt
to demonstrate dose effect.

Department of Anesthesiology
Grady Memorial Hospital
Atlanta, Ga.

2070 Haase, H. -J. Intensität und Aqui-
valenz neuroleptischer Wirkung und ihre
therapeutische Bedeutung. [Effectiveness
and equivalence of psycholeptic agents and
their therapeutic importance.] Nervenarzt,
1962, 33, 213-220.

Psycholeptic drugs act mainly on the extrapyramidal tracts which effect psychomotor

Journal of Neuropsychiatry, 1962, 4, 39-42.

A 4-point Target Symptom Rating Scale
(TSRS) was employed to evaluate several
different dimensions of clinical change in
29 schizophrenics (in- and outpatients),
aged 19-57 years, who received haloperidol
(1-5 mg t.i.d.) for 3 days to 3 months (mean
duration for. inpatients, 11.2 days), and 7
inpatient schizophrenics, aged 26-49 years,
who received chlorpromazine (100 mg t.i.d.
or q.i.d., average daily dose 370 mg) for
a mean duration of 10.5 days. Improvement
with haloperidol was significant in relation
to manifest anxiety, paranoid symptoms
and hallucinations; with chlorpromazine,
statistically significant improvement was
found in manifest anxiety, paranoid symptoms and structural thought disorder, etc.
Agitation and apathy also improved. Haloperidol was therapeutically comparable to
chlorpromazine. Extrapyramidal side effects of haloperidol were observed in 22
of the 29 patients: 9 had severe, principally
akinetic Parkinsonian manifestations and
5 displayed acute episodes of dystonic
movements. Therapy was discontinued in
3 outpatients and 1 inpatient. No gastrointestinal side effects occurred, but moderate hypotension was observed in 10 out of
17 patients. Drowsiness was reported by
5 patients. The therapeutic profile of haloperidol as examined by means of the TSRS
appeared to approximate that of chlorpromazine. Haloperidol did not exert an
analeptic effect on apathy and depression
in the schizophrenic patients under study.

Department of Psychiatry
Downstate Medical Center,
State University of New York
606 Winthrop Street
Brooklyn 3, N.Y.

2074   Lorenz, K., & Schmidt, G. Klinische
und elektroenzephalographische Beobachtungen bei und nach Chorea minor. [Clin-
ical and electroencephalographic observations during and after chorea minor.]
Deutsche Gesundheitswesen, 1962, 17, 35,
1499-1506.

Sixty-two chorea minor patients, 3-20 years
old (some with a medical history of somatic
or psychic disturbances before onset of

chorea) were treated conventionally. Sleep therapy was uniformly effective in 6 severe cases. Use of Fowler's solution frequently resulted in changes in the blood picture, the most frequent being leukocytopenia and, particularly granulocytopenia. Trihexyphenidyl seems to be beneficial. Endo- and myocarditis was observed in 44 patients (73%). Post-discharge examinations of 40 patients showed cardiac involvements in only 43%. Recidivism was high in comparison with other rheumatic conditions. Behavioral or physical disturbances were found in 31 of 43 discharged patients one year later, but onset of puberty was frequently a concomitant factor. However, 50% of the cases were damaged psychically or intellectually.

Kinderklinik
Medizinische Akademie
Dresden, Germany

2075 Horstmann, W. Erfahrungen mit einem barbituratfreien Schlaf- und Beruhigungsmittel bei jungen Kindern. Klinische und elektroenzephalographische Untersuchungen mit 2,4-Dioxo-3,3-diäthyl-5-methyl-piperidin (Noludar). [Experiences with a barbiturate-free hypnotic and sedative for small children. Clinical and electroencephalographic study with 2,4-dioxo-3,3-diethyl-5-methyl-piperidine (Noludar).] Münchener Medizinische Wochenschrift, 1962, 104, 603-608.

Methyprylon (Noludar) was used with a large number of clinical visits over a 5-year period, supplemented by records of 260 examinations performed on 226 children. It has proven useful as a sedative and hypnotic of medium duration with a wide range of clinical indications, including sedation of newborn with birth trauma, preparation for examinations (e.g., EEG'S, ECG'S). Only side effects noted are nausea and vomiting shortly after administration of the drug. No toxic effects have been noted with respect to hematopoiesis, renal and hepatic function, respiration, circulation, etc. Tolerance is good, so that dosages while perhaps requiring adjustment to individual needs, can be varied widely. Mean dosages are recommended by age groups, averaging ca. 30-35 mg/kg.

results were: 62 remissions, 101 satisfactory, 33 fair and 40 negative. A pilot
double-blind crossover study was made
with 8 patients; results for chlordiazepoxide versus placebo were: improvement-
4:1; aggravation of the condition followed
by some improvement-0:1; initial improvement followed by slight worsening-2:2; no
alteration-2:3, and progressive worsening-
0:1. The results of the double-blind study
did not warrant definite conclusions. The
only prominent side effect from chlordiazepoxide was daytime drowsiness.

Clinica Psychiátrica da Faculdade de
    Medicina de Lisboa
Lisbon, Portugal

2080 Katz, Robert A., Aldes, John H., &
Rector, Mina. A new drug approach to
muscle relaxation. Journal of Neuropsychiatry, 1962, 3, Suppl. 1, S91-S95.

Diazepam (25-40 mg/day p.o., parenteral
for 3-5 days in acute patients, then p.o.)
was administered to 84 patients, aged
20-77 years, with musculoskeletal disorders arising from trauma, neurological
orthopedic and arthritic diseases for an
average of 4 weeks. Outstanding symptoms
were muscle spasm and pain. Marked
improvement in 57 patients included diminished spasticity, alleviation of pain and
increased motion. A moderate response
occurred in 15, with adequate but not
remarkable improvement in spasticity and
pain, along with increased ambulation. A
minimal response was obtained by 4, and
4 failed to respond. Drowsiness occurred
with high doses of diazepam in elderly
patients. There were no indications of
toxic reactions or habituation, and laboratory data remained negative and within
normal range. Final evaluation was withheld in 4 patients. Diazepam has a definite place in the management of musculoskeletal disorders associated with emotional overtones.

Ben R. Meyer Rehabilitation Center
Cedars of Lebanon Hospital
Los Angeles, Calif.

2081 Vilkin, M.I., & Lomas, J.B. Clinical

815

experience with diazepam in general psychiatric practice. Journal of Neuropsychiatry, 1962, 3, Suppl. 1, S139-S144.

Diazepam (5 mg t.i.d. or q.i.d.) was administered to 83 patients (42 with anxiety
reactions, 23 severe agitated depression,
12 schizophrenic reactions and 6 chronic
alcoholics with anxiety), aged 14-78 years,
for more than 6 months. Improvement was
evaluated by the patient, his family and
physician. Several patients who manifested
immediate improvement received placebos
and experienced a return of symptoms
within a few days. Excellent results occurred in 28 patients, good in 20, fair in 21
and negative in 14. The most gratifying
results were obtained in anxiety reactions.
Mild to moderate depressions with agitation responded well, moderately depressed
and agitated patients responded to diazepam and imipramine [dosage unspecified].
Severely depressed patients required ECT.
Diazepam ameliorated anxiety in alcoholics.
The phenothiazines, especially trifluoperazine, are preferable in treating acute
schizophrenia. Side effects from diazepam
included dizziness and decreased coordination when performing athletic endeavors.

Westwood Hospital
Los Angeles, Calif.

2082   Collard, J. Clinical experience with
diazepam in neurosis. Journal of Neuropsychiatry, 1962, 3, Suppl. 1, S157-S158.

Diazepam (15 mg/day) was administered
to 25 neurotics (psychoneurotic depression,
anxiety, compulsion or conversion neurosis, etc.) with anxiety, psychic tension,
depression and psychosomatic symptoms
for 1-8 weeks. Symptoms and results were
assessed on a 0-4 point rating scale. Positive results were obtained in 68% of the
patients. Diazepam is a good anxiolytic in
moderate and mild cases of neurotic non-
melancholic anxiety. The drug also produces
symptomatic relief of psychic tension of
moderate intensity, but lacks the characteristics of a true antidepressant. Sleep was
normalized in 12 out of 13 cases. Excellent
inhibition of algesias, spasms and psychosomatic tachycardia was also observed.
In addition, mean anxiolytic activity indices

psychopathology, but 4 on diazepam deteriorated. Of those who improved, 6 received placebo, 6 chlorpromazine, 3 diazepam and 4 chlordiazepoxide.

Research Division
Central Islip State Hospital
Central Islip, N. Y.

2086   Borenstein P., Dabbah, M., & Blès, G. Etude électroencéphalographique de l' halopéridol. [Electroencephalographic study of haloperidol.] Annales Medico-psychologiques, 1962, 120, 1, 133-141.

Haloperidol 5 mg was administered i.p. once only to 32 patients (7 epileptics, 7 schizophrenics, 8 with behavioral problems, 10 miscellaneous) and EEG's taken 45-60 minutes later. Improvement, more stable alpha waves, was noted in 16, 3 retrogressed and 13 remained unchanged. Anomalies were noted in 7 cases, consisting of degraded points and pointwaves, and modifications of the theta and delta components where these had been present. Another 40 patients (15 schizophrenics, 10 delirium cases, 15 miscellaneous) were treated with an average dose of 3 mg haloperidol daily and EEG's were recorded for varying periods up to 3 months. No changes were registered in 10 cases, moderate changes in frequency and amplitude of basic activity were found in 8, improvement in the basic activity (with transitory and variable effects on the theta component) in 14 and retrogression was noted in 8 cases (both base activity and anomalous changes.) No epileptogenic effects were noted at the dosages used. The clinical symptomatic effects on the extrapyramidal system, the psyche and alertness were not reflected in the EEG's.

Hôpital Psychiatrique
Villejuif, Seine
France

2087   Borenstein, P., Dabbah, M., Blès, G.,& Roussel, A. Etude electroencéphalographique de l'aminotryptiline. [Electroencephalographic study of aminotryptiline.] Revue Neurologique, 1962, 106, 225-237.

Clinical studies
Abstracts 2088-2090
Aminotryptiline was administered parenterally in doses of 100 mg once only to
57 patients, including 33 epileptics, 13 with
behavioral disturbances, 7 depressed patients and 4 schizophrenics. Improvement
was noted in 10 epileptics and retrogression
(diffuse and bilateral point waves at 3-3.5
c/second) in 20 such cases; 10 nonepileptics showed improvement (regression of
dysrhythmic points, etc); 5 cases of depression experienced an increase in amplitude
and slowing of rhythm; effects on schizophrenics were variable. In 63 patients,
including 21 epileptics, 35 with depression
and 7 with behavioral troubles, all treated
over a long period of time the results
were as follows: during the first months
the effect of aminotryptiline on the EEG
tracings was variable, the most frequent
phenomenon in depression being a retardation of basic activity concomitant with an
increase of amplitude, while anomalous
points appeared in the behavioral patients.
Among epileptics isolated spikes, bilateral
synchronous point waves, slowing in alpha
rhythm, appearance of localized or diffused
theta and delta elements occurred. Anomalies would vanish, then occasionally reappear. The drug cannot be viewed as epileptogenic as clinical improvement was frequent and anomalies were suppressed. Side
effects consisted of anxiety symptoms and
functional disturbances during the 1st days,
asthenia, tremor, blurred vision, stammering, constipation, dry mouth, bulimia and
considerable weight gain. Prognosis on an
EEG-clinical basis is not yet possible.

Hôpital Psychiatrique
Villejuif, Seine
France

2088 Borenstein, P., Dabbah, M., Blès, G., &
Roussel, A. L'aminotryptiline dans les
épilepsies. Etude clinique et électroencéphalographique. [Aminotryptiline in epilepsy.
A clinical and electroencephalographic study.] Annales Médico-Psychologiques, 1962,
120, 1, 153-167.

Aminotryptiline was administered, usually
in oral doses of 50 mg t.i.d. to 23 epileptics
(20 male, 3 female). The frequency of crises,
psychomotor equivalents and absences decreased in 19 out of 23 cases, remained
unchanged in 1, and retrogressed in 3 cases.
Behavioral and character disorders were
lessened in 14 cases. Subsequent treatment

agent.] Der Nervenarzt, 1962, 33, 86-88.

Clinical investigation with MF 11 d, an experimental drug which consists of pipera-zine-phenothiazine combined with a central stimulant, were simultaneously undertaken independently in 4 hospitals. Of 180 patients treated, 140 were schizophrenics, 19 had endogenous depressions, and 21 were treat-ed for miscellaneous reasons. The daily dosage was 30-80 mg p.o., initially 10 mg t.i.d. or q.i.d. Most patients tolerated the drug very well. No significant effects were observed on the cardiovascular system. Blood counts and liver function tests showed no pathological changes. A distinct increase in weight was noted in most patients. The side effects were mostly parkinsonian in nature, and only occurred in 12-13%. The preparation is as efficacious as other piperazine-derivatives, but it is better tol-erated. Patients generally become more responsive, and a distinctly beneficial psy-chomotor-activating effect may be observ-ed. The results were very encouraging, particularly with catatonic schizophrenics. Therapeutic effects are equally valuable. Some patients however, proved resistant to the preparation.

Universitäts-Nervenklinik Würzburg
Würzburg, Germany

2092 Haase, H.J. Die Beeinflussung psy-chomotorischer Akitvität bei neurolepti-scher und antidepressiver Behandlung. [The influence of neuroleptic and antidepressant therapy on psychomotor activity.] Nerven-arzt, 1962, 33, 116-124.

The effects of chlorpromazine, prochlor-perazine, fluphenazine and thioperazine (do-sages: 438, 66, 13, 12, and 22 mg/day, respectively) on the behavior patterns of 96 predominantly schizophrenic patients were recorded for a period of 4524 days. The behavior of 39 patients with depressive psychoses, under treatment with imipra-mine, phenelzine, and nialamide was also recorded. Drug effects were measured with respect to increases and decreases in walk-ing activity, and increases or decreases in speech and other activity. The relationship of these changes to the increase or decrease of akathisia was evaluated statistically.

Neuroleptic drugs were found to have a distinctly more intense and direct effect than do the antidepressants on psychomotor activity; their influence appears to be exerted upon the extrapyramidal system.

Psychiatrische Klinik
Medizinische Akademie
Düsseldorf, Germany

2093 Mans, J., Cornil, & Ajzemberg. De l'interet de l'association systematique de la thiomucase aux neuroleptiques. [Significance of systematic combination of thiomucase with neuroleptics. Annales Médico-Psychologiques, 1962, 120, 1, 50-60.

A combination of the neuroleptic drugs (chlorpromazine, thioproperazine and levomepromazine) with thiomucase was injected i.m. into 37 psychiatric patients. When thiomucase is used in this fashion, the neuroleptic drugs diffuse very effectively, the beneficial clinical effect persists, and intraparenteral treatments can be continued for as long as the state of the patient renders it necessary. The pseudoinflammatory reactions, which hitherto had been a cause of difficulty when attempts were made to inject the drugs intramuscularly over longer periods of time, no longer occurred.

[No address]

2094 Gibbs, F.A., & Gibbs, E.L. Clinical and pharmacological correlates of fast activity in electroencephalography. Journal of Neuropsychiatry, 1962, 3, Suppl. 1, S73-S78.

Seventeen patients (16 schizophrenic and 1 mentally deficient) received chlordiazepoxide (60 mg/day), a chlordiazepoxide analogue (30 mg/day) or diazepam (30 mg per day) in randomized order for 10 days to determine therapeutic effects and EEG differences in waking and sleeping states. At effective dosages, the incidence of fast EEG activity was the same for all 3 drugs; 70% developed fast activity and 30% remained unchanged. No relationship was observed between EEG responses and thera-

Topeka State Hospital
Topeka, Kan.

2097 Sargant, William. The treatment of anxiety states and atypical depressions by the monoamine oxidase inhibitor drugs. Journal of Neuropsychiatry, 1962, 3, Suppl. 1, S96-S103.

Sixty patients with anxiety states received a combination of MAO inhibitors [(isocarboxazid, phenelzine, phenoxypropazine or iproniazid) dosages unspecified] and chlordiazepoxide, MAO inhibitors alone or chlordiazepoxide (10 mg b.i.d. or t.i.d.) alone. Fifteen patients, average age 41 years, responded best to MAO inhibitors alone. Good previous personalities characterized 87% of these patients, and precipitating factors were present in 73%. Severe depression was present in 13% and mild depression in 87%. Of the 28 patients, average age 42 years, who responded optimally to MAO inhibitors and chlordiazepoxide, 75% had good previous personalities and 43% had precipitating factors. Hysterical behavior was present in 43% and mild depression was manifested by 97%. Of the 17 patients, average age 41 years, who failed to respond to MAO inhibitors and chlordiazepoxide, only 25% had good previous personalities and 29% had adequate precipitating factors. Hysterical behavior was seen in 23%, but mild depression was observed in 94%. All patients who initially responded well to a combination of MAO inhibitor and chlordiazepoxide showed a return of symptoms when the MAO inhibitor was withdrawn and the patient was maintained on chlordiazepoxide alone. An MAO inhibitor combined with chlordiazepoxide will ameliorate cardiac neuroses, effort syndrome and hysterical hyperventilation syndrome within 7-10 days in patients so predisposed.

Department of Psychological Medicine
St. Thomas's Hospital
London, Great Britain

2098 Freund, J. Dennis. The place of insulin coma therapy in modern psychiatry. Journal of Neuropsychiatry, 1962, 3, 246-250.

A series of 2033 patients (71% paranoid schizophrenic, 14% catatonic, 5% pseudoneurotic, 8% schizoaffective and 2% miscellaneous) received insulin coma therapy. Results included full recovery in 1402 (69%), great improvement in 183 (9%), improvement in 102 (5%) and no improvement in 346 (17%). Of the 346 who failed to improve, 189 received ECT superimposed at the deep coma level. Of the 189, 168 (89%) recovered fully and 158 (11%) did not improve. A plethora of references allude to work done with insulin coma therapy since 1937.

Fairview Hospital
2828 South Prairie Avenue
Chicago, Ill.

2099 Mans, J., Cornil, J., & Ajzemberg, D. Essais therapeutiques du G. 22-355 chez les vieillards d'un service psychiatrique. [Therapeutic trials with G. 22-355 (imipamine) in older patients in a psychiatric clinic] Annales Medico-Psychologiques, 1962, 120, 2, 57-70.

Imipramine was administered to 41 geriatric patients, at an initial dose of 110 mg tablet per day, gradually increased to 5 or 6 per day according to the age of the patient or the gravity of the syndrome. The patients were classified as follows: 30 pure seniles, 4 premature seniles, and 7 miscellaneous cases with psychasthenia, depression, melancholia, in all of whom the depressive or melancholy aspect was dominant. Imipramine proved effective in combating emotional phenomena consisting of outbursts of laughing or weeping, in calming paranoids and depressives, while poor or indifferent results were registered in hypochondriacs and senile dementia cases. Generally speaking, advanced cases do not respond, while in less advanced cases contact is made easier, and the troubles of the patient become less painful.

[No address]

2100 Lairy, G. C. Action du Librium sur l'électroencéphalogramme. [Action of Librium (chlordiazepoxide) on the encephalogram.] Révue Neurologique,1962,106,152-156.

of 20 cc), and bemegride (0.5% solution - dose of 1 cc/10 kg, followed by 1 cc at 15 second intervals up to 100 cc maximum). The epileptic crises were filmed simultaneously with the recording of the EEG tracing. Comparative studies on the different activation and provocation techniques show considerable variation between the patterns evoked by different techniques. Even when it is known that a definite cortical and hemispheric pathology is present, proof of a definite epileptogenic focus is very chancy. Presence of a well-defined electrical focus which would permit good electro-clinical correlation is found in a very small number of cases, and is rendered difficult to ascertain by the differences between the different methods. Results presented here are of importance in the sense of demonstrating the need for sharpening techniques and methods for determining by means of electro-clinical correlation, the epileptogenic focus.

Laboratoire d'Electroencéphalographie
Hôpital Cantonal de Genéve
Geneva, Switzerland

2104   Detre, Thomas P., Feldman, Robert, G., Rosner, Burton, & Ferriter, Christine. Vibration perception in normal and schizophrenic subjects. Journal of Neuropsychiatry, 1962, $\underline{3}$, 145-150.

Vibrograms were traced by 9 acute schizophrenics, aged 18-30 years, and 31 normal controls employing the principle of the Bekesy audiometer in which the subject automatically traced his own threshold of vibration perception. No significant differences were observed in audiograms between normal and schizophrenic subjects. The average threshold of vibration perception was highest for the female schizophrenics and next highest for the schizophrenic males. Both were appreciably higher than the threshold curves for normal males and females. As a control measure, audiograms and vibrograms were determined over the same frequency range on 2 normal and 2 schizophrenic subjects. The normal and schizophrenic subjects had comparable audiograms while the vibrograms of the schizophrenics were distinctly different from those of the normals. Serial tests were

used to show the effects of fluphenazine
and trifluoperazine on vibratory sensitivity.
Minimal changes occurred in threshold
curves when normal subjects received the
drugs, but definite changes occurred in serial vibrograms of drug-treated schizophrenics. Clinical improvement was reflected
in a shift of the average vibration threshold
into the normal range. The audiometric
vibrogram may be useful in evaluating psychopharmacological drugs.

Department of Psychiatry
Yale University School of Medicine
New Haven, Conn.

2105 Lohrenz, John G., Levy, Leonard,
& Davis, John F. Schizophrenia or epilepsy?
A problem in differential diagnosis. Comp-
rehensive Psychiatry, 1962, 3, 54-62.

A 4-year-old girl with acute schizophrenia
and epilepsy received chlorpromazine (200
mg/day), diphenylhydantoin (100 mg t.i.d.
with a maintenance dose of 100 mg/day)
and phenobarbital (60 mg parenterally).
Aberrant EEG tracings necessitated maintenance therapy with diphenylhydantoin. The
significance of the EEG in differentiating
between epilepsy and schizophrenia is stressed as well as the importance of conservative management in such atypical cases.
Maintenance therapy aided complete recovery. A brief survey of pertinent literature is included.

Department of Psychiatry
McGill University
Montreal, Quebec
Canada

2106 Keller, Hans H. Ein weiterer Beitrag
zur medikamentösen Parkinson-Therapie.
[A further contribution to the drug therapy
of Parkinson's disease.] Münchener Medizinische Wochenschrift, 1962, 104, 510-513.

The effect of thenophenopiperidine (Sando-
sten) was measured separately for each
of a series of 11 symptoms of Parkinson's
disease. Results are based on 30 patients,
but additional studies confirm these findings. Treatment consisted of oral or i.v.
administration of thenophenopiperidine (2

2110 Tölle, Rainer, Die Behandlung endogener Psychosen mit Laevomepromazin
(Neurocil). [Treatment of endogenous psychoses with levomepromazine (Neurocil).]
Nervenarzt, 1962, 33, 178-180.

Eighty-three female patients with acute
schizophrenia, hebephrenia, defect schizophrenia and manic psychoses were given
levomepromazine orally 150-250 mg/day, in
severe cases 400 mg, rarely 500 mg/day
(generally only 2/3 of the dose of chlorpromazine required to give the same effect).
The treatment was ineffective in 11 acute
schizophrenics with paranoid hallucinations,
but was effective in 4 patients with considerable motor unrest but without delusions; it was very effective in the control
of convulsions. In 13 acute schizophrenics
with hebephrenic symptoms 400-500 mg/day
was necessary; results were good in 6
cases, moderate in 4, negligible in 3, and
generally were evident in 2-3 weeks. Results
were convincing in only 6 of 22 patients
with defect schizophrenia and were unfavorable in patients requiring continuous treatment, because of the exhausting effects of
levomepromazine. The drug, 100-200 mg/
day orally (initially 75-100 mg i.m.) favorably influenced the anxiety states of 10
patients (5 schizophrenic, 5 cyclothymic)
and inhibited delusions. It was relatively
ineffective in 7 depressed patients; only 3
patients were improved by high doses of
about 400 mg/day. Four cyclothymic-de-
pressed patients were unimproved. Treatment of 5 manic psychoses (3 cyclothymic,
2 miscellaneous psychotics) with levomepromazine gave good results. The principal
side effect was a pronounced decrease in
blood pressure resulting in collapse in
hypotonic patients and those with low blood
pressure. In general levomepromazine was
less effective in acute and chronic schizophrenia than the piperazine phenothiazine
derivatives.

Universitäts Nervenklinik
Tübingen, Germany

2111 Schmidt, & Van Ba, Nguyen. Traitement d'un malade par le prothipendyl C.I.H.
[Treatment of a patient with prothipendyl
C.I.H.] Annales Médico-Psychologiques,
1962, 120, 1, 147-152.

A 25-year-old male was admitted with delirium of several weeks duration. He was given 50 mg chlorpromazine by injection, followed by t.i.d. oral chlorpromazine, then 10 ECT sessions. Several weeks after such therapy the patient was switched to prothipendyl beginning with i.m. injections of 80 mg. Then injections were alternated with 50 mg tablets, later 50 mg prothipendyl tablets t.i.d. The patient showed good recovery within 2 weeks.

[No address]

2112 Náhunek, K. Die Behandlung endogener Depressionen mit Perphenazin und Trihexyphenidyl. Beziehung zur extrapyramidalen Symptomatologie. [Treatment of endogenous depression with perphenazine and trihexyphenidyl. Relationship to extrapyramidal symptomatology.] Acta Psychiatrica Scandinavica, 1962, 38, 108-116.

Sixty-eight patients with melancholia and involutional depression were treated with perphenazine or trihexyphenidyl on 1 of 3 dosage schedules. The 1st group of 26 patients was given 24-96 mg perphenazine and 6-12 mg trihexyphenidyl a day for 16-38 days. The 2nd group of 26 patients received perphenazine alone, 24-76 mg/day for 5 to 33 days; the 3rd "control" group of 16 patients received trihexyphenidyl alone (6-12 mg/day for 3-14 days). In the event of failure of treatment in the 2nd and 3rd groups, trihexyphenidyl was added to the treatment of the 2nd group and perphenazine to the 3rd. Results were evaluated by 2 doctors according to a modified Serejski classification as cured, markedly improved, partially improved, insignificantly improved, unimproved, or worsened. In the 1st treatment group who received the 2 drugs in combination, 16 patients were discharged, 4 were partially improved and 6 were unchanged. In the 2nd group, trihexyphenidyl was given to 23 patients when perphenazine proved ineffective; 3 of the patients were discharged on perphenazine alone and 13 when trihexyphenidyl was added. Nine patients improved partially with the drugs in combination, 1 slightly, 1 was unchanged and 2 were worsened. Of 16 patients who at first received only trihexyphenidyl, there was only 1 who showed slight

on the basis of duration of treatment, the drug appeared to be optimally effective at about the 3rd week of treatment. The most common side effects were malaise, pulse irregularities, hypothermia, Parkinsonism (resulting in cessation of treatment in 7 patients), nausea and vomiting (treatment discontinued in 5), insomnia, turbulence (discontinued in 10), convulsions (discontinued in 9), collapse and depression.

Psychiatrische Universitätsklinik
  Burghoelzli
Zurich, Switzerland

2115   Baruk, H., & Richardeau. Traitement d'un cas grave de dépersonnalisation avec troubles de la conscience par la phénelzine. [Treatment of a serious case of depersonalization with intellectual disorders with phenelzine.]   Annales Médico-Psychologiques, 1962, 120, 1, 950.

A male patient suffering from depersonalization, perceptual disorders (lack of time appreciation, etc.) and amnesia, who had an abnormal EEG, was greatly aided by treatment with phenelzine [no details].

[No address]

See also 1989, 2120, 2168, 2208, 2225, 2234

2116 Rabinowicz, Th., & Foroglou, G.P.
4. Lésions par intoxication aigue à l'imipramine. [4. Lesions caused by acute imipramine intoxication.] Schweizer Archiv
für Neurologie, Neurochirurgie und Psychiatrie, 1962, 90, 268-295.

A 59-year-old woman who had previously
been given ECT for depression committed
suicide through the ingestion of 182 25 mg
imipramine tablets. In the past, 1 of her
brothers and a sister had committed suicide.
Two days before her death she had begun
treatment with 9 tablets per day. Ten
hours after the toxic ingestion she was
found unconscious and entered the hospital
in a deep coma with total areflexia and
a drop in blood pressure; she died within
8 hours, having epileptic seizures. Imipramine levels in body fluids and organs
were (in mg%): plasma 0.2; urine 0.7;
bile 3.2; gastric contents 810; intestinal
contents 108; intestinal walls 5.1; heart
5.0; liver 23.0; spleen 40.5; muscles 3.5;
kidneys 9.50; thyroid 2.0; adrenals 17.6;
brain (average of 560 g): 11.3; gyrus centralis 10.7; nucleus caudatus 12.4; brain
stem 11.1; frontal lobe 10.3; basal ganglia
13.1; temporal lobe 11.2; occipital lobe
10.0; pons 12.6; thalamus 12.8; cerebellum
3.2. In the CNS (lower brain stem and
spinal cord were not available), the left
side was used for histological examination,
and severe lesions probably caused by
the product were found in the following
regions: putamen (partly), claustrum (partly), large neurons of the nucleus caudatus,
nucleus ruber, nucleus parasympathicus
of the 3rd cranial nerve, nucleus oculo-
motorius (III), nucleus motorius trigemini,
olivae bulbaris, certain hypothalamic and
thalamic nuclei and certain elements of
the reticular system. The following regions
were less severely involved: anterior part
of the gyrus uncinatus, a small part of
the reticular substance of the pons and
certain thalamic and hypothalamic nuclei.
A list of nuclei with slight lesions (probably
due to hypoxemia following circulatory
and/or respiratory failure) is presented.

Laboratoire de Neuropathologie
Institut d'Anatomie Pathologique
Université de Lausanne
Lausanne, Switzerland

presented showing a sample of poisonings
reported in New York City on 1 weekend.

[No address]

2121 Schmitt, Alfred. Besonderheiten bei
Vergiftungen mit "barbitursäurefreien"
Schlafmitteln. [Characteristics of poisoning
with "barbiturate free" sleeping potions.]
Nervenarzt, 1962, 33, 418-419.

Relatively small amounts (20-30 tablets) of
the socalled barbiturate-free drugs, including glutethimide, methyprylone and methaqualone have deleterious effects on circulation often greater than those caused by the
barbiturates. A specific effect of glutethimide is an increase in the likelihood of
convulsions. Four suicide attempts are
described in which methaqualone was the
drug taken, 2 of them with fatal outcome.
In each case 40-100 of these tablets were
taken. Symptoms included edema of the lung,
severe oxygen insufficiency, heart and circulatory failure.

Nervenklinik der Stadt und Universität
  Frankfurt
Frankfurt-am-Main, Germany
 See also 1988, 1991, 2046, 2154, 2158,
2159, 2161, 2171, 2173, 2190, 2197

2122 Dostalek, C., & Scheer, E. Über den Einfluss von Benactyzin und Atropin auf die bedingten Pupillenreflexe bei Katzen. [The influence of benactyzine and atropine on conditioned pupillary reflexes in cats.] Acta Biologica Medica Germanica, 1962, 8, 523-529.

Conditioned pupillary reflexes were formed in 5 cats. Light exposure of 1 eye served as a US which produced maximal miosis, while a tone was used as a CS. This sound stimulation did not effect any change of the pupils before the formation of a CR, not even when applied at 10-fold amplitude. During and after formation of the conditioned miosis, mydriasis also occurred. Atropine (25 µg/kg) and benactyzine (100 µg/kg), s.c., eliminated or reduced mydriasis and promoted the formation of the conditioned miosis. Here atropine caused a light miosis. The effects of atropine and benactyzine on the pupillary CR's were contrary to the effect upon the peripheral target organ.

Deutsche Akademie der Wissenschaften
Berlin, Germany

2123 Pihkanen, T., & Kauko, O. The effects of alcohol on the perception of musical stimuli. Annales Medicinae Experimentalis et Biologiae Fenniae, 1962, 40, 275-285.

Three blind piano tuners, 2 men and a woman, were tested for ability to determine pitch, loudness, rhythm and for tonal memory after the ingestion of alcohol. The dosage of ethanol was 1 g/kg given as a 20% solution in 2 divided doses: the 1st dose (0.75 g/kg) was taken slowly in the 1st hour and the 2nd (0.25 g/kg) during the 2nd hour. The Seashore Measures of Musical Talent was used in evaluation. The same subjects were given the test again a week later when sober for comparison. Alcohol caused disturbances in pitch and rhythm perception, and in tonal memory, but no distinct effect in respect to loudness perception.

Institute of Occupational Health
Helsinki, Finland

diazepoxide and chlorpromazine on a punishment discrimination. Psychopharmacologia, 1962, 3, 374-385.

Male Holtzman-Sprague-Dawley strain rats were conditioned to a punishment discrimination by simultaneously rewarding with food and punishing with shock, all lever responses made in the presence of a discriminative stimulus (tone). Shock intensity was either high or low, but stable during the tone periods. Various doses of each drug were administered i.p. in intervals of at least 2 weeks. On the high-shock control baseline, rats were given chlordiazepoxide in doses of 7.5, 15.0 and 30.0 mg/kg. These worked during tone periods and tolerated more shocks at 7.5 and 15.0 mg/kg, while 30 mg/kg produced side effects interfering with performance. On the low shock baseline, rats were given chlorpromazine in doses of 0.25, 0.5, 1.0, 2.0 and 3.0 mg/kg; these accepted less shocks during the tone period with a decrease in shocks related to an increase in dosage. This technique may be useful in investigating new compounds before clinical investigations.

Department of Psychopharmacology
Wyeth Laboratories, Inc.
Box 8292
Philadelphia 1, Pa.

2128 Scriabine, A., & Blake, M. Evaluation of centrally acting drugs in mice with fighting behaviour induced by isolation. Psychopharmacologia, 1962, 3, 224-226.

Aggressive male mice in which fighting behavior was induced by isolation, were used in pairs to compare the tranquilizing activity of chlorpromazine, chlordiazepoxide and meprobamate at 3 dose levels. Reduction in fighting time for pairs of mice was used for evaluation. Dose increase, limited to the level at which motor function was impaired, was comparable for mice treated with 4-8 mg/kg chlorpromazine, 20 mg/kg chlordiazepoxide and 200 mg/kg meprobamate i.p. Highest reduction in fighting time occurred with chlorpromazine and lowest with chlordiazepoxide. As an antifighting agent, chlorpromazine was 13.1 times more potent than chlordiazepoxide, and the latter was 8.3 times more potent than meprobamate. This method is considered efficient and precise for quantitative evaluation of potential tranquilizing agents.

Department of Pharmacology
Medical Research Laboratories
Chas. Pfizer & Co.
Groton, Conn.

2129 Grandjean, E., Battig, K., & Wanner, H.U. Die Wirkungen eines Narkotikums (Trichloräthylen) auf verschiedene Verhaltensreaktionen der Ratte. [The effect of an anesthetic (trichlorethylene) on various behavioral responses in rats.] Helvetica Physiologica et Pharmacologica Acta, 1962, 20, C25-C26.

The effect of inhalation of trichlorethylene vapors (200-1600 ppm, 4-8 hours/day for up to several months) on CAR's, swimming time, performance on Hebb's intelligence test, the climbing test and the T-maze, and spontaneous motility was studied in rats. At 200-800 ppm, sedative effects predominated under most test situations, but some tests revealed decreased inhibitions or increased motivation. At 1600 ppm, the effects were almost all sedative in nature.

Institut für Hygiene und Arbeitsphysiologie
Eidgenossische Technische Hochschule
Zürich, Switzerland

2130 Peterson, Ernest A., Haun, Kenneth, & Upton, Morgan. The effects of meprobamate, d-amphetamine, and placebo on disjunctive reaction time to taboo and nontaboo words. Psychopharmacologia, 1962, 3, 173-187.

To compare the effects of meprobamate and dexamphetamine, a study was made of response to lists of frequently occurring nontaboo words and taboo words, all of the same length and classifiable under animal, vegetable or mineral categories. Following a study of the response of 19 healthy males without medication, 72 subjects were tested in 12 drug sessions. In each group of 6, 2 were given meprobamate

2133   Shurtleff, Donald, Mostofsky, David, & DiMascio, Alberto. The effects of some phenothiazine derivatives on the discrimination of auditory clicks. Psychopharmacologia, 1962, 3, 153-165.

The effects of chlorpromazine, promethazine, perphenazine and trifluoperazine on discrimination of several standard auditory pulse rate frequencies was studied in 30 normal male subjects. Four groups of 5 subjects were each administered placebo and 1 drug at 4 dose levels: chlorpromazine and promethazine each at 25, 50, 100 and 200 mg; trifluoperazine and perphenazine each at 2, 4, 8 and 16 mg. Ten subjects were used as controls. The 3-category Method of Constant Stimuli was used to estimate the subject's sensitivity to auditory pulse frequency differences. Two measures were used for discrimination; the difference limen (DL) and the standard deviation (SD) of difference judgements. At both high and low standard frequencies, chlorpromazine impaired discrimination while promethazine impaired discrimination only at the higher frequency. Increases in the DL under the higher doses of chlorpromazine was related to a systematic increase in the use of equal judgements at these dose levels. Perphenazine and trifluoperazine did not impair discrimination, however, a "crescent"-shaped dose curve for DL's was noted on perphenazine, consistent with similar dose effects reported for other behavioral measures.

Department of Psychology
Boston University
Boston 15, Mass.

2134   Aston, Roy, Sekino, Eiji, & Greifenstein, Ferdinand E. Quantitation of drug effects upon conditioned avoidance behavior in the rat. Toxicology and Applied Pharmacology, 1962, 4, 393-401.

The effect of pentobarbital, chlorpromazine, propiomazine and reserpine upon conditioned avoidance behavior in rats were studied quantitatively using a modification of the technique of Cook and Weidley (1957). The depression of CAR's was found to be due both to a drug-indiced indifference (reduction of anxiety or loss of fear moti-

vated behavior), and to sedation, muscular
weakness and ataxia. At equipotent doses,
all tranquilizers were found to possess the
same degree of specific activity (reduction
of anxiety, etc.), while pentobarbital showed
much less specificity in this context. When
the influence of acutely administered reserpine was compared to the chronically administered drug, no qualitative differences
were seen as ptosis, lethargy and depression
were similarly observed.

Department of Anesthesiology
Wayne State University College of Medicine
Detroit, Mich.

2135 Buchel, Laïa, & Levy, Jeanne. II. -
Sur les propriétés neuroleptiques du tripéridol. [On the neuroleptic properties of triperidol.] Therapie, 1962, 17, 1063-1084.

Catalepsy induction was studied in mice
by means of injections of 0.5-5 mg/kg
triperidol i.p. or s.c., and in rats by oral
administration of 5-10 mg/kg. The higher
doses induced catalepsy. Subsequent tests
with i.p. and s.c. administration in rats
indicate similar results, young rats being
more sensitive to triperidol than older
animals. Caramiphene and trihexyphenidyl
at doses of 20 mg/kg are capable of
exercising a protective action against catalepsy induced by triperidol, while diethazine
is ineffective. At noncataleptic doses of
0.075-0.1 mg/kg, triperidol exercises a
depressant effect on investigative activity
as measured by the number of movements
per 5 minutes. At noncataleptic doses,
triperidol is antagonistic to dexamphetamine, in both species and for various
routes of administration, both in the sense
of calming hyperactivity induced by low
doses of amphetamine, and in protecting
the mice against the lethal effects of LD_{50}
doses of amphetamine. Triperidol is like-
wise antagonistic to caffeine and cocaine
as measured by effects on behavior and
activity patterns. At doses of 1 mg/kg
and higher, it tends to reduce mouse body
temperature, but less so than haloperidol.
At noncataleptic doses, triperidol potentiates sleep induced by chloral hydrate or
hexobarbital. The percentage of failures
in the chimney-climbing test is as great
with 1 mg/kg triperidol as with 4 times

version was not significantly correlated
with any of the measures of figural after-
effect.

Institute of Psychiatry
Maudsley Hospital
London, Great Britain

2139 Stewart, Jane. Differential responses based on the physiological consequences
of pharmacological agents. Psychopharmacologia, 1962, 3, 132-138.

Male hooded rats were trained to make
differential escape responses based solely
on the different physiological states brought
about by chlorpromazine, imipramine, prochlorperazine, acepromazine, perphenazine
and prothipendyl. The test drug, administered i.p., was never given more than
twice a week, and on days between test
drugs, daily trials were given under normal training conditions. Three groups of
10 animals each were used as follows:
2 groups were trained to differentiate
between saline and chlorpromazine while
the 3rd was trained to differentiate between
saline and imipramine. When responses
were well established, "test drugs" were
substituted for the "training drugs" in an
attempt to determine the degree of transfer of learned response from the "training
drug" to the "test drug". Chlorpromazine-
induced response transferred to acepromazine, perphenazine and prothipendyl, yet
there was no transfer from chlorpromazine
to prochlorperazine or to imipramine at
the doses studied. The imipramine-trained
response did not transfer to either chlorpromazine or acepromazine. The animal's
behavior is guided by a particular constellation of physiological changes, i.e., changes
in muscle tonus and body temperature.
Thus the present study could serve as a
starting point for a detailed study of the
comparative effects of the more complex
drugs used in this study with drugs known
to have more specific and limited physiological effects.

Ayerst Research Laboratories
P.O. Box 6115
Montreal, Quebec
Canada

2140 Kinnard, William J., Aceto, Mario
D.G., & Buckley, Joseph P. The effects of
certain psychotropic agents on the conditioned emotional response behavior of the
albino rats. Psychopharmacologia, 1962,
3, 227-230.

Conditioned emotional response (CER) was
used as a drug screening procedure in
male Wistar rats. A wide dosage range
was administered i.p.: chlorpromazine 0.5-
3.0 mg/kg, reserpine 0.5-0.6 mg/kg and
mephenoxalone 15-75 mg/kg. Dosage level
was kept below that producing motor depression; chlorpromazine was administered
in a motor depressant dose only when lower
doses did not produce attenuation in the
CER program. None of the drugs produced
an attenuation in the "anxiety" response.
Drug administration was repeated at intervals of 3-7 days with normal saline administered in intervals between tests. Animals
initially placed in a Foringer Rat Box

termination of the experimental period. Ascending paper chromatographic analysis showed that a mean of 75.2% radioactivity was associated with the T3 carrier spot; the remainder was associated mainly with iodide and mono- and diiodotyrosine. While the rats received enough reserpine to be "tranquilized", this dosage had no effect on the uptake and degradation of labeled-triiodothyronine by the nervous system, muscle or anterior pituitary lobe. Furthermore there was no indication that reserpine in any way interfered with iodide concentration by the thyroid subsequent to deiodination of T3 by other tissues in the intact animal.

Department of Anatomy
450 Carson Ave.
Brooklyn 3, N.Y.

2143 Kaumann, A.J., Coussio, J.D., & Izquierdo, J.A. Der Einfluss von Imipramin auf die Blutdruck- und Ekg-Wirkungen von Adrenalin, Noradrenalin, Hydroxytryptamin und Hypertensin. [The influence of imipramine on blood pressure and ECG activity by epinephrine (adrenalin), levarterenol (noradrenalin), hydroxytryptamine and angiotensin.] Medicina Experimentalis, 1962, 6, 1-13.

The influence of imipramine on the pressor and ECG responses to epinephrine, levarterenol, 5HT and angiotensin was studied in 20 pentobarbital narcotized dogs. In 4 dogs pretreated with reserpine 48 hours previously, the effects of imipramine, epinephrine and levarterenol were studied. The dosages employed were: 0.5-2.0 µmg/kg levarterenol monohydrate-ditartrate, 1.0-2.0 µmg/kg epinephrine chlorhydrate, 20.0 µg/kg serotonin creatinine sulfate, 0.2 µ/kg angiotensin, 5.0-10.0 mg/kg azamethonium (ganglionic blocking agent), 3.0 mg/kg imipramine and 250 µg/kg reserpine. Imipramine stimulates the heart rate and moderately influences cardiac repolarization. Epinephrine after imipramine causes variable hyperpressure responses while the ECG remains unaffected. Levarterenol after imipramine elicits a marked blood pressure rise and tachycardia with significant changes in repolarization. The pressure effects of 5HT and angiotensin are accentuated after imipramine, while no change in the

ECG was detected. In reserpinized dogs,
imipramine abolishes hypotension, restoring normal tension and exerting moderate
influence on cardiac repolarization. The
potentiation of levarterenol hypertension
after reserpine is still more accentuated
after imipramine, leading to tachycardia
and repolarization changes. Azamethonium
only slightly influenced the effects of the
other agents.

Cátedra de Farmacología Experimental
Facultad de Farmacia y Bioquímica
Buenos Aires, Argentina

2144   Anderson, Elvin L., Bellinzona, G.B.
Craig, Paul N., Jaffe, Gerald E., Janeway,
Katherine P., Kaiser, Carl, Lester, Bruce
M., Nikawitz, Edward J., Pavloff, Alex M.,
Reiff, Harry E., & Zirkle, Charles L.
Synthesis of phenothiazines. Arzneimittel-
Forschung, 1962, 12, 937-941.

Pharmacological and clinical data has shown
that substitution of the 4-methylpiperazine
group for the dimethylamino group in 10-
(3-aminopropyl)-phenothiazine derivatives
results in compounds with enhanced tranquilizing and antiemetic activities. Therefore, substituted piperazine derivatives of
2-chloro- and 2-trifluoromethyl-phenothi-
azines were synthesized and studied. Most
of the compounds (42), 4-substituted-piper-
azinylalkyl derivatives, are listed in tabular
form, replete with physical and analytical
data. Pharmacological data on thiopropazate and fluphenazine is reviewed. Complete data on all procedures required for
organic synthesis is included.

Research and Development Division
Smith Kline and French Laboratories
Philadelphia, Pa.

2145   Perényi, L., Csütörtök, L., Demet-
er, Magda, & Földes, I. Anwendung von
Ionaustauscher-Chromatographie zur spek-
trofluorometrischen Bestimmung des Sero-
tonins. [Use of ion-exchange chromatography for the spectrofluorometric determinations of serotonin.] Acta Physiologica
Academiae Scientiarum Hungaricae, 1962,
20, 12-13. [Abstract]

test to some animals. Others were given
10 U ACTH i.v. about 8 hours before the
test. The 1st 2 groups were selected for
anticipated antagonistic and synergistic effects in relation to thiopental. ACTH was
tried for possible protective effect. Negative results were obtained in relation to
experimental conflict, which appear due
mainly to the predominant effect of restrictive feeding in reducing the threshold.
In all tests amphetamine and ACTH produced no consistent effects while chlorpromazine caused a marked decrease in
the threshold. Rabbit barbiturate thresholds
seem to resemble those in man.

Department of Psychiatry
College of Medicine
State University of Iowa
Iowa City, Iowa

2150 Glow, Peter H. The antagonism of
methyl phenidate and iproniazid to bulbocapnine catatonia in the rat. Australian
Journal of Experimental Biology and Medical Science, 1962, 40, 499-504.

The effects of methylphenidate on spontaneous psychomotor activity (method of Dicker
et al. 1957) on bulbocapnine-treated male
hooded inbred rats were studied. Fifty
mg/kg bulbocapnine produces a complete
cessation of movement. Depending on the
dose strength of methylphenidate, there
is a stepwise corresponding increase in
the amount of spontaneous psychomotor
movement. The effect of this dosage of
bulbocapnine (50 mg/kg) is almost indistinguishable from those effects reported
with 5 mg/kg reserpine. Methylphenidate
(20-60 mg/kg) has some potency as an
antagonist to the catatoniclike action of
bulbocapnine, but iproniazid (25-100 mg/kg)
was ineffective.

Department of Psychology
University of Adelaide
Adelaide, Australia

2151 Russell, R.L., & Westfall, B.A. Alleviation of barbiturate depression by fat
emulsion. Anesthesia and Analgesia, 1962,
41, 582-585.

Lipomul (a 15% cottonseed oil emulsion, 1.5 g fat/kg) was infused i.v. into 10 male rats immediately following thiopental (20 mg/kg i.v.) administration, and 11 male rats which acted as controls received fat free Lipomul to compare the effect on duration of anesthesia. A 10% corn oil emulsion was administered to 10 male rats and 10 controls to determine the effect of corn oil emulsion on duration of thiopental anesthesia. Thiopental (30-100 mg per 100 ml) in buffered saline was added to brain slices pretreated with corn oil emulsion in order to measure the effects of the emulsion on oxygen consumption. In in vivo experiments with cottonseed oil emulsion, the mean duration of anesthesia for the control group was 13.6 minutes, while that for animals receiving emulsified cottonseed oil was 9.4 minutes. In animals receiving corn oil emulsion, mean duration of anesthesia was 8.1 minutes, while that for controls was 11.6 minutes. Differences in duration of anesthesia were statistically significant. In vitro, a thiopental concentration of 30 mg per 100 ml resulted in no change in oxygen consumption as compared with controls. However, a concentration of 100 mg/100 ml did depress the QO_2 significantly at the 60 and 90 minute intervals. The emulsion alone apparently acted as a stimulant to O_2 uptake by brain slices. The duration of thiopental anesthesia was decreased significantly in rats by an infusion of cottonseed oil and corn oil emulsions. The increased QO_2 of brain slices in the presence of corn oil emulsion is probably due primarily to the emulsifying agent, as neither corn oil nor a 5% glucose solution altered O_2 uptake in the absence of thiopental.

Department of Physiology and Pharmacology
University of Missouri School of Medicine
Columbia, Miss.

2152   Echlin, Francis A., & Battista, Arthur. Regional differences in the epileptiform electrical response of the unanesthetized cerebral cortex to acetylcholine. Neurology, 1962, 12, 551-559.

In 20 monkeys electrocorticograms were

lation and the livers of 2 of these were severely congested. Etryptamine was appreciably better tolerated than α-methyltryptamine. Further doses of etryptamine which were well tolerated orally by rats and dogs during subacute studies were 30-50-fold greater than the anticipated human therapeutic dose. Etryptamine appeared to be without significant cardiovascular toxicity in the dog. In rabbits, muscle irritation was essentially nil at 1 mg/kg and moderate at 10 mg/kg. Also daily p.o. doses of 10 mg/kg produced no effect on rat reproduction.

Research Laboratories
The Upjohn Company
Kalamazoo, Mich.

2155 Kato, R., Vassanelli, P., Frontino, G., & Bolego, A. Metabolism and distribution of carisoprodol in tissues and organs of the rats. Medicina Experimentalis, 1962, 6, 149-157.

The metabolism and tissue distribution of carisoprodol (150-200 mg/kg i.p.) was studied in female Sprague-Dawley rats. Assay was by the method of Hoffman and Ludwig and animals were sacrificed at various intervals after drug administration. The concentration of carisoprodol reached a maximum 20-30 minutes after injection with marked accumulation occurring in liver and kidney and little in muscle or brain tissue. Only 7.5% of injected carisoprodol was eliminated during 48 hours after administration, while 5.5% was eliminated within 12 hours postinjection. Within 5 hours after drug administration, carisoprodol concentration fell to 20% of that observed after 30 minutes. There was a low rate of excretion of the drug in either urine or feces. The biological half-life was about 3 hours. SKF 525 (25 mg/kg i.p.) inhibited carisoprodol metabolism in vivo and prolonged the duration of paralysis in these animals. In vitro experiments suggested that a liver microsomal enzyme (which required TPNH and oxygen) was largely responsible for the metabolism of carisoprodol.

Institute of Pharmacology
University of Milan
Milan, Italy

2156   Cahen, Raymond, Montagne, Jacqueline, Pessonnier, Jeanne, & Pessonnier, André. Etude pharmacologique de la 2-diéthylaminopropiophénone. I. Toxicité. [A pharmacological study of 2-diethylaminopropiophenone. I. Toxicity.] Thérapie,1962, 17, 373-412.

A comparative study of the acute, subacute and chronic toxicity of 2-diethylaminopropiophenone and its closely related analogue dexamphetamine in mice and rats showed that the lethal doses are 1.33-1.6 times as high for the new derivative as for dexamphetamine in mice and 2.13-2.8 times as high in rats (i.p. and p.o.). Addition of highly polymerized polyhydroxyethylenehydroxypropylene (M.W. = 8250) to provide sustained release had no apparent effect on toxicity, and long-term administration of the mixture to rats for 146 days (at levels up to 0.01% of the diet or 5% of the LD_{50}) produced no significant ill effects, only a slight inhibition of growth being seen at the highest dosage.

Centre de Recherches Lafon
Maisons-Alfort, France

2157 Benesová, O., Bohdanecký, Z., & Votava, Z. Electrophysiological comparison of the action of imipramine and propazepine. Psychopharmacologia, 1962, 3, 423-431.

Imipramine and its structural isomer propazepine were compared using 3 electrophysiological methods: bioelectrical activity of cortical and subcortical areas in rabbits with implanted electrodes, changes in the motor thresholds in rabbits with permanent epidural electrodes and self-stimulation in rats (Olds 1954, 1960). EEG records in cortical and subcortical areas (hippocampus, thalamus) in rabbits with implanted electrodes after the administration of both drugs (5 mg/kg i.v.) did not differ. Imipramine had a greater antagonistic effect to cortical desynchronization and subcortical synchronization evoked by physostigmine (0.1 mg/kg i.v.). The potentiation of thiopental anesthesia measured by motor threshold in rabbits with permanent epidural electrodes was greater after the administration of propazepine (2.5 mg/kg i.v.). Imipramine (1, 1.5 and 2 mg/kg i.p.)

pressure, spinal fluid pressure, intestinal tone and respiratory volume. The increase in spinal fluid pressure always appeared later than that in blood pressure, but the effect lasted a relatively long time [30-45 minutes]. At the point of maximal spinal fluid pressure, the rate and amplitude of the spinal fluid pulse reached a minimum, indicating a disturbance in cerebral circulation. This increase in spinal fluid pressure did not occur after i.v. reserpine. The increase in spinal fluid pressure produced by serotonin could be counteracted by LSD, the specific antagonist, but could not be prevented by antihistamines, sympathicolytic agents or anticoagulants. No 5HT could be detected in the brain or spinal fluid, even after i.v. injection of a large dose (1, 2 or 3 mg/kg), indicating that it is unable to pass the blood-brain-spinal fluid barrier.

Institute of Pharmacology
Medical University of Debrecen
Debrecen, Hungary

2161   Ferguson, Hugh C. Dilution of dose and acute oral toxicity. Toxicology and Applied Pharmacology, 1962, $\underline{4}$, 759-762.

Doses of 12 compounds (amphetamine, benactyzine diphenhydramine, mephenesin, pentobarbital, pentetrazol, phenylbutazone, potassium cyanide, etc.) were administered by stomach tube to groups of fasted Sprague-Dawley rats in volumes corresponding to 5, 2.5 and 1.25% body weight. The number of dead animals was recorded after 24 hours. These compounds were also administered to Swiss-Webster mice given in the water 4 hours before drug administration. Further LD_{50}'s for pentobarbital, potassium cyanide, procaine and sodium fluoride were established in mice at 5 and 1% body weight levels. Results show the same trend for all 12 compounds: the greater the dilution of the toxic dose, the greater the death rate. Dilution may alter not only toxicity, but also many other pharmacological responses and determinations.

Distillation Products Industries
Division of Eastman Kodak Company
Rochester 3, N. Y.

2162   Morillo, Arturo, Revzin, Alvin M., &
Knauss, Thomas. Physiological mechan-
isms of action of chlordiazepoxide in cats.
Psychopharmacologia, 1962, <u>3</u>, 386-394.

Acute and chronic experiments were performed on 18 cats in order to investigate
the action of chlordiazepoxide. With electrodes stimulating the lateral nucleus of the
amygdala and recording from the basal hippocampus, the magnitude and time course
of the produced changes upon the electrical
and behavioral responses were studied. The
effects upon the diffuse thalamocortical system were also investigated by stimulating
the nucleus centralis lateralis of the thalamus and recording the recruiting response
from the pial surface of the suprasylvian
gyrus. For acute experiments, chlordiazepoxide was used in single i.v. doses of
2, 5 and 10 mg/kg; in chronic study single
i.m. doses of 10 mg/kg were given. In the
chronic preparations, chlordiazepoxide
showed a strong depressant action on the
hippocampal response and a delayed "slow
motion" response to stimulation of the
amygdala. The diffuse thalamocortical system was unaffected. Results are interpreted
as indicating a site of drug action chiefly
at the amygdalohippocampal level.

Thudichum Psychiatric Research Labora-
   tory
Galesburg State Research Hospital
Galesburg, Ill.

2163   Hansson, Eskil, & Steinwall, Oskar.
Abnormal blood-brain passage of a quater-
nary phenothiazine derivative (S^{35}-labelled
Aprobit) induced by chemical agents. Acta
Physiologica Scandinavica, 1962, <u>54</u>, 339-
345.

Abnormal blood-brain passage of S^{35}-la-
beled Aprobit (aphenothiazine derivative)
was induced by regional brief perfusion of
Hg^{++}, cyanine dye 863 or unlabeled Aprobit
through rabbit cerebral vessels. The test
substance, radiochemically pure S^{35}-Apro-
bit was injected into the left cardiac ventricle after ligation of the thoracic aorta in
order to augment cranial concentration in
doses of 90-150 µc/kg body weight. Cerebral
uptake of S^{35}-Aprobit was recorded by
means of autoradiography and radioassay.

greater than 40 mg/kg produced a short
asymptomatic lag period (5-10 minutes),
which preceded tonic, clonic convulsions and
the Straub tail effect. Dosages in excess of
80 mg/kg produced brief convulsions which
rapidly terminated in death. Nalorphine (0.5
mg/kg s.c.) injected 10 minutes before dextropropoxyphene increased the LD50 to 105
mg/kg. Whereas animals not treated with
nalorphine died during the initial part of
the convulsant period, the nalorphine-treat-
ed animals survived with a proportionally
longer convulsant period. Three groups of
8 animals received dextropropoxyphene (65
mg/kg i.p.) followed by nalorphine (0.1-20
mg/kg s.c.) administered at the initial
convulsion to determine whether or not
nalorphine could antagonize established
convulsions. Convulsant time was diminished to 52% of controls with 0.1 mg/kg,
to 39.9% with 0.5 mg/kg and to 10.2% with
20 mg/kg. Generalized convulsions were
shown to be cerebral in origin.

Department of Pharmacology
University of Kansas Medical Center
Kansas City 3, Kan.

2167 Miller, Lowell D. The distribution,
metabolism, and excretion of phenyramidol
in the dog. Toxicology and Applied Pharmacology, 1962, 4, 190-199.

Phenyramidol determinations were made
on samples of dog urine, blood plasma and
tissue at various times after the administration of 150 or 200 mg/kg phenyramidol.
Paper chromatography and spectrophotometric analyses of the urine extract before
and after β-glucuronidase hydrolysis sub-
stantiated the presence of phenyramidol
glucuronide as a major metabolite. In anesthetized dogs, the circulating phenyramidol
disappeared rapidly from the blood stream
so that within 5 minutes after injection
most of the drug had been removed. Two
elimination pathways were noted: one via
the bile and the other in the urine. The
rate of urinary excretion was 10-15% of
a daily oral dose. Less than 1.5% of the
administered dose was present in the urine
in unmetabolized form and most of this
appeared within the 1st 24-hour period. After
i.v. (25 mg/kg) or oral administration, most
of the drug was retained by the muscle

mass whence it was slowly released back
into circulation for conjugation with glucuronic acid by the liver. Skeletal muscle
appears to act as a repository for the
administered drug.

Research Laboratories
Irwin, Neisler and Co.
Decatur, Ill.

2168   Erdmann, G., & Külz, J. Experimentelle Krämpfe durch INH und ihre therapeutische Beeinflussung, auch im Hinblick auf
INH-bedingte Veränderungen des EEG bei
Kindern. [Experimentally induced convulsions with isoniazid (INH) and their treatment, with special reference to INH-related
changes in the EEG of children.] Monat-
schrift für Kinderheil Kunde, 1962, 110,
123-125.

Oral doses of 200 mg/kg isoniazid induced
convulsions in mice, and led to death
within 1-2 hours. Doses of 50 mg/kg phenobarbital and 5-(2-butenyl)-5-ethyl barbituric acid (Kalypnon) successfully combated
the convulsant effects of isoniazid, but as
the dosage of phenobarbital was increased,
the mice died despite suppression of the
convulsions. Guayacolglycerineether in doses of 200 mg/kg suppresses INH-convul-
sions, and will prevent subsequent death.
In view of the effect of isoniazid on mice,
EEG's were obtained from 17 children receiving 10 mg/kg/day isoniazid for 3 days.
Of the 17, 6 showed signs of hyperventilation, including 2 cases of neurological or
psychic disorders, and 2 cases of suspected
cerebral attacks. Suspension of INH treatment or dosage reduction is recommended
in cases where EEG's reveal latent convulsive tendencies.

Universitäts Kinderklinik
Mainz, Germany

2169   Carlsson, Arvid, & Lindqvist, Margit.
In vivo decarboxylation of α-methyl-dopa
and α-methyl metatyrosine. Acta Physiologica Scandinavica, 1962, 54, 87-94.

α-Methyl DOPA and α-methyl metatyrosine
were administered to mice (400 mg/kg i.p.).
α-Methyl DOPA was also administered to

rat and dog studies.

International Research and Development
Corporation
Kalamazoo, Mich.

2172 Schievelbein, H., & Werle, E.,
Freisetzung von 5-Hydroxytryptamin durch
Nicotin [Release of 5-hydroxytryptamine by
nicotine.] Psychopharmacologia, 1962, 3,
35-43.

Nicotine (N) produces release of 5HT from
rabbit thrombocytes (phosphate buffer pH
7.3; 37°C; 50 min.). This effect increases
with increasing N-concentration. N at 1
mg/ml produces release of 58% of the
total 5HT present. Temperature changes
between 20 and 40°C have no effect on the
reaction. There is no release below pH
6.7. Above pH 6.9 the release increases
with increasing alkalinity. Sodium fluoride,
EDTAA, 2,4-dinitrophenol and iproniazid
(all at 0.001 mg/3 ml) did not affect the
reaction but Natriumazid [sodium acetate?]
produced slight inhibition. In a 10 times
higher concentration N accelerates release
of histamine from rat thrombocytes and
from mast cells. Urinary excretion of 5HIAA
increases in nonsmokers from 1.81 mg/24
hours to 3.03 mg/24 hours after smoking
of 5-10 cigarettes in a day. The possible
physiological significance of these observ-
ances is discussed.

Klinisch-Chemisches Institut
Chirurgische Klinik der Universität München
Munich, Germany

2173 Duchene-Marullaz, P., Busch, N., &
Vacher, J. Toxicité aiguë, actions analgésique et sédative générale de quelques
dérivés du crésotamide. [Acute toxicity,
analgesic and general sedative actions of
some cresotamide derivatives.] Thérapie,
1962, 17, 999-1004.

Eight substitution derivatives of cresotamide were studied for analgesic and sedative actions by means of electroshock pain
to the dental pulp of rabbits. Three doses
were used for each product: 250, 500 and
1000 mg/kg p.o. Also potentiation of pentobarbital narcosis was studied, using the

derivatives at 500 mg/kg p.o. and 100 mg/kg
i.p. in mice. Effects of temperature regulation were studied in rats at 4°C; little modification was effected. Mice were tested on
the turning rod 0.5 hours after the administration of 500 mg/kg p.o. doses. The LD_{50}'s
p.o. were 1-3 g/kg, except for the chloro-
benzyloxy derivative which at 3 g/kg did
not cause mortality. Most of the compounds
possess analgesic activity superior to that
of aspirin and sedative action is marked for
allyloxy, butoxy and methoxy derivatives.

Route de Marsat
Riom, Puy-de-Dome
France

2174 Buchel, L., Levy, Jeanne, & Tissier,
M. Contributionà l'étude pharmacologique
du Tripéridol (R. 2498). [Contribution to
the pharmacologic study of triperidol
(R 2498).] Thérapie, 1962, 17, 1053-1062.

The acute toxicity of triperidol was determined in Swiss mice i.v., i.p., i.m. and p.o.
(stomach tube), and in Wistar rats i.m. and
p.o. (stomach tube). LD_{50}'s for female mice
were i.v.-17.4 mg/kg (aqueous solution) and
18.4 mg/kg (aqueous solution containing
methyl and propyl paraoxybenzoates), i.p.-
35.8 mg/kg, i.m. 64.0 mg/kg and p.o. 98.8
mg/kg. In rats the addition of paraoxyben-
zoate did not modify results. Male rats were
more resistant to toxicity than females. The
i.m. LD_{50} in rats approximated 50 mg/kg
while the p.o. LD_{50} was approximately 3
times higher. In subacute 3-week and chronic 2-month toxicity studies (e.g., 2.5 mg/kg/
day p.o. in young rats, none lost weight or
died. Congestion of the hepatic veins after
3 weeks of treatment was noted at sacrifice.
After 2 months congestion of the meninges
and liver, with the presence of vacuolar cells
was noted. These alterations regressed
slightly after 2.5 months rest, and recovery is more marked in female than in male
rats. The blood formula was not modified
significantly in any instances.

15, rue de l'Ecole de Médecine
Paris VI°, France

2175 von Ledebur, I., Frommel, Ed., &
Béguin, M. Nalorphine antagonism to the

2178 Kelemen, K., Magyar, K., & Knoll,
J. Elektroenzephalographische Differenzierung von Sedato-Hypnotika und Major-
Tranquillantien. [Electroencephalographic
differentiation between sedative hypnotics
and major tranquilizers.] Acta Physiologica
Academiae Scientiarum Hungaricae, 1962,
20, 41-42. [Abstract]

The prolonged, reproducible, generalized
EEG arousal reaction produced by the
conditioned stimulus during the "spring
test" in rats could not be inhibited even
by high doses of sedatives or hypnotics
(e.g., 40 mg/kg phenobarbital), but was
prevented completely by low doses of the
major tranquilizers (e.g., 1 mg/kg reserpine). These results confirm the specificity
of the "spring test" for studies on the
major tranquilizers and indicate that the
nonextinguishing CR is facilitated by a
specific condition in the reticular formation
of the brain stem.

Institute of Pharmacology
Medical University of Budapest
Budapest, Hungary

2179 Kuhn, H.-F., & Friebel, H. Über
den Nachweis von "Physical Dependence"
bei Codein-behandelten Ratten. [Demon-
stration of "Physical Dependence" in co-
deine-treated rats. Medicina Experimentalis, 1962, 6, 301-306.

Male Wistar rats received s.c. injections
of codeine in increasing amounts for a
period of 8 weeks. The total amount injected per animal was 2.3 g/kg in 8 weeks.
After the last injection with codeine the
rats received s.c. 20 mg/kg nalorphine,
while another group of rats which received
the same amount of nalorphine had received
only 30 minutes prior to this injection an
initial dose of 22.2 mg/kg codeine. Both
groups were closely observed for 30 minutes after the injection, regarding reactions
such as stretching, scratching, chewing,
etc., on 1 hand, diarrhea, and increased
or decreased locomotor activity on the
other hand. Behavioral differences in the
2 groups were evident after 5 minutes. It
is without doubt that chronic treatment
with codeine produces in rats a condition
in which the injection of nalorphine brings

about a physical imbalance. The symptoms
of nalorphine-induced acute abstinence are
regarded as "physical dependence".

Pharmakologisches Institut
Universität Bonn
Bonn, Germany

2180 Carlsson, Arvid, & Hillarp, Nils-
Ake. Formation of phenolic acids in brain
after administration of 3,4-dihydroxyphen-
ylalanine. Acta Physiologica Scandinavica,
1962, 55, 95-100.

The formation of 3,4-dihydroxyphenylacetic
acid (DOPAC) and homovanillic acid (HVA)
in rabbit brain following i.v. injection of
DOPA (100 mg/kg body weight) was studied
to gain further knowledge of the role of
brain catechol-O-methyl transferase and
MAO. After varying periods of time following DOPA administration, animals were
killed and the brain was immediately removed and dissected. DOPAC was determined spectrophotofluorimetrically (by the
method of Rosengren, 1960). HVA was
estimated semiquantitatively by chromatography. As well, nialamide (100 mg/kg)
and reserpine (5 mg/kg) were given i.v.
20 hours before DOPA injections. When
DOPA was administered, large amounts
of DOPA and HVA accumulated rapidly
in the brain stem. This suggests that the
dopamine formed endogenously from DOPA
administration rapidly reaches sites of
MAO, where DOPAC is formed which in
turn reaches sites of catechol-O-methyl
transferase. The data also suggests that
the accumulated phenolic acids do not
easily escape from the brain to the blood.
The possibility of MAO being localized
within the amine producing cell and the
O-methyl transferase located extracellu-
larly in the vicinity of supposed receptors,
is discussed. In addition, iproniazid and
nialamide prevent the formation of DOPAC
from DOPA.

Department of Pharmacology
University of Göteborg
Göteborg, Sweden

2181 Walther, H. Die Wirkung von Anti-
cholinergica auf den Strychnintremor in-

when animals were pretreated with increasing doses of chlorpromazine. Intracerebral injection of minute amounts of nicotine caused immediate and violent convulsions in mice, directly related to nicotine dosage. Intracerebral CD_{50} of nicotine was found to be 1.0 ± 0.52 μg.

Department of Pharmacology
Medical College
Baroda, India

2183   Clouet, Doris H. The methylation of normorphine in rat brain. Acta Neurologica Scandinavica, 1962, 38, 26-27.

Morphine and codeine, and their demethylated nor-derivatives [See also Abstract 945] were isolated from rat tissue homogenates in incubation mixtures and identified by extraction followed by paper chromatography. In addition, when methyl donors labeled by C^{14} were used, the chromatographic strips were examined for radioactivity in a strip-counting autoscanner. Methionine labeled in the methyl group and reduced glutathione were incubated with normorphine, and morphine was recovered from the incubation mixture. Various liver preparations catalyzed the methyl action of normorphine, including the supernatant of 0.25 M sucrose homogenate after centrifugation at 10,000 gravities for 20 minutes. A brain fraction prepared in the same way as liver methylpherase was also effective in promoting normorphine methylation. With this brain preparation norcodeine was methylated to codeine and morphine was also recovered, presumably by 3-demethylation of codeine. When S-adenosyl-methionine (C^{14}-methyl) was substituted for methionine and the methionine activating enzyme, the pH optimum for the methylation of normorphine was 5.5. In vivo, no morphine methylation was demonstrated: methionine (C^{14}-methyl) was injected into the cisterna magna of the rat (0.5 μM containing 2.5 μc of C14), and 15 minutes later 0.5 μM normorphine was administered by the same route. The rats were killed 10 minutes later and labeled morphine isolated from these brains. Therefore, with normorphine, remethylation of morphine is a possible metabolic step.

New York State Research Institute for
  Neurochemistry and Drug Addiction
New York, N.Y.

2184   Winter, Charles A., & Flataker, Lars. Cage design as a factor influencing acute toxicity of respiratory depressant drugs in rats. Toxicology and Applied Pharmacology, 1962, 4, 650-655.

Young male rats received s.c. injections of morphine (18.75-150 mg/kg), anileridine (12.5-22.25 mg/kg) or pentobarbital (37.2-45 mg/kg) and were placed in open or shut cages. Two types of closed cages were used: 1 type with the bottom and 4 sides of sheet metal and the top of wire mesh, and the other type with the bottom and 1 wall of sheet metal, and the remaining 3 sides and top of wire mesh. The open cage consisted completely of wire mesh. When drugs were in effect and an animal was severely depressed, his nose would sometimes be pressed against a sheet metal surface and he would succumb, apparently in respiratory failure. More than a 10-fold increase in LD_{50} could be obtained by placing animals in open cages as compared to sheet metal cages. Cages of wire mesh with sheet metal reinforcements and solid corners gave intermediate mortality figures. In sheet metal cages, deaths could be prevented either by shielding with wire mesh or moving the animal whenever his nose was pressed against a solid metal corner. Differences of the kind described in rats were not observed in mice injected with morphine or anileridine, a fact explainable by the hypermotility observed in mice during the peak effect of these drugs in contrast to the quiescence in rats.

Merck Institute for Therapeutic Research
West Point, Pa.

2185   Horovitz, Zola P., Chow, May-I, & Carlton, Peter L. Self-stimulation of the brain by cats: effects of imipramine, amphetamine and chlorpromazine. Psychopharmacologia, 1962, 3, 455-462.

Cats with electrodes in the lateral hypothalamus or caudate nucleus, which were

trained through a self-stimulation procedure (Horovitz et al., 1962), were tested
3 times a week and given i.p. injections
of saline immediately before each 1 hour
session. Before the 2nd session each week,
various doses of imipramine (1-4 mg/kg),
dexamphetamine (0.1-0.5 mg/kg), or chlorpromazine (2.5-5.0 mg/kg), were substituted for the saline. Doses were given in
random order with at least 1 week intervening between drug injections. Dexamphetamine increased and chlorpromazine tended
to decrease the response of cats working
for stimulation of the caudate nucleus and
lateral hypothalamus. In contrast, imipramine increased responses maintained by
stimulation of lateral hypothalamic sites,
but did not have a comparable effect on
self-stimulation of the caudate. Thus, while
all drugs altered rates of response maintained by lateral hypothalamic stimulation,
only dexamphetamine and chlorpromazine
produced comparable results on self-stimulation of both sites. Several postulates
based on other studies are given for these
results, including the suggestion that the
site of imipramine activity differs from that
of dexamphetamine and chlorpromazine in
the cat, and imipramine activity may be
restricted to hypothalamic structures.

Squibb Institute for Medical Research
New Brunswick, N.J.

2186 Hoffmeister, F. Über cerebrale po-
lysynaptische Reflexe des Kaninchens und
ihre Beeinflussbarkeit durch Pharmaka.
[The cerebral polysynaptic reflexes in rabbits and their susceptibility to certain
drugs.] Archives Internationales de
Pharmacodynamie et de Thérapie, 1962,
139, 512-527.

The relation of pulse frequencies to strength
of threshold signal, effects of resection of
certain nerves, and effects of certain drugs
upon the threshold signal were studied on
more than 100 rabbits. The licking-reflex
response to electrical stimulation of the
upper incisors is extinguished by resection
of the CNS on the mesencephalic and
thalamic levels, but not on the prethalamic
level. The jaw-opening reflex caused by
electrical stimulation of the upper incisors
is unaffected even by resections in the

shocks. Marked reduction in the severity
of convulsions occurred at all dosage levels.
No benefit was observed in picrotoxin or
strychnine-induced seizures. The drug prevented development of the tonic extensor
component produced by electroshock treatment.

Department of Pharmacology
Medical College
Bikaner, India

2189 Dandiya, P.C., Sharma, P.K., &
Menon, M.K. Studies on central nervous
system depressants. Part IV. Structure-
activity relationship of some locally synthesized trimethoxy benzene derivatives.
Indian Journal of Medical Research, 1962,
50, 750-760.

Fifteen trimethoxy benzene derivatives,
differing from each other only in the
relative positions of the methoxy group
with respect to the side chain or in the
structure of the side chain, were synthesized. Their influence on barbiturate hypnosis in mice, spontaneous activity in rats,
CAR's in rats and effect on blood pressure
in morphinized and urethanized dogs was
studied. These compounds resemble reserpine and chlorpromazine in that they prolong
pentobarbital hypnosis. None of the compounds influenced spontaneous motor activity. Only 2 compounds, 3,4,5-trimethoxy
benzamide and its N-acetyl derivative were
effective in influencing CAR's in trained
rats. Most of the compounds caused a
lowering of blood pressure in dogs.

Department of Pharmacology
S.M.S. Medical College
Jaipur, India

2190 Knecht, M., & Bernhard, K. Intensi-
vierung der Demethylierung in vivo nach
Angewöhnung. [Acceleration of demethylation in vivo after habituation.] Helvetica
Physiologica et Pharmacologica Acta,1962,
20, C34-C35.

When rats were fed small doses of glutethimide for 3 weeks and methyl-labeled N-
methylglutethimide was then added to the
microsome preparations from the rats'

livers, measurement of the radioactivity
in the resultant formaldehyde showed that
demethylation was going on at a much
more rapid rate in the livers of habituated
rats than in control animals. These results confirm the postulate that the reason
for increased tolerance to drugs after
prolonged use is stimulation of the activity of the catabolic enzymes.

Physiologisches-Chemisches Institut
Universität Basel
Basel, Switzerland

2191 Knoll, J., & Knoll, Berta. Methode
zur tierexperimentellen Untersuchung von
antidepressiv wirkenden Mitteln. [A method
for animal experimentation with antidepressant drugs.] Acta Physiologica Academiae Scientiarum Hungaricae, 1962, 20,
41. [Abstract]

A procedure, based on the "spring test"
for the major tranquilizers, is described
for measuring the psychoenergetic activity
of the clinically effective antidepressants
in animals. While untreated rats generally
jump up from a 45°C hotplate in 10-120",
and those treated with reserpine (0.1 mg/kg)
fail to jump up and eventually die, those
given both reserpine and amphetamine (1
mg/kg), imipramine (5 mg/kg) or phenelzine (5 mg/kg) jump up even more rapidly
than untreated controls.

Institute of Pharmacology
Medical University of Budapest
Budapest, Hungary

2192 Bättig, K. Wirkungen von Amphäta-
min auf verschiedene Schwimmleistungen
der Ratte. [Effects of amphetamine on
swimming capacity in rats.] Helvetica
Physiologica et Pharmacologica Acta, 1962,
20, C15-C16.

The effect of amphetamine (1.5 and 4.0 mg
per kg) on swimming time carrying a
ballast of 10% of the body weight and on
swimming speed (time to swim 4 m either
free or against a load) was determined in
male rats. The average swimming capacity
was not improved by training but was
increased 20-30% by amphetamine. The

physiologische Unterschiede im Wirkungs-
mechanismus einiger Muskelrelaxantien.
[The electrophysiological differences in
the mechanism of action of some muscle
relaxants.] Acta Physiologica Academiae
Scientiarum Hungaricae, 1962, 20, 44-45.
[Abstract]

Recordings of the action potential of individual muscle spindle afferents had γ-
efferents isolated from the lumbar spine
(L5-S1) of cats showed that the activity
of the γ-efferents was inhibited for sever al
hours by 1 mg/kg of chlorpromazine but was
unaffected by Mydeton (10 mg/kg i.v.).
Neither drug had any effect on the muscle
spindle receptors, even at high doses.
Since Mydeton does not inhibit the monosynaptic patellar reflex and has no curariform activity, the muscular weakness after
Mydeton administration must be due mainly
to depression of the multisynaptic connections in the spine.

Institute of Physiology
Medical University of Szeged
Szeged, Hungary

2197 Werboff, Jack, & Dembicki, Eugene
L. Toxic effects of tranquilizers administered to gravid rats. Journal of Neuropsychiatry, 1962, 4, 87-91.

Reserpine (0.1 mg/kg s.c. in 3 divided
doses), chlorpromazine (6.0 mg/kg/day s.c.
in 3 divided doses), meprobamate (60.0
mg/kg/day s.c. in 3 divided doses) or
distilled water was administered to 89
gravid Sprague-Dawley rats during gestation on either days 5 through 8, 11 to 14
or 17 to 20. Daily observations for neonatal
mortality were made for 21 days from birth
through weaning. Weight was recorded at
regular intervals for 120 days. Mortality
was classified 3 ways; born dead, died on
days 1 through 21, or devoured by mother.
The 89 gravid rats delivered a total of 869
animals, 279 of which failed to survive.
Neonatal mortality with drugs administered
during the 1st trimester was: 27.1% with
reserpine,   43.9% with chlorpromazine,
48.0% with meprobamate and 19.2% with
controls. Drugs in the 2nd trimester yielded: 36.8% with reserpine, 11.7% chlorpromazine, 35.4% meprobamate and 10.6%

controls. Mortality figures for the 3rd trimester were: 25.0% reserpine, 61.6% chlorpromazine, 45.6% meprobamate and 7.3% controls. These tranquilizers administered to the gravid rat are toxic to the embryos and to the newborn. The largest contributor to the high neonatal mortality in the drug groups was the devoured by mother category. Reserpine and meprobamate-treated offspring weighed less than controls, while chlorpromazine-treated offspring weighed more than controls.

University of Madrid
Madrid, Spain

2198 van der Schoot, J.V., Ariëns, E.J., van Rossum, J.M., & Hurkmans, Th. M. Phenylisopropylamine derivatives, structure and action. Arzneimittel-Forschung, 1962, 12, 902-907.

Amphetamine (phenylisopropylamine) and a large number of its derivatives were tested, using spontaneous activity in mice (interruptions of photoelectric cell light beams per minute). A dose-effect curve was worked out for amphetamine at 10, 15, 20 and 25 μM/kg i.p. for use as a reference. Also several α-sympatholytic and β-sympatholytic compounds were used. The replacement of the phenyl ring in amphetamine by certain 5- or 6-membered rings is allowed. The binding of the amino group to a secondary carbon atom seems to be required. The chain between the amino group and the ring is restricted to 2 carbon units. The introduction of substituents results in a decrease or a loss of activity. A relatively wide variation of substituents in the side chain and even an incorporation of an amino group in the aliphatic ring is tolerated. The introduction of OH groups in the phenyl ring leads to a definite loss of activity. The introduction of other small substituents in the phenyl ring is tolerated in the para and meta positions. Substitution in the ortho position leads to a loss of activity. All reasonably active compounds have an amino group attached to a secondary carbon atom. For some compounds closely related to amphetamine, a direct action on cerebral catecholamine receptors is feasible, while for a number of N-substituted amphetamines and cocaine an indirect action

receiving morphine and neostigmine. Acta Pharmacologica et Toxicologica, 1962, 19, 286-292.

Morphine (700 mg/kg) and neostigmine (0.2 mg/kg) were given i.p. to morphine-tolerant and nontolerant male rats. Spontaneous death after i.p. injection of both drugs occurred 14-26 minutes later. For comparison, the rats given morphine alone were killed at about the same times as those at which the rats died from the combined injections. Morphine was determined in the brains of both groups. Neostigmine was not found to increase the amounts of brain morphine. The simultaneous i.p. administration of both drugs can lead to an erroneous determination of morphine. However this was overcome when paper chromatography was included in the analytical procedure and the error was not met with during the analysis of the brains of the tolerant rats.

Department of Pharmacology
University of Copenhagen
Copenhagen, Denmark

2203 Frahm, Margarete, Lübkens, K., & Soehring, K. Der Einfluss subchronischer Alkoholgaben auf die Barbiturat-Narkose von Meerschweinchen. [The influence of subchronic administration of alcohol on barbiturate narcosis in guinea pigs.] Arzneimittel-Forschung, 1962, 12, 1055-1056.

Ethyl alcohol solutions of 5, 10 or 15% were given to guinea pigs as the only source of liquid over a period of 14 days. The onset and duration of narcosis with pentobarbital (20 mg/kg), methitural (70 mg per kg) and hexobarbital (50 mg/kg) were measured at intervals of 7 days. The onset of narcosis is slightly prolonged in proportion to the concentration of alcohol ingested. In contrast, the duration of narcosis was considerably reduced in proportion to the concentration of alcohol in all 3 series of experiments. Measurements taken 14 days after discontinuation of the alcohol ingestion showed a return to normal values.

Pharmakologisches Institut
Universität Hamburg
Hamburg, Germany

2204   Pletscher, A., & Gey, K.F. Action
of imipramine and amitriptyline on cerebral monoamines as compared with chlorpromazine. Medicina Experimentalis,1962,
6, 165-168.

Wistar rats were pretreated with varying
doses of imipramine, amitriptyline and
chlorpromazine i.p. One hour later the
animals received 2 mg/kg reserpine or
100 mg/kg iproniazid s.c. Rats receiving
1 drug only or no drug at all served as
controls. Brain levels of 5HT or of 5HT
and levarterenol were determined 4 hours
after administration of iproniazid and reserpine respectively using spectrophotofluorometric methods. Furthermore, rats
pretreated with chlorpromazine or imipramine 1 hour before injection of 5HTP
were sacrified half an hour later and the
following procedures were carried out:
a/ immediate homogenization of the brains
and spectrophotofluorometric assay of 5HT
(5HT rise in vivo) and b/ incubation of the

2205 Vasbinder, H., & van der Sijde, H.R. Een gevoelige kleurreactie op imipramine. [A selective color reaction for impramine.] Pharmaceutische Weekblad, 1962, 17, 610-611.

Imipramine reacts in the diphenylamine test for nitrates and nitrites by forming a colorless solution in acidified (H$_2$SO$_4$) solutions and a dark blue color in alkaline solutions (NaNO$_3$). Also acidic and basic diphenylamine colors were given for chlordiazepoxide, haloperidol, hydroxazine, mephenesin, meprobamate, chlorpromazine, levomepromazine, mepazine, perphenazine, prochlorperazine, promethazine, promazine and thiazinaminum.

Gemeente Apotheek
Rotterdam, The Netherlands

2206 Kamp, W., Klijsen, J.B., & Ruward, R.H. De scheiding van enige barbitalen met behulp van een anionuitwisselaar op haarsbasis. [Separation of some barbiturates by means of anion exchange resins.] Pharmaceutisch Weekblad, 1962, 6, 889-894.

Separation of 11 barbituric acid derivatives was accomplished. About 50 mg of the barbiturates were dissolved in 10 ml 0.1 N NH$_3$ and passed through a 10 x 250 mm column of Dowex 1-X2 (100-200 mesh) in the acetate form. After washing with 3 x 10 ml water, the acids were eluted with 0.71 M NH$_4$COOH buffer solutions at pH 5.1, which contained different concentrations of methanol. A number of mixtures were analyzed, including Solutio Barbamini (allobarbital and barbital) and Iniectio Barbamini (acrobarbital and barbital).

Farmaceutische Laboratorium der
Rijksuniversiteit
Utrecht, The Netherlands

2207 van Haeringen, A. De bepaling van barbituren in bloed en urine. [The determination of barbiturates in serum and urine.] Pharmaceutisch Weekblad, 1962, , 173-190.

For the UV spectrophotometric determination of barbiturates in body fluids, extraction in an acid medium followed by the measurement of optical density at 240 mμ, at both pH 2 and pH 10 is the method of choice. Sulfonamides and salicylates may significantly interfere with the determination and these interferences are difficult to correct. With urine samples, careful purification and extraction is necessary. A method for quantitative determination in sera, and qualitative estimations in urine samples is given.

Klinisch Chemisch Laboratorium
Psychiatrische Inrichting "Dennenoord"
Zuidlaren, The Netherlands

2208 Fournel, J. Dosage de l'acide phénylpyruvique urinaire en présence de lévomépromazine (7.044 RP). [The assay of phenylpyruvic acid in the presence of levomepromazine (RP7-044).] Annales de Biologie Clinique, 1962, 20, 659-663.

An assay method was worked out for urinary phenylpyruvic acid in patients under treatment with levomepromazine. Phenylpyruvic acid was separated from levomepromazine by acidic ether extraction (the phenothiazines and their metabolites remained in the aqueous phase). Colorimetric determination is then made by means of the addition of ferric chloride (640 mμ). The method is sufficiently precise to evaluate phenylketonuria in oligophrenics treated with levomepromazine or other amines derived from phenothiazine.

Societé des Usines Chimiques Rhône-
Poulenc
Laboratoires de Recherches
Vitry-sur-Seine, France

2209 Bernsohn, Joseph, Custod, James T., Remenchik, Alexander P., & Talso, Peter J. High energy phosphate compounds in erythrocytes from schizophrenic and nonschizophrenic subjects. Journal of Neuro-psychiatry, 1962, 4, 22-27.

Samples of venous blood from 12 schizophrenic patients, 4 nonschizophrenic psychiatric patients and 6 clinically healthy subjects were used to measure the rate of

P^{32} incorporation by erythrocytes into
various high energy phosphate compounds
and to determine erythrocytic ATP levels.
Chlorpromazine [dosage unspecified] was
administered to psychiatric patients, and
all biological determinations were performed within 2-3 weeks of hospitalization. The
blood samples were incubated and centrifuged, after which blood nucleotides were
eluted; values were obtained for erythrocytic levels of inorganic phosphate hexo-
sediphosphate, ADP and ATP. Analysis of
variance on the resultant data revealed no
significant difference between the control
group and nonschizophrenics. Therefore,
these 2 groups were combined. No statistically significant differences occurred between schizophrenics and controls with
respect to inorganic phosphate, hexosedi-
phosphate and ADP. Comparison of the
schizophrenic group with the control group
revealed significant differences in ATP
level. Thus ATP accumulates in the erythrocyte of the schizophrenic at a rate in
excess of that in the normal persons.

Stritch School of Medicine
Loyola University
Chicago, Ill.

2210   Vander Kamp, Harry. Nuclear changes in the white blood cells of patients with
schizophrenic reaction. Journal of Neuropsychiatry, 1962, 4, 1-3.

Blood samples from 40 normal people
and 60 chronic schizophrenics was centrifuged, air dried, fixed and stained with
Masson's trichrome stain. Color photographs of the resultant slides revealed that
lymphocytic nuclei in schizophrenics stained black to dark purple and that chromatin
lacked even distribution, showed marked
variation in density and lacked an organized
pattern. These differences lacked clarity
when Wright's stain was substituted. The
Feulgen reaction also demonstrated the
difference in chromatinic density and in
distribution. The periodic acid-Schiff procedure indicated that more glycoprotein
granules were present in the cytoplasm of
the lymphocyte in the schizophrenic person
than in the normal individual. Consulting
hematologists and histochemists state that
variations may be anticipated in other blood

2215 Mukai, Akira, & Ejima, Tatsunori.
Studies on sialic acid (neuraminic acid) in
cerebrospinal fluid. Part 1: Total bial-
positive substance in cerebrospinal fluid
in schizophrenic subjects. Tohoku Journal
of Experimental Medicine, 1962, 77, 120-
127.

Bial-positive substance (total neuraminic
acid by Bogoch's 1958 method) was assessed
in CSF samples from 46 schizophrenics and
25 other patients with various mental disorders. Also the diphenylamine reaction
was used on protein-free (ethanol-precipit-
ated) CSF. In the schizophrenic subjects
the concentrations of neuraminic acid in
CSF averaged ca. 48.2, while in manic-
depressive psychoses it averaged ca. 46.0.
In the control group (neuroses) it averaged
ca. 46.0, while in mental and nervous disorders caused by somatic illness the figure
was 45.1 µg/ml. No tendency of the low
neuraminic acid concentration appeared in
schizophrenic subjects compared to the
control group or other mental and nervous
disorders. No characteristic relationship
could be established between the total
neuraminic acid and total protein or protein-
bound neuraminic acid in the CSF.

Department of Neuropsychiatry
Tohoku University School of Medicine
Sendai, Japan

2216 Jensen, Knud. Paper chromatographic determination of indoles in human
cerebrospinal fluid.   Acta Neurologica
Scandinavica, 1962, 38, 278-284.

CSF samples were obtained from a general
hospital and extracted with acetone-ether
after saturation with sodium chloride (Nakai
1958). The solvent residue was taken up in
methanol-acetone and used for paper chromatographic analysis of indoles. The amount
of indoles extracted from pooled fluid was
estimated semiquantitatively from the size
and intensity of the spots on the chromatogram. The following indoles could be detected in human CSF: tryptamine, indol-3-acetic
acid, tryptophan and 5 HIAA.

Neurochemical Research Unit
State Mental Hospital
Risskov, Denmark

2217 Bonta, I. L., Wijmenga, H. G., & Hohensee, F. The action of substance P and other brain extracts on the central nervous system. Acta Physiologica et Pharmacologica Neerlandica, 1962, 11, 265.

CNS depressant activity of crude preparations containing substance P [no details] were confirmed, using the exploratory behavior test and i.v. strychnine titration. However, other subfractions of hog-brain extracted according to methods employed for substance P, but devoid of ileum-contracting properties, displayed comparable inhibition of the CNS.

Pharmacological Research Department
N.V. Organon, Oss
Amsterdam, The Netherlands

2218 Rajeswaran, Ponnusamy, & Kirk, Paul L. Tranquillizing and related drugs: properties for their identification (part III). Bulletin on Narcotics, 1962, 14, 19-33.

X-ray diffraction has been successfully utilized with the study and identification of alkaloids, barbiturates, analgesics, sedatives and anticonvulsants. A total of 46 compounds were examined, using a copper-K α-radiation X-ray spectrometer equipped with a recording potentiometer. Phenothiazine derivatives; reserpine and related alkaloids; diphenyl methane derivatives; substituted butanediols; ureides, amides, hydrazines and related compounds, and miscellaneous compounds were detailed. Additionally UV spectrum absorption data on these drugs is given.

School of Criminology
University of California
Berkeley, Calif.

2219 Roberts, Eugene. Enzymology and function of the γ-aminobutyric acid system. Acta Neurologica Scandinavica, 1962, 38, 19.

Experiments were performed on laboratory animals in which correlations were sought between the electrophysiological measurements and GABA levels, and the activities of the related enzymes in various areas

tic acid and p-hydroxyphenylpyruvic acid do not form a product giving interference near 250 mμ in concentrations as great as 200 mg/liter. Also ascorbic acid interferes with the color reaction for 5HIAA when added to the buffer before the developer (ascorbic acid was capable of partial reduction of 1,4 benzoquinone-2-acetic acid to homogentisic acid).

Department of Medicine
University of Minnesota Medical School
Minneapolis, Minn.

2223   Paasonen, M.K., & Kivalo, E. The inactivation of 5-hydroxytryptamine by blood platelets in mental deficiency with elevated serum 5-hydroxytryptamine. Psychopharmacologia, 1962, 3, 188-192.

Blood was collected from mentally retarded children (mongolism, cerebral palsy and encephalopathy) or young adults and the inactivation of 5HT was measured by the disappearance of 5HT during incubation of platelet-rich plasma with or without 20 μg/ml tetrabenazine. The mentally defective patients were divided into 2 groups according to the 5HT content in serum. In the 1st ("normal") group were those with values < 200 ng/ml (6 mongolism, 4 cerebral palsy) and in the 2nd those with values > 200 ng/ml (7 cerebral palsy, 5 encephalopathy). The content of 5HT per platelet was twice as high in the 2nd than in the 1st group. When the platelet-rich plasma was incubated with tetrabenazine in vitro equal amounts of 5HT were liberated from platelets from both groups. During the liberation slightly more 5HT was inactivated in the 1st group than in the 2nd. The ability of platelets to inactive 5HT under these conditions does not explain the higher serum and platelet values found in some patients.

Department of Pharmacology
University of Helsinki
Helsinki, Finland

2224   Horita, A., & Weber, L.J. Dephosphorylation of psilocybin in the intact mouse. Toxicology and Applied Pharmacology, 1962, 4, 730-737.

Male mice received psilocybin (100 mg/kg i.p.) and psilocin (72 mg/kg i.p.), preceded in some instances by sodium β-glycerophosphate (45 mg) administered as a competitive substrate 5 minutes before drug administration. The mice were sacrificed at 5 minute intervals after which the brain, liver and kidney tissue was homogenized. Resultant homogenates were analyzed for psilocin content. Behavioral changes were recorded before sacrifice. After psilocybin injection, measurable amounts of psilocin occurred in liver and kidney tissue in 5 minutes and peak levels were observed in 10-20 minutes, while peak brain levels occurred in 25-30 minutes. Psilocin levels were highest in kidney tissue and lowest in brain. Animals treated with psilocybin evidenced piloerection, exophthalmos, hind-leg ataxia and depression which gradually disappeared in 3-4 hours. Pretreatment with sodium β-glycerophosphate markedly reduced the accumulation of psilocin in all tissues and attenuated behavioral effects. Tissue concentrations of psilocin after psilocin administration were considerably higher than those observed with psilocybin. Psilocin given to mice pretreated with sodium β-glycerophosphate yielded tissue concentrations which approximated those in normal psilocin-treated animals. Psilocybin was obviously dephosphorylated to psilocin in the intact mouse. Psilocybin exerts CNS effects only after dephosphorylation since the amount of brain psilocin is much lower after treatment with sodium β-glycerophosphate.

Department of Pharmacology
School of Medicine
University of Washington
Seattle 5, Wash.

2225 Culley, W.J., Mertz, E.T., Luce, M.W., Calandro, J.M., & Jolly, D.H. Paper chromatographic estimation of phenylalanine and tyrosine using finger-tip blood. Its application to phenylketonuria. Clinical Chemistry, 1962, $\underline{8}$, 266-269.

Using a paper chromatographic method for the determination of serum phenylalanine and tyrosine which requires 0.12 ml of serum from finger-tip blood, no deproteinization and no expensive equipment, 15

tonus of the closing muscle, and hence on periodic activity, were studied in *A. cygnea* by applying the substances to the cerebral ganglion and recording the activity of the posterior closing muscle. Serotonin, tryptamine, epinephrine and levarterenol were all able to terminate the prolonged tonic contraction of this muscle or to prevent onset of contraction; this was accompanied by a considerable increase in rhythmic activity. LSD produced a gradual but quite marked inhibition of muscle tone. These substances therefore seem to play a significant role in the regulation of the diurnal activity of this mussel.

Institute of Physiology
Medical University of Debrecen
Debrecen, Hungary

2229   Tsukada, Y., & Huszák, I. Enzymic activity related to neural function. I. Effects of environmental complexity and training on brain cholinesterase and brain anatomy in the rat. Acta Neurologica Scandinavica, 1962, 38, Suppl. 1, 57-58.

Thirty-one pairs (weaning littermates) of Berkeley S1 male rats were studied under either environmental complexity and training (ENCT) or in isolation (IC). In some cases a triplet was assigned to an intermediate social control (SC) environment. After 80 days the animals' brains were dissected, weighed and analyzed for cholinesterase activity. The ENCT animals showed 2.5% greater acetylcholine activity in both the cortex and the rest of the brain; they also showed a 5.8% greater cerebral cortex weight than IC rats. SC rats showed acetylcholinesterase and brain weight values intermediate between the rats from the other 2 conditions. Over 200 rats of 5 other strains gave similar results. Shorter periods were used in other experiments. Here the differences between ENCT and IC groups were decreased, but still significant. Finally, subjects in other experiments were denucleated at weaning to preclude a visual experience. Here over 400 animals were tested and again environmental stimulation resulted in demonstrable changes in brain chemistry.

Lawrence Radiation Laboratory
University of California
Berkeley, Calif.

2230   Ryan, Wayne L., Carver, Michael J.,
& Haller, James. Phenosulfonphthalein as
an index of drug ingestion. American Journal
of Pharmacy, 1962, 134, 168-171.

To determine drug ingestion, phenolsulfon-
phthalein (10-40 mg p.o.) was given to 4
normal males after which urine samples
were tested for phenol red every 2 hours
for 8 hours. A characteristic violet color
resulted in almost all cases, optimal results
being produced by 20 mg of dye. Then, 9
patients received dye mixed with reserpine
(0.25 mg), meprobamate (400 mg), promazine (100 mg) or phenobarbital (200 mg).
Urine samples were collected every 2 hours
and the depth and intensity of coloration
approximated that obtained when dye was
ingested without medication, although promazine decreased the rate of phenolsulfon-
phthalein excretion. The rapid rate of dye
absorption and excretion permits determination of drug ingestion within 2 hours.
Since the dye is yellow at a pH below 7.0,
the patient is unaware that a test is being
conducted. This test should enable clinicians
to reliably detect whether or not drugs are
being taken as directed.

Department of Biochemistry
Creighton University School of Medicine
Omaha, Neb.

2231   Chatagnon, C., & Chatagnon, P. Variations quantitatives des constituants lipid-
iques du sérum sanguin au cours d'une
thérapeutique par phénothiazine (Largactil).
[Quantitative variations in the lipid constituents of serum in the course of phenothiazine
(Largactil) therapy.] Annales de Biologie
Clinique, 1962, 20, 551-562.

Total fats, phospholipids, free and esteri-
fied cholesterol, total fatty acids, (esteri-
fied and nonesterified) and triglyceride
were measured in the sera of 2 women,
aged 40 and 57, and a control case, non-
medicated, aged 23 years. Dosages of
chlorpromazine (Largactil) were as high
as 900 mg/day. Chlorpromazine caused a

Action de la 5-hydroxytryptamine sur la
sécrétion in vitro des corticostéroides par
les capsules surrénales du Rat. [Action of
5-hydroxytryptamine on the in vitro secretion of corticosteroids by rat adrenal
glands.] Comptes Rendus Hebdomadaires
des Séances de l'Académie des Sciences
(Paris), 1962, 254, 3444-3445.

The adrenal glands of male rats were
removed and cut into quarters for incubation with and without 150 µg/100 mg 5HT.
Paper chromatography using tetrazolium
blue as a developer and UV light was
employed for the qualitative estimation
of corticosteroids. 5HT caused a clear
increase in steroid X_2 and aldosterone;
in contrast, steroid X_3, corticosterone and
11-dehydrocorticosterone concentrations
were not significantly affected. Serotonin
(5HT) has a limited selective action on
the genesis of corticosteroids. Quantitatively, the addition of 5HT caused 25-62%
increase in corticosteroids.

Faculté de Médecine et de Pharmacie
Université de Rennes
Rennes, France

2236 Put, T.R., & Meduski, J.W. The effect
of adrenalectomy on the 5-hydroxytrypt-
amine metabolism in the rat. Acta Physiologica et Pharmacologica Neerlandica,
1962, 11, 240-256.

Rats were adrenalectomized or sham-
operated on; at 3 weeks 90% survived. The
metabolism of 5HT was followed through
the assay of 5HIAA in 24-hour urine samples
and the assay of brain 5HT. There were 5
experimental conditions: untreated, sham-
operated, unoperated but given substitution
therapy, adrenalectomized, and adrenalectomized and substitution therapy. In substitution experiments the mixture Hydro-
Adreson Organon, 25 mg suspended in
1 ml, and DOCA Organon, 5 mg in 1 ml
oil were used, i.e., 150 and 350 µg DOCA,
and 150 and 350 µg Hydro-Adreson s.c.
The observed changes suggest a biphasic
type of metabolic response. The 1st postoperative phase (up to 24 hours after
surgery) is characterized by the immediate increase of urinary 5HIAA, and unchanged 5HT brain level and impairment

of the "binding - unbinding" and storage
mechanisms of 5HT. The 2nd postoperative
phase (24 hours after surgery) revealed
the impairment of the 5HT binding mechanism and its storage. A scheme is proposed
for the mechanism of binding and storage
of 5HT.

Department of Neurosurgery
University of Utrecht
Utrecht, The Netherlands

2237 Haefely, W., Thoenen, H., & Hürli-
mann, A. The effect of intraventricular
application of substance P preparations of
different purity. Medicina Experimentalis,
1962, 7, 245-249.

Fourteen pentobarbital-anesthetized cats
(cannulated in the right lateral ventricle)
were given intraventricular injections of
substance P in 3 grades of purity: 5, 200
and 2400 μ/mg. Negative results were obtained with highly purified substance P
by intraventricular administration in accord
with previous failure to find specific central effects after i.v. injection. Whether
the lack of activity is due to rapid inactivation or to the failure of substance P to
reach possible specific receptor sites in
the CNS cannot be decided at present.
Central effects of substance P, as reported
by various authors working with crude
preparations, may well be due to other
active principles present in extracts. The
crude extract had an initial stimulant effect
on the CNS followed by a depression, which
is also caused by equivalent amounts of
ammonium sulphate (the protein precipitating agent).

Department of Experimental Medicine
F. Hoffmann-LaRoche & Co., Ltd.
Basel, Switzerland

2238 Panagopoulos, K., Matsopoulos, K.,
Damigos, E., Kallistratos, G., Vavougios,
J., Gregoriades, G., & Pfau, A. Biological

ABBREVIATIONS

α-ketoglutarate	F	Fahrenheit scale
Zuckerman's Affect Adjustive Check List	FDA	Federal Drug Administration
adrencorticotropic hormone	FFA	free fatty acid
free choice	g	gram
adenosinediphosphate	GABA	γ-aminobutyric acid
morning	GABOB	γ-amino-β-hydroxybutyric acid
American Medical Association Article	HD	hypnotic dose
adenosinetriphosphate	5HIAA	5-hydroxindoleacetic acid
	5HT	5-hydroxytryptamine
Bell Adjustment Inventory	5HTP	5-hydroxytryptophane
British antiLewisite		
benzyl analogue of serotonin	i.a.	intrarterial
twice a day	ibid.	in the same place
bromolysergic acid diethylamide	i.e.	that is
	i.m.	intramuscular
blood urea nitrogen	IMPS	Lorr's Inpatient Multidimensional Psychiatric Scale
Celsius scale	i.p.	intraperitoneal
about	IPAT	Cattell's Institute for Personality and Ability Testing Anxiety Scale
conditioned avoidance response		
chronic brain syndrome		
cubic centimeter	IQ	intelligence quotient
Communicable Disease Center	IU	international unit
square centimeter	i.v.	intravenous
cubic centimeter		
S. Centre National de la Recherche Scientifique	kg	kilogram
central nervous system	K_i	Michaelis constant for an inhibitor
catechol-o-methyl transferase	K_m	Michaelis constant for a substrate
counts per minute		
counts per second		
conditioned reflex (response)	lbs	pounds
conditioned stimulus	LD	lethal dose
climbing time delay	LSD	lysergide
dichlorodiphenyl trichlorethane	μ	micron
deoxyribonucleic acid	μc	microcurie
3,4-dihydroxy-phenylalanine	μg	microgram
diphosphopyridinenucleotide	μl	microliter
reduced diphosphopyridinenucleotide	μM	micromolar
	m	meter
	M	molar
electrocardiogram	ma.	millamperes
electroconvulsive therapy	MACC	Motility Affect Cooperation Communication
editor		
effective dose	MAO	monoamine oxidase
ethylenediaminetetraacetic acid	MAS	Taylor Manifest Anxiety Scale
electroencephalogram	meq	milliequivalents
for example	ml	milliliter
electroretinogram	mμ	millimicron
electroshock treatment	mm	millimeter
and others	mM	millimolar
and so forth	mm^2	square millimeter

MMPI	Minnesota Multiphasic Personality Inventory
MPI	Maudsley Personality Inventory
MSRPP	Multidimensional Scale for Rating Psychiatric Patients
N	normal
NEFA	nonesterified fatty acid
NIH	National Institutes of Health
NIMH	National Institute of Mental Health
NINDB	National Institute of Neurological Diseases and Blindness
p	probability
PABA	para-aminobenzoic acid
PAH	para-aminohippuric acid
PBI	protein-bound iodine
pH	negative logarithm of hydrogen ion concentration
PM	afternoon and evening
p.o.	by mouth
ppm	parts per million
PRP	Psychotic Reaction Profile
q.i.d.	four times a day
refs.	references
Rf	ratio of the distance of dissolved substance to solvent distance
RNA	ribonucleic acid
ru	rat unit
s.c.	subcutaneous
S.D.	standard deviation
SGOT	serum glutamic oxaloacetic transaminase

SGPT

sic
SRA
SSAI

Suppl.

TAT
TCA
TD
TH
t.i.d.
TPN
TPNH

TSH

U
UR
US
USAF
USDHEW

USP
USPHS

UV

VA
viz.

WAIS

WHO
WPRS

in monkeys. Federation Proceedings, 1962, 2, 327. [Abstract]

955 Griesemer, Ernest C., & Gasner, Linda T. Altered DOPA antagonism of reserpine hypothermia by α-methyl DOPA. Federation Proceedings, 1962, 2, 333. [Abstract]

970 Sankar, D.V. Siva, Phippa, Edward, Gold, Eleanor, & Sankar, D. Barbara. Effect of LSD, BOL, and chlorpromazine on "neurohormone" metabolism. In: Sankar, D.V. Siva [Ed.] Some Biological Aspects of Schizophrenic Behavior. Annals of the New York Academy of Sciences, 1962, 96, Art. 1, 93-97.

978 Funderburk, William H., Finger, Kenneth F., Drakontides, Anna B., & Schneider, Jurg A. EEG and biochemical findings with MAO inhibitors. In: Sankar, D.V. Siva [Ed.] Some Biological Aspects of Schizophrenic Behavior. Annals of the New York Academy of Sciences, 1962, 96, Art. 1, 289-302.

996 Hartmann, H.A., & Muranis, L. Electonmicroscopic alterations of spinal motor neutrons produced by β-μ-iminodipropionitrile. Federation Proceedings, 1962, 2, 362.

1000 Burke, J.C., High, J.P., Laffan, R.J., & Ravaris, C.L. Depot action of fluphenazine (Prolixin): enanthate in oil. Federation Proceedings, 1962, 2, 339. [Abstract]

1002 Sackler, A.M., Weltman, A.S., Russakow, M., Sparber, S.B., & Owens, H. Endocrine effects of lysergic acid diethylamide on female rats. Federation Proceedings, 1962, 2, 416. [Abstract]

1006 Waddell, W.J. The metabolic conversion of secobarbital to 5-allyl-5-(3-hydroxy-y-1-methylbutyl) barbituric acid. Federation Proceedings, 1962, 2, 182. [Abstract]

1010 Malhotra, G.L., & Prasad, K. Effect of chlorpromazine and reserpine on the catechol amine content of different areas of the central nervous system of the dog. British Journal of Pharmacology and Chemotherapy, 1962, 18, 595-599.

1014   Yasuda, Manabu. Effect of reserpine on febrile responses induced by pyrogenic substances. Japanese Journal of Pharmacology, 1962, 11, 114-125.

1028   Curtis, D.R., & Davis, R. Pharmacological studies upon neurones of the lateral geniculate nucleus of the cat. British Journal of Pharmacology and Chemotherapy, 1962, 18, 217-246.

1029   Pscheidt, G.R. Demethylation of imipramine in male and female rats. Biochemical Pharmacology, 1962, 11, 501-502.

1170   McCusker, Kenneth, Ota, Kay Y., Michaux, William W., & Kurland, Albert A. Methyl analogue of phenmetrazine (McN-R-747-11); in the treatment of apathetic chronic psychotics. Current Therapeutic Research, 1962, 4, 6-11.

1227   Dormer, A. Eric. Tranylcypromine (Parnate). Lancet, 1962, 2, 162.

1491   Dwyer, Brian, & Gunner, B.W. Phenacetin cyanosis, barbiturate habituation and cardiac arrest. Medical Journal of Australia, 1963, 2, 13-14.

259   Karli, P. Action du méthaminodiazépoxide ("Librium") sur l'agressivité interspécifique Rat-Souris. [The action of chlordiazepoxide ("Librium") on interspecific agressiveness of rats and mice.] Comptes Rendus des Séances de la Société de Biologie et de Ses Filiales, 1961, 155, 625-627.

From 5 to 20 mg/kg i.p., the action of chlordiazepoxide (methaminodiazepoxide) on the aggressive behavior of male rats toward mice was practically negligible. Starting with 30-35 mg/kg, interspecific aggressiveness was abolished in most rats,

873

DEPOUTOT J C, 2029
DESIDERIO VINCENT, 2012
DETRE THOMAS P, 2104
DIETHELM OSKAR, 2003
DIMASCIO ALBERTO, 2133
DIXON H LORING, 2005
DORNETTE WILLIAM H L, 2055
DOSTALEK C, 2122
DUCHENE-MARULLAS P, 2173
DUNLOP EDWIN, 2023
DURLAND ALBERT A, 2053
DYRBERG V, 2004
ECHLIN FRANCIS A, 2151
EJIMA TATSUNORI, 2211, 2212, 2213,
   2214, 2215
EKBOM K A, 2056
EKSTROM NILS AKE, 2124
ELDER JOHN T, 1985
ELODI P, 2221
ERDMAN G, 2168
ESSIG CARL F, 2187
FELDMAN PAUL E, 2096
FELDMAN ROBERT G, 2104
FERGUSON HUGH C, 2161
FERRITER CHRISTINE, 2104
FINDLAY CHARLES W JR, 2041
FINK MAX, 2034
FISHER EDWARD, 2170
FISHER G W, 2006
FIUME SEBASTIANO, 2078
FLATAKER LARS, 2184
FLEURY C, 2148
FOLDES I, 2145
FONTAN M, 2234
FORD DONALD H, 2142
FORNEY ROBERT B, 2146
FOROGLOU G P, 2116
FOSSATI P, 2234
FOURNEL J, 2208
FRAHM MARGARETE, 2203
FRENTZEL A, 2089
FREUND J DENNIS, 2098
FREYBURGER W A, 2154
FRIEBEL H, 2179
FROMMEL ED, 2148, 2175
FRONTINO G, 2155
FUMAGALLI REMO, 2220
FUSTER JOAQUIN M, 2132
GAMBESCIA JOSEPH M, 2012
GEISSMANN P, 2022, 2029, 2101
GELLER IRVING, 2127
GENNERICH E, 2076
GEY K F, 2204
GIBBS E L, 2094
GIBBS F A, 2094
GLADTKE E, 2118
GLOW PETER H, 2150
GLUECK BERNARD C, 2016
GOFFAUX P, 2039

GOKHALE S D, 2182
GOLDBERG H D, 2125
GOLDBERG RONALD I, 2009
GOLDMAN DOUGLAS, 2001
GOODSON DAVID N, 2005
GRANDJEAN E, 2129
GRAY J E, 2154
GREEN HENRY D, 2005
GREGORIADES G, 2238
GREIFENSTEIN FERDINAND E, 2134
GREISMAN S E, 2165
GROH CH, 1995
GROSS J, 2014
GROSSI ENRICA, 2220
GRUENWALD FRANCES, 2053
GSCHLACHT V E, 2071
GULATI O D, 2182
GUTBUT TH, 2029
HAASE H J, 2070, 2092
HAEFELY W, 2237
HALLER JAMES, 2230
HANDCOCK K A, 2045
HANKOFF LEON D, 2073
HANNA CALVIN, 2021
HANSSON ESKIL, 2163
HARDY T K, 2040
HARMEL MEREL H, 2024
HARNEY MALACHI L, 1986
HASHKES HENRY R, 2043
HAUN KENNETH, 2130
HEINRICH K, 1983
HELBIG HANS, 2108
HELWIG H, 1991
HEYCK H, 2090
HICKS ROBERT G, 2068
HILLARP NILS-AKE, 2180
HIMWICH HAROLD E, 2120
HOFFMEISTER F, 2186
HOHENSEE F, 2217
HOLMES J W, 2059
HORITA A, 2224
HOROVITZ ZOLA P, 2185
HORSTMANN W, 2075
HSU B, 2035
HUDSPETH WILLIAM J, 2131
HUGHES FRANCIS W, 2146
HUKUHARA T, 2176
HULPIEU HAROLD R, 2146
HURKMANS TH M, 2198
HURLIMANN A, 2237
HUSEN JAN-HINNERK, 2042
HUSZAK I, 2229
HUTER K A, 2062
HYMAN YVETTE K, 2010
ITIL T, 2064
IZQUIERDO J A, 2143
JACOBZINER HAROLD, 2160
JAFFE GERALD E, 2144
JANEWAY KATHERINE P, 2144
JANKE HORST, 2038

875

SUBJECT INDEX
Numbers refer to abstracts
No abbreviations used as subject headings

ACEPROMAZINE
    EFFECT ON CARS IN RATS, 2139
ACETOPHENAZINE
    AS ANTIEMETIC, 2025
ACETYLATION
    METABOLISM OF CARBOHYDRATES AFTER BARBITURATES, 2238
ACETYLCHOLINE, 2170
    EFFECT ON EEG IN MONKEYS, 2152
ADDICTION, 1993
    COMPULSORY TREATMENT, 1986
    DETECTION WITH NALORPHINE, 1986
    IN THE UNITED STATES, 1986
ADENOSINE TRIPHOSPHATE, 2209
ADRENOCORTICOTROPIC HORMONE
    IN EPILEPSY, 1995
AGGRESSIVENESS
    IN CHILDREN, 2002
    IN MICE, 2128
AGITATION AS SIDE EFFECT, 2032, 2077
AGITATION TREATMENT, 2029, 2030, 2044
AGRANULOCYTOSIS AS SIDE EFFECT, 2074
AKINESIA AS SIDE EFFECT, 2070
ALCOHOL ETHYL
    EFFECT ON BARBITURATE NARCOSIS IN GUINEA PIGS, 2203
    EFFECT ON PERCEPTION OF MUSICAL STIMULI, 2123
    METABOLISM IN MICE, 2146
ALCOHOLISM ACUTE
    AMNESIA, 2003
ALCOHOLISM CHRONIC, 2003
    DELIRIUM, 2108
    WITH ANXIETY, 2081
ALKALOIDS
    DETECTION IN SALIVA AND URINE, 2231
ALPHAPRODINE, 2021
G-AMINOBUTYRIC ACID
    ENZYMOLOGY, 2219
AMITRIPTYLINE, 2023
    AS A SEDATIVE, 2039
    AS AN ANXIOLYTIC, 2039
    EFFECT ON CEREBRAL MONOAMINES, 2204
    IN BEHAVIORAL DISORDERS, 2087, 2088
    IN CYCLOTHYMIC REACTION, 2039
    IN DEPRESSION, 2087, 2109, 2065, 2066, 2071, 2078
    IN EPILEPSY, 2087, 2088
    IN MANIC DEPRESSION, 2109
    IN PARANOID HALLUCINATION SYNDROME, 2109
    IN SCHIZOPHRENIA, 2087, 2109
AMITRIPTILINE ANALOGUES, 2023
AMNESIA TREATMENT
    IN ACUTE ALCOHOLIC INTOXICATION, 2003
    WITH CHLORPROMAZINE, 2004
    WITH HALOPERIDOL, 2004
AMOBARBITAL, 2000
    CARDIOVASCULAR EFFECT IN RATS, 2193

CHILD, 2007
    HYPNOTICS AND SEDATIVES, 2075
    IMPLICATIONS WITH PSYCHOACTIVE DRUGS, 2002
    MENTALLY DISTURBED, 2001
    PSYCHOSIS, 2002, 2001
    TREATMENT OF EPILEPSY, 1995
CHIMNEY-CLIMBING TEST, 2135
A-CHLORALOSE, 2103
CHLORDIAZEPOXIDE, 2082, 2083
    ANTAGONISM BY NALORPHINE IN GUINEA PIGS, 2175
    AS POSTOPERATIVE MEDICATION, 2009
    AS PREANESTHETIC MEDICATION, 2060
    AS PREOPERATIVE MEDICATION, 2009
    EFFECT ON ANTICONVULSANT ACTIVITY IN RATS, 2187
    EFFECT ON CARS IN RATS, 2127
    EFFECT ON EEG WITH INTERMITTENT PHOTOSTIMULATION, 2100
    EFFECT ON PENTOBARBITAL ANALGESIA IN RATS, 2187
    EFFECT ON RIGHTING REFLEX IN RATS, 2187
    IN AGITATION, 2077
    IN ANXIETY, 2079, 2097
    IN CHOREO-ATHETOSIS, 2077
    IN DEPRESSION, 1996, 2097
    IN HALLUCINATIONS, 2096
    IN MENTAL RETARDATION, 2094
    IN OLIGOPHRENIA, 2077
    IN PSYCHOPATHIC PERSONALITY, 2085
    IN SCHIZOPHRENIA, 2085, 2094
    IN SPASTICITY, 2077
    IN THE TREATMENT OF ANXIETY COMPULSIVE REACTION, 1996
    IN TUBERCULAR PATIENTS, 2042
    PHYSIOLOGY IN CATS, 2162
    USED AT DELIVERY, 2014
    WITH MAO INHIBITORS IN ANXIETY, 2097
    WITH MAO INHIBITORS IN DEPRESSION, 2097
    WITH QUARZAN BROMIDE IN GASTROINTESTINAL DISORDERS, 2033
CHLORPERPHENTHIXENE
    EFFECT ON CARS IN RATS, 2139
CHLORPHENOXAMINE
    ANTAGONISM TO TREMORINE CONVULSIONS IN MICE, 2147
    TOXICITY DETERMINATION, 2158
CHLORPROMAZINE, 2045, 2070, 2159
    ANTAGONISM BY NALORPHINE IN GUINEA PIGS, 2175
    ANTAGONISM TO AMPHETAMINE TOXICITY, 2164
    ANTAGONISM TO NICOTINE CONVULSIONS IN RATS, 2182
    ANTAGONISM TO TREMORINE CONVULSIONS IN MICE, 2147
    AS ANTIEMETIC, 2004
    COLORIMETRIC ASSAY, 2205
    EFFECT ON ATTENTION RESPONSES IN CATS, 2153
    EFFECT ON AUDITORY DISCRIMINATION, 2133
    EFFECT ON BARBITURATE THRESHOLD DETERMINATION IN RABBITS, 2149
    EFFECT ON BEHAVIOR IN RETARDED CHILDREN, 2057
    EFFECT ON BRAIN SELF STIMULATION BY CATS, 2185
    EFFECT ON CARS IN DEER MICE, 2136
    EFFECT ON CARS IN MICE, 2124
    EFFECT ON CARS IN RATS, 2127, 2134, 2139
    EFFECT ON CEREBRAL MONOAMINES, 2204
    EFFECT ON CONDITIONED EMOTIONAL BEHAVIOR IN RATS, 2140
    EFFECT ON EEG IN CATS, 2196
    EFFECT ON FETUS AND NEWBORN, 2046

881

MOGENTISIC ACID
  INTERFERENCE IN 5HIAA DETERMINATION, 2222
MOVANILLIC ACID
  FORMED AFTER DOPA ADMINISTRATION, 2180
DRAZINES
  AS MAO INHIBITORS, 2227
HYDROXYINDOLE ACETIC ACID
  DETERMINATION, 2222
  EFFECT OF HYDRAZINES, 2227
  EXCRETION IN CRANIAL TRAUMA, 2234
  IN CFS, 2216
  THIN LAYER CHROMATOGRAPHY, 2233
HYDROXYTRYPTAMINE SEE SEROTONIN
HYDROXYTRYPTOPHANE
  EFFECT ON CEREBRAL MONOAMINES, 2204
  EFFECT ON SEDATIVE ACTION OF RESERPINE IN MICE, 2199
DROXYZINE, 2012
  AS PREANESTHETIC, 2069
  EFFECT ON EEG IN CATS, 2176
  IN CHILDREN, 2007
  WITH OXYPHENCYCLIMINE EFFECT ON GASTRIC ACID, 2012
OSCINE
  AMNESIC PROPERTIES, 2040
PERACTIVITY
  IN CHILDREN, 2002
PERERGIA TREATMENT, 2096
PERSOMNIA AS SIDE EFFECT, 2032
PERTENSION TREATMENT
  WITH IPRONIAZID, 1998
PERVENTILATION HYSTERICAL, 2097
PNOTICS
  IN SCHIZOPHRENIA, 2076
  IN SMALL CHILDREN, 2075
POCHONDRIA TREATMENT, 2031, 2099
POTENSION AS SIDE EFFECT, 2010, 2017, 2032, 2068, 2073, 2096, 2110
POTHERMIA AS SIDE EFFECT, 2114
STERICAL HYPERVENTILATION SYNDROME, 2097
EUM
  EFFECT OF SUBSTANCE P, 2217
IPRAMINE, 2023, 2083, 2159
  ANTAGONISM TO AMPHETAMINE TOXICITY, 2164
  COLORIMETRIC ASSAY, 2205
  EFFECT ON BLOOD PRESSURE, 2143
  EFFECT ON BRAIN LIPID METABOLISM, 2220
  EFFECT ON BRAIN SELF STIMULATION BY CATS, 2185
  EFFECT ON CARS IN RATS, 2139
  EFFECT ON CEREBRAL MONOAMINES, 2204
  EFFECT ON ECG ACTIVITY BY EPINEPHRINE, 2143
  EFFECT ON ECT ACTIVITY BY LEVARTERENOL, 2143
  EFFECT ON EEG IN RABBITS, 2157
  EFFECT ON SELF STIMULATION IN RATS, 2157
  EFFECT ON SPRING TEST IN RATS, 2191
  IN DEPRESSION, 2019, 2028, 2092, 2099, 2113
  IN ENURESIS, 2006
  IN LOCOMOTOR INERTIA, 2028
  IN MELANCHOLIA, 2099
  IN PSYCHASTHENIA, 2099
  IN PSYCHIATRIC GERIATRICS, 2028
  IN SENILITY, 2099

LEVOMEPROMAZINE
    COLORIMETRIC ASSAY, 2205
    IN ACUTE SCHIZOPHRENIA, 2110
    IN ENDOGENOUS PSYCHOSIS, 2110
    IN HEBEPHRENIA, 2110
    IN MANIC PSYCHOSIS, 2110
    IN PARANOID HALLUCINATIONS, 2110
LIBIDO DIMINUTION AS SIDE EFFECT, 2032
LIGHTHEADEDNESS AS SIDE EFFECT, 2084
LILLY 18947
    EFFECT ON ASCORBIC ACID SECRETION IN RATS, 2141
LILLY 32391
    EFFECT ON ASCORBIC ACID SECRETION IN RATS, 2141
LINGUOMANDIBULAR REFLEX
    IN RABBITS, 2186
LYSERGIC ACID DIETHYLAMIDE SEE LYSERGIDE
LYSERGIDE
    ANTAGONISTS, 1985
    EFFECT ON ATTENTION RESPONSES IN CATS, 2153
    NEURAL EFFECT ON CLAMS, 2228
MALAISE AS SIDE EFFECT, 2042, 2114
MALAMUD SANDS SCALE, 2085
MANIC DEPRESSIVE REACTION, 2000, 2008, 2058, 2114
MAST CELLS
    NICOTINE EFFECT ON 5HT RELEASE, 2172
MAUDSLEY PERSONALITY INVENTORY, 2138
MD 2028
    IN AGITATION, 2029
    POTENTIATION OF PHENOTHIAZINES, 2029
MELANCHOLIA TREATMENT, 2099
MENOPAUSE, 1989, 1990
MENTAL RETARDATION, 2094
    EEG, 2001
    EFFECT ON ENURESIS WITH IMIPRAMINE, 2006
MEPERIDINE, 2021
    AS PREANESTHETIC, 2069
MEPHENESIN
    COLORIMETRIC ASSAY, 2205
    EFFECT ON REFLEXES IN RABBITS, 2186
    TOXICITY DETERMINATION, 2161
MEPHENOXALONE
    EFFECT ON CONDITIONED EMOTIONAL BEHAVIOR IN RATS, 2140
    IN ANXIETY, 2032
    IN OBSESSIVE COMPULSIVE REACTION, 2032
    IN TENSION, 2032
MEPROBAMATE, 2082, 2083
    ANTAGONISM BY NALORPHINE IN GUINEA PIGS, 2175
    ANTAGONISM TO TREMORINE CONVULSIONS IN MICE, 2147
    COLORIMETRIC ASSAY, 2205
    EFFECT ON ASCORBIC ACID SECRETION IN RATS, 2141
    EFFECT ON BEHAVIOR IN RETARDED CHILDREN, 2057
    EFFECT ON EEG IN CATS, 2176
    EFFECT ON FIGHTING BEHAVIOR IN MICE, 2128
    EFFECT ON KINESTHETIC FIGURAL AFTER-EFFECTS, 2138
    EFFECT ON VERBAL DISJUNCTIVE REACTION TIME, 2130
    IN ACCIDENTAL POISONING, 2117
    IN CARDIOVASCULAR DISEASE, 2038
    IN CHILDREN, 2002
    TOXICITY IN GRAVID RATS, 2197

MORPHINE
     TRANSFORMATION IN VIVO INTO NORMORPHINE, 2200
MOTILITY, 2129, 2184
MOUSE, 2035, 2124, 2128, 2146, 2147, 2154, 2156, 2158, 2159, 2164,
            2168, 2169, 2173, 2174, 2182, 2184, 2189, 2194, 2199,
            2224, 2226
MUSCULOSKELETAL DISORDERS TREATMENT, 2080
MYDETON
     EFFECT ON EEG IN CATS, 2196
N 640, 2159
N 685, 2159
NALORPHINE, 2179
     ACTION ON RETICULAR SYSTEM, 2175
     ANTAGONISM OF MORPHINE INDUCED RESPIRATORY DEPRESSION, 2050
     ANTAGONISM TO DEXTROPROPOXYPHENE TOXICITY, 2166
     AS SEDATIVE, 2050
     EFFECT ON TRANQUILIZER INDUCED SLEEP IN GUINEA PIGS, 2175
     IN DETECTION OF OPIATE ADDICTION, 1986
     TRANSFORMATION IN VIVO INTO NORMORPHINE, 2200
NARCOTICS
     WORLD REQUIREMENTS, 1987
NAUSEA AS SIDE EFFECT, 2036, 2084, 2114
NAUSEA TREATMENT, 2043, 2059
     WITH CHLORPROMAZINE, 2004
     WITH FLUPHENAZINE, 2010
     WITH HALOPERIDOL, 2004
     WITH TRIFLUPROMAZINE, 2010
NEOSTIGMINE
     IN MORPHINE TOLERANT RATS, 2202
NEURAMINIC ACID
     ASSAY IN CSF SAMPLES, 2211, 2212, 2213, 2214, 2215
     IN CSF SAMPLES, 2211, 2212, 2213, 2214, 2215
NEUROLEPTICS
     EFFECTS ON PSYCHOMOTOR ACTIVITY, 2092
     IN PUERPERAL PSYCHOSIS, 2013
     WITH THIOMUCASE, 2093
NEUROSIS, 2052
NEUROSIS CLIMACTERIC, 2101, 2102, 1984
NEUROSIS CONVERSION REACTION, 2000
NEUROSIS OBSESSIVE COMPULSIVE REACTION, 2000, 2101, 1996, 2032
NEUROSIS PHOBIC REACTION, 2101
NEW YORK CITY POISON CONTROL CENTER
     REPORT, 2160
NIALAMIDE
     IN DEPRESSION, 2023, 2092, 2102
     IN MENOPAUSAL DEPRESSION, 2102
     IN NEUROSIS, 2102
     IN SCHIZOID DEPRESSION, 2102
     IN SCHIZOPHRENIC DEPRESSION, 2102
     PREVENTION OF 3,4-DIHYDROXYPHENYLACETIC ACID FROM DOPA, 2180
NICOTINE
     DETECTION IN SALIVA AND URINE, 2231
     EFFECT ON 5HT RELEASE, 2172
NICOTINE CONVULSIONS
     IN MICE, 2182
     IN RATS, 2182
NICOTINIC ACID
     ANTAGONIST TO LSD, 1985

PSYCHOPHARMACOLOGY ABSTRACTS is a publication of the
National Clearinghouse for Mental Health Information
of the National Institute of Mental Health. It is a
specialized information medium designed to assist the
Institute in meeting its obligation to foster and support laboratory and clinical research into the nature
and causes of mental disorders and methods of treatment and prevention. Specifically, this information
service is designed to meet the needs of investigators in the field of psychopharmacology for rapid and
comprehensive information about new developments and
research results.

PSYCHOPHARMACOLOGY ABSTRACTS is distributed gratis to
investigators doing research in psychopharmacology. It
is not available on a subscription basis. Requests
to receive the ABSTRACTS should be accompanied by a
brief statement of the research interests and scientific specialty of the investigator. Requests to receive the ABSTRACTS, address changes, and other communications should be addressed to:

> Psychopharmacology Abstracts
> National Clearinghouse for Mental
>   Health Information
> National Institute of Mental Health
> Bethesda 14, Maryland

(The text of PSYCHOPHARMACOLOGY ABSTRACTS is prepared
under contract with the Literary Division of Biological and Medical Services, Philadelphia, Penna.)

U. S. DEPARTMENT OF HEALTH, EDUCATION AND WELFARE
Public Health Service
National Institutes of Health
National Institute of Mental Health
Bethesda 14, Maryland

PSYCHOPHARMACOLOGY ABSTRACTS

Volume 2, Number 10

2239 Huxley, Julian. Psychometabolism. Journal of Neuropsychiatry, 1962, 3, Suppl. 1, S1-S14.

Schizophrenia is balanced psychometabolic morphism. About 19% of all people are schizophrenic; the disease appears to have a strong genetic basis and genetic theory indicates that such a clearly disadvantageous entity could not persist in a population unless it is balanced by a compensatory advantage. Biochemical studies indicate that adrenochrome or adrenolutin constitutes the genetically determined basis for schizophrenia. Perceptual anomalies tend to accompany biochemical abnormalities. Minimal doses of hallucinogens like mescaline, LSD and psilocybin exert similar dislocating effects on perception, which effects resemble acute transient schizophrenia. Work must be undertaken to determine whether psychotomimetics modify or enhance dreaming. Significant contributions to psychiatry and psychology include experimental work on mother surrogates, taste perception, pain sensitivity, manipulative behavior, the genetic basis for species awareness and the establishment of intraspecific emotional bonds. (40 refs.)

31 Pond Street
Hampstead N.W. 3
London, Great Britain

2240 Leconte, Maurice. Etude clinique et traitement du mutisme en médecine psychiatrique. [Clinical study and treatment of mutism in psychiatry.] Annales Médico-Psychologiques, 1962, 120, 2, 886-908.

Mutism in psychiatric patients may be voluntary, as in chronic delirium, (in which it may be motivated, or occur as an act of defiance, or in obedience to hallucinatory voices, or the result of excitational, discordant, or oligophrenic syndromes), or it may be involuntary as in hysterical, aphonic and aphasial syndromes. It tends to be complete in the melancholic, confusional, and catatonic stupor syndromes. It occurs in partial forms in melancholic, delirious, demential, oligophrenic, obsessional, and psychic-disequilibrium syndromes. Treatment should be both etiologic and symptomatic. Pentetrazol is indicated in post-confusional mutisms, in apathy, but may sometimes result in anxiety states. ECT and various narco-analeptic agents are often useful. Methamphetamine at 30 mg i.v. can be used for the exploration of mutism, since it augments the patient's speech and induces emotional discharge, but frequently the contraindications hypertension, arteriosclerosis and exophthalmic goiter are noted. Psychotherapy is helpful but more important in prophylaxis than in therapy. Further, a single case is presented in which chlorpromazine proved of benefit. In children, the drawing-test methods, accompanied by empathy and comprehension are also useful. (38 refs.)

Centre Psychiatrique Sainte-Anne
Paris, France

2241 Jermulowiecz, Z.W., & Turnau, Mag. A. Control and treatment of drug addicts in Israel. Bulletin on Narcotics, 1962, 14, 11-18.

With the establishment of the State of Israel in 1948 and mass immigration from the Arab countries, the problem of drug addiction assumed serious proportions in Israel. Lack of hospital facilities delayed treatment and in 1952 the Ministry of Health began to allocate drugs to addicts until they could be hospitalized. Finally, an institutional program was created. Thus far, 274 addicts have been hospitalized. Addicts are initially kept in a closed ward with psychotic patients and then transferred to a special ward. Addicts prefer the special ward and are highly motivated to recover rapidly. Success in initial weaning is largely attributed to chlorpromazine (initially 150 mg, then 400-500 mg/day). Group as well as individual psychotherapy is also of value. The most toxic drug among addicts is pethidine, which leads to epileptic seizures after use for 1-1½ years. Illiterates who were opium addicts since adolescence and those over 45 years of age who have never worked creatively are the most difficult to cure. At present, it is estimated that those who fail to relapse constitute 2-3% and prevention of addiction is far more successful than cure. (No refs.)

Government Hospital for Mental Patients
Bat-Yam, Israel

2242 Blazek, J., Spinkova, V., & Stejskal, Z. Analytik der Phenothiazinderivate. Übersicht. [Analysis of phenothiazine derivatives. A review.] Pharmazie, 1962, 17, 497-514.

Analytical methods for the determination of phenothiazine derivatives are presented. Three tables are given listing chemical names, formulas, generic names, and therapeutic use of phenothiazine derivatives not substituted in the ring, those substituted in the ring, and those not substituted at the nitrogen. An extensive list of synonyms for the various phenothiazine derivatives is also given. (218 refs.)

Staatliches Institut für Arzneimittel-
   kontrolle Prag
Prague, Czechoslovakia

2243 Linke, H. Möglichkeiten und Probleme der Psychopharmakotherapie im höheren Lebensalter. [Possibilities and problems of psychopharmacologic therapy in advanced age.] Zeitschrift für Arztliche Fortbildung, 1962, 15, 805-811.

Physiologic aging, frequently accompanied by psychological phenomena and emotional disturbances (due to arteriosclerotic and other organic changes) is expounded. Psychopharmacologic agents, often in combination with a sedative or a circulatory stimulant, play a vital role in the attempt to brighten the prolonged evening of life. Four most frequently occurring geriatric problems are: the manifold symptoms presented by retardation of psycho-physical agility; various forms of geriatric insomnia; treatment of psychomotor agitation and confusion, and treatment of depressive states of anxiety and mood disturbance. Successful treatment depends upon use of the proper psychotropic agents, good psychotherapeutic guidance and an environment free of stress and conflict. (No refs.)

Medizinische Klinik
Medizinische Akademie
Magdeburg, Germany

2244 Himwich, H.E., Morillo, Arturo, & Steiner, William G. Drugs affecting rhin-

spinal fluid upon the central nervous system. World Neurology, 1962, 3, 706-714.

Injections of various pharmacologically active substances (acetylcholine and cholinesterase inhibitors, 5HT, catecholamines, curare, tryptamine, potassium and calcium salts, CSF, LSD, morphine, reserpine, mescaline and chlorpromazine) into the lateral ventricle of conscious cats produces characteristic behavioral and neurologic effects, predominantly convulsions, muscular hypotonia, ataxia and stuporous states. These studies indicated that the periventricular region is an area of high pharmacologic sensitivity. Minute CSF drug concentrations produce profound effects on the CNS. A bioassay preparation may be used as an excitable organ in order to reflect the biological properties of CSF and as a means of measuring substances present in subthreshold concentrations. Acetylcholine is present in CSF and perfusates of the ventricular system. Specialized chemoreceptors in the walls of the 4th ventricle may provide the means by which pharmacologically active substances in CSF affect the CNS. (62 refs.)

Section of Neurology
Yale University School of Medicine
New Haven, Conn.

2247 Lancet. The premature persuaders. Lancet, 1962, No. 7222, 198-199. [Editorial]

All physicians in the United Kingdom have recently received a letter warning of the possible untoward effects of thalidomide. In New York, similar warning letters have preceded withdrawal of 7 drugs from the market (triparanol, zoxazolamine, erythromycin, triacetyloleandomycin, furaltadone, diazthazanine and amphenidone). A new drug should never be brought into general use unless it is clearly more effective than existing remedies. Drug efficacy can be determined only by properly planned controlled therapeutic trials. A feasible system should be inaugurated whereby clinical trials are performed by reliable groups of clinicians dealing primarily with such endeavors. (No refs.)

7, Adam Street, Adelphi
London W.C. 2, Great Britain

2248 Winkler, K., & Gröger, D. Neuere Arbeiten zur Biosynthese der Mutterkornalkaloide. [Recent literature on the biosynthesis of ergot alkaloids]. Pharmazie, 1962, 17, 658-670.

The review deals with papers published since 1950. Extensive experiments are discussed which, with the aid of isotopic labeling, have shown the incorporation of tryptophan and of a C5 derivative of "mevalonic acid" into ergot alkaloids, including LSD. Anthranilic acid and/or indole can be used as precursors during the biosynthesis of tryptophan. The transformation of certain alkaloids by chemical means is briefly outlined. Numerous formulas explain hypothetic and proven pathways. (98 refs.)

Pharmakognostisches Institut
der Martin Luther Universität
Berlin, Germany

2249 Dunlop, Edwin. The neurotic feeling of inferiority. Journal of Neuropsychiatry, 1962, 3, S79-S82.

Patients with reactive depression complicated by anxiety and depersonalization exhibiting hysterical behavior will often respond to antidepressant drugs, but about 75% require some additional medication, such as a phenothiazine, meprobamate or chlordiazepoxide, accompanied by nocturnal sedation. The necessary pot pourri of drugs makes delineation of drug-induced side effects difficult. Patients with classical neurotic depression respond very well to treatment with diazepam. After acute withdrawal therapy, alcoholics respond well to 30-40 mg of diazepam per day. Acute schizoaffective disorders show satisfactory improvement with diazepam but no convincing results have been obtained in acute paranoia or chronic regressed schizophrenia. (No refs.)

Fuller Memorial Sanitarium
South Attleboro, Mass.

2250 Branch, C.H. Hardin, Himwich, Harold, Feldman, Robert S., McConnell, James, & Shagass, Charles. Panel discussion. Journal of Neuropsychiatry, 1962, 3, S59-S61. [Discussion]

A panel discussion encompasses the following topics: comparison of averaging techniques with examination of raw EEG data, present evidence for MAO inhibition as an important factor in relieving depression, severe depression experienced 4-5 hours after an initial dose of meprobamate, interaction effects of psychoactive drugs, results obtained with excessive doses of pentobarbital, antidepressants and chlordiazepoxide, administration of chlordiazepoxide during conflict, conditioning in worms, biochemical fractionation of trained worms, the application of worm conditioning to the mentally retarded, rate or regeneration and cannibalization in worms, potential corroboration of the theory that acquired traits can be transmitted genetically, relation between breast feeding and intelligence, non-segmented worms and categorization of the phenothiazines. (No refs.)

[No address]

2251 Callaway, Enoch, Feldman, Paul, Towler, Martin L., Gibbs, Frederic A., Detre, Thomas P.,Collard, J., Katz, Robert & Shea, Paul A. Panel discussion. Journal of Neuropsychiatry, 1962, 3, S83-S90. [Discussion]

An extensive panel discussion provided elaboration on the following topics: the use of diazepam in adolescents, EEG changes with various phenothiazines, fast EEG activity secondary to alcoholism, transient drowsiness following diazepam ingestion, the anticonvulsant action of psychotropic drugs, the relationship of fast EEG activity and withdrawal seizures, relief of neuromuscular symptoms with diazepam or chlordiazepoxide, maintenance dosage in responsive depressed patients, large doses as a means of obviating the overstimulating effect of 2.5-5 mg doses of diazepam, muscle relaxant properties of diazepam, duration of diazepam therapy in depression to determine therapeutic efficacy, diazepam as an analgesic, incidence of suicide in relation to diazepam and chlordiazepoxide, alterations in dreams during diazepam therapy, the definite potentiating effects of diazepam on alcohol, automobiles and diazepam, and diazepam as an effective sedative. (No refs.)

[No address]

2256   Norton, Alan. The chemotherapy of
the major psychoses.   Guy's Hospital
Gazette, 1962, 76, 172-176.

The use of major tranquilizers (reserpine,
the phenothiazines and the piperazine phenothiazines), the thymoleptics (imipramine
and amitriptyline), the MAO inhibitors and
psychotomimetic drugs, in treating schizophrenia, manic and depressive psychoses
and some kinds of nonpsychotic depression
is discussed. (No refs.)

[No address]

2257   Mandel, P., & Weill, J.D. Nucléotides
du système nerveux central. [Nucleotides
of the central nervous system.] Journal de
Physiologie, 1962, 54, 199-267.

The constitution of nucleotides, methods of
separation and identification of free nucleotides, their biosynthesis, their role in
enzymatic mechanisms, and their physiological chemistry are reviewed. In relation
to nucleotide in vitro physiological chemistry, energy metabolism, ion exchange, the
relationship between acetylcholine and free
nucleotides and the effects of electric
stimulation are detailed. In vivo studies are
reviewed in regard to the generation of
nucleotides throughout growth, the reforma-
tion of free nucleotides, the effect of cerebral hyperactivity, convulsant agents and
electroshock, hypoxia, anoxia, anesthetics
and various pharmacologic agents. Among
the latter chlorpromazine and "promazine"
are noted as influencing the in vivo synthesis of DPN (Burton et al. 1958), but
evidence is insufficient for the formulation
of a valid hypothesis concerning phenothiazine mechanism of action. (533 refs.)

Institut de Chimie Biologique
Faculté de Médecine
Strasbourg, France

2258   DeProspo, Chris J. News and notes.
American Journal of Mental Deficiency,
1962, 67, 133-136.

The Guthrie test (which uses a few drops
of blood from a newborn's heel to detect
phenylketonuria) provides the basis for

inauguration of a new national program which may prevent mental retardation resulting from phenylketonuria and other inborn errors of metabolism. The Guthrie test will be utilized to screen some 400,000 newborn babies as of July 1, 1963 in cooperation with various health departments and hospitals. Once phenylketonuria is diagnosed, special diet arrangements can be instituted which will preclude development of the disease with its concomitant irreparable mental retardation. During 1960, the ferric chloride urine test detected more than 25 infants with phenylketonuria. Dietary treatment was promptly instituted to prevent mental retardation. (No refs.)

[No address]

2259 Peters, Rudolph A. Seminar on the physiology and biochemistry of disturbed brain function: Introductory statement. Journal of Neuropsychiatry, 1962, 4, 105-106.

Convulsions may be produced in pigeons by disrupting the Kreb's cycle at any number of points: thiamine deficiency or BAL prevent the oxidation of pyruvate to acetyl co-A, fluorocitrate inhibits triosephosphate dehydrogenase and lewisite inhibits the oxidative decarboxylation of α-ketoglutarate. In addition, injection of Cu^{++} into the subarachnoid space in pigeons rapidly produces convulsions and death by irreversibly inhibiting some component of pyruvic dehydrogenase. Irreversible convulsions follow injection of fluorocitrate into the subarachnoid space in pigeons. Convulsions induced by thiamine deficiency stop within 30 minutes if thiamine is injected into the brain. Internal changes in the nerve cell must therefore modify all subtle pharmacological reactions. (No refs.)

Department of Biochemistry
University of Cambridge
Cambridge, Great Britain

2260 Hagen, Paul B. Some current ideas on the biosynthesis and storage of simple amines and some consideration of their relationship to central nervous function. Journal of Neuropsychiatry, 1962, 4, 107-112.

Germane to CNS localization of simple amines, most levarterenol is located in the hypothalamus and most dopamine may be found in the basal ganglia. Levarterenol and dopamine are catecholamines of adrenergic nerves along with traces of epinephrine. Whether brain catecholamines are present in specialized amine storage cells or in neurones or glial cells remains a hypothetical question. Dopamine is in solution in the fluid cytoplasm, but epinephrine and levarterenol are located within special cytoplasmic storage granules as the adenine nucleotide salts. In mammals, 5HT is found principally in the argentaffin cells of the alimentary canal, but in brain tissue it is stored in granules of lower specific gravity than mitochondria. Acetylcholine is stored in brain vesicles. The function of GABA remains unknown at present, as does the function of taurine. (24 refs.)

Department of Biochemistry
University of Manitoba
Winnipeg, Manitoba
Canada

2261 Pletscher, A. Basic aspects of psychotropic drug action. American Journal of Mental Deficiency, 1962, 67, 238-244.

Rauwolfia alkaloids with sedative action (e.g. reserpine) and benzoquinolizine derivatives with sedative action (e.g., tetrabenazine) decrease the storage capacity for monoamines like 5HT, levarterenol and dopamine. Administration of α-methyldopa or 2-methyl 5HTP results in a fall of brain 5HT, levarterenol and dopamine through blocking monoamine formation by preventing decarboxylation of monoamine precursors. Irreversible (long acting) MAO inhibitors include hydrazine derivatives like iproniazid, isocarboxazid, pheniprazine, phenelzine, tranylcypromine, etc. Hormone derivatives like harmine and harmaline are short acting or reversible MAO inhibitors. Inhibition of MAO degradation by these drugs increases the brain content of various endogenous monoamines. Certain phenothiazines (chlorpromazine) and thioxanthenes (chlorprothixene) inhibit monoamine penetration through biological membranes. Thymoleptics like imipramine and amitriptyline may exert their influence by increasing the monoamine sensitivity of CNS receptor sites.

Medical Research Department
F. Hoffmann-La Roche and Co., Ltd.
Basel, Switzerland

2262 Schulte, W. Psychotherapeutische
Bemühungen bei der Melancholie. [Psycho-
therapy of melancholy.] Deutsches Medizinische Wochenschrift, 1962, 81, 2225-2231.

A distinction must be drawn between depressives and melancholics. The latter do
not feel "sad" but rather "indifferent",
"empty", "lifeless", etc. Indifference ex-
presses itself in a dull personality and care-
less grooming. Contact and therapy are
difficult because the physician is mistrusted
and considered incapable of understanding
the uniqueness of the patient's condition.
During the freer intervals the patient may
be brought to accept the melancholic phase
as part of his life and to place confidence
in the physician, who must also subsequently
be always available to fortify the patient
against his fear of reentering the external
world. Psychotropic drugs are useful but
doses must be carefully watched or the
patient may retrogress. (No refs.)

Universitäts Nervenklinik
Osianderstrasse 22
Tübingen, Germany

2263 Beskine, Harry. Psychiatric inpatient
treatment of adolescents. A review of clinical experience. Comprehensive Psychiatry,
1962, 3, 354-369.

This review of the residential psychiatric
care of adolescents includes historical background, nonhospital facilities, psychiatric
facilities, adolescent-adult wards versus
all-adolescent wards. problems in controlling aggressive, destructive and acting-out
behavior, and follow-up results. Admixture
of adolescent and adult patients seemed
helpful although there were some differences
of opinion. The dearth of systematic investigation into the problem of treating adolescents in psychiatric hospitals was noted.
Drug therapy is mentioned (i.e., phenothiazines) but no details were given. (51 refs.))

Massachusetts Mental Health Center
Boston, Mass.

2264 Weingärtner, L. Zur medikamentösen
Therapie Neu- und Frühgeborener [Drug
therapy of newborn and premature infants]
Zeitschrift für Ärztliche Fortbildung, 1962,
17, 969-972.

Newborn and premature infants require
often greatly reduced dosages of drugs,
unrelated to body weight. Thirteen potentially dangerous drugs, hormones and vitamins are listed, including opiates, atropine,
barbiturates and phenothiazines. Metabolic
processes required for excretion or detoxi-
cation are not fully developed in these
infants, and may easily be damaged by
drugs. The role of enzymes and the
significance of enzymatic defects are discussed in connection with certain hereditary
diseases. (No refs.)

Universitäts-Kinderklinik
der Martin Luther-Universität
Halle-Wittenberg, Germany

2265 Chatagnon, C., & Chatagnon, P. A.
Les drogues en gériatrie et en gériatrie-
psychiatrique. [Drugs in geriatrics and
psychiatric geriatrics.] Annales Médico-
Psychologiques, 1962, 120, 2, 231-242.

Utilization of hypocholesterolemics, anticoagulants, vasodilators, and rauwolfia derivatives in geriatrics necessitates great
attention to dosage requirements. Hormone
treatments and vitamin therapy are frequently useful, particularly in cases of
senile osteoporosis. A large number of
stimulants has been in vogue and on occasion, favorable results have been obtained
when placental or amniotic lyophilized extracts were used on depressive senile
patients. Tolerance to various sedatives
and hypnotics is lower in older persons,
and patients must be carefully observed for
certain secondary   symptoms such as
Cheyne-Stokes respiration or morphine-induced depression of the respiratory center.
Psychoactive drugs, particularly tranquilizers and ataractics are more dangerous to
older persons than is commonly realized,
and dosages should be minimal. Little is
known of their mechanisms of action or biochemical effects. Chlorpromazine is excreted, not stored within the body; its transitory

biochemical effects include higher erythrocyte sedimentation rate with concomitant variation of blood viscosity, lower fibrinemia and potassiemia. Large doses over a long period of time will cause slight weight loss and possible convulsions. (No refs.)

Hôpital de Maison-Blanche
Neuilly-sur-Marne, France

2266   Berger, F.M. The treatment of anxiety. A critical review. Journal of Neuropsychiatry, 1962, 4, 98-103.

Anxiety is an organic or functional disturbance of the brain rather than the mind since the mind is merely a manifestation of brain activity. Considerable evidence contradicts Freudian and Pavlovian concepts of anxiety. Psychologically, anxiety is manifested as a unitary factor which is neither a primary drive nor related to the general drive level. Deleterious anxiety may be ameliorated by 2 basic pharmacological drugs: meprobamate and chlorpromazine. Meprobamate, the drug of choice appears to act directly on anxiety, while chlorpromazine specifically counteracts hallucinations. (9 refs.)

Wallace Laboratories
Cranbury, N.J.

2267   LaVerne, Albert A. Compendium of neuropsychopharmacology. Preparations used in treatment of alcoholism. Journal of Neuropsychiatry, 1962, 4, 127-133.

Information on the drugs used in the CR treatment of chronic alcoholism is presented in tabular form replete with generic and trade names, type of drug and action, indications for use, therapeutic rating (effectiveness and toxicity, side effects, contraindications and cautions, recommended dosage and references). Drugs so elucidated include apomorphine, emetine, disulfiram, calcium carbimide, chlordiazepoxide, various phenothiazines, dexamphetamine, ACTH and other corticosteroids and insulin. (15 refs.)

[No address]

aspects. Illinois Medical Journal, 1962,
122, 264-268.

With regard to the moral implications of
the thalidomide tragedy, 4 physicians and
3 theologians tender their views on abortion and euthanasia. Of the physicians, 1
feels that the present laws should be
changed to legalize abortion for such specific cases, 2 others believe that many of
these children are of normal or high
normal intelligence indicating an excellent possibility of emotional and social
habilitation, and the 4th proposes that a
therapeutic abortion be performed if the
mother gives her consent after having
examined her religious beliefs. One theo-
logian would not censure the couple that
would decide upon legal abortion if the
decision were based upon sufficient medical advice and an earnest examination of
their motives. However, another asserts
that such abortion and euthanasia are utterly
immoral. An eminent Rabbi promulgates
the view that failure to prevent such births
would be nothing short of a sin against God
and man. (No refs.)

[No address]

2273   Lancet. Profession, government, and
drug industry. Lancet, 1962, No. 7229,
580-581. [Editorial]

In an address Louis Lasagna gave 8 reasons
for the present deplorable condition of the
American pharmaceutical industry and offered suggestions for improvement. In the
ensuing discussion, other physicians discussed the advent of continuously improved
phenothiazine drugs, the reliability of generic name drugs, the fact that doctors
kill more people than inferior drugs do
and that most American postgraduate medical education is carried out by the pharmaceutical industry. (No refs.)

7, Adam Street
Adelphi
London W.C. 2, Great Britain

2274   Lecks, Harold I., & Kravis, Lillian
P. Drug therapy of asthma. Bronchodilators.
Clinical Pediatrics, 1962, 1, 125-129.

Tables of bronchodilators used in asthma

therapy include tranquilizing drugs (chlorpromazine, prochlorperazine, promethazine, meprobamate, chlordiazepoxide and
hydroxyzine), bronchodilators (epinephrine,
ephedrine, ethyllevarterenol, ethylnorepin-
ephrine, etc.), expectorants, oral inhalation
therapy, sedatives (phenobarbital and chloral hydrate) and ACTH and corticosteroids.
(No refs.)

[No address]

2275   Macdonald, A.D. Habituation and addiction. Indian Journal of Physiology and
Pharmacology, 1962, 6, 165-173.

A general discussion is given on habituation
and addiction in Great Britain in relation
to incidence (reportedly much lower than
in the United States), prevention, treatment and classification of habit-forming
drugs. The responsibility of the pharmacist
as well as the medical doctor is emphasized.
Brief mention is made of the continued
dependency in Great Britain upon morphine
rather than synthetic analgesics which have
greater preference in the United States.
(7 refs.)

Department of Pharmacology
University of Manchester
Manchester, Great Britain

2276   Gilbert, Enid F. An evaluation of
some laboratory diagnostic tests in phenylketonuria. Clinical Proceedings, Children's
Hospital of the District of Columbia, 1962,
18, 328-332.

Laboratory procedures which may be employed in the diagnosis of phenylketonuria
include the ferric chloride test, Phenistix
test, dinitrophenylhydrazine test, 2-dimen-
sional chromatography and electrophoretic
studies. Elevated levels of serum phenylalanine with urinary excretion of abnormal
metabolites derived from phenylalanine,
tyrosine, ortho-tyrosine and tryptophan
constitute a definitive laboratory diagnosis.
Many other conditions, particularly hepatic
malfunction or insufficiency, can produce
positive urinary ferric chloride test findings. Negative urinary findings during the
neonatal period should be interpreted with

the progress of investigations. In notifying the FDA before undertaking clinical investigation with a new drug, manufacturers would be required to provide the following: a summary of all preclinical investigations, copies of all relevant data regarding preclinical information and experience with the drug and names and summaries of training and experience of all personnel who will participate in the investigation. The notice of proposal to amend regulations governing new drugs for investigational use is reprinted in its entirety. (No refs.)

Revere Publishing Company
New York, N.Y.

2281   Journal of New Drugs. Generic names of new drugs. Journal of New Drugs, 1962, 2, 252-254. [Editorial]

Generic names for psychoactive drugs newly adopted by the AMA-United States Pharmacopeia Nomenclature Committee include propenzolate, diazoxide, piperacetazine and thioridazine. Piperacetazine and thioridazine are both highly efficacious phenothiazine tranquilizers. (No refs.)

Revere Publishing Company
New York, N.Y.

2282   Journal of New Drugs. Drug amendments of 1962. Federal Food, Drug, and Cosmetic Act: a summary. Journal of New Drugs, 1962, 2, 314-320. [Editorial]

Major alterations in drug provisions of the Federal Food, Drug and Cosmetic Act encompass the following topics: quality manufacturing controls, requirement of proof of effectiveness for new drugs, prohibition of false or misleading labeling of new drugs; suspension or withdrawal of new drug approval on safety grounds, additional grounds for withdrawal of new drug approval, new drug clearance procedure and time limits for federal action, report on experience with new drugs and antibiotics on the market, requirements as to experimental drugs, strengthened factory inspection authority for prescription drugs, registration and periodic inspection of the establishments of drug manufacturers, standardization of nonproprietary drug names, drug names and ingredient formulas on labels and labeling, advertisements for the prescription drugs, batch certification of antibiotics, information to physicians on request, information to the Patent Office from the Department of Health, Education and Welfare, feed additives and effective dates. (No refs.)

Revere Publishing Company
New York, N.Y.

2283 Journal of New Drugs. New Federal regulations for the control of new drug testing in humans. Journal of New Drugs, 1962, 2, 373-376. [Editorial]

New regulations issued by the FDA are designed to strengthen and extend control over new drug investigations. An avalanche of objections from scientists resulted in division of the clinical investigation program into 3 arbitrary sections; phases 1 and 2 relate to clinical pharmacology of the drug, while phase 3 constitutes clinical trials. Reports of all phases must present design modifications in detail. Sponsors must promptly investigate and report any information associated with drug usage which is indicative of significant signs of toxicity. Alarming findings will necessitate discontinuation of clinical testing pending data evaluation. Ordinarily, investigators may withhold the names of volunteers of such information or patients. Extremely important new drugs may be utilized where necessary as lifesaving measures. Enough information must be provided on preclinical data to permit scientific review. Sponsors must discontinue shipments to any investigator who repeatedly or deliberately fails to maintain or proffer his records for inspection. Radioactive drugs for investigational use remain status quo provided they are shipped in accordance with AEC regulations. The full text of the regulations is reprinted for further elucidation. (No refs.)

Revere Publishing Company
New York, N.Y.

2284 Journal of New Drugs. New federal regulations for the control of new drug testing in humans. Journal of New Drugs, 1962, 2, 372. [Editorial]

and 200-450 μg/day orphenadrine, reduced finally to 4-12 mg/day reserpine and 200-600 μg/day orphenadrine. Good improvement was obtained in 15 cases, satisfactory improvement in 7 and no improvement in 7. Side effects were difficulty in accommodation, mild tremor, akathisia and restlessness, although 1 case did show a severe Parkinsonian syndrome. Some patients could not be given this combined treatment because of marked intolerance. In 1 older patient, not in the group of 29, treatment with reserpine and orphenadrine may have led to a fatal thrombosis.

Nervenklinik der Universität München
München, Germany

2288 Sherwood, J.N., Stolaroff, M.J., & Harman, W.W. The psychedelic experience. A new concept in psychotherapy. Journal of Neuropsychiatry, 1962, 4, 69-80.

LSD (100-200 μg p.o.) and mescaline (200-400 mg p.o.) were administered in a single session to 25 patients (5 with marital problems, 3 alcoholics, 9 with ineffectual personalities, 7 neurotics and 1 with homicidal tendencies) over a 5-month period. Drug ingestion was followed by a tripartite psychedelic experience characterized by the evasive stage, symbolic stage and stage of immediate perception, in which the patient undergoes complete revitalization of self-concept. Overall, 12 were considerably improved, 9 improved and 4 did not improve. The amount of improvement can generally be correlated with the subjects willingness to face himself during the LSD session, and with his acceptance of the abreactive material encountered as indicated by the extent to which he is willing to utilize this material. Optimally, sensitivity and awareness are heightened considerably.

International Foundation for Advanced Study
Menlo Park, Calif.

2289 Webb, H.E., & Lascelles, R.G. Treatment of facial and head pain associated with depression. Lancet, 1962, No. 7225, 355-356.

Phenelzine (15 mg t.i.d. or q.i.d.) and
imipramine (25-50 mg t.i.d.) were administered to 21 depressed patients with facial
and head pain of trigeminal origin (18
with trigeminal neuralgia and 3 postherpetic
neuralgia) and 10 with functional facial
and head pain. Of those with pain of organic
origin, 17 showed a marked response consisting of reestablishment of normal sleep
pattern, loss of apathy and listlessness,
and considerable pain relief. Of the 10 with
psychogenic pain, 8 responded to antidepressants with disappearance of pain.
Pain was apparently relieved by treating
the underlying depressive state.

Department of Neurology
St. Thomas's Hospital
London, S.E. 1, Great Britain

2290 Feer, H. Beeinflussung schizophren-
er Zustandsbilder mit Hypertensiva. [Effect
of hypertensive medication on schizophrenic
conditions.] Psychopharmacologia, 1962, 3,
99-104.

Twenty-seven patients (12 men and 15
women, aged 16-60 years) were treated
with levarterenol and Hypertensin by i.v.
infusion. All patients were schizophrenic
(15 catatonic, 8 paranoid, and 4 hebephrenic); 13 patients were in acute stages,
14 were chronically ill (more than 6 months).
The rate of infusion was 5-20 µg levarterenol and 0.5-2 µg Hypertensin per minute,
depending on the blood pressure. The duration of the infusion was 2.5-3 hours. For
control, 7 schizophrenic patients received
infusions of dioxyphenylalanine derivatives.
Following the infusions improvement was
observed in most patients; those in acute
phases reacted more favorably than chronic
patients. The infusions with dioxyphenylalanine derivatives had no effect. In some
patients the behavioral changes were quantitatively evaluated by the IMPA. The
morbidity index fell after successful infusion with levarterenol in 41%, with Hypertensin in 43%; in patients who did not
respond to the infusions in 13%, and in
the controls in 16%.

Psychiatrische Universitätsklinik
  Friedmatt
Basel, Switzerland

with anxiety, average age 38 years, for 2 weeks. Of the 50, 13 failed to complete the course of treatment. Assessment procedures included psychiatric progress reports, the Target Symptom Rating Scale (TSRS), AACL and a global psychiatric rating. The improvement rate for the placebo group was higher (47.6%) than that for the drug group (31.3%), but the difference was not statistically significant. Side effects of both agents were slight, including retardation, nausea, depression, diarrhea, irritability and nervousness. Pyrbenzindole was no more effective than placebo in relieving anxiety and depression and in producing global clinical improvement.

Kings County Hospital Center
Brooklyn, N.Y.

2295 Broussolle, P., & Rosier, Y. Nouvel essai du méprobamate: la forme injectable en thérapeutique hospitalière. [A new trial of meprobamate: the injectable form in hospital therapy.] Annales Médico-Psychologiques, 1962, 120, 1, 130-138.

Meprobamate (400 mg for 3 days, then 800 mg for 20-35 days) was injected into 29 female psychiatric patients, including 7 manic depressives, and 5 cases of senile dementia. Injections were given 1 hour before bedtime. Symptomatic relief of anxiety approximated that obtained with oral administration, while hypnogenic action was considerably greater. Complete disappearance of all abnormal anxiety occurred in 6 cases, great improvement in 11, partial improvement in 7 and failure in 5. Of the 7 depressed psychotics, 5 demonstrated complete or partial improvement. The 5 senile dementia patients showed a new interest in their surroundings. Favorable results appeared 5-6 days after initiation of treatment, duration of the therapy being 3 weeks. Prolongation of treatment beyond this point did not produce new benefits, while suspension of treatment at this point fails even after 2 months to result in any recurrence. However, parenteral treatment should be continued with oral administration of smaller doses. Minor, local side effects consisted of mild pains at the site of injection.

[No address]

2296 Gambs, Pouget, Champeau, Miribel, Marinier, & Auge. Aspects clinique et electroencephalographiques du traitement par le 71-62 R.P. [Clinical and electroencephalographical aspects of treatment with R.P. 71-62.] Annales Médico-Psychologiques, 1962, 120, 2, 410-417.

Sixty-three patients were treated for varying periods of time with R.P. 71-62, 50 mg/day p.o., initially increased by 25-50 mg increments until a mean daily dose of 150-200 mg was reached. The drug was injected in 3 cases. Mean duration of treatment was about 1.5 months, with a maximal hospital stay of 8 months. Most patients also received 50 mg/day levomepromazine. Barbiturates (50 mg in the evening) and symptomatic treatment of minor side effects were associated with R.P. 71-62 treatment. Important side effects included generalized epileptic crises and convulsions. Minor symptoms included dry mouth, hesitant speech, faintness on arising, constipation, and some instability. Results were as follows: controlled discharge-16 cases; improvement-27 cases; no effect-17; aggravation-3. EEG disturbances in order of severity were, slowing of appearance of slow delta waves with or without hyperpnea via sensitization and appearance of point waves. The EEG anomalies do not bear any unequivocal relationships to clinical symptoms.

[No address]

2297 Hackstock, H. Alkoholhalluzinose und Delirium tremens und deren Behandlung mit Vitaminen. [Alcohol-hallucinosis and delirium tremens and their treatment with vitamins.] Therapeutische Umschau, 1962, 19, 110-113.

Two forms of acute psychoses in chronic alcoholics are discussed: (a) the alcoholic hallucinosis and (b) delirium tremens. Thirteen hospitalized patients were treated; 9 suffered from delirium, 2 had hallucinosis and 2 were chronic alcoholics with severe liver damage. The average age was 55.5 years. The physical findings were comparable in all; all patients had liver damage. The patients were given extensive vitamin therapy. Chlordiazepoxide (75-90 mg p.o.)

noted, and some indication exists of damage to liver cells if treatment is continued beyond 6 months. Ambulatory treatment is advisable only when the symptoms, especially anxiety symptoms, indicate no danger of suicide attempts.

Hospital Ste-Antoine
Paris 12, France

2301 Büssow, H. Kombination neuroleptischer Mittel mit vegetativ wirksamen Substanzen. [Association of neuroleptic, drugs with substances having autonomic action.] Medicina Experimentalis, 1960, 7, 100-111; discussion 112-125.

Patients suffering from melanchlia were treated for a 6-8 day period with reserpine [dosage unspecified] or other neuroleptic drugs. After this treatment glutethimide was administered as an additive, at 125-250 mg 3-4 times per day. After a macimal latency period of 2 days, a change occurred, consisting of either increased somnolence or euphoria resembling inebriety, but these effects were transitory, being followed by favorable effects on the melancholic state. In many cases continued treatment with the combination made it possible for the patient to leave the hospital and even to return to work. Extreme cases were also favorably affected by the treatment, stupor being alleviated, and acute hyperkinesia being sedated. Success was also registered in the treatment of acute endogenous psychoses, agitational anxiety depressions, acute paranoid - hallucinatory psychoses, subacute toxic hallucinations, and epileptic emergencies. Paranoid and hallucinatory syndromes persist even after improvement of psyche and drive. The effect of the association is believed to be due to the anticholinergic properties of glutethimide, since the association of other neuroleptic drugs and with anticholinergic drugs has also proved efficacious. The use of a number of antipsycotic phenothiazines is expanded in the discussion.

Allgemeines Krankenhaus
Hamburg-Ochsenzoll
Hamburg-Langenhorn, Germany

2302   Borenstein, P., Dabbah, M., & Blès,
G.   Etude électroencéphalographique de
la thiopropérazine. [Electroencephalogra-
phic study of thioproperazine.]   Revue
Neurologique, 1962, 106, 238-243.

In 29 patients, EEG's taken after single
10 mg doses of thioproperazine disclosed the following. Based activity in the form
of a regular, well-structured, bilateral,
symmetric alpha wave with normal reactivity under hyperpnea but no intermittent
light stimulus 12 cases; regular alpha base
activity with short theta bursts, 10 cases,
5 of these also showing pointed dysrhythmias; reduced- amplitude irregular al-
phas, 3 cases; and 3 cases of theta base
activity. EEG's taken after a prolonged
treatment consisted of: 10 cases of regular
alpha base activity; base activity consisting of a regular alpha alternating with
or without pointed dysrhythmias, 5 cases;
3 cases of less abundant and less ample
irregular alpha base activity; and 1 case
of a less ample base alpha overlaid with
a large number of rapid rhythms. Cases
included hebephrenics, epileptics, hebe-
phrenic-catatonics, delirious psychoses,
and other various psychoses. No relationship could be discovered between clinical and EEG results.

Hopital psychiatrique
Veillejuif
Seine, France

2303   Straube, Wolfgang, & Melliwa, Helmut. Zur Dauerbehandlung extrapyramidal-
er Hyperkinesen mit Perphenazin. [The
permanent treatment of extrapyramidal hyperkinesia with perphenazine.] Nervenarzt,
1962, 33, 549-553.

Fifty-six hospitalized and ambulatory patients with various forms of chorea, extrapyramidal hyperkinesia, torsion spasm,
tic, were treated orally with perphenazine.
Adults received at the onset 8 mg t.i.d.
or q.i.d.; the dosage was increased and
regulated when improvement became evident. Children and young adults were started
on 4 mg b.i.d. or t.i.d.; the dosage was
increased to 20-24 mg/day. Outpatients
received not more than 16 mg per day;
others were hospitalized until the dosage

depressions; they did not show any signs of delirium but showed significant organic deterioration. The 2nd group consisted of 9 patients suffering from drug addiction hospitalized for withdrawal. In the latter group, the treatment was started after 3 weeks of complete drug abstinence. The average age of the patients was 48-86. The preparation was administered in the following manner: I) a series of 12 injections of Gerioptil during 4 weeks, with 3 injections weekly; II) a 2nd series for 4 weeks with 6 capsules Gerioptil plus H3 during the 1st week, and 3 capsules during the following 3 weeks; III) a 3rd series of 12 injections as in I). All patients tolerated the medication well; no significant changes in blood pressure and temperature were observed; no pathological changes in blood count and liver function tests were seen. The results were as follows: in group I (11) 1 excellent, 5 good, 1 satisfactory, 2 improved, 2 not improved; in group II (9) 5 good, 2 markedly improved, 1 satisfactory and 1 not improved.

[No address]

2306 Degkwitz, Rudolf. Uber die Imipraminwirkung bei Depressionen. [The effect of imipramine in depressions.] Nervenarzt, 1962, 33, 450-457.

Six-hundred-and-fifty hospitalized and 150 ambulatory patients were treated with imipramine. The patients were selected on the basis of 3 conditions: 1) only those forms of depression were chosen which did not necessitate sedation; 2) only those patients were selected who had not previously been treated with neuroleptic agents, with MAO inhibitors and ECT, and 3) the treatment had to be continued for a sufficiently long time without interruption. Imipramine treatment alone (75-350 mg) gave 70% good or fair improvement; imipramine in combination with a neuroleptic agent (75-150 mg/day) or ECT gave superior results, and the result of the treatment is seen in 90% of the cases in the 2nd or 3rd week of treatment. Side effects (10% necessitated the interruption of treatment) become evident in the 1st week of treatment (restlessness, increased depression, delirium, lip and tongue spasms).

Results are independent of sex but depend on age. The chances for improvement in patients over 30 years of age are considerably better. The success of the treatment is independent of the state of depression existing at the onset of treatment. Satisfactory treatment should not be abruptly discontinued.

Universitäts-Nervenklinik
Frankfurt am Main, Germany

2307 Flügel, F., & Itil, T. Klinisch-elektrencephalographische Untersuchungen mit "Verwirrtheit" hervorrufenden Substanzen. [Clinical-EEG investigations on delirium-producing agents.] Psychopharmacologia, 1962, 3, 79-98.

Psychotic-delirious conditions were induced with ethotrimeprazine (0.02-0.14 mg per kg i.m. and 0.06-0.25 mg per kg i.v.); phencyclidine (0.02-0.14 mg/kg i.m. and 0.04-0.25 mg/kg i.v.); diethylaminoethyl-phenobarbital (0.3-1.5 mg/kg i.v.); and phenylisopropyl-oxyacetic-dimethylamino-propylester (0.03 mg/kg i.v. and 10-15 mg orally). One-hundred-and-fifty-six investigations were carried out in 47 patients (26 endogenous depressions, 5 schizophrenics, 7 epileptics, 5 neurasthenics and 4 functional disorders). The following symptoms were observed with increasing dosage: fatigue, difficulty and/or inability to concentrate, disorientation, motor unrest, ataxia, equilibrium disturbances, illusions and hallucinations. The mental disturbances are parallel to disorganization of cortical activity in the EEG, which shows dissolution of alpha rhythm, decrease of voltage and appearance of slow waves and fast activity at the same time. The EEG differentiates these drugs clearly from the "hallucinogenic", and partly from the anticholinergic drugs. The possible therapeutic importance of drug-induced "exogenous" psychoses is pointed out.

Neuro-Psychiatrischen Klinik
Universität Erlangen-Nürnberg
Erlangen, Germany

2308 Grahmann, Hans, & Peters, Uwe H. Durch Psychopharmaka induzierte und pro-

vozierte Psychosen, ihre Psychopathologie
und ihre therapeutische Bedeutung. [Psy-
choses induced and precipitated by psychopharmacological drugs, their psychopathology and therapeutic importance.] Nervenarzt, 1962, 33, 398-430.

Psychotic conditions are sometimes precipitated by psychopharmacologic treatment. In 20 patients suffering from different
types of compulsive neuroses and from various depressions, psychosis or delirium
was intentionally precipitated. Chlorpromazine (100-700 mg i.d.), promethazine (25-
300 mg i.d.), chlorprothixene (415 mg i.d.),
thioridazine [no dosage given], and orphenadrine [no dosage given] were used, alone
or in combination. They were administered
initially in large doses which were rapidly
increased until delirium was reached. The
psychotic state was usually maintained for
2-5 days, up to 10 days. Two patients
showed excellent, 9 good and 3 doubtful
response: the results were negative in 9.
Some of the successfully treated patients
had previously not responded to psychopharmacological agents, convulsive drugs
and/or psychotherapy. Only cases without
organic disorders were treated; massage
of the lower extremities and physical exercise was carried out during the psychotic
stage. No side effects were experienced.
A larger [unidentified] number of patients
treated in the same manner did not respond with delirium.

Psychiatrische und Nervenklinik der
   Universität Kiel
Kiel, Germany

2309 Fiegel, Georg, & Kukwa, Dietrich.
Der regulative Effekt von Hydroxyzin auf
die Störungen der Herzrhythmik. [The regulating effect of hydroxyzine on cardiac
arrhythmia.] Therapie der Gegenwart,1962,
6, 284-287.

Hydroxyzine pamoate was administered to
67 patients with arrhythmia, caused by
functional dysregulation and characterized
by extrasystoles and tachycardia; 50 mg
t.i.d. p.o. was sufficient for the majority
of patients. In severe cases initial doses
of 300 mg were given. Two types of response are differentiated: 1) the extra-

effective sleep inducer than cyclobarbital.

Department of Medicine
The General Infirmary
University of Leeds
Leeds, Great Britain

2313 Fleming, Jack W., & Orlando, Robert. Effect of deanol on attention in the mentally retarded: A reaction time method. Journal of New Drugs, 1962, 2, 239-244.

In a double-blind procedure, deanol (75 mg per day p.o.) or placebo was administered to 32 institutionalized retardates, aged 12-25 years, for 55 days after the baseline period, after which the deanol group received 150 mg/day for another 37 days. Attention response to a light stimulus was measured during the last 2 weeks of the initial 3 week baseline period and during the final 2 weeks of the study. A distracting stimulus (orange light, buzzer or combination thereof) was presented simultaneously with a green light stimulus once during each block of 10 trials. Deanol effect was estimated by comparison of reaction time performance before and after drug administration, as well as between drug and placebo groups. Statistical analysis of mean reciprocal reaction times for all trials, distracting trials and trials following distraction revealed no evidence that deanol greatly improved attention, as reflected in overall reaction time. Some positive drug effect is indicated, however, by resistance to attention loss, as well as increased alertness or sensitivity to sudden, novel stimuli.

Rainier School
Buckley, Wash.

2314 Terry, James G., & Teixeira, Theodore C. Nalorphine testing for illegal narcotic use in California: Methods and limitations. Journal of New Drugs, 1962, 2, 206-210.

Nalorphine (3 mg) is injected s.c. in suspected narcotic users, before and after which pupillary size is measured by a pupillometer to the nearest 10th of a millimeter. During a standard clinic session, if the 2nd pupillary diameter exceeds the 1st by 0.25 millimeter or more, the test is considered positive and the patient is thoroughly examined for needle marks and other signs and symptoms of narcotic use. Patients are permitted to leave the clinic if the pupil remains the same size or constricts. In California, parolees receive 5 tests per month while probationers receive 2. Physical similarities are observed in clinic design. Nalorphine clinics are located throughout the state of California. One of the detriments of the nalorphine test is that too much emphasis is placed on pupillary measurement with no additional evidence of narcotic use. The test should be considered only as a diagnostic aid. Correlation of the pupillary test in 419 subjects with chemical tests of urine revealed that pupillary tests agreed with the chemical tests in 85% of the cases, 339 having been negative and 18 positive by both procedures. The chemical tests were more sensitive in 28 instances. Nalorphine induced side effects which occur in 5-10% of those tested include dizziness, lightheadedness, tiredness, peripheral vascular effects, ataxia and euphoria. Nalorphine testing is effective as a restrictive procedure.

Santa Rita Rehabilitation Center
Pleasanton, Calif.

2315 McCusker, Kenneth, Ota, Kay Y., Michaux, William W., & Kurland, Albert A. N-(2,5-dimethyl-1-pyrrolyl)isonicotinamide in the treatment of the inactive chronically psychotic patient. Journal of New Drugs, 1962, 2, 232-238.

In the 1st portion of a 2-part study, 39 men (31 schizophrenics, 6 mental defectives with psychosis and 2 CBS), aged 27-64 years, average duration of hospitalization 19.0 years, received placebo or N-(2,5-dimethyl-1-pyrrolyl)isonicotinamide (SQ-3242) (50 mg q.i.d. for 2 weeks, 100 mg t.i.d. for 2 weeks and 100 mg q.i.d. for 1 week) on a randomly assigned double-blind basis for 5 weeks, followed by a 2 week medication free observation period. Routine laboratory analyses were performed before and after treatment. Patients were evaluated on a double-blind basis by

means of the MACC Behavioral Adjustment Scale, the Psychotic Reaction Profile (PRP) and weekly clinical interview assessments by 3 psychiatrists. The 2nd phase of the study involved administration of SQ 3242 (100 mg q.i.d. for 1 week, 100 mg t.i.d. for 2 weeks with 200 mg at bedtime, 200 mg t.i.d. with 100 mg at bedtime for 1 week and 200 mg q.i.d. for 1 week) for 6 weeks to 9 men (7 chronic undifferentiated schizophrenics and 2 mental defectives with psychosis, average age 47.3 years, who were members of the placebo group in the 1st phase of the study. One psychiatrist evaluated patient response. Analysis of covariance for MACC and PRP scores yielded no significant differences. No decisive therapeutic effect was observed from the drug in the 1st or 2nd phase. Moderate slurring of speech and other basal ganglion symptomatology occurred in 3 patients with medium to high drug dosage. Seven dropouts were observed in toto.

Research Department
Spring Grove State Hospital
Baltimore 28, Md.

2316 Kurland, Albert A., McCusker, Kenneth, & Michaux, William W. Clinical trial of haloanisone with hospitalized psychiatric patients. Journal of New Drugs, 1962, 2, 352-360.

Haloanisone (15-150 mg/day p.o.) was administered to 30 patients (2 acute undifferentiated schizophrenics, 9 paranoid schizophrenics, 2 schizoaffective schizophrenics, 1 manic-depressive, 2 depressive reactions, 1 alcoholic, 1 adolescent adjustment reaction, 1 acute brain syndrome and 1 CBS) for 5 weeks. Patients were evaluated by 2 psychiatrists at weekly intervals. Results revealed that 3 (10%) were markedly improved, 2 (7%) moderately improved, 12 (40%) minimally improved, 9 (30%) essentially unchanged and 4 (13%) worse. Side effects occurring in 20 patients were primarily extrapyramidal in nature and generally reversible with appropriate medication. Severity of side effects precluded further treatment in 5. Physical and laboratory observations yielded no evidence of serious toxic effects. Statistical analysis revealed significant differences in sex and

2318 Sörgel, H.-J. Klinische Erfahrungen mit dem Psychotonikum Centedrin. [Clinical investigation with the psychotonic "Centedrine".] Deutsches Gesundheitswesen, 1962, 7, 256-259.

Twenty-eight hospitalized and ambulatory patients were treated with Centedrine [sic: methylium piperidyl-phenylacetum hydrochloricum; related to piperylone]. Twelve of these patients were suffering from endogenous depressions, 4 displayed depressive-paranoid symptoms due to cerebral arteriosclerosis, 5 had involutional depressions, 4 had developed organic complaints due to neuroses of long standing; 2 suffered from functional dysregulation, and 1 was in a narcolepsy-like condition. The treatment was initiated with 1-2 tablets b.i.d., and was increased to 1-2 tablets t.i.d. The duration of treatment was 2-8 weeks for hospitalized patients, and up to 3 months for ambulatory patients. The effect was very good in 12 patients, good in 11, fair in 4 and insignificant in 1. Frequent laboratory investigations of blood and urine revealed no pathology. Withdrawal of the medication had no negative effects.

Nervenklinik der Medizinische Akademie Erfurt, Germany

2319 Lereboullet, J., Benoit, Ph., & Ledoux, M. Action anxiolytique du chlordiazépoxide. [Anxiolytic action of chlordiazepoxide.] Thérapie, 1962, 17, 1005-1009.

Thirty-five mixed cases including some cases of cranial trauma were treated with oral doses of chlordiazepoxide (30-100 mg per day). Rarely the drug was used i.m. The common dosage was 30-40 mg/day and maintenance 20-40 mg/day. In some cases chlordiazepoxide was associated with other antidepressants or neuroleptics. Where anxiety was the chief component, 11 cases, excellent results were obtained in 5 and definite improvement in 6. The drug suppressed the anxiety of depression but not depression per se. Reactions with psychotic states were poor. Tolerance was excellent. One case of digestive disorder, and 1 case of erythematous eruption occurred.

Hospice de Bicêtre, Kremlin-Bicêtre Seine, France

2320 Madalena, J.C. O emprêgo do clor-
protixeno (RO 4-0403) na psicose maníaco-
depressiva. [The use of chlorprothixene
(RO4-0403) in manic-depressive psychosis.]
O Hospital, 1962, 61, 199-200.

Success was obtained in 4 cases of manic
excitation with suppression of crises within
48 hours through the i.m. use of 30 mg
chlorprothixene in the morning and afternoon.

Psiquiatria do Hospital da Ordem Terceira
de S. Francisco da Penitência
Universidade do Brasil
Rio de Janeiro, Brazil

2321 Dos Santos, Oswaldo. Resultados
clínicos do uso da trifluopromazina em
esquizofrênicos com mais de dois anos de
doença e submetidos a vários tratamentos.
[Clinical results on trifluopromazine in
schizophrenics ill for more than 2 years
and submitted to various treatments.] Revista Brasileira de Medicina, 1962, 19,
574-578.

Five schizophrenic hospitalized women,
including 3 paranoid reaction were treated
with trifluopromazine, initially 10 mg i.m.,
then 50 mg tablets, both t.i.d. Doses were
raised until maximum daily dosage reached
300-600 mg for 10-23 days. The onset of
extrapyramidal reactions in these patients
was correlated with improved mentation
in all cases. Insomnia, anxiety, iron deficiency anemia, amenorrhea, galactorrhea
and vomiting were noted as side effects
as well as slight hypotension in 1 case.
Complementary treatment consisted of barbiturate, B-complex vitamins, iron sulphate
and an antispasmodic. Total remissions
were obtained in 3 patients and partial
remissions in 2. These results were superior to those obtained previously in these
patients using fluphenazine or chlorpromazine.

[No address]

2322 Nagle, Gilberto J. Tratamento da
úlcera péptica gastro-duodenal pela as-
sociação do brometo de clidinium à Clor-
diazepoxida. [The treatment of gastro-
duodenal peptic ulcer with the combination

In the 1st condition results were 6 excellent and 1 good, in the 2nd 3 excellent and 1 good, and in ulcer patients 3 excellent and 1 good. Also, 3 cases of tension headache were treated with alleviation and diminution of crises.

Soc. Gastrenterol.
Rio Grande do Sul
Brazil

2327 Medrado, Valdir C., & Conde, Daisy. Avaliação clínica e experimental de um nôvo analéptico: 3-metil-7-metoxi-8-dimetilaminometil-flavona. [Clinical and experimental evaluation of a new analeptic: 3 - methyl - 7 - methoxy - 8 - dimethylamino-methyl-flavone. O Hospital, 1962, 62, 1077-1090.

3-Methyl-7-methoxy-8-dimethylaminomethyl-flavone was studied for acute toxicity (i.p. in rats), convulsant activity, analeptic activity in rats in comparison with other respiratory stimulants, and action on respiration, blood pressure, heart rate, ECG and EEG, the latter in dogs. In rats the LD_{50} is 5.3 mg/kg while the CD_{50} is 4.9 mg/kg. Pentobarbital treated rats were used in tests of analeptic activity: when compared to nikethamide, pentetrazol and Micoren, the analeptic activity of 3-methyl-7-methoxy-8-dimethylaminomethyl-flavone was greater, There were no changes in blood pressure and heart rate after i.v. administration in dogs, while the depth of breathing was markedly increased. Further there were no significant effects in the EEG. One hundred patients scheduled for dilatation and curettage were selected for clinical evaluation and 50 of these were anesthetized with pentobarbital (8-10 mg/kg). The 2nd group of 50 was given a preliminary dose of 0.16 mg/kg of a new analeptic before pentobarbital administration, and a 2nd dose was applied near the end of the operation. Results were encouraging, i.e., marked increase in pulmonary ventilation. The drug showed advantages in relation to the resuscitation of asphyxiated newborns, and newborns depressed by anesthetic and analgesic drugs.

Universidade da Bahia
Bahia, Brazil

2328   Dos Anjos, Edgar Soares. O clor-
protixeno em psiquiatria de ambulatório.
[Chlorprothixene in the psychiatry of ambulatory patients.] O Hospital, 1962, 62,
739-745.

Of 12 patients treated with chlorprothixene,
3 were paranoid schizophrenics while the
others were suffering from various types
of neuroses. The drug was given in the
form of 15 mg tablets, 15-45 mg per day,
sometimes combined with psychotherapy.
Results with the 3 schizophrenics were
considered excellent in relation to the
suppression of hallucination and improved
behavior. With 6 cases of anxiety results
were: 3 excellent, 2 good and 1 poor, while
with the 3 remaining cases, obsessive-
compulsive reaction, results were 1 excellent and 2 good. That is, improvement
occurred in 11 out of the 12 cases. Side
effects were practically absent (drowsiness in some patients at the beginning of
treatment).

Psiquiatra do I.A.P.I.
Rio de Janeiro, Brazil

2329   Pünder, Norma de Araújo. Contribui-
ção ao estudo da síndrome pré-menstrual.
[Contribution to the study of the premenstrual syndrome.] O Hospital, 1962, 62, 857-
864.

The combination 1 mg fluphenazine, 2.5 mg
benzhydroflumethazide and 500 mg KCl
was administered to 15 patients with premenstrual syndrome, aged 18-41 years.
Nine had previously been unresponsive
to hormonal or antispasmodic therapy.
Seven cases received the combination for
4 successive months and the 8 others
received it alternating 1 month on drug
and the other on placebo for the 4 months.
Treatment was always initiated 10 days
preceding expected menstruation. After 4
months, 4 were in complete remission,
and 3 had markedly improved. No toxicity
was recorded.

[No address]

2330   Marques, Jamerson Rodrigues, Lino,
Renato, Freitas, Abelardo, & Luiz, Augusto

following year revealed no evidence of autonomic imbalance, improvement in peripheral neuropathy and amelioration of other symptoms.

Smith Kline & French Laboratories
15th & Spring Garden Sts.
Philadelphia, Pa.

2334   Vestre, Norris D., Hall, Wilson B., & Schield, Burtrum. A comparison of fluphenazine, triflupromazine, and phenobarbital in the treatment of chronic schizophrenic patients: a double-blind controlled study. Journal of Clinical and Experimental Psychopathology & Quarterly Review of Psychiatry and Neurology, 1962, 23, 149-159.

Ninety-three hospitalized schizophrenics were randomly assigned to triflupromazine, fluphenazine and phenobarbital on a double-blind basis for 12 weeks. Average daily dosage reached by the end of the period was: 130 mg triflupromazine, 10 mg fluphenazine and 130 mg phenobarbital. The PRP and MMPI were used before, after 4 and 12 weeks of treatment. The 2 phenothiazines were more effective than phenobarbital; 5 patients dropped from the study were in the phenobarbital group. On the basis of the PRP, triflupromazine was superior to phenobarbital, while fluphenazine was not. No difference in the overall effectiveness of the 2 phenothiazines was found. The difference between fluphenazine and phenobarbital was detected in "thinking disorganization", where triflupromazine was superior to phenobarbital. Also, the side effects were very infrequent, i.e., parkinsonism.

VA Hospital
St. Cloud, Minn.

2335   Burner, M., Bieri, J., & Calanca, A. Bilan préliminaire de l'essai du traitement des dystonies neuro-végétatives par un médicament organo-magnésien, le Cirtonal-N. [Preliminary evaluation of therapy of autonomic dystonias with an organic magnesium drug, Cirtonal-N.] Praxis, 1962, 7, 187-190.

Forty-five patients, suffering from autonomic dystonias, including alcoholics, neurotics and schizophrenics, were treated
either with organic magnesium, Cirtonal-N,
i.v. (34 patients), or with placebos (11
cases). Of those receiving the drug, definite
improvement was noted in 6, good results
obtained in 21, doubtful effects in 3, and
no effect in 4. Only 5 of the 11 patients
receiving placebos reported good results,
the remaining being either doubtful or
zero. Injections were well tolerated.

Policlinique Psychiatrique
Universitaire de Lausanne
Lausanne, Switzerland

2336 Lanter, R., Weil, J., & Roth, M.
Note à propos de l'utilisation diagnostique
et thérapeutique des drogues hallucinogènes
(mescaline-L.S.D. 25). [Note on the diagnostic and therapeutic use of hallucinogens
(mescaline-LSD 25).] Annales Médico-
Psychologiques, 1962, 120, 2, 244-252.

Fourteen patients, institutionalized sex per-
verts and recalcitrant chronic alcoholics,
were placed under hallucinogenic therapy.
All of these subjects shared certain personality traits, namely, impulsiveness, avidity,
and "orality". Patients received either
mescaline (600-1400 mg) orally or by
injection, or LSD (100-800 mg) or an
association of the latter with apomorphine,
this combination being administered to
alcoholics. Generally the hallucinogens can
constitute an important adjunct to other
therapeutic methods. The reaction to mescaline seems to be more marked than to
LSD. Typical reactions are stupor with
inhibition and mutism, or agitation. Subjects report greater suggestibility, analogous to that of hysterical states. Their
diagnostic value so far has resided in
their reinforcement of latent psychotic or
neurotic symptoms.

[No address]

2337 Delachaux, A., & Schwed, S. A propos
de l'utilisation du Tofranil dans un service
de gériatrie de réhabilitation fonctionnelle.
[On the use of Tofranil in a geriatric
rehabilitation clinic.] Praxis, 1962, 23,

2340 Borenstein, P., Dabbah, M., Blès, G., Roussel, A., & Rosemberger. Etude clinique et électroencéphalographique de l'éthy-benzatropine (1) (U.K. 738 ou tropéthydry-line) utilisée en administration exclusive. [Clinical and EEG study of ethybenzatro-pine (U.K. 738 or tropethydryline) used by itself.] Annales Médico-Psychologiques, 1962, 120, 1, 288-295.

Thirty-eight male patients (10 schizophren-ics, 10 epileptics with behavioral and char-acter disorders and 18 miscellaneous psychotics) were treated with methylbenz-tropine [sic: ethybenzatropine (20 mg/day, i.m., i.v. or i.p.)] for a total of 1079 days, mean duration of therapy varying from 11-20 days in 14 cases, and 20-40 days in 19 cases. In 16 patients, side effects included mydriasis, visual fatigue, dry mouth, asthenia, daytime somnolence, urine retention and autonomic disturbances. Neurological sequelas were rare and mild. No psychic effects were noted in 22 cases, some improvement in 10, and aggravation in 8. After drug administration no EEG modification was noted in 27, clearcut amelioration of alpha-base activity in 14, and accentuation or exacerbation or pre-viously existing anomalies in 9. EEG tracings after a prolonged period of treat-ment were generally the same as those obtained after a single dose. The drug is not epileptogenic, but remains "active" in almost half of the convulsive disorders.

Centre de Médecine Psycho-Somatique
Hopital Psychiatrique de Villejuif
Villejuif, France

2341 Goldstein, Leonide, Murphree, Henry B., Sugerman, A. Arthur, Pfeiffer, Carl C., & Jenney, Elizabeth H. Quantitative electro-encephalographic analysis of naturally oc-curring (schizophrenic) and drug-induced psychotic states in human males. Clinical Pharmacology and Therapeutics, 1962, 4, 10-21.

Drohocki's integrator was used in this study made up of 3 parts: the character-istics of the quantified EEG of normal subjects without drug and after placebo; measurements obtained from EEG's of male chronic schizophrenics, and effects on EEG's of LSD administered to normal subjects and schizophrenics. Analysis of the quantified EEG of the left occipital lead of 21 normal male subjects revealed an average coefficient of variation in electrical energy of 15.4%. In 25 male chronic schizophrenic patients, the mean coefficient of variation was 8%. Placebo administration did not produce any significant change in either group. In the normal men, oral dosage with 0.3 µg/kg LSD produced a 33% decrease in variability without significant change in the mean energy content of the EEG. When the LSD dose was increased to 1 µg/kg, a 25% decrease in variability and 23% reduction of the energy content of the EEG followed. In schizophrenic patients, LSD at 1 µg/kg orally did not affect the mean energy content but produced a 47% increase in variability. The EEG of male institutionalized chronic schizophrenics tends to be hyperregulated. Similar hyperregulation is produced in normal volunteers by threshold and larger doses of LSD.

Bureau of Research in Neurology and
    Psychiatry
New Jersey Neuropsychiatric Institute
Princeton, N.J.

2342   Kameda, Hideaski, Hidaka, Yasuhiko, & Furukawa, Tadayuki. Changes in electroencephalogram following administration of chlordiazepoxide. Folia Psychiatrica et Neurologica, 1962, 16, 15-22.

EEG changes following administration of chlordiazepoxide (20-40 mg/day) were studied in 13 patients (9 epileptics, 2 epileptoid character disorders and 1 each head trauma and encephalomalacia), aged 6-20 years, for 1 week to 57 days. Marked improvement was shown by 6 patients, moderate improvement by 5 and no change or no evaluation in 2. A decrease of high-voltage paroxysmal dysrhythmia was associated with clinical improvement. Paroxysmal activity provoked by activating procedures like photic stimulation, hyperventilation and i.v. injection of bemegride was considerably reduced following drug administration. Fast waves, about 20 per second, increased predominantly in the frontal and central regions in most cases. This suggested a

dementias, 10 manics, 11 acute delirious psychotics, 27 with chronic delirium and 55 schizophrenics). The side effects of thioproperazine were remarkably attenuated by combination therapy. Only 2 excitomotor crises occurred, akinetic-hypertonic syndrome in only 16% of the cases, tremor in 24% and hyperkinetic syndrome in 6%. Daytime somnolence affected only 27%. Autonomic effects were mild and only occurred in 9%, while hypotension was encountered in 40%. Weight increases were noted in 53%, amenorrhea in 8 and galactorrhea in 15. A "down hill" syndrome was noted in a few aged persons, heralded by loss of weight. Cessation of therapy or dosage reduction is indicated for such persons.

Hopital psychiatrique
Saint-Egrève, France

2347   Lanternier, J. A propos d'un nouvel anti-convulsant l'alpha-éthyl-alpha-méthyl-succinimide. [A new anticonvulsant drug: a-ethyl-a-methyl-succinimide.] Pédiatrie, 1962, 17, 173-178.

Ethosuximide (a-ethyl-a-methyl-succinimide; 4-6 250 mg capsules/day) was administered to 44 children (12 petit mal with absences but without generalized crises, 14 with I.Q. varying from 75-100, including both generalized crises, absences of the petit mal type, and myoclonia. Seven of these patients were photosensitive and 18 remaining cases were encephalopaths) for 4-5 weeks. Concomitantly, dione medication was slowly decreased, but barbiturates were maintained. Of the petit mal cases, 11 showed complete clinical and EEG normality, while the 12th evidenced 50% improvement. Of the 14 centra-encephalics, 100% clinical improvement was observed along with 70-90% EEG improvement. Improvement was more rapid and complete in those who were not photosensitive. In the 18 encephalopaths considerable amelioration of clinical and electrical convulsions was noted. Side effects were generally slight, consisting of somnolence, vertigo and headaches at the start of treatment. In addition about half the children displayed anorexia, nausea, and gastric pains accompanied by vomiting and loss of weight.

931

However, these effects continued only 15-
30 days and then stopped abruptly.

7, rue de Castries
Lyon 2, France

2348 Jacob, Elizabeth, Marie, Claude,
Thévenot, Jean-Pierre, & Dauxois, Fran-
çoise. Contribution à l'étude du 7843 R.P.
(Majeptil) dans la schizophrénie. [Contribu-
tion to the study of RP 7843 (Majeptil) in
schizophrenia.] Annales Médico-Psychologiques, 1962, 120, 1, 139-144.

Thioproperazine (Majeptil) was administered to 17 chronic schizophrenics, aged
25-55 years, with excellent results (possibility of discharge and adequate social
readaptation) obtained in 3 cases, good
results in 3, some improvement in 4,
negligible results in 5, and 2 were aggravated. A battery of psychological tests
was administered to 11 patients. These
included Wechsler-Bellevue or Stanford-
Binet intelligence tests, Heuyer-Baille
Motor-Development tests, Seguin tests, etc.
Comparison of psychological test results
and retests generally confirmed the modifications of schizophrenic structure mentioned above.

[No address]

2349 Fouks, Lainé, Mathis, Ferrant, Riou,
& Bouchet. Note sur l'utilisation clinique
de la dixyrazine. [Note on the clinical use
of dixyrazine.] Annales Médico-Psychologiques, 1962, 120, 1, 392-399.

Dixyrazine is a methylated piperazine phenothiazine derivative. Clinical doses (35
mixed cases) were 50-100 mg/day for
neuroses and mild depressions, and 150-
200 mg/day for endogenous depressions
and other psychoses. In depression, it
was frequently combined with phenelzine,
or imipramine. Side effects are generally
mild, consisting of excito-motor troubles,
slight hypotension, and diminished alertness. Neuroleptic psychomotor effects are
frequently noted, but antiparkinsonian drugs
(trihexyphenidyl and orphenadrine) generally alleviate the condition rapidly. Somnolence tends to occur in neurotic children and

93

for 4 months. Treatment was considered completely successful in regard to skin discoloration, while no conclusion could be drawn with respect to the effect upon mental illness.

Prefectural Mental Hospital "Yukyuso"
  Nagaoka
Niigata Ken, Japan

2354   Gover, Douglas M. Thioridazine and chlorprothixene in the management of anxiety in tuberculous patients. American Revue of Respiratory Diseases, 1962, 85, 587-590.

Thioridazine (25-300 mg/day p.o.), chlorprothixene (25-300 mg/day p.o.) or placebo was administered on a double-blind basis to 24 patients, aged 37-78 years, with anxiety states, for 90 days. Drugs were alternated every 30 days. Satisfactory to excellent results were obtained with thioridazine and chlorprothixene in 70 and 75% of the patients, respectively. Side effects for both active drugs included dry mouth, drowsiness, bitter taste, headache, vertigo, insomnia, etc. No correlation was observed between dosage and side effects or dosage and overall response. All patients had withdrawal symptoms or side effects from the placebo. A similar trial was conducted in 28 men with anxiety secondary to tuberculosis, utilizing thioridazine (average dose 135 mg/day p.o.), chlorprothixene (average dose 148 mg/day p.o.) and placebo. Good to excellent results occurred in 75% of the patients with both active drugs while all patients reacted to placebo within 48 hours with relapses into insomnia, restlessness and anxiety. Thioridazine was tested for 33 days and chlorprothixene for 39. Side effects were minimal.

701 North Walnut
Springfield, Ill.

2355   Inose, Tadashi, Makino, Toshio, Sakai, Masao, Kobayashi, Hideo, Kajiwara, Akira, & Tsuda, Masatoshi. Use of dehydroepiandrosterone in psychiatric treatment. Preliminary report. Yokohama Medical Bulletin, 1962, 13, 37-45.

Dehydroepiandrosterone Δ^5-androsten-3-βal-17-one) was used in treatment of 104 psychiatric cases, mostly schizophrenia, neurosis and depression. The initial daily dose was 15-30 mg, in some cases up to 50 mg, in male patients; and from 6-20 mg, in some cases 30 mg, in females. Treatment was usually for 2 months but in some continued 6 months of more. No immediate changes were noted, but from 1-3 weeks responses occurred: 31 cases showed marked improvement, 16 mixed response, 37 no response and 20 cases were aggravated. Desirable changes were: brighter and milder attitude, more active and less withdrawn behavior, etc. Undesirable responses were: impulsiveness and aggressivity, including restlessness and increased erotic behavior. For 56 males, 16 were markedly improved, 8 had mixed responses, 21 no response and 11 were worse. For 48 females, responses were ibidem. 15, 8, 16 and 9. In schizophrenia, patients with immature personalities showed better response than others, while in depression those in a prolonged depressive state showed good responses. Physical changes such as masculinization, etc. were not noted. Urines were assayed for the β-fraction of 17-ketosteroids in 28 cases, and 18 of these showed a low β-fraction value, below 5% of the 17-ketosteroids.

Department of Neuropsychiatry
Yokohama University School of Medicine
Yokohama, Japan

2356 Arruda, Elso. Observações clínicas com um análogo do clordiazepóxido-O Ro 5-2807. [Clinical observations on an analog of chlordiazepoxide-RO 5-2807.] O Hospital, 1962, 62, 937-955.

Twenty-five mixed cases, including 8 epileptics and 7 cases of anxiety, were treated with diazepam (RO 5-2807), 10 mg b.i.d. or t.i.d. Drowsiness sometimes necessitated the reduction to 10 mg/day. The compound is more active than chlordiazepoxide. Besides somnolence, side effects included nausea, lassitude, cold sweating and rare visual disturbance. Tolerance is, in general, less than that for chlordiazepoxide. Treatment lasted up to 4 months, usually 2-3 months. Results in 8 cases out of the 25 were considered good and in 9 fair. In epilepsy, results were good in 5, average in 3 and negative in 1 with some EEG improvement, but without regular correlation between clinical and EEG findings.

Departamenta de Psiquiatria
Universidades do Brazil
Bahia, Brazil

2357 Adams, Peter, Stephens, B.T., & Kilpatrick, G.S. Transaminase activity after codeine administration. Postgraduate Medical Journal, 1962, 38, 348-349.

Thirteen patients were studied before and after 2 grains of codeine i.m. Codeine administration did not affect SGOT or SGPT activity, except in one patient where there was an increase in transaminase activity. This evidence is in contradiction to that of Foulk and Fleischer (1957).

Royal Infirmary
Cardiff, Great Britain

2358 Favier, M., Ramel, P., & De Toffol, M. Intérêt du méprobamate injectable en milieu psychiatrique. [The role of injectable meprobamate in the psychiatric milieu.] Lyon Médical, 1962, No. 48, 1125-1130.

Six alcoholics, 4 agitation, 4 psychotic, 9 neurosis with minor or moderate depression and 6 melancholia cases were treated with 1-4 i.m. injections of 400 mg meprobamate per day, later changing over to oral administration after the sedation of acute phenomena. The melancholia cases were treated with combined therapy - meprobamate with imipramine. Injectable meprobamate provided very satisfactory results in neurosis, minor or moderate depression and the acute manifestations of alcoholism. Some success was obtained in melancholia with the meprobamate-imipramine combination, but results were insufficient in major states with intense anxiety. Other types of psychoses remained unmodified.

[No address]

2359 Cox, Erwin M., & Lougheed, J.C.

ansiedade. (Nota sôbre o uso da Flufena-
sina). [Some implications of the pharmacologic therapy of anxiety. (Note on the use
of fluphenazine).] O Hospital, 1962, 61,
137-146.

Theoretical and practical implications of
the role of fluphenazine in the suppression
of anxiety are discussed and 7 cases are
presented. Improvement in the suppression
of anxiety and quarrelsomeness was obtained on a daily dosage of 1 mg fluphena-
zine/day, maintained over long periods,
e.g., 6 months. This therapy aided in
improving and maintaining psychotherapeutic measures.

Instituto Raul Soares
Belo Horizonte, Brazil

2362 Madalena, J. Caruso. Ensaio tera-
pêutico com o clordiazepoxido no alco-
olismo. [Therapeutic trial with chlordiazepoxide in alcoholism.] O Hospital, 1962,
62, 69-94.

Seventy-one male hospitalized patients in
withdrawal were treated with chlordiazepoxide in 6 groups. Group A constituting
54.9% of the patients received only chlordiazepoxide; Group B constituting 15.4%
received only chlorpromazine; Group C,
8.4%, was given chlordiazepoxide combined
with chlorpromazine and Group F, 4.2%,
received no treatment. All daily dosage
was: 125 mg chlordiazepoxide and 150 mg
chlorpromazine, in 3 divided doses; the
maximal dose of the 1st drug was 200 mg
per day and for chlorpromazine 300 mg
per day. Duration of observation was 7-20
days. Chlordiazepoxide had higher efficiency than chlorpromazine and standard treatment. However, this drug does not seem
indicated in alcoholics with a psychotic
background in view of possible reactivation
of psychotic disturbances.

Pavilhão São José
Universidade do Brasil
Rio de Janeiro, Brazil

2363 Hartocollis, Peter. Drunkenness and
suggestion: an experiment with intravenous
alcohol. Quarterly Journal of Studies on

Clinical studies
Abstracts 2364-2365

Alcohol, 1962, <u>23</u>, 376-389.

In a study of drunkenness and suggestion, as it is virtually impossible to mask alcohol in beverages, the i.v. root was chosen in experimentation with 15 subjects, all male psychiatric residents, aged 26-36 years. Their drinking habits were known and the group only included casual or moderate drinkers. Ethanol was injected, 1 ml/kg, as a 10% dilution in isotonic saline. This dose should produce a blood alcohol concentration of 0.1%, in the range regarded as putting an individual "under the influence." The infusion lasted about an hour. Emotion, speech and action were rated on a 5-point scale. A great deal of curiosity about the unknown agent was expressed, and more than a few made the right guess. Behavioral and subjective change was universal though not uniform. Subjects could look and feel drunk whether or not they knew or thought they were under the influence of alcohol. Behavior was difficult to evaluate; in most cases it changed towards elation and excitement followed by quieting, relaxation, sleep or stupor. Subjective reports included apprehension and bewilderment, parasthesia, peculiar taste, dyplopia, dysarthria and disturbed proprioception, feelings of depersonalization, irresponsibility, euphoria and gregariousness, timelessness, fatigue and depression. More elation, aggression and boisteriousness was noted when groups were tested compared to the testing of individuals.

VA Hospital
Topeka, Kan.

2364   Marx, H., & Krüger, H. Neue Gesichetspunkte in der neuroleptischen Behandlung akuter und chronischer Psychosen. Bericht über die klinische Prügung neuen Thiaxanthenderivates. [New viewpoints in the neuroleptic treatment of acute and chronic psychoses. Report on the clinical investigation of a new thiaxanthen-derivative.] Nervenarzt, 1962, 10, 469-472.

One-hundred-and-twenty-one patients who were hospitalized were treated with chlorperphenthixene (Fifty-one were acutely and

ed i.v. This solution contained: 2 g calcium glucuronate, 10 g sodium glutamate, 10 g cysteine, 10 g glycine, 10 g succinic acid, 0.5 g ascorbic acid and 1 g d-calcium pantothenate. The control group consisted of 51 cases and delirium tremens lasted 4.4 days while the treated group, 70 cases, had delirious attacks lasting 2 days. The amino acid treated subjects received a total of 9.025 mg (average 129 mg) of promazine and 720 cc (average 10 cc) of paraldehyde by way of adjunct therapy. In contrast, the control patients received a total of 1.297 cc (average 26 cc) of paraldehyde, 28 g (average 0.5 g) of bar- biturates, 445 IU (average 91 U) of insulin, and 851 ounces (average 17 ounces) of whiskey. Free serum amino acids, the effect of stress on these acids, hepatic insufficiency and miscellaneous pathologies were assayed. Depletion of amino acids was characteristic of delirium tremens. The more serious the delirium, the greater the depletion of these essential blood ele- ments. In further experimentation it was found that the amino acids sodium glutamate, arginine and arginine-glutamate and an amino acid sugar−n-acetyl-d-glucosamine− may be employed for the prevention or treatment of delirium tremens.

Division of Surgical Research
Department of Surgery
Harlem Hospital Center
New York, N.Y.

2368 Hill, Harris E., Haertzen, Charles A., & Davis, Howard. An MMPI factor analytic study of alcoholics, narcotic ad- dicts and criminals. Quarterly Journal of Studies on Alcohol, 1962, 23, 411-431.

MMPI profiles were obtained on institu- tionalized groups of alcoholics, narcotic addicts, and criminals, each sample being composed of 200 subjects. Application of the principal axes technique of factor analy- sis was made to the scale T-scores isolated 5 factors. Available factor analytic pro- grams which were adapted to the IBM-650, accommodating approximately 45 variables, were used. Three of these were sufficiently well defined to produce predictable and stable personality configurations. The 1st factor, labeled "undifferentiated psychopath" and interpreted as indicating un-complicated social deviance, was characterized by a single "spike" on the Psychopathic Deviate Scale. Small, statistically significant but nondiagnostic differences were found—criminals produced slightly greater loadings on this factor. Factor 2 was bipolar: The composite profile for the positive $_{Pole}$ was much the same "double spike" (psychopathic deviate-hypomania) pattern as was found previously in narcotic addicts; it was labeled "primary psychopath." The negative pole was labeled "neurotic psychopath, depressed," since it showed considerable elevation on the neurotic triad, especially on depression, and on the Psychopathic Deviate Scale. While both factors showed strength in the 3 criterion groups, small but again nondiagnostic differences were found. The criminals were more numerous on the positive pole, the alcoholics more numerous on the negative pole, and the addicts were intermediate in factor loadings. Factors 3, 4 and 5 produced further evidence for the presence of classic psychopathologies, but with clear indications of social deviance (psychopathic deviate elevation) in all. Suggestions were made with regard to the adoption of certain modes of adaptation by the social deviant and for further research in the addictions.

Addiction Research Center, NIMH
Lexington, Ky.

2369 Helou, Horacio Antonio. Tratamiento combinado de hipnosis y trifluoperazine en diversas afecciones psicosomáticas. [Combined treatment of hypnosis and trifluoperazine in various psychosomatic diseases.] Día Médico, 1962, 34, 951-952.

Eighty-three cases of neuroses, phobias and psychoneuroses were treated with hypnosis and trifluoperazine. Excellent results were obtained in 80% of the patients, who demonstrated marked and rapid improvement. Trifluoperazine (2-4 mg/day, in 2 or 3 doses) notably favored recovery, diminishing psychic tension and favoring adaptation to environment. Tolerance was excellent and the few side effects that were noted were transitory.

Hospital Politicial "Bmé. Chukruca"
Buenos Aires, Argentina

ance was noted: galactorrhea, oligomenor-
rhea and amenorrhea. A tendency to gain
weight was troublesome, particularly to
female patients. The effect of the drug
was excellent on 13 acute neurotic depressions, 7 of whom were able to return to
work, while considerable improvement was
noted in the remaining 6. Partial success
was recorded with 7 acute melancholics.
Of 28 schizophrenics, 15 failures were recorded, and 13 moderate to good improvements. Only 3 failures, and 16 partial to
total successes were noted in 19 chronic
delirium cases. Out of 11 feeble minded
patients, 3 were failures and 8 evidenced
partial to considerable improvement; 8
oligophrenics were unresponsive, revealing
only 2 who improved. Treatment was successful in 40%. Thioridazine is indicated
in all acute states, in systematic deliria,
and comprehensive depressions.

Hopital,
Sotteville-les Rouen, France

2374   Girard, J.P. Essais cliniques d'un
nouvel antiallergique, l'homochlorcyclizine.
Effets sur l'élimination urinaire du métabo-
lite de la sérotonine. [Clinical trials of a
new antiallergic, homochlorcyclizine. Effects on the urinary excretion of the metabolite of serotonin.] Therapeutische Umschau, 1962, 19, 50-53.

Forty-three cases of allergy, including
asthma, drug dermotoxicites, ulcerative
colitis, etc. were treated with homochlorcyclizine (100 mg p.o. and 60 mg parenterally; once it was administered as an
aerosol). Duration of treatment was from
some days to a month. Urinary 5HIAA was
assayed by the technique of Udenfriend et
al. Fourteen showed good improvement and
16 average improvement. Side effects were
nausea, drowsiness, anorexia and headaches.
Tolerance was excellent. In asthma cases,
homochlorcyclizine caused a slight increase
in urinary 5HIAA, while in rheumatism
5HIAA excretion was lessened.

Clinique universitaire de médecine interne
    de Genéve
Geneva, Switzerland

2375   Bitter, Tobias. Tratamento das cef-
aléias pós traumáticas com um antagonista
da serotonina. [Treatment of posttraumatic
headaches with a serotonin antagonist.]
Revista Brasileira de Medicina, 1962, 19,
543-544.

Methysergide was used i.m. in 10 cases
of posttraumatic headache at a dose of 1
mg every 8 hours and at half this dose for
children (2). Placebos were not used but
the patients did not know the nature of the
medication; evaluation was made by solici-
ting information daily. Methysergide provided relief of pain from headaches without
the production of side effects.

Departamento de Neurologia
Santa Casa de Misericórdia
Rio de Janeiro, Brazil

2376   Puech, J., Robin, Ch., Richet, L., &
Tetart, A. Effets du N. benzyl beta chlor-
propionamide (Posedrine) sur les anomalies
caractérielles de sujets épileptiques ou
présentant des perturbations du tracé E.E.G.
[The effects of N-benzyl-β-chlorpropiona-
mide (Posedrine) on character disorders
in epileptic subjects or those presenting
abnormal EEG's] Presse Médicale, 1962,
70, 1015-1018.

Thirty-six cases, 31 below 18 years of age
and 5 adults, showing character disorders,
behavioral disorders or psychotic abnormalities were treated with 4-9 tablets of
beclamide (Posedrine) per day. Duration of
treatment was 3-22 months. There were 14
cases of epilepsy. Fifteen out of the 36
cases improved markedly (41%) and 7 (19%)
improved slightly, i.e., 60% of the cases
improved. The number of epileptic seizures
was decreased but mental status rarely
improved. In nonepileptics, EEG's were
improved, particularly those demonstrating
a tendency toward epilepsy.

[No address]

2377   Schwaar, Robert. Essais de tolérance
de la méphénoxalone (OM-518) sur le tractus
digestif. [Tolerance trial of mephenoxalone
(OM-518) on the digestive tract.] Therapeutische Umschau, 1962, 19, 165-168.

in 1 case. Of the 7 cases, 5 obtained
excellent results, 1 good results and the
other was unaltered.

Hospital Pedro II (S.N.D.M.)
Rio de Janeiro, Brazil

See also 2240, 2241, 2262, 2265, 2269,
2382, 2463, 2489, 2512, 2523, 2527.

2380 Gardner, Alvin F., Gross, Sheldon G., & Wynne, Larry E. An investigation of gingival hyperplasia resulting from diphenylhydantoin sodium therapy in seventy-seven mentally-retarded patients. Experimental Medicine and Surgery, 1962, 20, 133-158.

An extensive review of the literature on gingival hyperplasia due to diphenylhydantoin therapy preceded an investigation of 77 mentally retarded patients who received diphenylhydantoin (7.5 grains/day). Some degree of gingival hyperplasia was shown by 78%, spastic patients exhibiting a higher percentage than others. Gingival hyperplasia showed no sex predilection and was more prevalent among those under 30 years-of-age. Neither dosage increase nor duration of therapy affected the degree of hyperplasia, and the prodromal period had to elapse before hyperplasia reached its peak. Degrees I and II were the most prevalent forms of hyperplasia, and the most severe, Degree III, was least prevalent. While patients with relatively normal occlusion had the greatest incidence of hyperplasia, the more serious the malocclusion the greater the degree of hyperplasia. Frequent proper, adequate brushing may decrease the degree of hyperplasia, but it will not eliminate it. Although calculus does not appear to affect the degree or act as a predisposing factor, it may influence an already established condition. No definite cure is known, and the etiology remains obscure.

Department of Pathology
Baltimore College of Dental Surgery
Dental School
University of Maryland
Baltimore 1, Md.

2381 Périn, M., Conte, Gamerman, J., & Salet, J. Hépatite aiguë mortelle au cours d'un traitment par l'iproniazide (marsilid). [Fatal acute hepatitis during iproniazid therapy (Marsilid).] Bulletins et Mémoires de la Société Médicale des Hôpitaux de Paris, 1962, 113, 13-20.

A female patient, aged 49 years, with severe jaundice and symptoms resembling those of choledocic lithiasis died within 48 hours after admission, despite treatment with antibiotics, hydrocortisone, arginine, vita-

mins and liver extracts. Autopsy revealed necroticizing hepatitis, which had developed over a 3-week period with hypertrophy of the hepatic cells. The patient had been under treatment for a chronic depression, most recently with iproniazid, which had been instituted shortly before the jaundice had appeared. Clinically, the case is similar to Rokitansky's disease, and a viral origin cannot be completely obviated. Iproniazid may have been responsible since the presiding psychiatrist had observed 2 other cases of icterus (benign) out of 50 patients so treated. Morbidity rates indicate that icterus in iproniazid patients is possible, its frequency, (1 in 2000) being about double that of the population at large.

[No address]

2382 Buisson, M., Collier, G., Armand-Laroche, J. L., Szymonowicz, R., & Bouchard, J. M. A propos de crises d'épilepsie survenues au cours de traitements par le tartrate d'alimémazine (6549 R.P.) ou théral' Lène. [Epileptic seizures occurring during treatments with alimemazine tartrate (RP 6549) or Theralene.] Annales Médico-Psychologiques, 1962, 120, 1, 775-781; discussion 781-782.

Of the 30 patients who had received alimemazine (mean dose 100 mg t.i.d.) 8 experienced epileptic crises which ceased with suspension of alimemazine therapy. Vitamin B deficiency, secondary to isoniazid therapy is believed responsible for the rapid onset of crises in 2 of these patients. Another 2 had a history of epilepsy, but convulsive phenomena had never occurred in the hospital prior to theralene administration. Another 2 had a family history of encephalopathy, but 2 had no pathological antecedents capable of explaining the crises, and their EEG's were within normal limits. The above figures refer to women only since none of the 38 male patients on the drug experienced these crises. Alimemazine is currently being continued, but phenobarbital (50 mg/day) is being administered as prophylaxis. No further crises have been noted.

[No address]

2383 Frankland, A.W. Skin testing and desensitization to drugs. Proceedings of the Royal Society of Medicine, 1962, 55, 46-48.

Patch testing has frequently been used to detect drug sensitivity to various allergens. It is imperative to differentiate among true allergic reactions, irritant reactions and nonspecific false positive reactions. Sunlight has been known to act nonspecifically in atopic individuals who exhibit no abnormal response to tests for photosensitivity, such as a woman treated with promethazine who developed hemorrhagic vascular eczema on her hands along with photosensitivity. The immediate type wheal response and passive transfer tests for demonstrating Prausnitz-Küstner antibodies are very rarely of value in finding causal agents in allergic drug reactions. Desensitization procedures, although arduous, must sometimes be undertaken.

[No address]

2384 Ffrench Devitt, R.E., & Kenny, Shelia. Thalidomide and congenital abnormalities. Lancet, 1962, No. 7226, 430.

Within 8 months 3 cases of phocomelia, 2 with duodenojejunal stenosis, were observed in South Down and Armagh, a region where no such case had arisen for at least 8 years. Further consultation revealed that thalidomide (100 mg/day) had been ingested by the 3 mothers, 2 of whom took the drug from the 5th to the 13th week of pregnancy, while the 3rd took it throughout pregnancy.

South Down Hospital Group
Newry, County Down
Great Britain

2385 Schaefer, Suzanne. Toxicity from drug overdosage in an eleven-year-old boy. Clinical Pediatrics, 1 962, 1, 103-104.

An 11-year-old boy ingested 17 tablets of chlordiazepoxide (425 mg) and 1-1/2 gr. of secobarbital after which he rapidly became deeply comatose with pinpoint pupils, absent deep tendon reflexes and a weak pulse. At the time of admission there was no suspicion of chlordiazepoxide intoxication, and general supportive therapy included caffeine (3-1/2 grains by i.v. drip), stomach aspiration, i.v. glucose solutions, penicillin and chloromycetin. Chlordiazepoxide was not detected by laboratory tests and the diagnosis was suggested only by questioning the family. Pentetrazol (7 cc i.v.) injections did not help. However, 36 hours after chlordiazepoxide ingestion the boy regained consciousness. Within 3 days he was able to be discharged.

[No address]

2386 Pick, Edgar. Adrenaline and schizophrenia. Lancet, 1962, No. 7227, 487.

A 50-year-old man who received a prophylactic tetanus antitoxin experienced an immediate anaphylactic reaction with severe hypotension, convulsions and loss of consciousness. Epinephrine (1 mg s.c. adrenalin) resulted in rapid recovery. However, shortly after recovery he became incredibly suspicious and anxious. Within 1 hour his behavior was normal and he had slight amnesia for his previous reaction. This paranoid reaction to an epinephrine injection apparently constituted an emotionally charged response in a predisposed person.

[No address]

2387 Clemmesen, C., Myschetzky, A. and Lassen, N.A. Forced diuresis in treatment of severe salicylate poisoning. Lancet, No. 7221, 1962, 162.

Forced diuresis was used in a series of 31 consecutive cases of severe salicylate poisoning, with only 1 fatality (recurrence of cerebrovascular disease in a patient with recent apoplexy). Few complications were encountered. Diuresis is being utilized in Denmark to treat severe meprobamate poisoning. Essential adjunctive therapy includes symptomatic supportive treatment counteracting respiratory, circulatory and infectious complications. Proper assessment of the efficacy of diuretic treatment in salicylate intoxication is predicted upon the determination of blood and urinary drug

Department of Psychiatry
University of Leeds
Leeds 2, Great Britain

2388 Sezgin, Ziya, Bosworth, David, & Frost, Harold M. Effect of Marsilid on diaphyseal lamellar rabbit bone. Henry Ford Hospital Medical Bulletin, 1962, 10, 209-216.

Experimentation in rabbits was prompted by the observation that iproniazid-(Marsilid) treated-patients appear to show abnormal bone qualities at the operating table. Eight out of 10 rabbits received iproniazid (10 mg/kg/day by stomach tube for 3 months, while 2 acted as controls to determine the effect of iproniazid on diaphyseal lamellar bone. All were healthy when sacrificed at 6 months of age with no evidence of liver damage. Sections of the tibia and femur from iproniazid-treated animals revealed considerable micropetrosis, a decrease in internal cortical remodeling and an increase in the number of necrotis in osteocytes. Then, 52 rabbits received tetracycline p.o. by gavage for 2 weeks followed by 2 weeks of abstinence and another 2 weeks of tetracycline treatment. Of this group, 26 also received iproniazid, 3 mg/kg/day for 6 weeks. Iproniazid-treated animals showed retardation of internal bone remodeling, and both groups indicated that tetracycline produced an unequivocal decrease in osteoid formation and rate of mineralization. Iproniazid decreased the rate of circumferential lamellar apposition. Oral tetracycline labeling proved to be completely unsatisfactory in labeling rabbit bone. In a 3rd experiment, 15 rabbits received tetracycline labels, 200 mg/kg i.p. on the 1st day of 3 successive weeks. Iproniazid (25 mg/kg/day) was given to 6 animals for 1 week and cortisone (50 mg/kg/day) was given to 3 animals for 1 week. Two of the iproniazid-treated animals died during the experiment and the remainder were sacrificed 1-9 days after termination. Gross and histological liver damage was observed in the 2 who died prematurely. Bone sections in the remaining iproniazid-treated animals revealed an increase in osteocyte death, little active periosteal bone formation, few osteoid seams and little fuchsin-permeable bone. Those sacrificed a week or more after the experiment manifested very active periosteal new bone formation. Cortisone-treated animals revealed almost total arrest of new bone formation. Cortisone-treated animals sacrificed well after the experiment showed, after a week or so, greatly augmented new bone formation (rebound) with very active periosteal appositional activity. The effects of iproniazid may have resulted from an endogenous increase in cortisone secretion accruing from experimental stress.

[No address]

2389 Moore, Henry W. Toxicity of phenothiazine tranquilizers. Journal of the South Carolina Medical Association, 1962, 58, 485-486.

A severely dehydrated 12-year-old girl received prochlorperazine (10 mg every 4 hours) suppositories for vomiting and diarrhea. Vomiting ceased, but bizarre facial contortions, oculogyric crisis, trismus, hypertonic extremities and various other extrapyramidal symptoms were manifested. Side effects disappeared after 12 hours of forced i.v. fluids to correct dehydration.

Columbia, S.C.

2390 Helmchen, H., & Hippius, H. Unerwartete neurologische Begleiterscheinungen der Pharmakotherapie von Psychosen. (Prinzipielle Bemerkungen anhand kasuistischer Beispiele). [Unexpected neurologic symptoms during treatment of psychoses with psychopharmacologic drugs.] In: Kranz, H., & Heinrich, K. [Eds.] Neurolepsie und Schizophrenie. [Neurolepsy and Schizophrenia] Stuttgart: Georg Thieme Verlag, 1962, 77-84; discussion 84-87.

One manic-depressive and 2 paranoid patients were treated with orphenadrine (2 tablets i.d.), and with perazine (300-550 mg i.d.). During this treatment, Oppenheim, Gordon and Babinski reflexes developed with orphenadrine, and ataxia of upper and lower extremities, spastic paralysis of both lower extremities and fecal and urinary incontinence on perazine. All of these symptoms disappeared after cessation of treatment. In all cases very slight neuro-

al disturbances were noted at the time mission which developed during treat-
into the above discribed symptoms. tent and minor pathologic disposition e CNS may have been activated by the administration and may have produced

the well-defined reversible symptoms.

[No address]

See also 2245, 2247, 2272, 2298, 2341, 2415, 2444, 2470.

2391   Leikola, Anto. Influence of stress on alcohol intoxication in rats. Quarterly Journal of Studies on Alcohol, 1962, 23, 369-375.

Four-month-old rats of both sexes were stressed by forcing them to swim in a large cask of water at 34-36°C. They soon learned how to float without effort, and therefore an 8 g weight was attached to their tails so that they had to swim actively—generally 10 minutes exhausted them. Fasted rats were administered a 30% ethanol solution immediately or 30 minutes before swimming, and in 1 experiment alcohol was given i.p. as a 10% solution. The doses were 3.6, 4.5 and 5.0 mg/g p.o. and 2 mg/g i.p. Levels of intoxication were tested on an inclined plane. The intoxication level of stressed rats was much lower than that of unstressed controls. When alcohol was administered orally, the blood alcohol also was lower in the stressed animal; after i.p. injection blood alcohol level was the same in stressed and unstressed rats. However the stressed rats were less intoxicated than controls with corresponding blood alcohol levels. With i.p. administration at the same blood alcohol level 90 minutes after the injection, the degree of intoxication in stressed animals was only about 40% of that in controls. Intoxicated rats could recover when subjected to swimming tests, though this was transitory. No convincing explanation for the intoxication—diminishing effect of stress can yet be given. A possible explanation is the influence of adrenal hormones released during stress.

Research Laboratories of the State
  Alcohol Monopoly
Helsinki, Finland

2392   Masserman, Jules H. Drugs, brain and behavior; an experimental approach to experimental psychoses. Journal of Neuropsychiatry, 1962, 3, S104-S113.

Following preliminary control observations for 2-10 months 152 cats and 48 monkeys (African vervet and Mangebey, American spider and rhesus) were trained to respond to a specific stimuli by pressing 1 of 2 reward levers. Experimental neuroses were

chlorpromazine during conditioning and re-training, but not before the transposition test, showed a much more impaired per-formance than controls. Chlorpromazine acts as a CNS sedative, reducing the intensity of association formed during con-ditioning so that impaired memory and transposition ability results.

Zoologische Institut
Universität Münster
Münster, Germany

2395 Rodgers, David A., & McClearn, Gerald E. Mouse strain differences in preference for various concentrations of alcohol. Quarterly Journal of Studies on Alcohol, 1962, 23, 26-33.

Tap-water and 6 concentrations of alcohol, 2.5-15%, in 2.5% increments were given ad lib to C57BL, BALB/c, C3H/2 and ACrgl/3 strains of mice, approximately a year in age. The amount of liquid con-sumed from each cylinder was recorded daily for a period of 3 weeks. The C57BL strain showed the highest preference for the 12.5% solution and a progressive in-crease over the 3 weeks in the proportional amount of alcohol consumed. The C3H/2 strain showed a progressive shift in pre-ference from lower concentrations during the 1st 2 weeks to a pronounced peak preference for 10% alcohol during the 3rd week. The BALB/c and A/3 strains tended to avoid all concentrations of al-cohol, preferring water. This preference for water, initially pronounced, tended to increase. Strain differences in change in alcohol consumption from the 1st to 3rd week were related to initial strain differ-ences in preference. Alcohol preference of mice is suggested as influenced by a multiple-allele or a multiple-gene system or both.

Cancer Research Genetics Laboratory
University of California
Berkeley, Calif.

2396 Purdy, Maud B., & Lee, Jordan G. The effect of restricted food intake, thi-amin deficiency and riboflavin deficiency on the voluntary consumption of ethanol by the albino rat. Quarterly Journal of Studies on Alcohol, 1962, 23, 549-556.

Paired litter-mate rats were allowed a choice between water and 15% ethanol. They were fed a normal diet ad lib. for 6 days to establish normal intakes. One member of each pair was then shifted to a ration devoid of thiamine (11 pairs) or riboflavin (8 pairs) and paired feeding was begun. As food intake decreased, the level of vitamin intake was maintained at levels established during the initial feeding period. After 24 days on the thiamine experiment, or 56 days on the riboflavin experiment, each animal was given 6 g per day of the complete ratio for a 5-day period, then returned to ad lib. consumption of the complete ration for 20 days. Significant mean intrapair increases in alcohol intake produced by lack of thiamine or riboflavin were not evident. Deficient and paried nondeficient groups increased their alcohol consumption above the norms established during the initial feeding period. These differences were significant only in the males paired with riboflavin-deficient males, females paired with thiamine-deficient females and the thiamine-deficient females. Alcohol intake increased when the previously missing vitamin was added and food intake limited. These increases held true above the final 5 days of depletion in previously thiamine-deficient but not in riboflavin-deficient animals. Ad lib. feeding of the complete ration restored intakes to the initial value. Increases in alcohol intake were due to decreased food intake resulting in tissue loss, and not to thiamine or riboflavin deficiency. The thiamine or riboflavin deficient rat is less able to utilize alcohol and therefore consumes less than when given the vitamin with restricted food intake.

Department of Chemistry
Louisiana State University
Baton Rouge, La.

2397   Feuer, G., & Broadhurst, P.L. Thyroid function in rats selectively bred for emotional elimination. III. Behavioral and physiological changes after treatment with drugs acting on the thyroid. Journal of Endocrinology, 1962, 24, 385-396.

and delayed response training for a concealed food reward. The LSD was given in i.p. doses of 25-100 µg/kg, 0.25-1 mg per kg psilocybin, 0.25-1 mg/kg psilocin. After LSD, cats adopted a wide-based "kangaroo" position with the tail extended, and exhibited staring, head shaking, and sprawling with claws extended. There was a loss of normal affective responses. These seizure-like episodes were seen in EEG records in a quiet environment; they were maximal in amplitude and were longest in duration in the dorsal hippocampal and entorhinal cortex, appearing variably in the thalamus and in the midbrain reticular formation. These seizures seemed critically dependent on reduction of visual and auditory sensory influences. At higher LSD doses, seizures persisted in a well-lit environment and disrupted a delayed response when the seizure episode encroached on the period when a discriminative performance was required. Unlike visual and auditory stimuli, the ingestion of food during the action of LSD was frequently associated with wave and wave-and-spike seizure activity, confined in some instances to hippocampal and amygdaloid systems. Tolerance to LSD appeared with doses repeated at more frequent intervals than 7-10 days. Psilocybin and psilocin resembled LSD in their general effects but did differ in both the brevity of their action and in the frequent occurrence of severe autonomic reactions. Included among these severe autonomic reactions were vomiting, micturition, and finally, pupillary dilatation. The relationship of all of these findings to physiologic mechanisms in the memory trace and to the various problems of sensory deprivation is discussed.

Brain Research Institute
Department of Anatomy
University of California
Los Angeles, Calif.

2399 Bignami, Giorgio. Influenza della l-tiroxina e del metilitiouracile sul condizionamento e la ritenzione nel ratto. [Influence of l-thyroxine and methylthiouracil on conditioning and memory in the rat.] Rendiconti Istituto Superiore di Sanità, 1962, 25, 165-175.

CAR's (shuttling response) were developed in male Wistar rats in a modified Warner automatic programmed shuttle cage. Four groups were developed: controls, 0.2 mg/kg l-thyroxine s.c., 0.1% methylthiouracil in the drinking water for 14 days and methylthiouracil plus thyroxine for 14 days. Hypothyroidism while not affecting acquisition during any day's trials, retards retention as measured on the early trials of successive daily tests. Injections of l-thyroxine did not significantly modify the behavior of otherwise treated rats. In hypothyroid rats, however, injections of thyroxine not only eliminated the impairing effects of the deficiency, but seemed to facilitate both acquisition and retention in early trials in comparison to control rats.

Laboratori di Chimica Terapeutica
Istituto Superiore di Sanità
Rome, Italy

2400 Latané, Bibb, & Schachter, Stanley. Adrenalin and avoidance learning. Journal of Comparative and Physiological Psychology, 1962, 55, 369-372.

Fifty naive male rats were trained in a modified Miller-Mowrer shuttle box. After each injection the rat was allowed to explore the box with the guillotine door lifted in order to check the possibility that epinephrine (adrenalin) may influence activity level and thus artifactually affect avoidance learning. Avoidance conditioning trials (light followed 5 seconds later by a grid floor shock) began 55 minutes after the injection and the number of crossings was recorded. Three injection conditions were: placebo 0.5 ml peanut oil, weak epinephrine (adrenalin) 0.0125 mg/100 g and strong epinephrine 0.25-0.50 mg/100 g. Rats injected with a weak dose of epinephrine learned a CAR more quickly and effectively than placebo runs, and rats given a heavy dose were significantly poorer learners than the weak epinephrine rats and not significantly better than the placebo rats. The relationship between epinephrine dosage and avoidance learning is nonmonotonic.

Columbia University
New York, N.Y.

2401 Barry, Herbert, III., Miller, Neal E., & Tidd, Gail E. Control for stimulus change while testing effects of amobarbital on conflict. Journal of Comparative and Physiological Psychology, 1962, 55, 1071-1074.

Male Sprague-Dawley rats were trained in the Bailey and Miller (1962) telescope alley. After some preliminary training the rats were given 3 days of approach training in the alley, followed by 9 days of approach-avoidance training, using increasing shocks. Food-approach versus avoidance of shock at the goal was tested with hungry rats under 20 mg/kg amobarbital and placebo. Approach performance in the conflict situation was also increased by the shift to a novel condition regardless of whether it was to drug or placebo. This effect of the shift disappeared as soon as shocks were experienced under the novel condition.

Yale University
Hartford, Conn.

2402 Boissier, Jacques R., & Simon, Pierre. La réaction d'exploration chez la Souris (Note préliminaire). [Exploratory reaction in mice. (Preliminary note).] Thérapie, 1962, 17, 1225-1232.

A test for the study of psycholeptic drugs is described. The number of holes in a board which are explored by a mouse in a given time under given conditions is recorded. The board is 40 x 40 x 1.8 cm and there are 16 3 cm diameter holes, regularly spaced. The reduction of the number of holes explored after the injection of a drug demonstrates a psycholeptic effect. The parameter for controls in 5 minutes was ca. 41.2. Two drugs (given in mg/kg i.p.) were used to exemplify the technique; with 0.25 chlorpromazine the figure was ca. 35.8, with 0.5 29.4, with 1 21.6 and with 1.5 17.7. With meprobamate, 25 the parameter was ca. 33.2, with 50-32.5, with 100-27.4 and with 150-17.5.

15, rue de l'Ecole de Médecine
Paris, France

2403 Miller, Robert E., & Ogawa, Noruya. The effect of adrenocorticotrophic hormone (ACTH) on avoidance conditioning in the adrenalectomized rat. Journal of Comparative and Physiological Psychiatry, 1962, 55, 211-213.

Sixty-seven male Carworth rats were maintained on an ad lib. diet, and after adrenalectomy on 1% saline. Avoidance training was conducted in a 2-compartment apparatus (Murphy and Miller 1955). One week after the adrenalectomy the avoidance-conditioning procedure was begun. One of the 2 randomly selected groups was given 5 mg/kg ACTH i.m., while the other group received a placebo injection. Animals receiving the hormone were significantly slower to extinguish the CAR than were animals which received the placebo. This supports the hypothesis that ACTH has important extra-adrenal effects on behavior.

School of Medicine
University of Pittsburgh
Pittsburgh, Pa.

2404 Fox, Stephen S. Self-maintained sensory input and sensory deprivation in monkeys: a behavioral and neuropharmacological study. Journal of Comparative and Physiological Psychology, 1962, 55, 438-444.

Four Macaca assemensis and four M. nemestrina were used in the investigation of sensory input levels, maintained by the monkey bar-pressing for light rewards. For period of light deprivation a 3 x 3 x 4 foot box was constructed with the addition of a compartment to house 2 mesh-colored 60-watt bulbs. Three experiments were conducted relating to deprivation, adaptation and pharmacology. In Experiment 1, constant and regular rates of response were observed to occur when the response was bar pressing for 0.5 seconds of light. Rate increased with increasing sensory deprivation. In Experiment 2, by partially compensating with light during the test for the need for light produced by deprivation, rates of response were decreased for all deprivation durations. In Experiment 3, injected amphetamine (3 mg/kg) increased

Institute of Psychiatric Research
Indiana University Medical Center
Indianapolis, Ind.

2406   Plotnikoff, N., Reinke, D., & Fitzloff,
J.   Effects of stimulants on rotarod performance of mice. Journal of Pharmaceutical Sciences, 1962, 51, 1007-1008.

After being trained for rotarod performance
for 6 minutes, 9 groups of mice received
amphetamine (1.25-10.0 mg/kg i.p.), 13
received pheniprazine (2.5-20.0 mg/kg i.p.)
and 9 received caffeine (5.0-20.0 mg/kg
i.p.). Thirty minutes postinjection rotarod
performance was observed for 1 hour to
determine drug effects at 3 different rotarod speeds. A dose response relationship
was observed with amphetamine. Performance was enhanced in 50% of the animals
(ED_{50}) by amphetamine at 2.8 ± 0.4 mg/kg
for the A speed, 1.9 ± 0.4 mg/kg for B
speed and 5.1 ± 0.5 mg/kg for the C speed.
Pheniprazine significantly increased the
mean performance time at all 3 speeds,
with ED_{50} doses at 6.0 ± 0.8 mg/kg for A,
7.0 ± 1.3 mg/kg for B and 6.5 ± 0.8 mg/kg
for C. At C speed, pheniprazine was ineffective in 30 minutes but exerted a
pronounced effect in 2 hours. Caffeine
produced no significant improvement in
performance at any speed.

Stanford Research Institute
Menlo Park, Calif.

2407   Levine, Seymour, & Soliday, Stanley.
An effect of adrenal demedullation on the
acquisition of a conditioned avoidance response. Journal of Comparative and Physiological Psychology, 1962, 55, 214-216.

In order to test theories concerned with
anxiety, conditioned fear and avoidance
learning which contain the hypothesis that
discharge of the sympathetic nervous
system is an integral part of fear mediated
behavior, male hooded rats were divided
into 2 groups, demedullated and non-
operated. CAR's were developed in an
automatic all-metal Miller-Mowrer type
shuttle box. The CS was the sound of a
buzzer, 10 seconds followed by the US, a
0.3 ma. shock. The US was terminated when

the animal left the grid and the CS continued as long as the US was on. Sixty-second intertrial intervals were used. There were no overall significant differences in this system. A 2nd experiment using variations [undisclosed] of the 1st system, i.e., "much more efficient training procedures", showed that demedullates made significantly fewer CAR's than did controls.

Department of Psychiatry
Stanford University
Palo Alto, Calif.

See also 2307, 2363, 2368, 2448, 249

PHARMACOLOGY

2408 Thienes, C.H., Cangelosi, J., & Skillen, R.G. Nicotine and thyroid effects on adrenal catecholamines. Proceedings of the Western Pharmacological Society, 1962, 5, 5-6.

Nicotine (7 mg/kg s.c.) or saline was injected into rats 45 minutes before bilateral adrenalectomy. Biochemical assay of the homogenized adrenals revealed a loss of 55% levarterenol and 30% epinephrine in the nicotine treated groups, with bioassay values of 57% and 26%, respectively. In chronic studies, rats received nicotine injections (0.5-3.75 mg/kg b.i.d.) or saline for 1-4 months. The chronic nicotine groups showed increase in adrenal weight, and epinephrine and levarterenol content, with doubled concentration of the latter. A challenge dose of nicotine (7 mg/kg) in chronic nicotine groups caused some loss of epinephrine and levarterenol, but significantly less than that noticed in acute experiments. This dose of nicotine had no effect on catecholamine concentration in chronic saline groups. Stress accruing from repeated injections may cause catecholamine release masked by compensating increased synthesis. Increase in adrenal weight and catecholamine content suggests an increase in catecholamine storage and synthesis. Studies on thyroid effect on adrenal catecholamines showed a decrease in catecholamine concentration in hyperthyroid and an increase in hypothyroid animals.

Institute of Medical Research
Huntington Memorial Hospital
Pasadena, Calif.

2409 Chatagnon, C., & Chatagnon, P. Recherches sur le rythme d'élimination urinaire, chez l'humain, de chlorpromazine. [Studies on the urinary excretory rhythm for chlorpromazine in humans. Biological and statistical considerations.] Annales de Biologie Clinique, 1962, 20, 75-84.

Free and conjugated chlorpromazine in the blood and urine of 3 patients was studied colorometrically for up to 39 consecutive days. Oral dosage increased from 25 to 900 mg/day then decreased to 0. Highly comparable curves were obtained for the

3 subjects. Excretion stopped when the drug was dropped; there was no accumulation of the compound in the body. Deviations noted in the 3rd case were due to renal pathology.

Laboratoire Central de Biologie
Biologie Nerveuse de Maison-Blanche
Neuilly-sur-Marne, S.-et-O.
France

2410 Palamos Salas, T. Recherches expérimentales et histo-pathologiques sur l'imipramine. [Experimental and histopathologic research on imipramine.] Annales Médico-Psychologiques, 1962, 120, 1, 850.

Chronic and acute experiments with imipramine [dosage unspecified] were made with fish, guinea pigs, pigeons, cats, mice, rabbits and monkeys. Violent imipramine-induced spasms in fish and epileptic crises in monkeys could be reduced with pyridoxine. After chronic treatment diffuse lesions were noted in the brains of animals, with degeneration of Nissl substance and sclerosis. These changes due to chronic intoxication could not be detected by clinical signs. In contrast, 1 monkey died with little evidence of brain lesions following an epileptic seizure in the course of acute experiments with massive doses.

[No address]

2411 Remmer, H., & Siegert, M. Kumulation und Elimination von Phenobarbital. [Accumulation and excretion of phenobarbital.] Archiv für Experimentelle Pathologie und Pharmakologie, 1962, 243, 479-494.

Phenobarbital was administered to dogs (40-100 mg/kg i.v. or 30-61 mg/kg p.o. per day). Plasma levels, determined by UV spectrophotometry, were used to estimate excretion. The rate of excretion is 26.5% per day after a single i.v. dose. After oral administration excretion is delayed for 1-2 days, proceeding afterwards at a similar rate as after i.v. injection. Prolonged administration gradually increases the plasma level to a maximum, and accelerates excretion to a maximum of 47-61% per day. This high rate was never noted after a single dose. The increased rate of excretion is due to increased oxidation.

Pharmakologisches Institut
der Freien Universität Berlin
Berlin, Germany

2412 Kehl, R., & Czyba, J.C. Sur l'action galactogène de la réserpine chez la lapine. [The galactogenic action of reserpine in rabbits.] Journal of Physiology, 1962, 54, 356-357.

Reserpine (0.25-1 mg/day) was injected into 29 juvenile and 66 adult rabbits. Lactation was followed daily. In juveniles, reserpine only caused increased lactation when the rabbits are given concomitant estrogenic treatment. Of the 66 adult females, only 41 showed lactation. Seasonal variation is evident and more positive in the summer; animals under artificial light respond more than those kept in the dark. Some animals which do not respond to reserpine may respond after estrogenic treatment or pinealectomy, but ovariectomized animals do respond. Lactation in normal animals appeared 3-15 days after the beginning of treatment and spontaneously ceased 3 weeks after the cessation of reserpine administration.

Chaire d'Histologie et Embryologie
Faculté de Médecine
Lyon, France

2413 Matthies, H., Decsi, L., & Schmidt, J. Über den Mechanismus der Narkosebeeinflussung durch Iproniazid. [On the mechanism of the effect of iproniazid on narcosis.] Biochemical Pharmacology, 1962, 11, 502-504.

Iproniazid (IPN) was injected i.p. (360 μM per kg) into mice, either 2 or 48 hours before the i.p. (400 μM/kg) administration of hexobarbital. Duration of anesthesia, and content of hexobarbital and MAO of the entire brain were determined. IPN administered 2 hours before hexobarbital doubled the duration of narcosis; IPN injected 48 hours before hexobarbital reduced the duration of sleep about 30%. IPN-treated mice showed higher hexobarbital and lower MAO content than untreated controls, regardless of effect on sleeping time. The narcosis-prolonging effect, but not the shortening effect, is caused by inhibition of hexobarbital breakdown.

Pharmakologische Institut
Medizinische Akademie
Magdeburg, Germany

2414 Frommel, Ed., Vincent, D., Fleury, C., Schmidt-Ginzkey, J. Analgesia, neurovegetative system, cholinesterase and monoaminoxydase. Archives Internationales de Pharmacodynamie et de Thérapie, 1962, 139, 470-475.

Using the dental pulp pain method in guinea pigs, the following sympathomimetics were injected s.c.: epinephrine, levarterenol, oxydrine, ephedrine, amphetamine and dexamphetamine. A series of parasympathomimetics including acetylcholine were also used, and finally, as blocking agents, cholinesterase and neostigmine. Sympathomimetics, having per se an analgesic effect, are very susceptible to degradation by MAO, therefore the analgesic effect is slight; also these substances exercise an inhibitory action towards MAO, which is highest for amphetamine. Parasympathomimetics having analgesic action fall into 2 classes: those readily inactivated by cholinesterase and those which are resistant. Carbaminoylcholine is resistant and shows the highest analgesic effect, while, logically, acetylcholine is the least active. Nitrocholine, carbaminoylcholine and neostigmine show inhibition of cholinesterase, neostigmine being the most active. Thus the more substance resists enzymatic degradation, the more analgesic it is.

Institute of Experimental Therapeutics
Faculty of Medicine
University of Geneva
Geneva, Switzerland

2415 Pfleger, K., Rummel, W., Seifen, E., & Rottman, W. Zur Frage nach der

Ursache des erhöhten Erythrocytenzerfalls unter Phenacetin. [On the causes of the high decomposition rate of erythrocytes under phenacetin administration.] Medicina Experimentalis, 1962, 6, 105-112.

Rabbit blood was removed from an ear artery, defibrinated, washed and centrifuged. The centrifuged erythrocytes were then placed in an ice-cold Tyrode solution and tested. Phenacetin, phenetedin, acetanilid and aniline, in concentrations up to 5×10^{-3} m/l had no influence upon the potassium and sodium distribution or on glycolysis in rabbit erythrocytes in vitro. Nitrosobenzene (4×10^{-8} m/l) and p-ethoxy-nitrosobenzene (4×10^{-4} m/l) produced a loss of potassium and a gain of sodium and the lactate formation is decreased; The comparison of the methemoglobin produced and the potassium lost in the presence of nitrosobenzene and sodium nitrite makes it evident that no quantitative correlation is present. The measurement of K and Na influx and efflux by means of K^{42} and Na^{22} indicates that nitroso compounds have no influence on active transport but increase passive permeability.

Pharmakologische Institut der Universität
Homburg/Saar, Germany

2416 Kohli, R.P., Sareen, K., Amma, M.K.P., & Gujral, M.L. Anticonvulsant action of indolin-2,3-dione (Isatin). Indian Journal of Physiology and Pharmacology, 1962, 6, 145-149.

Rats used to study the anticonvulsant spectrum of indolin-2,3-dione received the following tests: maximal electroshock seizure threshold (Sareen et al. 1962), minimal electroshock seizure threshold, hyponatremic electroshock seizure threshold, psychomotor seizure threshold, pentetrazol seizures (80 mg/kg s.c.), strychnine (1.5 mg per kg) or picrotoxin (7.5 mg/kg), neurotoxicity studies (Swinyard et al. 1952) and studies on blood pressure and respiration in anesthetized animals. Indolin-2,3-dione manifested anticonvulsant activity in maximal electroshock seizure and hyponatremic electroshock seizure tests in rats with respective ED_{50}'s of 83.7 and 183.3 mg/kg.

It was ineffective in minimal electroshock seizure threshold, psychomotor and pentetrazol tests. High protective indices with lack of side effects warrant further clinical trials.

Department of Pharmacology
K.G. Medical College
Lucknow, India

2417 Hano, Józef, Giełdanowski, Jerzy, & Kędzierska, Lidia. The action of 5-hydroxypropylbarbituric acids on the central nervous system. Archivum Immunologiae et Therapiae Experimentalis, 1962, 10, 353-367.

The chronic action of 5-allyl-5-(β-hydroxy-γ-iodo)-propylbarbituric acid (D_1) and 5-allyl-(β-hydroxypropyl)-barbituric acid (D_1H) on the CNS of mice, rabbits, dogs and humans. The preparations were administered to animals in doses of 0.4-0.5 g/kg during 2-3 weeks. The human experiments were conducted with volunteers who took D_1H as tablets only. Sleeping time after phenobarbital and barbital was shortened, and, to a smaller degree, after hexobarbital. After chloral hydrate and ether shortening of the time required for narcosis was not observed. Both compounds prolonged sleep, more after phenobarbital and hexobarbital than after the administration of barbital. The weakest synergistic action occurred after ether and chloral hydrate, preparation D_1 being somwhat more active. D_1 was the stronger antagonist to convulsions induced by pentetrazol, strychnine, picrotoxin and amphetamine. In nontoxic doses it prevented pentetrazol convulsions and strychnine convulsions in 1/3 of the animals; convulsions after amphetamine were delayed and picrotoxin convulsions were unaffected. D_1H only delayed or partially suppressed pentetrazol and picrotoxin convulsions, not affecting strychnine convulsions. It also acted paradoxically by stimulating amphetamine convulsions, both in regard to time of onset and intensity. This is probably due to the ease with which D_1H is converted into allylvalerolactone, which passes into the CSF and 1st paralyzes cortical inhibition, thereby facilitating amphetamine stimulation. In determining the effects of both compounds on central hypothermia induced by LSD administration, D_1H had hypothermic activity whereas D_1 had no effect. Compulsory motility in mice in a roller cage showed that both compounds inhibited motility. Maze experiments showed a degree of disorientation. Neither compound had any antiemetic effect (against apomorphine i.m. injections in dogs). EEG studies with cortical and hippocampal leads in rabbits showed that D_1H had an effect similar to that of reserpine. Thirty persons were subjected to the Raven test; 20 of them took 100 mg D_1H t.i.d. for 15 days. The test was given before and on the last day of treatment. Mental efficiency was not altered, either in relation to speed or precision. D_1H is considered a tranquilizer.

Department of Pharmacology
School of Medicine
Wroclaw, Poland

2418 Boissier, J.R., & Pagny, Jeannette. Etude pharmacologique d'une phénothiazine neuroleptique, la thiéthylpérazine ou GS 95 (Torécan). III. Action antivomitive-Discussion générale. [Pharmacological study of a phenothiazine neuroleptic, thiethylperazine or GS 95 (Torecan). III. Antiemetic action-General discussion.] Medicina Experimentalis, 1962, 6, 320-326.

Vomiting was induced in dogs by the injection of 100 μg/kg apomorphine s.c., 15 μg/kg ergot alkaloids i.v. or 10 mg/kg copper. The antiemetic activity of thiethylperazine was marked at 10 μg/kg and 300 μg/kg doses practically suppressed all vomiting. This dose is much lower than that needed for sedation. Its antiemetic activity is slightly greater than that of prochlorperazine and markedly superior to that of chlorpromazine. Apparently there is no necessary relationship between catatonic and antiemetic effects for phenothiazines. Activity-structural substitutant in position 3 and the fixed substitutents are attached to the extranuclear nitrogen in certain piperazine and sulphur derivatives.

Faculté de Médecine de Paris
Institut de Pharmacologie
Paris, France

chemistry, 1962, *9*, 477-486.

Fasted female rats injected i.p. with 1 ml saline containing [1-C^{14}] α-amino isobutyric acid (AIBA) were studied. Specific activities ranged from 8-16 μc/mg. Animals were decapitated after 40 minutes or 4 hours and tissues examined via digestion and CO_2 liberation in scintillometer. Drugs were injected i.p. either before or simultaneously with the radioactive amino acid. Substances used were trypsin, trypan red, β-lactoglobulin, starch, physostigmine, acetazolamide, pentetrazole, mescaline, iproniazid, reserpine, chlorpromazine, levarterenol and 5HT. Some of these were included because of reported influence on the blood-brain barrier. Many agents were found effective in depressing AIBA uptake in short-term experiments (40 minutes), but even repeated injections of active drugs were found ineffective in 4 hour experiments. The possible involvement of the neurohormones in brain transport is also discussed.

Biochemical Research
  Laboratories
The Institute of Living
Hartford 2, Conn.

2423 Biljani, J.C., Gulati, O.D., Gokhale, S.D., & Joseph, A.D. An investigation of the antibarbiturate action of treburon. Indian Journal of Physiology and Pharmacology, 1962, *6*, 129-136.

In a series of tests in which 3 different doses of treburon were tested against a fixed dose of the agonist (preliminarily determined as the amount which would produce 100% anesthesia in almost all animals). Groups of pigeons and rats were used. In most trials groups of 10 animals were used, pigeons i.v. injected and rats i.p. injected. Agonists were: thiopental (20 mg/kg), pentobarbital (30 mg./kg), phenobarbital (100 mg/kg). The results of a large treburon dose (120 mg/kg) was also studied as well as the possible antidepressant action of helparin and picrotoxin. Thiopental, pentobarbital and phenobarbital were antagonized respectively by treburin at: 30 and 45 mg/kg; 30, 60 and 90 mg/kg, and 60, 90 and 120 mg/kg. For paraldehyde, treburin (30, 60 and 90 mg/kg) did not significantly reduce the duration of anesthesia. Heparin (10 mg./kg) did not antagonize these drugs while picrotoxin (0.05 mg/kg) antagonized phenobarbital. The antibarbiturate effect of treburin was dose related, best against thiopental and least against phenobarbital. The lack of effectiveness against paraldehyde indicates that treburin may have a specific antibarbiturate effect, possibly mediated through competition for a common site in the CNS. Further tests, however, are necessary to confirm this. High doses of treburin had no convulsive action and in view of the hazards of currently available analeptic agents, further study of treburin is indicated.

Department of Pharmacology
Medical College
Baroda, India

2424 Viljanto, J., Isomäki, H., & Kulonen, E. Effect of aminoacetonitrile, iproniazid and semicarbazide on the tensile strength of experimental granulation tissue. Acta Pharmacologica et Toxicologica, 1962, 19, 191-198.

Implantation and measurement of tensile strength as described by Viljanto and Kulonen (1962) was made in 421 Wistar rats fed test substances 7 days following implanatation. Both aminoacetonitrile (25, 50 or 100 mg/100 g) and semicarbazide (25 mg/100 g) decreased tensile strength in developing granulation tissue. A similar but probably less specific effect was observed following administration of iproniazid (2, 5 or 10/100 g). The weight and nutritional state of the animal were important factors in the production of tensile strength. While normally tensile strength developed slowly in aminoacetonitrile-treated animals but hydroxyproline production was not inhibited to the same degree. The total nitrogen in the granulation tissue rose most rapidly in the controls before collagen synthesis. In aminoacetonitrile treated animals the nitrogen content of the granulation tissue persisted at the 5th day level.

Department of Medical Chemistry
University of Turku
Turku 3, Finland

2425 Soulairac, A., & Soulairac, M.L. Effets de l'administration chronique de réserpine sur la fonction génitale du rat mâle. Modifications du comportement sexuel, du tractus génital et altérations du système nerveux central. [The effects of chronic reserpine administration on the genital function of the male rat; modifications in sexual behavior, the genital tract and alterations in the central nervous system.] Annales Endocrinologie, 1962, 23, 281-292.

The sexual behavior of male rats was studied after reserpine administration: 25 μg/100 g/day for 15 days, and 60 μg per 100 g per day for 4 days. At the low dosage reserpine markedly increased the number of ejaculations and significantly decreased the number of intromissions preceding each ejaculation. At high dosage the drug modified sexual behavior in a similar manner at the 2nd day but 2 days later the animals were in a stuporous state and all tests were negative; 5 days after cessation of treatment normal sexual behavior returned. The testes deteriorate at the interstitial level with fibrocytic involution and the efferent canal shows marked reduction in the columnar height of its epithelium. In the CNS, neuronal deterioration is particularly clear in the lateral mammalary nuclei of the hypothalamus. This localized neurotoxic action of reserpine provides one possible explanation for the effect of this compound on male genital functions.

Laboratoire de Psychophysiologie
Faculté des Sciences
Université de Paris
Paris, France

2426 Otsuka, Yasuo, Sakai, Fuminori, Sakuma, Akira, Saji, Yoshiaki, Nakanishi, Suehiro, & Sawabe, Takashi. Central effects of phencyclidine hydrochloride (Sernyl). Japanese Journal of Pharmacology, 1962, 12, 104-110.

Phencyclidine's central action was studied in cats. Immediately after 1-2 mg/kg i.v., the animals lost the righting reflex, respiration became irregular and inspiratory spasticity prominent. Nystagmus and mydriasis, knee jerk reflex exaggeration and the presence of the tonic neck reflex were noted. Three to 12 hours after injection heavy ataxia with a peculiar shaking of the head was noted. The anesthetic dose was estimated to be 1.7 mg/kg. In curarized cats, cortical and subcortical EEG activity, multiple spikes and/or fast wave bursts were alternately superimposed on the background with marked changes in the suprasylvian gyrus and hippocampus. Phrenic volleys were depressed and markedly prolonged. Blood pressure was slightly elevated following an initial drop. When a 1% solution of phencyclidine was topically applied to the cortical surface near the electrodes, high-voltage waves were periodically reported, most frequently observed in the anterior sigmoid gyrus. The periodicity of these waves was closely related to that of a phrenic volley. Patterns were considerably modified by transection of the brain stem at various levels.

Department of Pharmacology
Faculty of Medicine
University of Tokyo
Tokyo, Japan

2427 Arvay, A., Nyiri, I., Rakosi, M., & Buris, L. Contribution à l'étude des modifications du fonctionnement de l'adénohypophyse par des substances pharmacologiques. [Effect of certain pharmacological substances on changes in the functioning of the adenohypophysis.] Annales d'Endocrinologie, 1962, 23, 186-199.

Female rats received p-oxy-acetophenone (POA), p-oxy-propiophenone (POP), o-oxy-propiophenone (OOP), p-oxy-butyrophenone (POB), o-oxy-chalcone, resacetophenone, chlorpromazine and phenobarbital, 20-40 mg per day, chlorpromazine p.o. and all others injected. o-Oxy-chalcone, resacetophenone and POB increase the duration of estrus, and with administration of POB, most animals were in a state of permanent estrus. OOP, POP and POA increased the intervals between estrus cycles and

frequently caused a state of permanent diestrus. After 3-4 weeks the animals were decapitated. POB increases while POA and POP decrease the percentage of Schiff-positive cells, which indicates production and inhibition of gonadotropin respectively. The drugs generally induced thyroid hyperfunction; POB, POP and POA immediately, and chlorpromazine after a brief period of hypofunction. POB causes endometrial hyperproliferation and the intensification of Graafian follicle maturation. POA inhibits maturation. Reduction in levels of endogenous estrogenic compounds following POA, POP, chlorpromazine and phenobarbital administration is accompanied by increased production of thyrotropic hormone, luteinizing hormone and luteotropic hormone.

Institute of Organic Chemistry
Debrecen, Hungary

2428 Romanowski, W., & Monnier, M. Influence de GABA et du thiosemicarbaside (TSC) sur l'activité électrique du cerveau du lapin. [Influence of GABA and of thiosemicarbazide (TSC) on the electrical activity in the rabbit brain.] Acta Physiologica Polonica, 1962, 13, 399-406.

Seven rabbits received i.v. injections of 6-20 mg/kg thiosemicarbazide (TSC). Tremors of the paws and clonic and tonic convulsions were noted at the lower doses, death intervening at doses of 14-20 mg/kg. GABA injection had no effect on TSC-induced symptoms. Heart action was slowed down during the 1st 10 minutes and again after 2 hours. Large 2-3 cps delta waves appear in the cortex, the number of spindles increases-the hippocampus is activated. Convulsions were preceded by abnormal synchronization of the activity of the hippocampus, caudate nucleus and the median thalamus. Administration of GABA (2 mg/kg i.v.) resulted in the replacement of the TSC tracing by an arousal pattern with desynchronization of the neocortex and synchronization of the archicortex and subcortex. High frequency stimulation of the mesenceph-

alic reticulum also induces similar reactions. Stimulation of the median thalamus
under TSC increases the cortical recruiting potentials. The substance also increases
the cortical potentials of hippocampal origin
and the excitability of the hippocampus.

Institut de Physiologie
Université à Bâle
Basel, Switzerland

2429 Fleming, William W. Supersensitivity of the cat heart to catecholamine-induced
arrhythmias following reserpine pretreatment. Proceedings of the Society of Experimental Biology and Medicine, 1962, 111,
484-486.

Reserpine (0.1 mg/kg/day i.p.) was administered to 26 cats for 7-28 days to
produce maximal depletion of heart levarterenol. Cats were then pithed under ether
anesthesia, after which they received consecutive single injections of levarterenol
or epinephrine (0.01-100 µg/kg i.v.) until
cardiac arrhythmias were observed. Ventricular premature systoles and extrasystoles constituted the initial arrhythmias,
followed in some instances by ventricular
tachycardia or fibrillation. Threshold doses
(appearance of 1st cardiac arrhythmia)
were established for reserpine. Statistical
significance of sensitivity change was determined by Chi-square analysis. Reserpine
treated animals showed significantly greater sensitivity to levarterenol and epinephrine than did controls. Dose-response
curves for positive chronotropic and pressor effect were shifted slightly to the
left, indicating supersensitivity after the
7, 14, 21 and 28 day reserpine treatments.
Sensitivity to levarterenol and epinephrine
induced arrhythmias becomes progressively greater with increasing length of reserpine treatment.

Department of Pharmacology
West Virginia University Medical Center
Morgantown, W. Va.

2430 Faure, J. La phase "paradoxale"
du sommeil chez le Lapin (ses relations
neurohormonales). [The "paradoxical"
phase of sleep in the rabbit (its neuro-

failed to prevent release of heart levarterenol.

Experimental Therapeutics Branch
National Heart Institute
Bethesda, Md.

2433 Boissier, Jacques R. Pharmacologie
des anorexigènes. [Pharmacology of anor-
exigenics.] Thérapie, 1962, 17, 803-825.

Four dogs were trained to eat 1 meal
per day within a 30-minute period. After
2 weeks of training, the dogs received
1 mg/kg amphetamine 1 hour before feeding time. After 30 minutes, the remaining
food was weighed. Amphetamine administration was stopped, and the dogs continued
on the same diet for another 2 weeks.
Modifications of this experiment in which
dogs were allowed to feed at will but
were given amphetamine at stated intervals
during the day were also conducted, as
were experiments on rats subjected to
a similar regimen. These results, and
some obtained with rats indicate that amphetamine is truly anorexigenic, and that
its action is greater in adults than in the
young. Tachyphylaxis occurs after a certain
period. When medication is stopped and
resumed at a later time, the anorexic
effect recurs. In the treatment of obesity
with the wide range of amphetaminelike
agents available, these compounds act as
a sort of psychotherapy they are psychoanaleptic adjuncts to conventional management, i.e., diet restriction, etc.

Institut de Pharmacologie
15 rue de l'Ecole de Médecine
Paris 6, France

2434 Ernst, A.M. Experiments with an
O-methylated product of dopamine on cats.
Acta Physiologica et Pharmacologica Neer-
landica, 1962, 11, 48-53.

To test the supposition that the hypokinetic
rigid syndrome could be suppressed by
administration of phenylethylamine or by
DOPA, 20 cats were injected with bulbocapnine 15 mg/kg and 20 cats administered
papaverine 35 mg/kg. When catatonia was
fully established (20 minutes after the 1st

injection) 6 animals of each group were
used as controls and 7 animals were injected with either 80-100 mg/kg phenylethylamine or 100 mg/kg DOPA. Papaverine
treated cats gained full motility after 30
minutes and controls remained catatonic
about 1 additional hour. The bulbocapnine
treated animals did regain the free motility
of their heads 10 minutes after phenylethylamine or DOPA and were able to look
behind but could not move either forelegs
or hindlegs. Their catalepsy disappeared
almost at the same time as the catatonia
of the controls. As well, 2 groups of 20
cats each were injected with 60 mg/kg
3,4-dimethoxy-phenylethylamine and 50 mg
per kg mescaline respectively. Six control
animals of each group were catatonic for
1.5 to 2.5 hours while 7 animals of each
group administered 100 mg/kg phenylethylamine and 7 animals injected with DOPA
regained motility within 30 minutes. As
the O-methylated products could easily
pass the blood-brain barrier, contrary
to dopamine itself, the disturbance in dopamine metabolism does not necessarily take
place exclusively in the brain but may,
for instance, also originate in the liver.
Further, in human patients phenomena of
the hypokinetic rigid type may be caused
by O-methylation of dopamine in the para
position as supported by the antagonistic
effects of phenylethylamine and of DOPA
on cats pretreated with O-methylated products of dopamine.

[No address]

2435 Mercier, J., & Dessaigne, S. Etude
psychopharmacologique et neurophysiolo-
gique d'un dépresseur médulaire, myoré-
solutif: le 2-(4-chlorophenyl)-3-methyl-4-
metathiazanone-1-dioxyde (Win 4692-Tran-
copal). [Psychopharmacological and neurophysiological study of a muscle relaxant
and medullary depressor: chlormezanone
(Win 4692 - Trancopal.] Anesthesia Analgesia, 1962, 19, 603-626.

The LD_{50} for chlormezanone was determined
in mice as 514 mg/kg i.p. The hypnotic
dose is 250 mg/kg in mice, and 175 mg/kg
in rats. Motor activity is slightly affected
in mice at 100 mg/kg and in cats at
200 mg/kg. The drug decreases motor

2438 Titus, E.O., & Spiegel, H.E. Effect of desmethylimipramine (DMI) on uptake of norepinephrine-7H^3 (NE) in heart. Federation Proceedings, 1962, $\underline{22}$, 179.

Cat heart slices which normally take up levarterenol-7H^3 to levels which are 3-5 times those obtained in buffer do not concentrate the labeled levarterenol when 10^{-6} M demethylimipramine (DMI) is added with partial inhibition at 10^{-10} M. Radioactive levarterenol in mouse heart 1 hour after i.v. administration of 10 μg/kg is 15.1 mμ/g in controls and 4.5 mμ/g in animals receiving 10 mg/kg DMI 1 hour before levarterenol. DMI appears to compete with levarterenol for sites of uptake, since a 250% increase in levarterenol dosage results in normal DMI uptake in mice. DMI does not deplete levarterenol. Reserpine (0.1 mg/kg) administered 1 hour after levarterenol depletes heart radioactivity to 19% of controls. The competitive relationship between the levarterenol and levarterenol inhibitors may govern the capacity of these drugs to deplete levarterenol.

National Institutes of Health
Bethesda, Md.

2439 Eechaute, W., Lacroix, E., Leusen, I., & Bouckaert, J.J. L'Activité du cortex surrénalien sous l'influence de la réserpine et de l'iproniazide. [The activity of the adrenal cortex under the influence of reserpine and iproniazide.] Archives Internationales de Pharmacodynamie et de Thérapie, 1962, $\underline{139}$, 403-414.

Male rats were separated into 5 groups. Two groups received 5 mg/kg reserpine, 1 group received 3 mg/kg, controls in these groups receiving 0.5 ml saline, all i.p. These 3 groups, who had received the "acute treatment" were killed 3, 9 and 20 hours after administration of the single dose. One group received 2.5 mg/kg reserpine for 4 days and the 5th group 1 mg/kg for 10 days. These were sacrificed 4 hours after the final reserpine injection. Some animals received single doses of 100 mg/kg iproniazide i.p. 6 hours before reserpine administration. Both acute and chronic treatments produced a marked

and prolonged increase of plasma corticosterone levels and of the steroid production
by the adrenals in vitro. Pretreatment with
iproniazide prevented, in both acute and
chronic conditions, the adrenocortical response to reserpine. On the other hand,
reserpine did not appear to block adrenocortical response to acute cold stress
(4°C for 60 minutes).

Laboratoires de Physiologie
Université de Gand
Gand, Belgium

2440 Luštinec, K. The effect of some
drugs on oxygen consumption in rats under
basal conditions and during cold stress.
Physiologia Bohemoslovenica, 1962, 11,
343-350.

The effects of the following drugs (mg/kg
i.p.) on basal oxygen consumption was
studied in rats: phenobarbital (150), pentobarbital (15, 30 and 45), urethane (1.5-2),
mephenesin (40 and 80), pentamethonium
(90), chlorpromazine (20), promethazine
(20), reserpine (5), and yohimbine (20);
the following were used s.c.: chloral hydrate
(600 mg/kg), dihydroergotoxin (0.4), quinine
(130) and amidopyridine (140). Oxygen consumption was measured by a modification
of the Regnault-Reiset system of indirect
calorimetry. Artificial respiration was
maintained during the use of narcotics.
For cold stress the metabolimeter was
immersed in a mixture of ice and water.
Here nearly all substances had a depressive
effect which was usually the same, if not
greater than that for classic artificial-
hibernation producing substances such as
chlorpromazine. The effect of reserpine is
slight even though high doses were used;
that of dihydroergotoxin which is used in
lytic cocktails instead of chlorpromazine
is doubtful. Synergism between hibernation
producing substances is evident during cold
stress, whereas it is not present at ambient
temperatures. At 26°C, none of these drugs
decreased basal metabolism if this is defined as oxygen consumption during sleep.
These drugs act nonspecifically and do not
affect biological oxidation.

Institute of Industrial Hygiene and
    Occupational Diseases
Prague, Czechoslavakia

tracheal tube) was studied in rats. Animals were killed 15, 30 and 60 minutes after drug administration. Similar experiments were performed on dogs with 25 mg imipramine i.p. The dogs were sacrificed after 30 minutes, 2, 4 or 24 hours. Total activity of exhaled carbon dioxide in rats over a 24-hour period varied between 26 and 42% with an average of about 34%. Short-term activity amounted to less than 0.5% after 15 minutes, and about 5% after 1 hour. Total and specific activities were measured in different parts of the brain, liver, kidneys, gall bladder, blood, urine, musculature and various adipose tissues. More than half the imipramine is absorbed within 15 minutes after oral administration, followed by rapid demethylation. Imipramine may be detected in an unchanged or partially (1-2%) changed form in the CNS. Specific activity was highest in the cerebrum.

Physiologische-Chemische Institut
Universität Basel
Basel, Switzerland

2444 Murphy, M. Lois. Teratogenic effects in rats of growth inhibiting chemicals, including studies on thalidomide. Clinical Proceedings, Children's Hospital of the District of Columbia, 1962, 18, 307-322.

Thalidomide (2 g/kg i.p. in 1 or 2 doses) was administered on day 12, or days 11 and 12, or 12 and 12, to 16 pregnant rats. Abnormalities resulted in 2 litters, complete resorption in 1, more than 50% resorption in 3 and normal litters in 10. Various cancer chemotherapeutic agents (alkylating agents and antimetabolites) were also administered i.p. in 1 or more doses of 0.05- greater than 2500 mg/kg/day to pregnant rats on days 9, 10, 11, 12 or 17 of gestation. Results indicated that 1 injection administered from day 9 to day 14 resulted in malformed appendages, brains, palates, lips, viscera, tails and bones. Comparative dosages are proffered in tabular form for LD_{50}'s in adult rats, minimal LD_{100}'s in fetuses, teratogenic doses and maximal doses which gave neither resorption nor teratogenic effects in fetuses. In contrast to statistics obtained with thalidomide, cancer-inhibiting drugs produce abnormalities at teratogenic dosages in over 90%

of embryos.

Division of Experimental Chemotherapy
Sloan-Kettering Institute for Cancer
   Research
New York, N.Y.

2445   Lecomte, J., & Troquet, J. Antagon-
isme entre salicylate de soude et brady-
kinine chez le rat. [Antagonism between
sodium salicylate and bradykinin in the
rat.] Archives Internationales de Physiologie et de Biochimie, 1962, 70, 735-737.

In anesthetized rats, 1 of the common
carotid arteries was separated without
vagotomy and blood pressure recorded
manometrically. All substances were injected i.v., usually in divided doses. Seventeen agents, including promethazine, BOL
and phenylbutazone, were tested against
$0.5-2.0 \mu g/100$ g bradykinin. All substances
except sodium salicylate (25-50 mg/100 g)
had no effect. Sodium salicylate almost
completely countered the marked drop in
blood pressure caused by bradykinin.

Institut Léon Fredericq
Université de Liège
Liège, Belgium

2446   Charpentier, Jean. Analyse de l'action analgésique de la morphine chez le
rat par une nouvelle méthode quantitative.
[Analysis of the analgesic action of morphine in the rat by new quantitative
methods.] Comptes Rendus Hebdomadaires
des Séances de l'Academie des Sciences,
1962, 255, 2285-2287.

Morphine was injected i.p. into male rats
at 4, 8 and 16 mg/kg. Twenty to 50 minutes after injection the reaction threshold
to electric tail shock, as a function of
voltage (0-150 volts), and increased the
central excitability after a 75 volt shock
were assayed. Central excitability decreased as follows (mg/kg): 4-16%, 8-
51% and 16-29%; the latter result seems
to be due to the fact that the excitability
of the animal is already much diminished
by the 1st shock.

most active as a muscle relaxant. Trans-
cinnamyl carbamate produced permanent
excito-motor syndrome, while cis-cinnamyl
carbamate had only sedative action.

Faculté de Médecine
Paris, France

2451 Kusch, T., Heinrich, I., & Hofmann,
H. Der Einfluss von Metrazol auf die
Dynamik der Ascorbinsäure bei Ratten.
[Effect of Metrazol on ascorbic acid meta-
bolism of rats.] Acta Biologica et Medica
Germanica, 1962, 8, 538-542.

Pentetrazol (Metrazol; 5 mg/100 g) was
administered s.c. to mature rats, producing convulsions. The animals were decapitated 1 hour later and the ascorbic
acid content of adrenals and liver determined. The ascorbic acid content of the
liver did not change, while that of the
adrenals rose from ca. 2838 µg/g to ca.
3596 µg/g.

Institut für Pharmakologie
Friedrich-Schiller-Universität
Jena, Germany

2452 Truitt, Edward B., Duritz, Gilbert,
Morgan, Ann M., & Prouty, Richard W.
Disulfiramlike action produced by hypo-
glycemic sulfonylurea compounds. Journal
of Studies on Alcohol, 1962, 23, 197-207.

Male rats received tolbutamide and chlorpropamide (65-250 mg/kg i.p.) 1 hour before
ethanol injection (1 g/kg i.p.) to determine
the resultant disulfiramlike increase in
blood acetaldehyde. Cats and dogs received
epinephrine (1 γ/kg i.v.), tolbutamide
(200-250 mg/kg i.v.), chlorpropamide (250
mg/kg i.v.), disulfiram (100-250 mg/kg/day
for 3 days), calcium carbimide (25 mg/kg
p.o.) and insulin (5 U/kg i.v.) at various
intervals. Tolbutamide produced markedly
increased blood acetaldehyde levels in rats.
The vasopressor phase of blood pressure
response in cats injected with acetaldehyde
was deeper by an average of 16.4 mm,
whereas a similar response to epinephrine
was unchanged by tolbutamide. Insulin failed
to alter the response to acetaldehyde or
epinephrine, but a dose of glucose sufficient

to correct the hypoglycemia reversed the
tolbutamide-induced potentiation of the
hypotensive phase. Bradycardia of vagal
origin occurred during the depressor phase
of acetaldehyde after tolbutamide injection.
Chlorpropamide also actively potentiated
acetaldehyde vasodepression. The cardiovascular changes appear to be caused by
interference with some glucose dependent
function which is affected by tolbutamide
but not by insulin.

Department of Pharmacology
University of Maryland School of Medicine
Baltimore, Md.

2453 Melson, F. Weitere pharmakologische Untersuchungen einiger Derivate des
1,3-Dioxolans. II. [Further pharmacological
investigations of some derivatives of 1,3-
dioxolan. II.] Acta Biologica et Medica
Germanica, 1962, 8, 381-386.

K 161 (2-p-chlorphenyl-2-methyl-4-hy-
droxymethyl-1-3-dioxolan; 100-200 mg/kg)
potentiates the hypnotic effect of barbiturates in mice. It diminishes the mortality
due to administration of strychnine, pentetrazol and picrotoxin and diminishes aggressive behavior among male mice; this
latter effect is slightly less than that of
meprobamate. It reduces anxiety of rats
exposed to electroshock to the same degree
as meprobamate. K 161 is considered a
tranquilizing agent.

Institut für Pharmakologie
Friedrich-Schiller-Universität
Jena, Germany

2454 Hodes, Robert. Electrocortical synchronization resulting from reduced proprioceptive drive caused by neuromuscular
blocking agents. Electroencephalography
and Clinical Neurophysiology, 1962, 14,
220-232.

Gallamine (2-4 mg/kg i.v.) produced electrocortical synchronization in 24 cats which
was maintained for many hours. Cessation
of gallamine results in rapid synchronization of desynchronized brain potentials
with injection of minute amounts (0.25-
0.50 mg/kg) of barbiturate. Synchronization

the 1 γ level, showed no lethal effect, was
not abolished after pancreatectomy, and
did not elevate blood pressure. No significant changes in respiratory quotient were
seen, with the exception of temporary
reduction immediately at the start of epinephrine or levarterenol infusion.

Institut für Pharmakologie und Toxikologie
Humboldt-Universität
Berlin, Germany

2458 Flanagan, T.L., Reynolds, L.W., Novick, W.J., Lin, T.H., Rondish, I.M., &
Van Loon, E.J. Biliary and urinary excretion patterns of chlorpromazine in the
dog. Journal of Pharmaceutical Sciences,
1962, 51, 833-836.

In bitches, 200 mg chlorpromazine dissolved in 10 ml of saline was administered
intraduodenally by cannula. Bile samples
were obtained at 1-hour and urine samples
at 2-hour intervals for a period of 8-10
hours following drug administration. Each
sample was analyzed individually for "free"
and "bound" chlorpromazine and chlorpromazine sulfoxide by the method of Flanagan
et al. (1959). In other experiments the dogs
received 200 mg chlorpromazine/day p.o.
for 2-14 days. Also chlorpromazine (25 mg
per kg) containing about 60 μc of S^{35} was
injected into the duodenum and urine samples collected. Based on chromatography
and UV analysis, chlorpromazine and its
sulfoxide undergo 2 types of binding. Strong
alkaline treatment hydrolyzed 1 type while
treatment with β-glucuronidase hydrolyzed
both types. In urine the concentration of the
bound phenothiazines liberated by alkaline
hydrolysis was 2-3 times as great as the
free material. In bile, the concentration of
this type of bound chlorpromazine and
chlorpromazine sulfoxide was 10-15 times
greater than the free forms of the compound.

Research and Development Division
Smith Kline & French Laboratories
Philadelphia 1, Pa.

2459 Bircher, Rudolf P., Kanai, Tatsuya,
& Wang, S.C. Intravenous, cortical and
intraventricular dose-effect relationship of
pentylenetetrazol, picrotoxin and deslano-

side in dogs. Electroencephalography and Clinical Neurophysiology, 1962, 14, 256-267.

The dose-route-effect relationship of 0.5-10 mg/kg pentetrazol, 0.5-2000 μg/kg picrotoxin and 1-300 μg/kg deslanoside administered i.v., subarachnoidally on the cortex, in the lateral ventricle, the 3rd and 4th ventricles, was determined in dogs with cannula or catheter chronically implanted in various brain areas. Pentetrazol and picrotoxin produced EEG convulsive discharges when given i.v., cortically or intraventricularly. Pentetrazol acted most rapidly and picrotoxin least rapidly. Deslanoside produced convulsive discharges only when applied cortically or intraventricularly. Cardiac arrhythmias were produced with all 3 drugs, as was an increase in blood pressure accompanied by tachycardia.

Department of Pharmacology
College of Physicians and Surgeons
Columbia University
New York, N.Y.

2460 Stumpf, Ch., Petsche, H., & Gogolak, G. The significance of the rabbit's septum as a relay station between the midbrain and the hippocampus. II. The differential influence of drugs upon both the septal cell firing pattern and the hippocampus theta activity. Electroencephalography and Clinical Neurophysiology, 1962, 14, 212-219.

Septal cell activity and hippocampal EEG's were studied in 15 unanesthetized, curarized rabbits treated i.v. with 0.25 mg/kg eserine, 30 mg/kg hexobarbital, 3 g/kg urethane, 0.1 mg/kg LSD, 0.5 mg/kg scopolamine and 3-6 mg/kg nicotine. Eserine and nicotine induced β-units in the septum to discharge in bursts which were synchronous with the hippocampal theta waves. Low doses of hexobarbital and scopolamine diminish theta rhythm and burst frequency of β-units, while high doses abolish theta rhythm and replace regular burst pattern with an irregular firing pattern, indicating depression of the limbic subcortical regions. LSD acts directly on the hippocampus, abolishing theta rhythm without

manifested by 75% of the epileptics, 40% of the schizophrenics and 6% of the depressives.

Department of Clinical Neurophysiology
Institute of Psychiatry
The Maudsley Hospital
London, Great Britain

2464 Wada, Toyoji, Goto, Akira, & Fukushima, Yutaka. Megimide-metrazol (M-M) activation in clinical electroencephalography. Electroencephalography and Clinical Neurophysiology, 1962, 14, 408-410.

A megimide (90 mg)-pentetrazol (metrazol) (200 mg) activation technique (4 cc i.v. followed by 1 cc every 15 seconds for 1 minute and 30 seconds) was combined with routine photic stimulation, after which 1 cc was injected every 15 seconds during light flashing procedures in 103 epileptics, 58 schizophrenics and 57 neurotics. Positive activation constituted a burst of abnormal discharges during seizure activity. Positive results were obtained in 95% of the epileptics, 55% schizophrenics and 46% of the neurotics. Differences between epilepsy and schizophrenia or neurosis are very significant. The average threshold value for megimide-pentetrazol activation in epilepsy in about 0.2 cc/kg in comparison with that for megimide (0.9 mg/kg) and for pentetrazol (2.0 mg/kg). With pentetrazol-photic activation the average threshold was as follows: 5.4 mg/kg in epilepsy, 6.1 mg/kg in schizophrenia and 6.8 mg/kg in neurosis. Following bursts of abnormal discharges clinical seizures were produced in 58 epileptics. Side effects included nausea, facial congestion, palpitation, dizziness, flushing, tremor, vomiting, tinnitus and pain in the extremities. The technique appears efficacious.

Department of Neuropsychiatry
Hirosaki University School of Medicine
Hirosaki, Japan

2465 Selldén, Ulla. The role of hyperventilation in the initial electroencephalographic responses to activation with megimide. Electroencephalography and Clinical Neurophysiology, 1962, 14, 368-375.

In conjunction with EEG studies, 12 people
(9 normal, 1 epileptic, 1 amnesiac and 1 with
multiple sclerosis), aged 20-51 years, received PCO_2 determinations in arterial
blood ($PaCO_2$) at rest and during megimide
(40-150 mg i.v.) activation. $PaCO_2$ determinations were also made during and after
voluntary hyperventilation in 10 subjects,
to establish whether hyperventilation might
be implicated in initial EEG response to
megimide activation. A slight rise in ventilation accompanies megimide activation.
Since this response is not significant, it
may be ignored as a source of error when
initial EEG responses to megimide activation are evaluated.

Laboratories for Clinical Physiology and
Clinical Neurophysiology
Sahlgrenska Sjukhuset
Göteborg, Sweden

2466 Kanai, Tatsuya, Misrahy, George, &
Clark, Leland C. Neuropharmacological
effects of O-methylbufotenine. Federation
Proceedings, 1962, 21, 322. [Abstract]

Minutes after the injection of 0.5 mg/kg
parenteral or intraventricular injections
of 5 μ/kg O-methylbufotenin cats are apprehensive, show autonomic overactivity,
ataxia, catatoniclike postures and mixed
reactivity to sensory stimuli. These effects
are reduced by lobotomy, section of optic
nerves, tranquilizers and anesthetics. De-
cortication or decerebration suppresses
hyperventilation. EEG shows high amplitude
slow waves and increased arousal responses. Cortical evoked responses to sensory stimuli increase; threshold of midbrain to electrical stimuli drops; and coch-
lear threshold and behavior of Purkinje
cells do not change significantly. Response
to pain is diminished. Small doses induce
tachycardia and increase blood pressure;
large doses cause the opposite effect. Pressor responses are elicited by tactile and
sound stimuli, but not by pain. Bufotenin,
in conjunction with methionine, may induce
changes similar to O-methylbufotenin.

Memorial Childrens Hospital
Los Angeles, Calif.

on the influence of meprobamate on hepatic function.] Thérapie, 1962, 17, 303-310.

Dogs were given massive doses of meprobamate, 0.10-0.15 g/kg (about 3 times the maximal therapeutic dose equivalent to 9 g per day in man) for 3 months. This dosage was then established as the approximate threshold limit for liver tolerance.

Université de Toulouse
Toulouse, France

2471 Clifford, Donald H., Good, Archie L., & Stowe, Clarence M. Observations on the use of ataractic and narcotic preanesthesia and pentobarbital anesthesia in bears. Journal of the American Veterinary Medical Association, 1962, 140, 464-470.

Intramuscular injection of large doses of promazine (8.8 mg/kg) and pethidine (22 mg per kg) were not effective preanesthetics in the North American bear. Morphine (4.4 and 8.8 mg/kg i.m.) was effective prior to pentobarbital anesthesia. Promazine (4.4 and 8.8 mg/kg) potentiated morphine. Suggested doses are 8.8 mg/kg morphine and 4.4 mg/kg promazine.

Division of Veterinary Surgery and
    Radiology
College of Veterinary Medicine
University of Minnesota
St. Paul, Minn.

2472 Casier, H. Accumulation of alcohol metabolites in the form of total lipids and fatty acids in the organism. Quarterly Journal of the Studies on Alcohol, 1962, 23, 529-548.

Groups of mice were given injections of 0.3, 0.6, 0.9 ml of a 33% alcohol solution, corresponding in radioactivity to 1.2, 2.4 and 3.6 μc. The amounts of alcohol were correspondingly 1.25, 2.5 and 3.75 g/kg. For comparison of the fixation of alcohol metabolites with that of sodium acetate equimolar doses of alcohol and acetate were injected. When a daily dose of 0.3 ml alcohol was administered for 8, 15 and 21 days respective amounts of alcohol metabolites reached 3-6 times as high a value

as after the administration of a single
dose. Probably a condensation or combination occurs between acetaldehyde and acetyl
CoA with the formation of cholesterol and
lipids. Hence the origin of the fixed metabolites derived from alcohol should be
different from the origin of fixed metabolites derived from acetic acid.

Institut J.F. Heymans de Pharmacodynamie
Ghent, Belgium

2473   Cadell, T.E., Harlow, H.F., & Wais-
man, H.A. EEG changes in experimental
phenylketonuria.   Electroencephalography
and Clinical Neurophysiology, 1962, 14,
540-543.

Five rhesus monkeys were raised from
the 5th day of life on a diet of whole
cow's milk or powdered milk which contained 0.25 g phenylalanine/100 ml. After
2 weeks the concentration was increased
to 0.5 g phenylalanine/100 ml. Daily intake
was ca. 2.75 g. Electrodes were implanted
and recordings made with the animals
restrained in a supine position. A photo-
stimulator was used. The predominance
of slow activity in the phenylketonuric
(PKU) monkey seems to agree partially
with EEG findings in humans with phenylketonuria. Slow activity is not constant,
merely predominant. Ordinarily EEG's contain 3/ second spikes and waves. Sleep
was induced in 3 PKU monkeys by 50 mg/kg
amobarbital i.p., and records taken in sleep
did not show any petit mal type discharge.
Two of the 5 animals have had grand mal
seizures with tonic-clonic contractions in
all extremities. PKU animals had a reduced
following response to photic stimulation and
showed a trend toward greater deficits in
following with increasing age.

Department of Psychology
University of Wisconsin
Madison, Wis.

2474   Dai-Xuong, N., Duchêne-Marullaz,
Vacher, J., & Buu-Hoï, N.P. Activité anti-
monoamineoxydase de divers dérivés des
nicotinyl- et isonicotinylhydrazines. [Anti-
monoamine oxydase activity of various
nicotinyl and isonicotinyl hydrazines.]

reserpine 1 mg/kg for 8 days. Injection of reserpine causes profound sleep for 15-20 hours, diminishing considerably the opportunity for feeding. Growth inhibition is merely parallel to degree of inability to feed.

Laboratoire de Physiologie Animale
Faculté des Sciences
Clermont-Ferrand, France

2479 Higuchi, Hideo, Matsuo, Takaaki, & Shimamoto, Kiro. Effects of methamphetamine and cocaine on the depletion of catecholamine of the brain, heart and adrenal gland in rabbit by reserpine. Japanese Journal of Pharmacology, 1962, 12, 48-56.

One mg/kg methamphetamine or 2 mg/kg cocaine was injected i.v. 1 hour before the administration of 1 mg/kg reserpine in intact rabbits. Brain, heart and both adrenals were taken and their homogenates assayed for epinephrine and levarterenol. Both drugs depressed the levels of catecholamine in central and peripheral organs, the effect being more marked in the brain tissues. During the decrease of central catecholamines, the animal showed motor and sympathetic excitement. The i.v. injection of 1 mg/kg to rabbits pretreated with 1 mg/kg methamphetamine reestablished levarterenol brain content in the 1st half hour of reserpine administration. During this reestablishment, the animal showed motor excitement. When the same reserpine treatment was applied following cocaine, levarterenol in brain tissue did not become reestablished, but decreased sharply. A similar decrease of catecholamine was observed in the atria and adrenal glands.

Department of Pharmacology
Faculty of Medicine
Kyoto University
Kyoto, Japan

2480 Tuchmann-Duplessis, H., Gabe, M., & Mercier-Parot, L. Diminution du produit de sécrétion hypothalamo-neuro-hypophysaire après injection de réserpine. [Diminution of hypothalamo-neuro-hypophyseal secretory product after reserpine in-

jection.] Annales d'Endocrinologie, 1962,
23, 65-77.

Histology of the hypothalamo-hypophyseal
neurosecretory path in rats after 50-75 μg
per day reserpine for 1-10 days revealed
a reduction in neurosecretory production
(using fuchsin-paraldehyde). This did not
appear related to electrolyte balance. Evidence favors direct action for reserpine
on the hypothalamo-hypophyseal complex.

Laboratoire d'Embryologie
Faculté de Médecine
45, rue des Saints Pères
Paris, France

2481   Ochs, S., Dowell, A.R., & Russell,
I.S. Mescaline convulsive spikes triggered
by direct cortical stimulation. Electroencephalography and Clinical Neurophysiology, 1962, 14, 872-884.

The cortices of rabbits and cats were
exposed after anesthesia; stimulating pulses
were applied with bipolar electrodes. Mescaline (a small drop of 1% solution placed
on the cortex at the site of the recording
electrode) was effective in producing convulsive activity in both the intact cortex
and in cortical island preparations. Driven
spikes were found in a number of cortical
regions, including frontal regions of the
rabbit and suprasylvian gyrus of the cat,
in addition to the visual cortex of the
rabbit. Spikes could be elicited in the acute
and chronic cortical island preparations.
The latency of the spike may be short
and the response gives the false appearance
of an exaggerated direct cortical response
(DCR) or the latency may be longer than
100 milliseconds varying with stimulus
strength. The DCT usually decreases in
size after mescaline application and does
not appear to be casually related to the
spike. GABA rapidly blocks both the DCR
and the spike, producing an inversion of
the DCR, but not the spike. Mescaline
spikes can be blocked by i.v. pentobarbital,
while DCR remains. Direct intracortical
action of pentobarbital to depress mes-
caline-sensitized intracortical neurons is
thereby indicated.

Indiana University School of Medicine
Indianapolis 7, Ind.

Experimental, 1962, 14, 47-59.

The in vitro MAO inhibitory potential of a series of compounds designated HM-, was assayed with rabbit liver homogenates and in vivo MAO inhibition was determined spectrofluorometrically by levarterenol and 5HT concentrations in tissues of rats and mice in acute and chronic trials. Methphendrazine (HM-11) was the best inhibitor, increasing the basal level of amines in vivo. Intravenous methphendrazine did not alter either the hypertensive response of epinephrine, or vasomotor reflexes. In the frog, methphendrazine showed hardly any cardiac reaction. The LD_{50} in the mouse is 38.7 mg/kg and in the rat 91 mg/kg. Administered to the rat at lethal or sublethal doses, methphendrazine produced restlessness, exopthalmia, hydriasia, tremor, excitability and death by respiratory paralysis. It did not produce hemic, hepatic, renal or pulmonary degeneration nor did it produce anorexia. Spontaneous motility in the rat was increased 30%, against 500% increase for amphetamine. Reserpine stupor in rats was negated by pretreatment with methphendrazine, and tryptamine convulsions were greatly potentiated.

Consejo Superior de Investigaciones
    Científicas
Instituto de Farmacología Experimental
    Sección de Madrid
Madrid, Spain

See also 2255, 2357, 2388, 2398, 2406, 2486, 2488, 2501, 2506, 2531.

2486 Ankermann, Horst. Zum Problem der stoffwechselsenkenden Wirkung des Adrenalins. [The mechanism of the metabolism-reducing action of adrenalin.] Acta Biologica et Medica Germanica, 1962, 8, 609-616.

Intravenous infusion with small amounts of epinephrine (adrenalin; 1.5 γ/minute/100 g) into rats increased oxygen consumption and blood pressure. Additional infusion of the sympatholytic phentolamine [2-(N-p-Tolyl-N-m oxygenyl-aminomethyl)-imidazoline] (3 γ/minute/100 g) did not change the accelerated metabolic rate but prevented the rise of blood pressure. Large doses of epinephrine (3.8 γ) reduced the oxygen consumption to about half the norm in 12 out of 16 rats. Simultaneous infusion of phentolamine (7 γ) produced in all (8) rats an almost 2-fold increase in oxygen consumption, although this dosage of phentolamine without epinephrine does not significantly alter the metabolic rate. Also, the metabolic effect may be caused solely by its pressor effect.

Institut für Pharmakologie und Toxikologie
Humboldt-Universität
Berlin, Germany

2487 Schmidt, Joachim, & Matthies, Hansjürgen. Über einen zentralen Serotonin-Noradrenalin-Antagonismus. [Central antagonism of serotonin and noradrenalin.] Acta Biologica et Medica Germanica,1961, 7, 107-109.

Injection into the cerebrum of either 5HT (serotonin) or levarterenol (noradrenalin) significantly prolonged duration of hexobarbital anesthesia (100 mg/kg i.p.) in mice. Simultaneous injection of both 5HT and levarterenol slightly shortened the anesthesia. Duration of anesthesia was reduced by injection of 5HT into the cerebellum; this effect was cancelled by the simultaneous injection of levarterenol. Dopamine showed the same effects as levarterenol; DOPA was without influence.

Pharmakologische Institut
Medizinische Akademie Magdeburg
Magdeburg, Germany

2488 Lee, Joseph C. Effect of alcohol injections on the blood-brain barrier. Quarterly Journal of Studies on Alcohol, 1962, 23, 4-16.

Of 21 rabbits receiving ethanol injections in the left common carotid artery, 7 got 2 cc of 30% solution, 8 received 2 cc of 7.5-45% solution and 6 received 4-10 cc of 30% solution, after which they were sacrificed at various intervals. Radioautographic studies with radioactive iodinated bovine albumin were used to detect changes in cerebral vascular permeability. The healthy cerebral blood vessels were impermeable to albumin molecules and trypan blue particles. Injections of alcohol produced a transient increase in cerebral vascular permeability to these molecules. Death ensued after injection of 10 cc alcohol solution at greater than 45% concentration. Radioautographs became very intense after 1 hour and declined markedly within 6 hours. Radioactivity was very pronounced in the thalamus, hypothalamus and amygdaloid nuclei, but less so in the cerebral cortex. Spread of radioactivity was observed in the opposite cerebral hemisphere along the corpus callosum, hippocampus and massa intermedia. Apparently alcohol influences neuronal metabolism which in turn produces an alteration in the blood-brain barrier.

Department of Anatomy
University of Saskatchewan
Saskatoon, Saskatchewan
Canada

2489 Holmberg, Maj Britt, & Jansson, Bengt. A study of blood count and serum transaminase in prolonged treatment with amitriptyline. Journal of New Drugs, 1962, 2, 361-365.

Amitriptyline (usually 50-100 mg/day) was administered to 100 depressed patients aged 10-79 years for an average of 6.1 months following 2 months pretreatment. Laboratory tests, including SGPT, white blood count and differential counts were performed once a month for the duration of treatment. Of necessity chlorpromazine was administered to 10%. About 84% of the patients showed obvious improvement in

Medizinische Universitätsklinik Erlangen
Erlangen, Germany

2491 Davis, Charles S., Jenkins, Glenn L.,
Knevel, Adelbert M., & Paget, Charles.
Synthesis of some N- and S-substituted
derivatives of 2-aminobenzenethiol. Journal of Pharmaceutical Sciences, 1962, 51,
840-842.

Ten N- and S-substituted derivatives of 2-
aminobenzenethiol (2-(2'-diethylaminoeth-
ylamino) benzenethiol, 2,2-pentamethylene-
benzothiazoline, etc.) were prepared by
various synthetic techniques as intermediates in the synthesis of analogues of the
phenothiazine tranquilizers. A new synthesis for preparing the benzothiazine ring
is reported and cleavage of the 2,2-penta-
methylenebenzothiazoline ring with alkylating agents is discussed.

Research Laboratories
School of Pharmacy
Purdue University
Lafayette, Ind.

2492 Mellinger, Theodore J., & Keeler,
Clyde E. Chromatography and electrophoresis of phenothiazine drugs. Journal of
Pharmaceutical Sciences, 1962, 51, 1169-
1173.

Through separation techniques, electrophoresis, paper chromatography and thin-
layer chromatography were used in order
to differentiate 19 phenothiazine compounds
(chlorpromazine, perphenazine, prochlorperazine, etc.) and 4 similar compounds
(imipramine, chlorprothixene, isothypendyl
and prothypendyl). Electrophoresis produced fast and distinctive migration of
these compounds, but tailing interfered
with the usefulness of this technique. Paper
chromatography proved to be a valuable
and easy means of separating these drugs.
Thin-layer chromatography with silica gel
showed the most accurate separation of
phenothiazine compounds. Chromatography
in combination with color reaction or fluorescence permitted good differentiation of
the various phenothiazine tranquilizers.

Milledgeville State Hospital
Milledgeville, Ga.

2493 Blake, Martin I., & Siegel, Frederick
P. Analysis of phenobarbital elixir by an
ion exchange and nonaqueous titration procedure. Journal of Pharmaceutical Sciences, 1962, 51, 944-946.

Phenobarbital, secobarbital, amobarbital
and pentobarbital elixirs were analyzed
by passing an aliquot through a strongly
basic anion exchange resin, followed by
elution with acetic acid in ethanol. Barbiturate assay was completed by evapor-
ating the solvent, dissolving the residue
in dimethylformamide and titrating with
sodium methoxide in benzene-methanol.
Recovery was far in excess of that obtained with standard procedures.

College of Pharmacy
University of Illinois
Chicago, Ill.

2494 Brochmann-Hanssen, E., & Svendsen, A. Baerheim. Separation and identification of sympathomimetic amines by gas-
liquid chromatography. Journal of Pharmaceutical Sciences, 1962, 51, 938-941.

Amphetamine, mephentermine, epinephrine, levarterenol and various other sympathomimetic amines were subjected to
gas chromatographic analysis on low-
loaded columns. All compounds save phenylephrine and synephrine could be separated
on a column of silicone rubber SE-30.
Many of the amines reacted with ketones
to produce sharp, symmetrical peaks on
the gas chromatogram. Ephedrine and
pseudoephedrine can be separated and
identified on the basis of the difference in
the rate of reaction with acetone. Certain phenolic amines were difficult to gas
chromatograph because of adsorptive effects. Monophenolic amines yielded good
chromatograms as ketone derivatives.
Catecholamines gave optimal results after
acetylation and treatment with hexamethyl-
disilazane before chromatography.

University of California School of Pharmacy
San Francisco, Calif.

2495 Mabry, C. Charlton, Nelson, Thomas
L., & Horner, Frederick A. Occult phenyl-

ECT seems to reflect a change in the metabolic condition of the liver.

Department of Neuropsychiatry
Tottori University School of Medicine
Tottori, Japan

2500 Culley, W.J., Saunders, R.N., Mertz, E.T., & Jolly, D.H. Effect of phenylalanine and its metabolites on the brain serotonin level of the rat. Proceedings of the Society for Experimental Biology and Medicine, 1962, 111, 444-446.

Wistar rats were placed on diets supplemented with 7% phenylalanine, 4.5% phenylpyruvic acid, 3% 5-hydroxyphenylacetic acid or 4% phenylacetic acid. Chromatographic analysis of brain samples revealed that serotonin levels were depressed most effectively by supplementing the diet with 7% phenylalanine. Phenylpyruvic acid diminished brain serotonin levels less effectively, while phenylacetic acid and o-hydroxyphenylacetic acid did not produce significant alterations in brain serotonin levels.

Mental Retardation Research Laboratory
Muscatatuck State School
Butlerville, Ind.

2501 Batrinos, M.L., De Verbizier, J., Moncuit, M., & Courjaret, J. L'excrétion de la FSH au cours du traitement par la lévomépromazine. [Excretion of FHS during levomepromazine treatment.] Revue Françaises Etudes Clinique et Biologique, 1961, 7, 521-523.

Urinary excretion of FSH was assayed in 6 physically normal women, aged 28-39 years. These psychiatric patients were receiving 300 mg levomepromazine p.o. daily. Assay was made before treatment and repeated from the 10th to the 30th day, and then was continued from the 31st to the 90th day of treatment. Assay was made through injecting an alcohol precipitate of urine into 18 day old mice and noting the increase in uterine volume (Batrinos 1959); normal values are 5-25 mouse units. No systematic alteration in FSH was noted. Apparently levomepromazine does not disturb the genital cycle.

Hôpital Broussais
Paris, France

2502   Itoh, Tadao, Matsuoka, Masami, Nakazima, Kazuhiko, Tagawa, Kunio, & Imaizumi, Reiji.   An isolation method of
catecholamine and effect of reserpine on
the enzyme systems related to the formation and inactivation of catecholamines in
brain. Japanese Journal of Pharmacology,
1962, 12, 130-136.

DOPA, dopamine and levarterenol in guinea
pig brains can be easily separated by
Duolite C-25 resin column chromatography
and measured fluorometrically. The animal
received 15 mg/kg reserpine i.p. Additionally Glenner's (1957) histochemical methods
were used on brain slices, demonstrating
an activating effect on MAO by reserpine
in all brain areas, especially the hypothalamus. Dopamine and levarterenol were
proven to be synthesized from DOPA by
brain homogenates in vitro. The activities
of DOPA carboxylase and dopamine β-
oxydase were increased by reserpine administration, as is true of MAO activity.
Increased enzymic activity related to the
formation and activation of catecholamines,
caused by reserpine administration, resulted in an increase in total acid catechols
in the brain.

Department of Pharmacology
Osaka University Medical School
Osaka, Japan

2503   Speck, Louise B. Effects of massive
X-irradiation on rat electroencephalograms
and brain serotonin. Journal of Neurochemistry, 1962, 9, 573-574.

EEG's of unanesthetized Sprague-Dawley
rats were made with implanted phonograph
needle electrodes before and after X-
irradiation. Whole body irradiation was
delivered at 98.4 r/minutes for 4500, 9000
or 20000 r. Decreased 5HT (serotonin)
levels were found immediately after exposure to 9000 r and 18 hours after 4500 r,
coinciding with EEG slowing and lethargy.
Later 5HT levels returned to normal even

esterase and butyrylcholinesterase in the human brain. Journal of Neurochemistry, 1962, 2, 559-572.

Acetylcholinesterase and butyrylcholinesterase were examined in human brains obtained at autopsy. The substrates were acetylcholine (ACh), acetylthiocholine iodide, butyrylcholine iodide (BuCh), butyrylthiocholine iodide and acetyl-β-methylcholine chloride (MeCh). Several inhibitors including 1,5-bis (4-allyldimethyl ammonium phenyl) pentane-3-1 dibromide and (2-hydroxy-5-phenyl benzyl) trimethylammonium (bromide) dimethylcarbamate were used. There were no marked differences in the hydrolysis rates of acetylcholine, butyrylcholine and acetyl-β-methylcholine in the various cortical areas, as determined by respirometry and Koelle's (1955) histochemical method. In the gray matter, acetylcholinesterase (AChE) activity was consistently higher than butyrylcholinesterase (BuChE) activity. While AChE activity paralleled the total ChE activity, there was relatively little variation found in the BuChE activity of various areas. The increasing order of AChE activity was: cerebral cortex, cerebellar cortex, thalamus, globus pallidus and caudate nucleus. No marked differences were found in the AChE activity of the various areas of the cerebral cortex. The AChE activity of the white matter of the internal capsule was higher, while that adjacent to the cortical areas was lower, than that of the cortical gray matter. BuChE activity in the white matter was considerably higher than in the gray matter. Hydrolysis activity curves of ACh and MeCh by human gray matter homogenates were similar to those obtained for their hydrolysis by human red cells. The BuCh hydrolysis activity curve for white matter homogenates was similar to that obtained in plasma. B.W.-284C51 at 10 μM selectively inhibited the AChE of both the human brain and red cell. The inhibitory effect of 0.05 μM RO2-0683 on the hydrolysis of BuCh by human brain homogenates was less than that on human plasma. With the histochemical method, the specific staining caused by AChE activity was primarily present in a granular pattern in the protoplasm of the neurons. The nuclei were free of specific staining. The distribution of ChE activity in the white matter was diffuse.

Department of Anesthesiology
Mercy Hospital
Pittsburgh, Pa.

2508 Häggendal, J. On the use of strong
exchange resins for determinations of small
amounts of catecholamines. Scandinavian
Journal of Clinical and Laboratory Investigations, 1962, 14, 537-544.

Epinephrine and levarterenol can be separated from dopamine by being passed through
a strong cation exchange column which
tends to hold back their 3 o-methylated
derivatives. Using Dowex 50 and Amberlite
CG-120, complete separation of levarterenol, epinephrine, normethanephrine, metanephrine, and dopamine was possible in
1 run by eluting with HCl. Destruction of
catecholamines can be controlled by means
of antioxidant and chelating agents. Columns of thoroughly purified strong cation
exchange resins were found to give off
fluorescent material which can interfere
with determinations.

Department of Pharmacology
University of Göteborg
Göteborg, Sweden

2509 Nukada, Tadaatsu, Matsuoka, Masami, & Imaizumi, Reiji. The effect of long-
term administration of pyrogallol on the
metabolism of catecholamines. Japanese
Journal of Pharmacology, 1962, 12, 57-61.

Male rabbits were injected with 20 mg/kg
pyrogallol/day s.c. for 5 weeks. Also male
rats were given 50 mg/kg pyrogallol/day
for 5 weeks, the observation period extending for 10 weeks. Column chromatography,
modified after Nakajima (1960), was used
for the determination of urinary catecholamines. The rate of excretion of o-methylated derivatives of catecholamines in the
urine decreased briefly during the administration, but after longterm treatment with
pyrogallol it returned to normal. Daily
treatment with pyrogallol increased the
rate of excretion of free catecholamines and
the rate reached a maximum after 3 weeks.
Longterm treatment with pyrogallol tends

longer chain acids resembled that of the
shorter chain acids in the following respects; effects on spinal reflexes were
absent in decerebrate cats and present
in spinal preparations; the effect on flexor
monosynaptic responses was reduced following strychnine administration, and the
effect on flexor monosynaptic responses
was abolished by conditioning volleys of
high threshold afferent fibers from extensor muscles. GABA produced depression
of extensor motorneurons with increased
membrane potential and facilitation of flex-
or motorneurons with decreased membrane
potential. A long chain omega-amino acid
depolarized extensor motorneurons and hy-
perpolarized flexor motorneurons. Some
polysynaptic potentials were changed by
GABA injection without appreciably changing monosynaptic spike potential and inhibitory postsynaptic potentials from the
antagonistic muscle afferent fibers. Some
interneurons were depressed and others
were facilitated by GABA. Significant effects of GABA were not found in Renshaw
cells. Apparently, short chain omega-amino
acids selectively depress certain spinal
interneurons, while longer acids activate
these same interneurons.

Department of Pharmacology and
   Physiology
Yamaguchi Medical College
Ube City, Japan

2514 Miyake, Hiroshi, Miyazaki, Masatoshi, & Imaizumi, Reiji. Determination of
urinary 3,4-dihydroxymandelic acid (DOMA).
Japanese Journal of Pharmacology, 1962,
12, 163-165.

A method for the determination of urinary
3,4-dihydroxymandelic acid (DOMA) is described based on alumina adsorption, fractionation with anion exchange resin and
extraction coupled with a conversion reaction of DOMA to protocatechu aldehyde
followed by development and optical reading at 495 mμ as well as paper chromatography. By this method 10 rabbits were
examined in related to 24-hour DOMA
excretion; the mean was ca. 720 μg/50 mg
creatinine.   Under the same conditions
levarterenol, insulin, reserpine, iproniazid,
pyrogallol and acetylcholine were adminis-

tered s.c. Respective increases in DOMA excretion after these drugs was 74, 168, 66, 38, 37 and 144%. The effect of electrical stimulation of rabbit hypothalamus was also studied; before stimulation DOMA μg per 50 mg creatinine was 10.4, while after stimulation 31.3 and blood glucose before and after figures were 88 and 110 mg%. Results are parallel to those for VMA excretion (Miyaki 1961). A substantial portion of endogenous epinephrine and of levarterenol may undergo oxidative deamination as the 1st metabolic step. Assay of DOMA represents another approach to inquiry on endogenous levels of epinephrine and levarterenol.

Department of Pharmacology
Osaka University Medical School
Osaka, Japan

2515 Miyake, Hiroshi, Yoshida, Hiroshi, & Imaizumi, Reiji. Determination methods for urinary 3-methoxy-4-hydroxymandelic acid and 3,4-dihydroxymandelic acid. Japanese Journal of Pharmacology, 1962, 12, 79-92.

The method of Sandler and Ruthven (1959) was modified for the determination of urinary vanilmandelic acid (VMA; 3-methoxy-4-hydroxymandelic acid) and 3,4-dihydroxymandelic acid (DOMA). The 3 additions to the original method were: the use of a Dowex, 1 x 2 (0.5 x 10.0), 2 step dilution and the use of a buffer blank. Urine samples were studied from normal male and female subjects, diurnal and nocturnal periods, and before and after a delivery. VMA did not exist in sulfate and glucuronide conjugates. VMA excretion values for 20 normal adults were: daytime ca. 9.9 μg DOMA/10 mg creatinine, while at night the corresponding value was about 4.2 μg. The pattern at parturition was characterized by a very high peak found in the 30 minute urine sample taken 150-180 minutes after delivery. In rabbits, DOMA values more than doubled after s.c. administration of either insulin or levarterenol.

Department of Pharmacology
Osaka University Medical School
Osaka, Japan

induced pathology.

Laboratorium voor Experimentele
   Geneeskunde
Rega Instituut
Universitaire Klinieken St. Rafaël
Louvain, Belgium

2520 Smith, Elizabeth R.B., & Weil-Mal-
herbe, H. Metanephrine and normetanephrine in human urine: method and results.
Journal of Laboratory and Clinical Medicine, 1962, 60, 212-223.

The amount of metanephrine and normetanephrine excreted were assayed through:
hydrolysis of urine at pH 1, passage through
an alumina column, electrodialytic desalt-
ing, incubation with sulfatase and adsorption of amines on a cation exchange resin.
The final eluate of the 2 amines was estimated fluorometrically on the principle
of the trihydroxyindole methods. Metha-
nephrine is oxidized at pH 3 and both
amines are oxidized in a separate aliquot
at pH 8. This method is able to estimate
0.02 μg metanephrine and 0.2 μg normetanephrine per sample. The mean 24-hour
excretion of metanephrine was 80 μg and
that of normetanephrine about 160 μg.
Although 4-hour excretion rates showed
definite diurnal variations in some individuals, these variations were not consistent
and their mean values, with 1 exception,
did not significantly deviate from the excretion rate calculated for the entire 24-
hour period. Variations in metanephrine
and normetanephrine excretion during successive 4-hour periods showed a highly
significant correlation.

Clinical Neuropharmacology Research
   Center
NIMH
Saint Elizabeths Hospital
Washington, D.C.

2521 Jérôme, Henri. Anomalies du méta-
bolisme du tryptophane dans la maladie
mongolienne. [Anomalies of tryptophan
metabolism in mongolism.] Bulletins et
Mémoires de la Société Médicale des Hôpitaux de Paris, 1962, 113, 168-172.

Determination of the α-amine nitrogen (Sör-
enson method) and total nitrogen (Kjeldahl
method) on 31 mongolian and 21 control
children showed no differences in the 24-
hour urine determinations of total nitrogen,
while the α nitrogen was significantly different in the mongolian children. The levels
of α-amine nitrogen and total nonprotein
nitrogen in the blood are higher in mongoli-
ans. The difference was, however, not
statistically significant. Mongolian children
excrete less creatinine than do normal
children of the same age, but the difference
in slope of the regression lines is not
statistically significant. Tryptophan metabolism tests show that mongolian children
excrete less 5HIAA, 3 indole acetic acid
(IAA) and xanthurenic acid, while the cy-
nurenine excretion is the same. The catabolism of 5HT to 5HIAA seems to be
normal in mongolian children. The deficit
in 5HIAA, IAA, xanthurenic acid elimination
in these children may be due to 1 of 2
causes: a higher renal threshold, or loss
of equilibrium of the intermediate metabolism.

Institut de Progenèse
15, rue de l'Ecole de Médecine
Paris 6°, France

2522   McLennan, H. Some effects of the
catecholamines on spinal cord reflexes.
Journal of Neuropsychiatry, 1962, 4, 125-
126.

Since systemic administration of epinephrine inhibits spinal reflexes, further
work was done to determine the effects of
topically and systemically administered
catecholamines (epinephrine, levarterenol,
and dopamine) on the spinal cord. Brain
extracts and dopamine shared a similarity
of action. Dopamine might bear some re-
semblance to the transmitter substance
active at inhibitory synapses; effects are
differently engendered than those which
follow topical application when produced
after systemic catecholamine administration. Stimulation of points in the bulbar
reticular formation inhibit spinal reflexes.
This inhibition may be blocked by dichloro-
isoproterenol (DCI) and strychnine but is
unaffected by dibenzyline or chlorpromazine. In an attempt to localize the site of

chemical method and conform to published figures. The method is simple, reliable, economical and adaptable to handling large numbers of samples.

[No address]

2527 Allgén, L.G., Izikowitz, S., Ordell, Inga-Britt, & Salum, Inna. Clinical biochemical studies in delirium tremens and other acute psychiatric sequels of alcohol abuse. I. Serum iron. Quarterly Journal of Studies on Alcohol, 1962, 23, 40-51.

The serum iron level was studied in 123 male alcoholics with delirium tremens and in 211 male patients with allied conditions in acute and convalescent stages. During the acute stage the group mean values of serum irons were below normal in more serious conditions (delirium tremens). The lowest mean value in any patient was 15 μg/100 ml. There was a steady decrease of group mean values (μg/100 ml) from the milder conditions to the more severe ones. Syndrome B_1 ca. 142.9, syndrome B_2 ca. 136.3, syndrome C 114.6, DT_1 ca. 80.5, DT_2 ca. 60.6 and DT_3 ca. 51.6. In the milder conditions there was a high percentage of abnormally high values, the highest mean being 305 μg/100 ml. In some cases a rapid decrease in the serum iron level was noted at an early stage. High serum iron values disappeared during convalescence. Among other causes, acute liver cell damage has been considered as possibly responsible for the hypersideremia and stress-induced changes in iron kinetics as possibly responsible for the hyposideremia.

Beckomberga Hospital
Bromma 4, Sweden

2528 Wallenius, Gunnar, Zaar, Bertil, & Lausing, Endel. A rapid method for determination of barbiturate in serum or urine. Scandinavian Journal of Clinical and Laboratory Investigation, 1962, 15, 252-256.

Serum (0.2 ml) or urine is soaked into an upper filter rod (CS 719 from Cigarette Components Limited, London) and 0.3 ml of Hg reagent solution [acidifed Hg $(NO_3)_2$] is pipetted into a lower filter rod; 0.3 ml dithizone solution is pipetted into a graduated test tube and the extraction column is fitted into the top of the tube. Chloroform is now slowly pipetted into the column on top of the sample-containing filter until a volume of 5 ml is drained down into the tube. Extraction takes about 1.5 minutes. Depending upon the amount and nature of the barbituric acid derivative, the color of the dithizone solution will turn from green to orange allowing spectrophotometric assay at 605 mμ.

Department of Clinical Chemistry
University Hospital
Uppsala, Sweden

2529 Brown, J.K., Malone, M.H., Stuntz, D.E., & Tyler, V.E. Paper chromatographic determination of muscarine in *Inocybe* species. Journal of Pharmaceutical Sciences, 1962, 51, 853-856.

A relatively simple paper chromatographic method was developed quantitatively to determine muscarine content in small dried samples of mushroom tissue in order to establish relative toxicity. This technique entailed duplicate spotting with suitable quantities (3-100 μl) of the purified extract on a buffered chromatogram. The chromatogram developed with Thies and Reuther's reagent to determine the minimum amount of extract which formed a detectable orange-red spot. Actual quantities applied varied according to the concentration of muscarine in the extract. If subsequent chromatograms verified initial observations, the quantity of extract producing a detectable muscarine spot was considered equivalent to 6 μg of muscarine. Concentrations of muscarine in dried carpophores were calculated from the resultant data. Application of the procedure to 34 species of *Inocybe* revealed detectable quantities of muscarine ranging from 0.01 to 0.80% in ca. 75%. No significant relationship was found between muscarine distribution and species differences.

College of Pharmacy
University of Washington
Seattle 5, Wash.

possible genetic nature of the lesion.

Department of Biochemistry
University of Western Ontario
London, Ontario
Canada

2534 Langer, Ella. Present and projected testing for phenylketonuria. Journal of the Maine Medical Association,1962,53,69-70.

The Division of Maternal and Child Health in Maine now conducts ferric chloride tests on infants and older children to screen for unsuspected phenylketonuria. Detection of a case is promptly followed by institution of a low phenylalanine diet to prevent mental deficiency. Of 3 cases detected early, 2 have manifested obvious I.Q. improvement. Eventually, it is hoped that hospital screening of newborns by the blood phenylalanine-agar diffusion tests will eventually replace the urine screening test in older children. Aspirin and some tranquilizers produce false positive results in the ferric chloride test.

Division of Maternal and Child Health and
    Crippled Children's Services
Augusta, Me.

2535 Lyons, J. Robert. Inhibition of mitochondrial ATP-ase and ATP-P_i exchange activity with Tofranil. Aviation and Medical Acceleration Laboratory Report, 1962, 6206,1-14.

Using Warburg manometry, in concentrations of 10^{-4}M and higher, imipramine inhibited phosphorylation and O_2 uptake in mitochondria (rat liver). An almost complete block of O_2 uptake and phosphorylation was observed with 10^{-3}M imipramine. A decrease in P/O ratio was observed with increasing imipramine concentrations. A decrease in the amount of ATP split with increasing concentrations was also observed, i.e., 10^{-6}-10^{-3}M imipramine. At 10^{-3}M imipramine caused ca. 50% inhibition of ATP-ase activity and the amount of ATP split approached O as the concentration of inhibitor increased. When the Mg/ATP molar ratio was kept constant at 0.13, imipramine was proven to cause noncompetitive inhibition of ATP-ase activity in mitochondria. Imipramine apparently competes with a site on the mitochondria which the substrate uses in order to participate in the reaction. Blocking ATP metabolism may prevent the cells from having an energy source available to maintain a normal potential difference across the membrane. If a presynaptic neuron did not release enough transmitter substance to cause the depolarization of the postsynaptic neuron, the postsynaptic neuron would not fire, but if the membrane potential of the postsynaptic neuron is lowered, then it may still be fired by a weaker transmitter. On the other hand the inhibitory in vitro effects described may have no bearing on drug action and merely represent toxicity.

Aviation and Medical Acceleration
    Laboratory
Johnsville, Pa.

2536   Beauvallet, M., Fugazza, J., & Solier, M. Nouvelles recherches sur les variations saisonnières de la noradrénaline cérébrale. [New studies on seasonal variations in cerebral levarterenol (noradrenalin).] Journal de Physiologie, 1962, 54, 289-290.

Periodically, the brains were removed and extracted from adult Wistar rats kept under the same conditions and temperatures for a year. Assay was made fluorometrically. The peak was 0.52 µg/g levarterenol in October, at the low 0.13 µg/g in June. The curve is presented below.

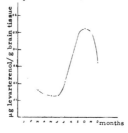

α-ketoglutarate	HD	hypnotic dose
Zuckerman's Affect Adjective Check List	5HIAA	5-hydroxyindoleacetic acid
	5HT	5-hydroxytryptamine
adrenocorticotropic hormone	5HTP	5-hydroxytryptophane
free choice		
adenosinediphosphate	i.a.	intraarterial
morning	ibid.	in the same place
American Medical Association	i.e.	that is
Article	i.m.	intramuscular
adenosinetriphosphate	IMPA	Lorr's Inpatient Multidimensional Psychiatric Scale
British antiLewisite	i.p.	intraperitoneal
benzyl analogue of serotonin	IPAT	Cattell's Institute for Personality & Ability Testing Anxiety Scale
twice a day		
bromolysergic acid diethylamide	I.Q.	intelligence quotient
blood urea nitrogen	IU	international unit
	i.v.	intravenous
Celsius scale		
about	kg	kilogram
conditioned avoidance response	K_i	Michaelis constant for an inhibitor
chronic brain syndrome	K_m	Michaelis constant for a substrate
cubic centimeter		
convulsive dose	lbs	pounds
centimeter	LD	lethal dose
square centimeter	LSD	lysergide
cubic centimeter		
Centre National de la Recherche Scientifique	μ	micron
	μc	microcurie
central nervous system	μg	microgram
catechol-o-methyl transferase	μl	microliter
counts per second	μM	micromolar
conditioned reflex (response)	$m\mu$	millimicrons
conditioned stimulus	M	molar
Climbing Time Delay	ma.	milliamperes
	MACC	Motility Affect Cooperation Communication
dichlorodiphenyl trichloroethane		
3, 4-dihydroxy-phenylalnine	MAO	monoamine oxidase
diphosphopyridineucleotide	MAS	Taylor Manifest Anxiety Scale
reduced diphosphopyridine-nucleotide	meq	milliequivalents
	ml	milliliter
	mm	millimeter
electrocardiogram	mm^2	square millimeter
editor	MMPI	Minnesota Multiphasic Personality Inventory
effective dose		
ethylenediaminetetraacetic acid	MSRP	Multidimensional Scale for Rating Psychiatric Patients
electroencephalogram		
for example		
electroretinogram	N	normal
and others	NEFA	nonesterified fatty acid
and so forth	NIMH	National Institute of Mental Health
Fahrenheit scale		
free fatty acid	p	probability
	PAH	para-aminohippuric acid
gram	PBI	protein-bound iodine
γ-aminobutyric acid	pH	negative logarithm of the hydrogen ion concentration
γ-amino-β-hydroxybutyric acid		

Pi	inorganic phosphate	TAT
P.M.	afternoon and evening	TH
p.o.	by mouth	t.i.d.
ppm	parts per million	TPN
PRP	Psychotic Reaction Profile	TPNH
q.i.d.	four times a day	TSH
refs.	references	U
Rf	ratio of the distance of dissolved substance to solvent distance	UR US
RNA	ribonucleic acid	USAF
ru	rat unit	USDHEW
s.c.	subcutaneous	USP
S.D.	standard deviation	USPHS
SGOT	serum glutamic oxaloacetic transaminase	UV
SGPT	serum glutamic pyruvic transaminase	VA
sic	exactly as found	viz.
SOSAI	Springfield Outpatient Symptom and Adjustment Index	WAIS
SRA	Science Research Associates	WPRS
Suppl.	supplement	

MCLENNAN H, 2522
MCMURRAY W C, 2533
MEAD WALTER R, 2352
MEDRADO VALDIR C, 2327
MEDUSKI J W, 2510
MEIRELLES PAULO, 2331
MELLINGER THEODORE J, 2492
MELLIWA HELMUT, 2303
MELMON KENNETH, 2432
MELSON F, 2453
MERCIER J, 2435
MERCIER-PAROT L, 2480
MERLIS SIDNEY, 2254
MERTZ E T, 2500
MEULEPAS E, 2519
MEYER J E, 2287
MEYER LUIZ, 2325
MICHAUX WILLIAM W, 2315, 2316
MICHEL J, 2293
MILLER NEAL E, 2401
MILLER ROBERT E, 2403
MIQUEL I, 2485
MIRIBEL, 2296
MISRAHY GEORGE, 2466
MIYAKE HIROSHI, 2514, 2515
MIYAZAKI, 2514
MOHYUDDIN F, 2533
MONCUIT M, 2501
MONNIER MARCEL, 2428, 2469
MONTANO CASTELLANOS R, 2372
MOORE HENRY W, 2389
MOREL P, 2371
MORGAN ANN M, 2452
MORILLO ARTURO, 2244
MULLER M, 2462
MUNEOKA A, 2513
MURPHREE HENRY B, 2341
MURPHY M LOIS, 2444
MUSTALA O O, 2437
MYERS ARLO K, 2393
MYSCHETZKY A, 2387
NAGLE GILBERTO J, 2322
NAKANISHI SUEHIRO, 2426
NAKAZIMA KAZUHIKO, 2502
NELSON THOMAS L, 2495
NICHOLSON A N, 2483
NOBLES W LEWIS, 2496
NORTON ALAN, 2256
NOVICK W J, 2458
NUKADA TADAATSU, 2509
NYIRI I, 2427
OCHS S, 2481
OGAWA NORUYA, 2403
OLIVEIRA JOSE DOMINGUES, 2331
ORDELL INGA-BRITT, 2527
ORLANDO ROBERT, 2313
OTA KAY Y, 2315
OTSUKA YASUO, 2426
OUACHI S, 2339
PAGET CHARLES, 2491

PAGNY JEANNETTE, 2418, 2419, 2450
PALAMOS SALAS T, 2410
PALEY HERBERT M, 2294
PASCALIS G, 2351
PENTTILA O I, 2437
PERIN M, 2381
PETERS RUDOLPH A, 2259
PETERS UWE H, 2308
PETSCHE H, 2460
PFANNMULLER B, 2490
PFEIFFER CARL C, 2341
PFLEGER K, 2415
PICK EDGAR, 2386
PLETSCHER A, 2261
PLOTNIKOFF N, 2406
PLUVINAGE R, 2523
PORTELLA JARBAS M, 2361
POSTERNAK J M, 2421
POTTS WILLIS J, 2272
POUGET, 2296
POULOS G L, 2405
PRIGOT AARON, 2367
PROCTOR RICHARD, 2254
PROUTY RICHARD W, 2452
PRULHIERE, 2478
PUECH J, 2376
PUNDER NORMA DE ARAUJO, 2329
PURDY MAUD B, 2396
PUT T R, 2510
RAHMANN H, 2394
RAKOSI M, 2427
RAMEL P, 2358
RATHBUN J C, 2533
RATOUIS ROGER, 2450
REINKE D, 2406
REMMER H, 2411
REYNOLDS L W, 2458
RIBEIRO SILVA ANTONIO, 2361
RIBEIRO SILVA IVAN, 2361
RICHET L, 2376
RIOS OSCAR, 2420
RIOU, 2349
ROBIN CH, 2376
RODEN THOMAS P, 2367
RODGERS DAVID A, 2395
ROMANOWSKI W, 2428, 2469
RONDISH I M, 2458
ROSEMBERGER, 2340
ROSIER Y, 2295
ROSSITER R J, 2533
ROTH M, 2336
ROTTMAN W, 2415
ROUFFIAC R, 2470
ROUQUETTE J, 2518
ROUSSELL A, 2340
ROUX G, 2470
RUDORFER LEON, 2294
RUESCH JURGEN, 2253
RUMMEL W, 2415
RUPHI M, 2421

998

999

1001

1013

ychopharmacology
BSTRACTS

vol. 2 no. 12
1962

DEPARTMENT OF HEALTH, EDUCATION, AND WELFARE
Public Health Service

PSYCHOPHARMACOLOGY ABSTRACTS is a publication of the
National Clearinghouse for Mental Health Information
of the National Institute of Mental Health. It is a
specialized information medium designed to assist the
Institute in meeting its obligation to foster and support laboratory and clinical research into the nature
and causes of mental disorders and methods of treatment and prevention. Specifically, this information
service is designed to meet the needs of investigators in the field of psychopharmacology for rapid and
comprehensive information about new developments and
research results.

PSYCHOPHARMACOLOGY ABSTRACTS is distributed gratis to
investigators doing research in psychopharmacology. It
is not available on a subscription basis. Requests
to receive the ABSTRACTS should be accompanied by a
brief statement of the research interests and scientific specialty of the investigator. Requests to receive the ABSTRACTS, address changes, and other communications should be addressed to:

> Psychopharmacology Abstracts
> National Clearinghouse for Mental
>   Health Information
> National Institute of Mental Health
> Bethesda, Maryland 20014

(The text of PSYCHOPHARMACOLOGY ABSTRACTS is prepared
under contract with the Literary Division of Biological and Medical Services, Philadelphia, Penna.)

U. S. DEPARTMENT OF HEALTH, EDUCATION, AND WELFARE
Public Health Service
National Institutes of Health
National Institute of Mental Health
Bethesda, Maryland 20014

Psychopharmacology Abstracts

Volume 2, Number 11

leptics; the tranquilizing effect.] Concours
Médical, 1961, 83, 6761-6762; 6764.

Nervous sedatives or tranquilizers are
drugs directed against anxiety from multiple causes. Among the older drugs, barbiturates still have their indications. Among
the newer neuroleptics in wide application
are: hydroxyzine, glutethimide, meprobamate, chlordiazepoxide, thioridazine, levomepromazine and benactyzine. Some of
these are used in high dosages in the
treatment of psychoses. (No refs.)

Clinique Neuropsychiatrique
Faculté de Toulouse
Toulouse, France

2541 Chih-fan, Ch'eng, & Ch'i-shan,
Chang. Some early records of nervous and
mental diseases in traditional Chinese medicine. Chinese Medical Journal, 1962,
81, 55-59.

The history of nervous and mental disease
in the Chinese classics and medical literature from ancient times through the
Ming and Ch'ing Dynasties (1368-1911)
is briefly reviewed. During the T'ang dynasty various attempts were made to classify these aberrations. The major contribution to the study of these diseases was
made by Wang K'en-t'ang of the Ming
Dynasty who explicitly categorized insan-
ity as composed of schizophrenia, mania
and seizures. In the 11th century nervous
and mental diseases were differentiated
from organic diseases. Various treatments
used in addiction and acupuncture included:
Epedra sinica, Siler divar icatum, alm-
ond, Atractylis ovata and gypsum in the
7th century and drugs derived from mercury, musk and ox bezoar, introduced in
the 12th century. (10 refs.)

Department of Medical History
Peking Medical College
Peking, China

2542 Batrinos, M.L., & DeVerbizier, J.
L'action de la chlorpromazine sur le système endocrinien. [Action of chlorpromazine on the endocrine system.] Revue
Française d'Etudes Cliniques et Biolo-

giques, 1962, 7, 87-97.

Clinically chlorpromazine may produce galactorrhea and disturbances in the menstrual cycle, usually amenorrhea. ACTH secretion in response to stress is suppressed; however the daily output of adrenal hormones does not seem to be affected, nor are thyroid hormone plasma levels. Its action is predominantly central, affecting the supraepiphyseal regional inhibiting centers which control pituitary secretion; there is also some direct effect on other endocrine glands. Simultaneous effect on different areas makes the evaluation of action difficult. In laboratory animals chlorpromazine at high doses has the following actions: a/ transitory stimulation of ACTH secretion; a partial depression of ACTH release in response to stress; no effect on exogenous ACTH, b/ disturbance of the sexual cycle tropins, c/ induction of mammary gland development and stimulation of secretion, d/ inhibition of TH secretion and direct depression of thyroid uptake of radioactive iodine, e/ increase of water retention following hydration both by stimulating ADH production and by facilitating its peripheral action, f/ neutralization or reversal of the hypertensive action of epinephrine without hindering other actions (the hypertensive action of levarterenol is also neutralized) and g/ hyperglycemic effects. (149 refs.)

Hôpital Broussais
Paris, France

2543   Stevenin, L. Les rapports de la psychothérapie et de la psychopharmacologie au Congrés de psychothérapie de Vienne (août 1961). [Reports on psychotherapy and psychopharmacology at the Vienna Psychotherapy Congress, August, 1961.] Annales Médico-Psychologiques, 1962, 120, 1, 849.

The association of psychotherapy with drug treatments in psychoses diminishes the number of relapses, and frequently in neuroses drugs are indispensable for the reduction of anxiety. The integration of psychotherapy with medical and pharmacological treatments was promulgated by a number of speakers. The author and Benoit suggested 3 therapeutic means of approach; narcoanalysis, weck analysis and dream analysis

phenylketonuria. Phenylketonuria has been induced in rats and mice. A phenylalanine-free diet initiated immediately after birth will frequently obviate development of mental retardation. Optimal results accrue from maintenance of the diet for a sustained period of time, even for life. (64 refs.)

Biochemical Laboratory
Pineland Hospital and Training Center
Pownal, Me.

2549 Eyres, Alfred E. Observations on psychiatry in certain areas of the Orient and the Middle East. Journal of Neuropsychiatry, 1962, 3, 171-176.

A description is given of the psychiatric facilities observed in a 6 week trip taken by the Eastern Psychiatric Research Association. Fifteen member psychiatrists visited Japan, Hong Kong, Thailand, India and Israel. In Japan, ECT has frequently been replaced by drug therapy. Methamphetamine addiction is a serious problem in Japan, while Thailand has numerous opium addicts. Thailand boasts treatment regimens for the mentally ill which include psychotherapy, pharmacotherapy and ECT. Psychiatric facilities are abysmal in India, with ECT constituting the mainstay for treatment. Israel enjoys good medical facilities, with ECT, insulin shock therapy and pharmacotherapy readily available for good psychiatric care. (No refs.)

Eastland Center Professional Building
17800 East Eight Mile Road
Detroit 36, Mich.

2550 Denber H.C.B., & Rajotte, P. Brèves considérations méthodologiques sur l'évaluation clinique des médicaments psychotropes. [Brief methodologic considerations on the clinical evaluation of psychoactive drugs.] Comptes Rendus du Congrés des Médecins Aliénistes et Neurologistes (Montpellier, 10-15 July, 1961), 1962, 370-373; discussion 374. Montpellier: A. Coueslant.

Among the various parameters which must be taken into account in the evaluation of psychoactive drugs are the population of the patients, hospital conditions and the personality of the investigator. The use of objective techniques such as double-blind, crossover, etc. are of aid in obtaining better comparisons. Emphasis is placed on the evaluation of haloperidol, butyrylperazine and chlorprothixene. In the discussion Fouks noted that chemotherapy allows contact with the patient and thereby increases the chances of psychosocial therapies. (13 refs.)

[No address]

2551 Heymans, C. Considérations sur l'interprétation des effets de l'électrochoc chez l'organisme réserpiné. [Considerations on the interpretation of electroshock effects in the reserpinized body.] Bulletin de l'Académie Royale de Médecine de Belgique, 1962, 2, 142-146.

The importance of peripheral catecholamine depletion caused by reserpine, without exclusion of the possibility of central action by the alkaloid, in relation to its utility in ECT, is reviewed. ECT causes hypertension in the normal animal through excitation of the vasoconstrictor centers. In the reserpinized animal, excitation of vasoconstrictor centers cannot act on the peripheral vessels because reserpine has depleted catecholamines at this level and thereby blocks peripheral vasoconstrictive adrenergic transmission. Marked prolonged apnea following ECT in the reserpinized animal is essentially due to the marked and prolonged reserpinized-induced drop in blood pressure. (15 refs.)

[No address]

2552 Finney, D.J. Placebomania and the interpretation of clinical trials. Journal of New Drugs, 1962, 2, 327-332.

Statistical interpretation of clinical trials falls prey to the following hazards: investgators inept in the more sophisticated aspects of statistical analysis, application of inappropriate statistical tests, arithmetic errors, inherent group differences, extraneous factors and failure to recognize efficacy of treatment. Other problems include an erroneous hypothesis, overcomplicated trial design, misinterpretation of

Pharmacopeia Nomenclature Committee are the following psychoactive drugs: pargyline, levamfetamine and hydroxyphenamate. (No refs.)

660 Madison Avenue
New York 21, N.Y.

2557 Journal of New Drugs. Generic names of new drugs. Journal of New Drugs, 1962, 2, 63-64.

Thalidomide and amphecloral are among the generic names for drugs which have recently been adopted by the AMA-United States Pharmacopeia Nomenclature Committee. Assignment of a generic name does not imply endorsement of the drug. (No refs.)

660 Madison Avenue
New York 21, N.Y.

2558 Shepherd, Michael, & Wing, Lorna. Pharmacological aspects of psychiatry. Advances in Pharmacology, 1962, 1, 227-276.

The multitudinous ramifications of pharmacology in psychiatry are based upon optimal methods of studying psychotropic drugs such as animal studies (which encompass motor functions, perception and discrimination, learning, memory and reasoning, emotion and motivation, fear and conflict), and studies in human subjects. Classification and description of psychotropic drugs include the major tranquilizers (the phenothiazines, reserpine and its congeners and the butyrophenones), the minor tranquilizers (phenothiazines and diphenylmethane derivatives), sedatives, centrally acting anticholinergics, thymoleptics (amphetamine, phenothiazine analogues and MAO inhibitors), psychotomimetic drugs (mescaline, LSD, cholinergic blocking agents and phencyclidine), transitional compounds (chlordiazepoxide and thioxanthene derivatives). Chemical interpretations of mental aberrations have resulted in proferring of postulates like the adrenaline-adrenolutin hypothesis and analogous serotonin metabolism as etiological factors in mental illness. Other relevant topics include the quantitative effects of psychotropic drugs on humans, and the role of clinical studies related to psychotropic drugs. (287 refs.)

Institute of Psychiatry
Maudsley Hospital
London, Great Britain

2559 Committee on Public Health, New York Academy of Medicine. The importance of clinical testing in determining the efficacy and safety of drugs. Journal of New Drugs, 1962, 2, 135-151.

The quest for new products led the pharmaceutical companies to embark upon research and development programs which have had almost incredible ramifications. Growth and expansion have necessitated federal controls, and the FDA once again has seen fit to impose more stringent regulations to protect the American consumer. Many profound alterations have been made in the Food, Drug and Cosmetic Act, including development of a new set of regulations for the pharmaceutical advertising industry. A report by the Professional Committee of the Pharmaceutical Manufacturers Association includes the following topics: deliberations on clinical testing, present quality of clinical testing, adequacy of supply of qualified clinical testers, utilization of available investigators, past attempts toward organization and new proposals. (28 refs.)

[No address]

2560 Friend, Dale G. Clinical evaluation of new drugs. Journal of New Drugs, 1962, 2, 152-159.

In clinical testing, the nature of the drug undergoing study largely predicates the type of evaluation program which will be carried out. Once sufficient animal toxicity testing and preliminary human testing have been performed, the drug is ready to be utilized by the clinical investigator. All drug investigations in patients should be initiated in the controlled atmosphere of hospital practice. Individual subjects should be carefully determined for each preparation. Interpretation of information secured from clinical evaluation requires a high degree of

accuracy and insight. New drugs should not be introduced into medicine unless they possess definite, proven merit. (1 ref.)

Peter Bent Brigham Hospital
Boston, Mass.

2561 Marks, John. Placebomania. Journal of New Drugs, 1962, 2, 71-77.

Clinical assessment of new drugs should encompass a pilot study or screening device followed by a thorough clinical trial where indicated. Controlled trials are most efficacious when double-blind or placebo methods are instituted as safeguards to maintain drug anonymity. Study designs now in vogue include the crossover, Latin square or incomplete block test. Legal and ethical problems may often be obviated in new drug testing merely by substituting standard therapy in lieu of the placebo. Placebomania results from erroneous hypotheses, incorrect criteria for assessment of results, extraneous biasing factors, excess faith in double-blind trials, complicated data collection procedures, negative effects of intervals between active drug administration, dearth of comprehension regarding statistical analysis, ignorance of randomization procedures and effects derived from standard therapy which influence trial results. Careful clinical observation will never be replaced by the placebo. (2 refs.)

[No address]

2562 Paget, G.E. Toxicity tests: a guide for clinicians. Journal of New Drugs, 1962, 2, 78-83.

Toxicity tests are useful to predict what will happen when a compound is given to human beings. Such predictions may be quantitative; an estimate of what drug dosage will cause an effect, or qualitative; what effect will occur with a given dose. In animals, the only important quantitative consideration which exists in toxicity testing is the way in which animal data are to be extrapolated from species to species. Toxicity tests most readily detect severe universal poisons which are likely to cause clinical catastrophes. Regardless of how

St. John's University
Jamaica, Long Island
N. Y.

2564 Sanchez F. Murias, D. Benjamin.
Tranquilizantes en médicina. [Tranquili-
zers in medicine.] Annales de la Real
Academia Nacional de Médicina, 1962, 79,
95-146.

Delay's classification and that of Lattanzi
techniques of evaluation, effects on behavior (including spider web building, nest
building activity in rats, aggressiveness in
monkeys, induction of fear in rats and aggressiveness in monkeys, induction of fear
in rats and aggressiveness of Siamese
fighting fish), conditioning experiments,
the study of reflexes (righting reflex, rotarod, traction, rotating cylinder, etc.), action
on the lower centers of the CNS, action
on the electrical activities of the brain,
interaction with convulsants, morphine,
lysergide (LSD), and with hypnotics and
general anesthetics, the mechanism of action (relationships to 5HT), modification in
oxytoxic response, interaction with novocaine and similar agents, and side effects
are reviewed. (78 refs.)

[No address]

2565 Diseases of the Nervous System.
Investigation of thalidomide deformities.
Diseases of the Nervous System, 1962,
23, 455. [Editorial].

Dr. Charles H. Frantz, orthopedic consul-
tant to the area Child Amputee Center
of the Michigan Crippled Children Commis-
sion, Grand Rapids, Mich., has been selected to aid Germany in solving problems created by the recent birth of 3,500-
5,000 thalidomide babies. He will investigate the deformities caused by thalidomide
and the methods devised by German scientists in fitting infants with prosthetic
devices. (No refs.)

[No address]

2566 Jerome, Joseph B. Selecting generic
names for new drugs. Journal of New Drugs,

1962, **2**, 276-282.

The A.M.A. and U.S. Pharmacopeia have
established the A.M.A.-U.S.P. Cooperative
Program under the auspices of a joint
Nomenclature Committee to facilitate the
adoption of acceptable generic names for
drugs. Specific procedures must be followed, in keeping with the concepts of sim-
plicity of generic name and maintenance
of relationship in nonproprietary names in
chemically related drugs used within a
given therapeutic area. Manufacturers are,
of course, closely consulted by the Committee in order to arrive at a decision
which is suitable to all concerned. Family
names like the tetracyclines, sulfonamides
and penicillins present horrendous nomenclature problems which must be simpli-
fied. Some names will be retained despite their cumbersome aspects since they
have been universally adopted. The general principles for guidance in devising international nonproprietary names for pharmaceutical preparations are presented in
tabular form. (No refs.)

[No address]

2567   Cole, Jonathan O. Evaluation of drug
treatments in psychiatry. Journal of New
Drugs, 1962, **2**, 264-275.

Close attention must be paid to all aspects
of the milieu in order to assure validity
in clinical trials of psychoactive drugs
like chlorpromazine and reserpine, which
have been in use for 10 years. Multitudinous factors influence the outcome of
a given study, and all must be considered
in the final evaluation. Drugs encourage
far more flexibility than psychotherapy
and permit utilization of biochemical changes to determine pharmacological effect.
The observational acumen and clinical
judgement of the investigator and his team
are of paramount importance in establishing adequate evaluation procedures. Work
with chronic schizophrenics poses many
difficult problems. Such individuals are
generally drug resistant and non-coopera-
tive, with a poor initial prognosis. However,
such patients exist in a controlled atmosphere under constant supervision. In acute
schizophrenia, studies reveal few differ-

PC 603, a monamine oxidase inhibitor, and amitriptyline, a derivative of the dibenzo-cyclo-heptadines.] Annales Médico-Psychologiques, 1962, 120, 1, 144.

Improvement in basic EEG rhythm in depressive states, absence of clinical epileptic seizure provoking activity, the appearance or aggravation of generally transitory abnormalities in the EEG tracings of epileptics with an absence of correlative aggravation in the clinical picture are noted for both amitriptyline and PC 603 (p-chlorophenoxyacetic isopropylhydrazine) [dosages unspecified]. The problem of criteria of psychotonic activity in the EEG is still current. EEG aggravations caused by psychotonics, however transitory and fluctuating, are often paradoxically in opposition to successful clinical results. (No refs.)

[No address]

2572 Northwest Medicine. Thalidomide. 1962, 61, 651. [Editorial]

The recent tendency toward more stringent drug regulations resulting from the thalidomide furor is decried on the basis of the deleterious effects of excessive governmental intervention in industry. Invectives are hurled at the President, Dr. F. Kelsey, and the government in general. (No refs.)

Northwestern Medicine
500 Wall St.
Seattle 1, Wash.

2573 Soulairac, A., Halpern, B., Grisoni, F., Brunhès, M., Frélot, Cl., Geier, S., & Ochonisky, J. Intéret des échelles de J.R. Wittenborn en récherche clinique psychiatrique. [The Wittenborn scales in clinical psychiatric research.] Annales Médico-Psychologiques, 1962, 1, 354-389.

Use of the Wittenborn scales as an aid in the objective description of psychic states and the effect of various drugs upon them is illustrated by profile for 5 examples out of 31 schizophrenics who had received various treatments [dosages unspecified] and were subsequently treated with chlorprothixene, followed by haloperidol therapy. Condition composed were: profile before treatment, after a month of chlorprothixene, a month after the chlorprothixene therapy and 3 out of the 5 cases after 1 month of haloperidol. These profiles indicate that objectivization of clinical observation is possible and useful in treating psychic stages. (5 refs.)

Centre Psychiatrique Ste-Anne, Paris, France

2574   Borel, A. Champignons, noyau indolique et psychisme. [Mushroom, the indole nucleus and psychism.] Journal des Sciences Médicales de Lille, 1962, 80, 119-130.

Amanita muscaria is toxic but generally not fatal. It induces disturbances of vision, auditory and visual hallucinations, amnesia, gaiety, and affects the parasympathetic system. Mexican hallucinogens include peyotl, *Datura* sp., *Rivea corymbosa* and *Sophora secundiflora*, as well as various *Psilocybe* and *Stropharia*. The active principles of these drugs have been isolated by extraction and analyzed chromatographically. These are 4-hydroxy-dimethyl tryptamine, and the phosphorylized derivatives of this compound (in position 4). Psychic effects include visions consisting of garish sights overlaid on steep streets and buildings. Ability to think and to remember is only slightly affected. *Panaeolus* fungi have similar effects. LSD, at doses of 0.5-2 mg/kg creates agitation, vertigo, semi-ebriety, characterized by extreme activity of the imagination. LSD had an indole structure. Dimethyltryptamine is hallucinogenic, as are also various methyl tryptamines, and also those derivatives which are obtained by phosphorylization on the 4th carbon atom. 5HT (serotonin), which is also an indole compound, may induce hallucinations and convulsions by slowing oxygen passage through the brain. Both LSD and psilocybin are used in anxiety neuroses and obsessive states for the facilitation of recall, particularly of early childhood traumas.

[No address]

2575   Lange, P. Über die Rolle der γ - Aminobuttersaure im Zentralnervensystem [The role of GABA in the central nervous system.] Zeitschrift für Ärztliche Fortbild-

Center of Alcohol Studies
Rutgers University
New Brunswick, N. J.

2580 Remmen, Edmund, Cohen, Sidney,
Ditman, Keith S., & Frantz, John Russell.
Psychochemotherapy.   The   Physician's
Manual. Los Angeles: Western Medical
Publications, 1962, Pp. 152.

This book is written as a guide to the
general practitioner. Mental illness, the
classification and diagnosis of mental illness, modern concepts on its biochemical
nature and information on psychotropic
drugs are presented. Copious miscellaneous
information is detailed on diagnostic aids
and sites of drug action with an emphasis
on dosage schedules for patients in private
practice. (317 refs.)

Western Medical Publications
Los Angeles, Calif.

2581 Brooks, Clyde. The new role of
the general practitioner in the treatment
of mental cases with the new psychobolic
drugs. Louisiana State Medical Society,
1962, **114**, 291-293.

Tranquilizers should be renamed psychobolic drugs, a classification which encompasses reserpine and thioridazine as typical examples. Improvements in psychiatric
training will result in greater treatment
of mental patients on an outpatient basis.
Reserpine (2.5 mg/ml parenterally) is advocated as the drug of choice, despite
side effects which include slow pulse and
hypotension. Mental patients may be treated
by psychotherapy, ECT or medical therapy,
including psychoactive drugs. Maintenance
therapy with reserpine (2-4 mg/day p.o.
interspersed with 5 mg i.m., b.i.d.) is
highly efficacious. (No refs.)

Alabama State Hospitals
Tuscaloosa, Ala.

2582 Dorfman, Wilfred. Depression and
psychosomatic illness. Southwestern Medicine, 1962, **43**, 195-197.

Obesity, coronary disease and rheumatic disorders are cited as conditions which may coexist with depression. In relation to treatment, the 2 major factors are the nature of the depression and the orientation etc. of the therapist. ECT, psychotherapy and pharmacotherapy all have their exponents. Neurotic or reactive depressions are best handled by psychotherapy. In some cases antidepressants may act as synergists in psychotherapy and provide greater acceptability. Some of the new drugs can eliminate ECT or cut down the number of treatments. These newer drugs include phenelzine, isocarboxazid, nialamide, imipramine and amitriptyline. Amitriptyline is preferable when high levels of anxiety accompany the depression. Difficulties in drug evaluation are noted. (10 refs.)

Department of Psychiatry
Maimonides Hospital of Brooklyn
Brooklyn, N.Y.

2583 Lasagna, Louis. Some explored and unexplored psychological variables in therapeutics. Proceedings of the Royal Society of Medicine, 1962, 55, 773-776.

Considerable psychological variation accounts for discrepancies in response to various medication. Most healthy volunteers treated with amphetamine or opiates are euphoric and mentally stimulated by amphetamine but a minority react with depression and sedation. Differential responses to morphine and heroin follow an analogous pattern. The toxicity of CNS stimulants is markedly enhanced in animals placed in a crowded environment. A doctor's tendency to innovate is based upon his individuality and his social position among other doctors. Psychological and sociological variables must be taken into consideration in drug evaluations. (20 refs.)

Johns Hopkins University
School of Medicine
Baltimore, Md.

2584 Gerecke, K., & Koch, K. Über den Verkehr mit Betaubnugsmittein. IV. Mitteilung. [Traffic in narcotics. IV. Communication.] Pharmazie, 1962, 12, 205-214.

cium carbimide and antidiabetic sulfonamides like tolbutamide. (28 refs.)

Alcoholism and Drug Addiction Research
    Foundation
Toronto, Ontario
Canada

2589 Gerscovich, José. Sub-coma insu-
línico. [Insulin sub-coma.] Revista Brasileira de Medicina, 1962, 19, 684-686.

The history of insulin coma therapy is
presented and contrasted to the technique
of insulin sub-coma therapy. Objectives,
contraindications (cardiac, hepatic or renal
disorders, or diabetes) clinical and laboratory test preparation for treatment,
adjunct and the technique itself, as well
as complications and secondary shock are
elucidated. (No refs.)

Sociedade Brasileira de Psiquiatria,
Neurologia e Medicina Legal
Rio de Janeiro, Brazil

2590 Medical Science. Poisons and Mental
Function. Medical Science, 1962, 12, 64-69.
[Editorial]

Compounds such as atropine, scopolamine
and some related synthetic drugs used in
the treatment of parkinsonism cause mental
and behavioral abnormalities through their
effect on acetylcholine. On the other hand,
substances like physostigmine, diisopropyl
fluorophosphate and some weed killers
increased acetylcholine amounts by inhibiting or destroying cholinesterase, and these
caused similar mental changes. Chronic
heavy mental poisoning, e.g., mercury, may
also mimic endogenous psychiatric disorders. Unsaturated indoles can cause depersonalization and sometimes hallucinations. One of these, LSD, occurred in
ergot, the fungus which grows on rye.
Carelessly made rye flour may cause epi-
demics of psychosis among those who eat
the bread made from it. Bufotenin and
its phosphate ester psilocybin are also
unsaturated indoles, occurring in mushrooms. Another of this type is harmine,
related to reserpine and yohimbine. Adrenolutin is also an unsaturated indole that

causes mental changes; spoiled epinephrine contains it. When sprayed into the airways in large amounts it may produce psychosis. The nonindolic hallucinogens, mescaline and marihuana, are noted. Barbiturates may cause excitement and confusion, particularly in elderly patients. Adrenosteroids often cause some degree of euphoria and may in some instances produce melancholia or schizophrenialike psychoses. Commonly used tranquilizers may cause severe stubborn depressions, e.g., the prolonged use of reserpine in hypertension. (No refs.)

227 S. 6th St.
Philadelphia, Pa.

2591 Connell, P.H. The amphetamines -
I. Medical World, 1962, 96, 18-20.

Amphetamines in clinical use today include ephedrine, epinephrine, levarterenol, deoxyphedrine and phenmetrazine. Related compounds which are effective anti-depressants include nialamide and tranylcypromine. Metabolic pathways remain nebulous, but relatively large amounts of the original dose are excreted unaltered in the urine. All amphetamines exert a general stimulating effect on the CNS coupled with a euphoriant action, appetite suppression and narcotic antagonism. Amphetamines appear to effect the reticular arousal system in the brainstem. Mild, undesirable side effects include dry mouth, insomnia, palpitations, headache, impotence, etc. With regard to CNS activity dexamphetamine is the most potent compound. (No refs.)

Newcastle General Hospital
Newcastle-on-Tyne Great Britain

2592 Hope, Justin M. The anxiety state.
Medical World, 1962, 96, 9-15.

Anxiety states encompass periodic acute attacks, headache, nervousness, palpitation, irritability, diffuse fear, sexual maladjustment, choking or smothering, trembling, precordial or chest oppression, dizziness, precordial or chest pain and fainting. Few positive findings are detected by physical examination. Anxiety is of unknown etiology. Differential diagnosis must include

In almost all instances of acute disturbance, a fundamental etiological factor is
that the patient himself is very frightened
or even panicky. Those around the patient
may demand that the doctor "do something immediately." The physician's role
is to allay anxiety and establish trust.
One first step is getting him to assent
to some medication such as 3.75-7.5 grains
of amobarbital or $\frac{1}{4}$ grain of morphine
i.m. After some quieting, 25-50 mg chlorpromazine is useful; blood pressure should
be observed and the patient watched for
a hypotensive reaction. The synergism
between a barbiturate and a phenothiazine
is useful. If force is indicated, a show of
force may suffice. The legal status of
the doctor is noted. (No refs.)

Minneapolis General Hospital
Minneapolis, Minn.

2598 Lesse, Stanley. Placebo reactions
in psychotherapy. Diseases of the Nervous
System, 1962, 23, 313-319.

Placebo reactions in general encompass
pure placebos (inert compounds), placebo
(drug or procedure), placebo effect (reaction), and positive or negative placebos.
The largest and most enduring number of
positive placebo reactions are obtained by
physicians who are optimistic and promul-
gate strong convictions with regard to the
anticipated positive response to be elicited
from a given drug or procedure. A similar
patient attitude is instrumental in evoking
this positive response. The forces which
determine manifestation of a placebo reaction play a vital role in determining the
final results in any psychotherapeutic
procedure. In evaluation procedures, the
question of spontaneous remissions must
also be considered. (No refs.)

Neurological Institute of New York
Department of Neurology
Columbia University
New York, New York

2599 Rice, Carl O. Tranquility and tranquilizers. Minnesota Medicine, 1962, 45,
1025. [Editorial]

Before the advent of tranquilizers, the word tranquility meant a calm state of mind. Now the search of tranquility appears to be the province of neurotics, psychopaths and others of unstable makeup. Perhaps the individual for whom tranquilizers are often prescribed is normally and temporarily distraught at various life situations. (No refs.)

[No address]

2600 Connell, P.H. The amphetamines - II. Medical World, 1962, 96, 106-111.

Amphetamines are used clinically for narcolepsy, parkinsonism, epilepsy, barbiturate poisoning, drug addiction, alcoholism, psychopathic states, behavior disorders in children, enuresis and depression. Drugs should be administered in a manner which minimized side effects and all patients should receive frequent reassessments. The most serious consequence of amphetamine administration is addiction. Other side effects include a "schizophrenic type" of psychosis, shock and collapse and the omnipresent risk of suicide. Amphetamine toxicity resembles alcohol intoxication and should not be so misdiagnosed. A hypersensitivity to sympathomimetics or any condition encompassing Reynaud's phenomenon contraindicates amphetamine administration. (15 refs.)

Newcastle General Hospital
Newcastle, Great Britain

2601 Aldridge, M.S. Open Way Psychotherapy Clinic. Medical World, 1962, 96 463-467.

The Open Way Clinic in London, England provides expert psychotherapy at low cost, with an analytically oriented staff, objective attitude and emphasis on drug utilization combined with psychotherapy. Drugs like chlorpromazine are essential adjuncts to other types of therapy. Psychotherapy is never used merely for the purpose of placation. Most patients pay a minimum fee and attend the clinic twice a week. Similar clinics are sorely needed.

Open Way Psychotherapy Clinic
London, Great Britain

2602 Cunningham, John J. Alcoholism. Minnesota Medicine, 1962, 45, 1029-1035.

The incidence and nature of alcoholism, alcoholism, alcohol addiction, withdrawal signs and symptoms and treatment are reviewed. Adrenal cortex extract in delirium tremens, with later suppression of craving for alcohol is cited, along with the use of glutamine as a nutritional supplement, again suppressing the urge to drink. (No refs.)

[No address]

2603 Romano, John. Psychiatric research and medicine. Medical World, 1962, 96, 281-287.

Psychiatric research appears to lag behind that undertaken in other areas of medicine. Psychiatric training aids fledgling physicians to achieve a higher degree of insight and critical perceptiveness. Psychiatry has contributed much to medicine, particularly psychoanalytic theory, where the unitary concept and team approach have been very valuable. The family doctor eases patients through the many crisis periods in their lives. The functions of the family doctor are diagnostic and judgmental, preventive, therapeutic, integrative, investigative and educational. The prevailing tendency to rely on tranquilizers as panaceas must be critically scrutinized. Treatment of psychotics with insulin shock, ECT, pentetrazol chemical sleep has not produced direct therapeutic benefit, except for ECT in depression. While more understanding of neural organization is needed, there is evidence of beginning relatedness in studies in animals and men between behavior, learning etc.

University of Rochester
Rochester, N.Y.

2604 Sussex, James N. Drugs used in psychiatric treatment. Medical Record and Annals, 1962, 55, 225-229.

pounds. Carbromal is an acylated urea, and is still used as a sedative. However, diethylacetamide and carbamide compounds can, if used over a long time, produce confusion and other difficulties. Barbiturates are highly effective and new ones are constantly being added. Barbiturates may be divided into four classes, based upon the duration of their effects: long-acting, average duration, short and ultra-short. Tolerance is increased by changes in the barbituric acid ring proper. Administration methods of various sedatives and hypnotics has been improved through the development of the sustained-release tablets. Tranquilizers are a development of the 1950's, meprobamate being the most prominent example. Phenothiazines and reserpine are detailed. Work with antihistamines has led to the development of phenothiazines with psychosedative effects. While psychotherapeutic drugs are extremely valuable they should be dispensed with proper precautions as prescription drugs, and not as over-the-counter items. (No refs.)

[No address]

2607 Hoch, Paul H., & Zubin, Joseph. [Eds.] The future of psychiatry. New York: Grune & Stratton, 1962. Pp. 1-271.

Multiple disciplinary cooperation in psychiatry is stressed. Neurochemistry may in the next decade further the understanding of behavioral disorders. More objective criteria are becoming available in the experimental laboratory which supplement the judgement of the clinician. Various new techniques and electronic devices are now promoting progress in psychiatry, and particularly in psychopharmacology. The 4 parts of the book are entitled: future of neurophysiologic and neurochemical approaches; future of psychologic, social and educational approaches; future of conceptual systems; and future of genetic, developmental, and organic approaches. (313 refs.)

Department of Mental Hygiene
State of New York
New York, N.Y.

2608 Evarts, Edward V. Speculations concerning future applications of neurophysiologic techniques to psychiatric research. In: Hoch, Paul H., & Zubin, Joseph [Eds.] The future of psychiatry. New York: Grune & Stratton, 1962. Pp. 1-10.

Previously, psychiatric problems have been refractory to solution by neurophysiological techniques, but these same techniques, especially the EEG, have been successfully applied to research on behavioral disturbances. Very revealing studies have been performed concerning evoked responses in patients with behavioral disorders. The EEG permits detection of electrical periodicities, which in turn may be correlated with relevant behavior. Much information has been gleaned from evoked potentials in animals using LSD, chlorpromazine and reserpine. (18 refs.)

Laboratory of Clinical Science
NIMH
Bethesda, Md.

2609 Waelsch, Heinrich. The future of neurochemistry and psychiatry. In: Hoch, Paul H., & Zubin, Joseph [Eds.] The future of psychiatry. New York: Grune & Stratton, 1962. Pp. 11-18.

The biochemist is searching in the mentally ill patient for metabolic reactions concomitant with mental phenomena. General reactions such as energy metabolism and specialized ones such as the metabolism of nitrogen compounds and nucleic acids or lipids are of special interest, e.g., the work of Rolf Gjessing on nitrogen metabolism in periodic catatonia. Much of the future biochemical research in psychiatry will be taken up by the search for abnormal metabolites and hypotheses involving the inborn errors of metabolism. Pharmacology and psychopharmacology will become a branch of neurobiology once they are able to interpret drug action in terms of changes in cellular metabolism. (7 refs.)

New York State Psychiatric
   Institute
New York, N.Y.

2614 Roessler, Robert, & Greenfield, Norman S. [Eds.] Physiological correlates of psychological disorder. St. Paul: University of Wisconsin Press, 1962. Pp. 1-281.

The papers in this volume were originally presented at a conference entitled "Physiological Correlates of Psychological Disorder" held at the University of Wisconsin, August 29-31, 1961. Reports are included from laboratories studying the relationship between intermediate carbohydrate metabolism and schizophrenia, adrenocortical function and anxiety, autonomic nervous system variables and psychological measures, and from laboratories active in elucidating psychological factors in somatic disease. Abstracts for 11 of the 15 chapters are presented in this issue of Psychopharmacology Abstracts, i.e., those chapters dealing with psychoactive drugs. (481 refs.)

Department of Psychiatry
University of Wisconsin Medical Center
Madison, Wisc.

2615 Malamud, William. Introduction: major trends in twentieth-century psychiatric research. In:Roessler, Robert, & Greenfield, Norman S. [Eds.] Physiological correlates of psychological disorder. St. Paul: University of Wisconsin Press, 1962. Pp. 3-11.

Cannon's concept of homeostasis, defined as a mechanism which enables organisms continually subjected to wide environmental variations to maintain a constancy of conditions within their own systems, offers a natural basis for the study of physiological correlates of psychological disorder. (11 refs.)

[No address]

2616 Tourney, Garfield, Frohman, C. E., Beckett, Peter G.S., & Gottlieb, Jacques S. Biochemical mechanisms in schizophrenia. In: Roessler, Robert, & Greenfield, Norman S. [Eds.] Physiological correlates of psychological disorder. St. Paul: University of Wisconsin Press, 1962. Pp. 13-28.

Biochemical investigations on intermediary carbohydrate metabolism in schizophrenics and control subjects reveal significantly higher ATP turnover rates in schizophrenics, coupled with an inability to mobilize ATP as an adaptive response to an insulin stressor. Findings for specific ADP activity paralleled those for ATP. The AMP levels of chronic schizophrenics were significantly lower under basal conditions than those of controls. Further metabolic studies indicate that more glucose is metabolized by Emden-Meyerhof glycolysis than via the monophosphate shunt. Schizophrenia may actually be identified biochemically on the basis of results obtained from the lactate-pyruvate ratio for chicken erythrocytes incubated with glucose. The elusive plasma factor isolated from schizophrenics is an α-globulin or a prosthetic group attached to an α-globulin. (14 refs.)

College of Medicine
Wayne State University
Detroit, Michigan

2617 Ax, Albert F. Psychophysiological methodology for the study of schizophrenia. In: Roessler, Robert, & Greenfield, Norman S. [Eds.] Physiological correlates of psychological disorder. St. Paul: University of Wisconsin Press, 1962. Pp. 29-43.

Biochemical measures and physiological variables related to the autonomic nervous system were examined in schizophrenics by means of the polygraph, GSR, ballistocardiograph, etc. Most schizophrenics do not evidence an epinephrine-like response to the stress of pain apprehension. Far more work is indicated to insure validity of statistical variables. Sensory deprivation studies pose the question of whether schizophrenia constitutes a distortion of self perception or environmental perception. Recent work utilizes the polygraph to study empathy. (27 refs.)

Lafayette Clinic and College of Medicine
Wayne State University
Detroit, Michigan

sponses to normal stress were ascertained by means of the Nowlis-Green Adjective Check List, and quasi-naturalistic studies relied on responses to arousing or bland commercial movies. Hormone levels were also determined with the subject under hypnosis. Initial hospitalization produced an immediate elevation in urinary 17-hydroxycorticosteroids. Modifications in response were also influenced by group background, past experience and the effects of immediate circumstances surrounding admission. (18 refs.)

Department of Psychiatry
Stanford University School of Medicine
Palo Alto, Calif.

2622   Persky, Harold. Adrenocortical function during anxiety. In: Roessler, Robert, & Greenfield, Norman S. [Eds.] Physiological correlates of psychological disorder. St. Paul: University of Wisconsin Press, 1962. Pp. 171-191.

Bliss determined plasma hydrocortisone levels during anxiety states in a number of patients. Acutely disturbed patients showed a mean hormone level 70% greater than normal subjects. Disruptive anxiety produces the greatest increases in hormone level. Eleven of the 46 steroids which have been isolated from the adrenal cortex have been shown to be true metabolic products of hydrocortisone. The relation between urinary steroid excretion values and tension levels were significantly and negatively related to tension estimates. These findings depend upon increased 17-ketosteroid production or a diminished rate of disposal. Also possible are increased sensitivity to ACTH stimulation or increased corticotropin production. Apparently, emotional arousal leads to adrenocortical activation. (43 refs.)

Indiana University Medical Center
Indianapolis, Ind.

2623   Oken, Donald. The role of defense in psychological stress. In: Roessler, Robert, & Greenfield, Norman S. [Eds.] Physiological correlates of psychological disorder. St. Paul: University of Wisconsin

Press, 1962, 193-210.

Defenses and related adaptive mechanisms are inextricably bound to the stress response, to the extent that defenses are crucial factors in determining stress responses. Rating scales were developed with full 3 scales; one which deals with the intensity and primivity of defense, a second which separately quantifies defenses operating at the perceptual level and a scale which gauges the extent of adaptive coping behavior. A scale to determine "Situational Cathexis" was also developed. Application of these scales to experimental data provides a far better understanding of the stress reaction. More precise rating scales are badly needed. (11 refs.)

Institute of Psychosomatic and Psychiatric
   Research and Training
Michael Reese Hospital and Medical Center
Chicago, Ill.

2624 Graham, David, T. Some research on psychophysiologic specificity and its relation to psychosomatic disease. In:Roessler, Robert, & Greenfield, Norman S. [Eds.] Physiological correlates of psychological disorder. St. Paul: University of Wisconsin Press, 1962. Pp. 221-238.

In corroboration of the postulated concepts of psychosomatic specificity and psychophysiologic specificity, several studies were carried out to determine the relation between disease and attitude as revealed by initial interviews with hospitalized patients. Attitudinally, the difference between predicted and unpredicted choice responses was significant. Patients with specific diseases were shown a group of cartoons, only 1 of which pertained to a given disease Verbal choice responses to the cartoons reveal that subjects tend to accept or deny their relevant cartoons, with a difference which corresponds roughly to intelligence level. Some normal subjects were hypnotized and then given attitudinal suggestions compatible with hives, essential hypertension and Raynaud's disease. Results, based upon skin temperature curves, were statistically significant.

University of Wisconsin Medical Center
Madison, Wis.

Apparently Dr. Frances Kelsey's stead-
fastness which prevented the thalidomide
tragedy from striking the American public
indicates that present FDA laws are stringent enough to protect the public and they
really do not need extensive revamping.
Greater cure will undoubtedly be exercised
by pharmaceutical companies in the future
to preclude any such catastrophe. The
Pharmaceutical Manufacturers Association
has allocated funds for establishing a Com-
mission on Drug Safety to investigate European problems associated with the thalidomide tragedy. (No refs.)

The Hearst Corporation
1790 Broadway
New York 19, N.Y.

2630   Miller, Ernest C. Functional depression, its recognition and management. Journal of the Louisiana State Medical Society,
1962, **114**, 285-290.

The diagnosis of depression must differentiate between normal depression (grief
and sadness) and pathologic depression
(with insomnia, anorexia, weight loss and
vegetative changes). Involutional psychotic
reaction also poses a diagnostic problem.
Psychotic depressions are best managed
with ECT, chlorpromazine and other phenothiazines, hydrazine derivatives (MAO inhibitors), imipramine and trifluopromazine.
Dexamphetamine may also be efficacious.
Toxicity is frequent with psychoactive
drugs. Isocarboxazid (10-20 mg/day), imipramine (25-150 mg/day) and nialamide
are also highly recommended. The general
practitioner should always feel free to seek
outside help when treating a patient with
psychotic depression. (13 refs.)

Lake Charles Mental Health Treatment
   Center
Lake Charles, La.

2631   New Medical Materia. Librium. New
Medical Materia, 1962, **4**, 60. [Editorial]

Chlordiazepoxide (Librium; 10 mg t.i.d.
or q.i.d.) was administered to 29 patients
by Brodie and Dow (Portland, Ore.) as an
anticonvulsant for 1-18 months. Of the

29, 3 manifested practical seizure control, 3 showed temporary practical control and 13 had a temporary reduction in the number of seizures. Chlordiazepoxide had no effect in 5 patients and 5 became worse. Behavior improved significantly in 2 children with marked mental impairment. Side effects constituted drowsiness or constipation. (1 ref.)

The Hearst Corporation
1790 Broadway
New York 19, N.Y.

2632   New Medical Materia. Ensidon. New Medical Materia, 1962, 4, 60. [Editorial]

Kristof et al. (Montreal, Quebec) administered piperazinoiminostilbene (Ensidon; 150-200 mg/day) to 18 depressed males, aged 37-66 years, for 6-63 days. Results included 10 much improved, 5 improved and 3 relatively unimproved. Ensidon was most efficacious in decreasing depressed effect, sad facial expression, impaired appetite and anxiety, while exerting least effect on apathy, agitation, irritability and decreased sexual interest. (No refs.)

The Hearst Corporation
1790 Broadway
New York 19, N.Y.

2633   New Medical Materia. Quantril. New Medical Materia, 1962, 4, 58. [Editorial]

Benzquinamine (Quantril; 150-1400 mg/day) was administered by Feldman (Topeka, Kan.) to 66 refractory patients (55 schizophrenics, 9 CBS and 2 psychotics with mental deficiency) for an average of 106 days. Significant improvement was shown by 53% of the schizophrenics and 67% of those with CBS. No response was obtained in the 2 mentally retarded patients. Side effects were limited to mild, transient hypotension in 3 patients. (No refs.)

The Hearst Corporation
1790 Broadway
New York 19, N.Y.

2634   New Medical Materia. Sparine. New

acologists, physiologists and biologists who meet at Maison Nationales de Charenton, Ecole des Hautes Etudes, Paris. Papers are devoted to the history of psychopharmacology, methods of analysis and reporting, animal psychopharmacology, clinical applications and tests of psychotropic drugs (prochlorpemazine, acetopromazine, thioproperazine, alimemazine, promazine, imipramine, centrophenoxine, buterophenone derivatives and hydrazines), and neuro-, psycho-, and physiologic, and biochemic studies . Summaries of all papers appear in this issue of Psychopharmacology Abstracts. (85 refs.)

Laboratoire de Psycho-Pathologie Expérimentale
Ecole Pratique des Hautes Etudes
Paris, France

2639   Schuhl, P.M. Les débuts de la psychopharmacologie dans l'antiquité grecque. [The beginnings of psychopharmacology in Greek antiquity.] In: Baruk, Henri, & Launay, Jacques [Eds.] Annales Moreau de Tours. Tome I. Mémoires récents sur la psychopharmacologie. -- Annals of Moreau de Tours. Volume I. Current memoirs in psychopharmacology. Paris: Presses Universitaires de France, 1962. Pp. 3-8.

The use of drugs and psychoactive drugs in Greek antiquity is discussed with particular reference to the Odyssey. The use of various roots and flowers, etc. for the treatment of mental disease, and especially anguish, is elucidated. Mention is also made of Plato's role in pharmacodynamic investigation. (6 refs.)

La Sorbonne
Paris, France

2640   Baruk, H. La vie et l'oeuvre de Moreau de Tours. [The life and work of Moreau de Tours.] In: Baruk, Henri, & Launay, Jacques [Eds.] Annales Moreau de Tours. Tome I. Mémoires récents sur la psychopharmacologie. -- Annals of Moreau de Tours. Volume I. Current memoirs in psychopharmacology. Paris: Presses Universitaires de France, 1962. Pp. 9-14.

Joseph Moreau de Tours was born in 1804 and after early education at Ecole de Médecine de Tours became an intern at Charenton in Paris in 1826. His thesis was written in 1830 on delirium, i.e., "monomania." He traveled in the Middle East and studied the effects of marihuana, concluding that its psychotomimetic effects were in some way related to the natural production of delirium. He experimented with marihuana, both on himself and volunteers. This work precedes narcoanalysis, and Moreau de Tours is considered an initiating figure in the development of psychopharmacology. (No refs.)

Laboratoire de Psycho-Pathologie Expérimentale
Ecole Pratique des Hautes Etudes
Paris, France

2641 Collet, C.-G. Candidature de Joseph Moreau (de Tours) au Prix Montyon de l'Académie des Sciences en 1846. [The candidature of Joseph Moreau (de Tours) for the Montyon Prize of the Académie des Sciences in 1846.] In: Baruk, Henri, & Launay, Jacques [Eds.] Annales Moreau de Tours. Tome I. Mémoires récents sur la psychopharmacologie. -- Annals of Moreau de Tours. Volume I. Current memoirs in psychopharmacology. Paris: Presses Universitaires de France, 1962. Pp. 15-21.

In 1846, Moreau presented a paper "Du hachisch et de l'aliénation mentale" to the Académie des Sciences in competition for the Montyon Prize. Marihuana-induced hallucinations were compared to those caused by different opiate preparations, belladonna, alcohol, etc. The germ of the concept of narcoanalysis sprang from the mind of Joseph Moreau from 1837-1845, following his experiences in Egypt and other areas of the Middle East. (1 ref.)

Laboratoire de Psycho-Pathologie Expérimentale
Ecole Pratique des Hautes Etudes
Paris, France

2642 Baruk, H. L'expertise et les décrets récents en psychopharmacologie. [Report

general system (particularly hepatic and renal functions), and publish observations on biological tests and assay methods; endow sufficiently qualified psychiatric hospitals with the means of following their patients with all the resources of modern medicine. (No refs.)

Société Moreau de Tours
Maison Nationale de Charenton
Paris, France

2646 Coirault, R. Les examens biologiques et l'expertise des drogues psychotropes. [Biological examinations and report on psychotropic drugs.] In: Baruk, Henri, & Launay, Jacques [Eds.] Annales Moreau de Tours. Tome I. Mémoires récents sur la psychopharmacologie. -- Annals of Moreau de Tours. Volume I. Current memoirs in psychopharmacology. Paris: Presses Universitaires de France, 1962. Pp. 39-42.

The difficulties inherent in extensive biological testing of mental patients under drug therapy are outlined. Aside from common laboratory tests, variations in electrolytes, enzymatic variations, oxidases, transaminases, dehydrogenases, etc. catecholamine assays and changes in hormone excretion, as well as bioelectric tests (neuromuscular excitability, electromyography, study of the myotactic reflex, ECG and EEG, etc.) should be followed. Difficulties in interpretation, e.g., the meaning of a hypopotassemia, are also elucidated. (No refs.)

Société Moreau de Tours
Maison Nationale de Charenton
Paris, France

2647 Baruk, H., Launay, J., & Perlès, R. Les phénothiazines et la psychiatrie. [Phenothiazines in psychiatry.] In: Baruk, Henri, & Launay, Jacques [Eds.] Annales Moreau de Tours. Tome I. Mémoires récents sur la psychopharmacologie. -- Annals of Moreau de Tours. Volume I. Current memoirs in psychopharmacology. Paris: Presses Universitaires de France, 1962. Pp. 45-62.

The chemical structure of phenothiazine

and relationships to animal experimentation are reviewed. Potentiation of narcosis and analgesia, hypothermia, antiserotonin activity in vitro, the traction test, the Winter and Flataker test, tests for CR's, antiapomorphine activity and catalepsy, experimental catatonia, and the deJong and Baruk test are emphasized. Psychomotor, ergographic and ECG modifications, as well as those in other bioelectrical tests are outlined. Information is presented on chlorpromazine, prochlorpemazine, thioproperazine, levomepromazine, acetomepromazine and alimemazine, with emphasis on work in monkeys. Classification scheme of Decourt and that of Courvoisier, Lambert and Revol is presented along with Baruk and Launay's scheme. (No refs.)

Société Moreau de Tours
Maison Nationale de Charenton
Paris, France

2648 Courvoisier, S., & Lambert, P.-A. Essai de classification pharmacologique et clinique de certains neuroleptiques à structure phénothiazinique.[Pharmacologic and clinical classification of some phenothiazine neuroleptics.] In: Baruk, Henri, & Launay, Jacques [Eds.] Annales Moreau de Tours. Tome I. Mémoires récents sur la psychopharmacologie. -- Annals of Moreau de Tours. Volume I. Current memoirs in psychopharmacology. Paris: Presses Universitaires de France, 1962. Pp. 63-72.

The sedative, depressive, antiapomorphinic and cataleptic qualities of chlorpromazine, methopromazine, alimemazine, levomepromazine, prochlorpemazine, thioperazine, promazine and acepromazine are reviewed. (No refs.)

Société Moreau de Tours
Maison Nationale de Charenton
Paris, France

2649 Courvoisier, S. Expérimentation animale de la prochlorpémazine. [Animal experimentation and prochlorpemazine.] In: Baruk, Henri, & Launay, Jacques [Eds.] Annales Moreau de Tours. Tome I. Mémoires récents sur la psychopharmacologie. -- Annals of Moreau de Tours.

Emotion, mentation, will, human expression through writing and speaking, Platonic versus Aristotelian concepts of space, perception and sensory organs, and underlying mechanisms are expounded. (No refs.)

Société Moreau de Tours
Maison Nationale de Charenton
Paris, France

2654 Cahn, Th., & Houget, J. Mise en évidence de la défense de l'organisme dans la réponse à de faibles quantités d'hormones. Généralités possibles de ce processus. [Evidence of body defenses in response to low amounts of hormones. Possible properties of this process.] In: Baruk, Henri, & Launay, Jacques [Eds.] Annales Moreau de Tours. Tome I. Mémoires récents sur la psychopharmacologie. -- Annals of Moreau de Tours. Volume I. Current memoirs in psychopharmacology. Paris: Presses Universitaires de France, 1962. Pp. 299-302.

Constitutional genetic differences in relation to responses to hormone administration is reviewed, e.g., the variation in glycemia from 1 species to another in response to epinephrine or insulin. The work of Claude Bernard and followers is elucidated. The heterogeneity of the body and equilibrium system, with reference to Le Chatelier's equilibrium principle, are noted. The role of pharmacological agents in displacing equilibria is commented on and the necessity for judicious analysis on the eventual role of a drug is stressed. (No refs.)

Société Moreau de Tours
Maison Nationale de Charenton
Paris, France

2655 Cahn, Th. Modèles électroniques et fonctionnement de l'organisme. [Electronic models and the functioning of the body.] In: Baruk, Henri, & Launay, Jacques [Eds.] Annales Moreau de Tours. Tome I. Mémoires récents sur la psychopharmacologie. -- Annals of Moreau de Tours. Volume I. Current memoirs in psychopharmacology. Paris: Presses Universitaires de France, 1962. Pp. 303-308.

The regulation of metabolic reactions is compared to the activity of electronic machines. The great differences between organ activity and activity on the molecular level are stressed. Memory and the problem of inscription in relation to CNS liasons are noted in reference to computer construction. (No refs.)

Société Moreau de Tours
Maison Nationale de Charenton
Paris, France

2656 Cahn, Th. Sur la pensée et ses connexions avec l'organismes. [On thinking and its connections in the system.] In: Baruk, Henri, & Launay, Jacques [Eds.] Annales Moreau de Tours. Tome I. Mémoires récents sur la psychopharmacologie. --Annals of Moreau de Tours. Volume I. Current memoirs in psychopharmacology. Paris: Presses Universitaires de France, 1962. Pp. 309-315.

The inherent independence of human thought allows analysis of the events in the environment. The fragility of cerebral function as indicated by intoxication, damage from fever or diseases is evident. Dialects, language and logic and their development from Plato through Descartes to the present are outlined. (No refs.)

Société Moreau de Tours
Maison Nationale de Charenton
Paris, France

2657 Cahn, Th. Sur l'activité métabolique des organismes. [On the metabolic activities of organisms.] In: Baruk, Henri, & Launay, Jacques [Eds.] Annales Moreau de Tours. Tome I. Mémoires récents sur la psychopharmacologie. -- Annals of Moreau de Tours. Volume I. Current memoirs in psychopharmacology. Paris: Presses Universitaires de France, 1962. Pp. 316-321.

The role of biology as a science in the theoretical and practical examination of metabolism is discussed. (No refs.)

2662 Binning, Rex, Watson, W.R., Samrah, M., & Martin, Esmee. Premedication for adenotonsillectomy. British Journal of Anaesthesiology, 1962, **34**, 812-816.

A total of 121 children aged 2½-8 years, received quinalbarbital (6 mg/kg), 120 received promethazine and chlorpromazine (0.8 mg/kg each), 135 received trimeprazine (4 mg/kg) and 80 received atropine (0.9 mg/kg) on a double-blind basis as premedication for adenotonsillectomy. Atropine (0.9 mg) was administered p.o. to all patients to dry up secretions. Preoperative vomiting occurred in 47%. Two-thirds of the quinalbarbital treated patients were asleep on arrival in the anaesthetic room, and 57% vomiting occurred postoperatively. With promethazine and chlorpromazine, only 25% of the children were asleep at the time of induction, and 36% postoperative vomiting ensued. With trimeprazine, 2/3rds of the patients were awake during induction. Trimeprazine is the most efficacious premedication to date available for younger children facing an inhalational induction.

Royal Alexandra Hospital for Sick Children Brighton, Great Britain

2663 Cross, Thomas N. A ten-year study of the inpatient population of the adult psychiatric service. University of Michigan Medical Bulletin, 1962, **28**, 37-40.

From 1950-1960, 3 samplings of data culled from the Adult Service of the Neuropsychiatric Institute of the University of Michigan Medical Center reveal a progressive increase in the number of emergency admissions and of patients with more serious illnesses. In 1950, 21 patients received ECT while only 2 received ECT in 1960. In 1960, of 89 patients receiving tranquilizers or antidepressants, 73 were treated with phenothiazine derivatives or similar drugs and 16 took antidepressants. Inpatient populations tend toward fewer patients with neuroses and more with psychoses, necessitating profound alterations in treatment, teaching and research activities.

Department of Psychiatry
University of Michigan Medical Center
Ann Arbor, Mich.

2664 Munson, Wayne M., & Jenicek, John A. Effect of anesthetic agents on patients receiving reserpine therapy. Anesthesiology, 1962, **23**, 741-746.

A total of 58 patients received reserpine (1-5 mg parenterally) to determine drug effects on response to anesthesia. Therapy was maintained in 42 until 5 days before surgery. In the control series, 16 were withdrawn from therapy within 8 days of surgery. Neurocirculatory instability was demonstrated by 9 out of 16 in a previous series, 13 out of 26 in the present series and 7 out of 16 in the control series. The control series revealed no significant decrease in the incidence of severity of hypotension during induction of anesthesia. Rauwolfia derivatives need not be discontinued before anesthesia and surgery, as drug withdrawal does not insure prevention of circulatory stability

Anesthesia and Operative Service
Brooke General Hospital
Brooke Army Medical Center
Fort Sam Houston, Tex.

2665 Hankoff, Leon D. Treatment comparison and the placebo effect. Diseases of the Nervous System, 1962, **23**, 39-40.

Positive placebo responses were observed in a hospitalized 29-year-old woman with apathy, confusion and tenseness. A 34-year-old man with recurrent uncontrolled bizarre thoughts received meprobamate (200 mg as needed), thiopropazate (5 mg t.i.d.) and chlordiazepoxide (50 mg t.i.d.) for varying periods of time. Considerable improvement was observed with chlordiazepoxide. A 43-year-old woman with acute delusional episodes responded well to a daily regimen of meprobamate (400 mg b.i.d.), pyribenzamine (50 mg t.i.d.) and a belladonna-barbiturate mixture t.i.d. Substitution of placebos for meprobamate resulted in subjective feelings of dizziness, nausea, blindness and numbness around the mouth. An inert or active psychopharmacological a-gent may precipitate a variety of responses depending upon clinical conditions and other factors.

Department of Psychiatry
State University of New York
Downstate Medical Center
Brooklyn, N.Y.

2666 Yi-Yunh Hsia, David, Rowley, William, & Raskin, Nathaniel J. Clinical management of phenylketonuria. Quarterly Bulletin of Northwestern University Medical School, 1962, **36**, 25-32.

A low-phenylalanine diet was administered to 12 phenylketonurics, below 3 years of age at initial diagnosis in order to prevent or minimize mental retardation. The diet was maintained for 324 months, and good biochemical control was sustained. Four of the 5 children who began the diet before the age of 6 months are normal intellectually. In contrast, 6 out of 7 whose diet began after 1 year of age are retarded. A general increase was observed in intellectual growth rate among the 6 who were retested. Mental deficiency can be prevented or controlled by institution of a low-phenylalanine diet before age 6 months. A national program is in progress to screen newborn infants for phenylketonuria at 3-4 weeks of age.

Department of Pediatrics and Neurology
    and Psychiatry
Northwestern University Medical School
Evanston, Ill.

2667 Powell, L.W., & Schonell, M.E. The role of bemigride in the treatment of barbiturate overdosage: results of a controlled study. Medical Journal of Australia, 1962, **1**, 551-552.

Bemigride (1 g i.v.) or saline was administered to 102 patients, average age 39.9-40.8 years, presented with barbiturate overdosage (greater than 50 grains). Mephentermine or albumin was given to raise blood pressure. Physicians recorded level of consciousness, pupillary and tendon reflexes, pulse rate, blood pressure and respiratory rate. Only 1 death occurred. Resuch as anorexia, flatulence or insomnia, is recommended. This had 2 advantages over most of the tranquilizers, hypnotics, etc.: it is inexpensive and never causes stuffy nose, dry throat or thirst.

112 Willison Road
Carlton, New South Wales
Australia

2670 Alexander, Daniel D. Observations in the use of Tindal. Diseases of the Nervous System, 1962, 24, 351.

Fifty-six patients, 49 women and 7 men, were treated with acetophenazine (Tindal). Fifty of the patients were 50-95 years of age and 22 of these were 70-80. Twenty-six had organic brain disease. The majority took 20 mg acetophenazine t.i.d., and a few took 20 mg t.i.d. or only once. Sixty-eigh⁺ percent showed definite improvement, 25% did not change and 7% were not as well as when they had been treated with other drugs. The greatest improvement was observed in psychomotor activity; 31 overactive patients then became noticeably quieter. Improvements were noted in personal appearance, social relationships, clearer speech, etc. The mood of 10 depressed patients became elevated, although 2 others showed no change. The only adverse hematological reaction was leukopenia in 1 patient. Five patients complained of drowsiness and 1 instance of drooling was noted.

Danvers State Hospital
Hathorne, Mass.

2671 Cohen, Harry. Treatment of chronic regressive refractory schizophrenia. Diseases of the Nervous System, 1962, 24, 335-339.

Hydroxyzine (100-500 mg t.i.d., p.o.) was administered to 40 chronic refractory female schizophrenics, aged 23-70 years, for 10-12 weeks. Minimal improvement was observed in 12.5%, indicating that hydroxyzine is not particularly suited for severely regressed, poorly motivated patients. Side effects occurred in 95%, including ataxia, restlessness, tremor, grand

mal seizures, drowsiness, etc. At the most
economic therapeutic dosage level, however, there were few side effects.

Brooklyn State Hospital
Brooklyn, N.Y.

2672 Clarke, Edward T. Observations on
Benizol therapy in general practice. Ninety
senile patients. Medical Record and Annals,
1962, **55**, 186-189.

Ninety senile or arteriosclerotic cases
(47 ambulatory), aged 56-93 years and
averaging 77 years, were treated for 12
weeks with Benizol (100 mg pentetrazol
and 50 mg nicotinic acid). Dosage varied
from 1 or 2 tablets or teaspoonsful t.i.d.
Improvement percentages were: appearance
77, personal habits 74, physical condition
91, sociability 76, depression 74, feeling
95, memory 79, work habits 63, eating
habits 71 and sleep patterns 80. Twenty
cases were not so tabulated and were
clinically rated: 14 very good, 5 good and
1 no improvement. Slight flushing of the
skin in some patients due to nicotinic acid
was the only side effect; in 4 cases with
high blood pressure some slight change
towards normal was recorded.

3801 Kirby Drive
Houston, Tex.

2673 Dorfman, Wilfred. A short-acting
anaesthetic in psychiatry. Diseases of the
Nervous System, 1962, **23**, 276-278.

Methohexital (8-10 cc of 1% solution i.v.)
was administered to 75 patients before
ECT, for a total of 650 injections over
a 14-month period. In addition, 38 patients
received methohexital as a method of narcoanalysis. With methohexital, the patient
recovered completely within 15-30 minutes.
In narcoanalysis, patients emerge from
anesthesia in a more receptive state. Rapid
symptom removal was frequently accomplished for psychosomatic symptoms
under methohexital narcoanalysis.

1921 Newkirk Avenue
Brooklyn 26, N.Y.

2679 Collard, J., & Kerf, J. Le traitement de l'anxiété névrotique par le valium. [Treatment of neurotic anxiety with Valium.] Encéphale, 1962, **51**, 571-573.

Eighteen cases of psychoneurotic depression, 5 cases of anxiety, 4 of obsessional neurosis and 1 conversion reaction (total 28) were treated with an optimal average of 15 mg/day diazepam (Valium) in 3 divided doses. Two were cured, 5 markedly improved, 14 showed improvement and 8 slight improvement with no failures. The side effects were drowsiness in 22% and some slight euphoria.

Clinique Psychiatrique
Université de Liège
Liège, Belgium

2680 Langston, William B., Jr. Psychotic and psychoneurotic states. Treatment with chlordiazepoxide. Southwestern Medicine, 1962, **43**, 295-298.

Chlordiazepoxide (10-75 mg/day) was administered to 130 psychiatric patients aged 16-75 years, with a variety of psychotic and psychoneurotic disorders. Dosage was usually 10 mg, 2, 3 or 4 times daily and the duration of treatment was from 1 day to 5 months. Seventy patients received adjunctive therapy with iproniazid, mescopalamine, isocarboxazid, glutethimide and chlorpromazine. Responses were excellent in 22.2%, good in 38.1% and fair in 11.1%. Thirty-six percent showed no improvement. In anxiety reaction 8 out of 12 had excellent response, while in depression only 5 out of 44 had an equivalent response. Side effects were infrequent; ataxia was observed in 6 patients, drowsiness in 8 and one patient developed a skin rash. It was necessary to discontinue medication in only 2 patients.

703 North 6th St.
Longview, Tex.

2681 Caldwell, William G. The treatment of premenstrual tension and dysmenorrhea with a non-narcotic analgesic. Southwestern Medicine, 1962, **43**, 68-74.

A 128 cases of premenstrual tension (abdominal water retention 121, headaches

93, etc.) and 248 cases of dysmenorrhea
(severe cramps 227, low back pain 172, etc.),
aged 16-48 years, were treated with Fiorinal (50 mg butalbital, 200 mg acetylsalicylic
acid, 40 mg caffeine and 130 mg phenacetin).
Forty-two cases had pelvic pathology and 21
of these received surgical treatment. Fifty-
three patients suffered from both premenstrual tension and dysmenorrhea. One-
hundred and fifty-four were unmarried, 94
married, 51 having borne 1 or more children. An initial dose of 2 Fiorinal tablets
taken at the 1st sign of symptoms, followed
at 4 hour intervals with 1 or 2 tablets,
proved the most efficient dosage schedule.
Dosage requirements were 1-12 tablets
given over a 2 day period; the overall
average dosage was 4-6 tablets. Individuali-
zation permitted a reduction of dosage in
137 cases. No side effects were noted in
any of the patients. One-hundred and ninety-
four cases whose symptoms varied from
very severe to moderate obtained excellent
to good results.

Department of Clinical Research
St. Anne's Hospital
Los Angeles, Calif.

2682 Guyotat, J., & Hochmann, J. Situation
actuelle du 8228 R.P. en thérapeutique
psychiatrique. Apropos de 32 nouveaux cas.
[The present position of RP 8228 in psychiatric therapy; on 32 new cases.] Lyon
Médicale, 1962, **43**, 777-783.

Levophacetoperazine (RP 8228; 5-10 mg/
day p.o.) was used in the treatment of 32
adults, 21 ambulatory and 11 hospitalized.
Among ambulatory patients, 5 had excellent
results, 1 an average result and the rest
were dropouts, cured of either their ailment
or their doctor. Among the hospitalized
group excellent results were obtained in 2
(asthenia and exhaustion neurosis) and good
results in 8. One failure, depression in an
Algerian immigrant, was recorded. After
eliminating dropouts, excellent results were
obtained in 40%, good results in 50% and
failure in 10% of the remaining 18 patients.

Clinique Neuro-Psychiatrique et d'Hygiène
   Mentale
Université de Lyon
Lyon, France

2688 Rabe, F., Penin, H., & Matthes, A. Erfahrungen mit Ospolot in der Epilepsiebehandlung. [Some experiences with Ospolot in the treatment of epilepsy.] Deutsche Medicina Wochenschrift, 1962, 87, 953-959.

Ospolot is a sulfonamide derivative (N-(4'-sulfamyl-phenyl)-butansultam-(1-4). Two-hundred and thirteen patients (47 children under 14 years of age) with psychomotor attacks with or without grand mal seizures were treated; with few exceptions observations were continued for at least 6 months. Dosage: for children 1½-5, adults 2-15 tablets daily (mostly ½-3, and 4-6, respectively) [amount unspecified]. Of 57 patients with isolated psychomotor attacks 10% remained free of attacks and 30% were improved; 53% could not be improved and in 7% the attacks occurred more frequently. The treatment was even less effective in 89 cases of combined psychomotor attacks and grand mal. The effect of Ospolot on the minor attacks of petit mal, Jacksonian epilepsy, or adversive or cortical epilepsy (29 cases) was not significant. Sixteen percent of 40 patients with grand mal epilepsy could be relieved of attacks; a result which is clearly inferior to that of other antiepileptic agents. Side effects were noted in 75% of the patients: paresthesia in 38%, tachypnea and hyperpnea in 30%, cardiovascular symptoms in 7%, and gastrointestinal symptoms in 14%. Loss of weight was seen in 8% and various functional disturbances in 24%. For these reasons, Ospolot is contraindicated for persons with vasomotor lability, with hyperthyroidism or arterial hypertonia. In 14% of the patients the treatment resulted in abnormal excitation. Due to the insignificant anti-epileptic effect, and the high percentage of side effects, Ospolot is not recommended as treatment of choice for psychomotor attacks or grand mal seizures. Under certain conditions, however, it is useful as an adjuvant.

Nervenklinik der Universität Heidelberg Heidelberg, Germany

2689 Tölle, Rainer. Über zwei Piperazinderivate des Phenothiazins. [Two piperazine phenothiazine derivatives.] Nervenarzt, 1962, 10, 457-462.

Twenty-nine acute and chronic schizophrenics, 19-55 years of age, were treated

with prochlorperazine (60 to 120-200 mg/
day/p.o.). The results were excellent in 6
cases, good in 6 and questionable in 4.
Improvement did not seem to depend on
dosage and appeared usually within the 1st
3 days of treatment. Side effects were seen
in 62% of the patients; dyskinetic and hyperkinetic symptoms appeared most often within the 1st 3 days, psychic disturbances
similar to Korsakow's syndrome after 3-4
weeks. Thirty-six schizophrenics, mostly
acute cases, received thioproperazine (30-
90 mg i.m. daily during the 1st 3 days,
later 60-140 mg/day/p.o.). Therapeutic results were favorable; side effects similar
to those experienced with prochlorperazine
occurred in 48% of the patients. The side
effects could greatly be reduced by simultaneous administration of beperidene. Patients with severe schizophrenic defects
showed the poorest response.

Privatklinik Christophsbad
Göppingen, Germany

2690 Wachsmuth, R. Fluphenazin - mehr
als ein neues Psychopharmakon. [Fluphena-
zine - more than a new psychopharmkon.]
Nervenarzt, 1962, 10, 466-469.

One-hundred and sixty-one hospitalized patients treated with fluphenazine were investigated in regard to over-all clinical effect
and drug influence on target symptoms
examined. The medium standard dosage was
3-6 mg/day p.o. or i.m.; no patient was
treated less than 4 weeks. The patients
suffered from schizophrenia, hebephrenia,
catatonia and paranoia. The average age
was 33-41 years and 124 subjects were men.
The drug was generally well tolerated; it
is compatible with barbiturates and antidepressants and ECT. Effects were very
good in 68 patients, good in 50, moderate in
20 and uncertain in 14. No effect was noted
in 9 patients. There were no toxic or cardiovascular side effects. Overdosage leads to
extrapyramidal symptoms; i.m. administration not infrequently leads to hyper-
kinetic-dystonic syndrome.

Westfälische Landeskrankenhaus
Gütersloh, Germany

2696 Weil, Andre A. EEG observation in
narcoleptic adults. Diseases of the Nervous
System, 1962, 23, 279-283.

EEG tracings of 21 narcoleptic subjects (15
narcoleptic attacks only, with concomitant
cataleptic episodes and 3 with sleep paralysis), aged 17-54 years, were analyzed and
records were obtained during free intervals
and narcoleptic attacks. Characteristic
findings in 76% included low voltage theta
patterns corresponding to physiological
states of drowsiness. Persistent EEG
drowsiness patterns were noted in 7 subjects (33%) even during vigorous hyperventilation. Administration of deoxyephe-
drine or amphetamine i.v. produced waking
records with good alpha spindling. EEG
observations seem to implicate a reversible
disturbance in the brain-stem reticular
activating system.

Huron Road Hospital
Division of Neurology
Cleveland, Ohio

2697 Oybir, Fahrettin. Trifluoperazine in
chronic, withdrawn schizophrenics. (A
double-blind study). Diseases of the Nervous
System, 1962, 14, 348-350.

Trifluoperazine (2-20 mg b.i.d., p.o.) or
placebo was administered on a double-
blind basis to 29 chronic female schizophrenics (average duration of illness 24
years), average age 57 years, for 6 months.
Results were rated by means of 75-item
symptomatologic profiles. Eighteen were
granted grounds priviliges because of their
obvious improvement. Patients showed increased sociability, communicativeness and
activity, with emphasis on greater accessi-
bility to group and occupational therapy.
Hallucinations and interpersonal relations
were particularly improved. Controllable
side effects included restlessness, anorexia,
parkinsonian reactions, excessive thirst,
allergy, perspiration and dysphagia.

State Hospital for Mental Diseases
Howard, Rhode Island

2698 Haynes, Elmer, Blanchette, James,
& Gericke, O.L. Experience with chlor-

diazepoxide in Huntington's chorea. Diseases of the Nervous System, 1962, **23**, 326-328.

Chlordiazepoxide (30-150 mg/day) was administered to 9 patients with Huntington's chorea, aged 32-62 years, for several weeks. Anxiety symptoms decreased and mild euphoria was noticeable. Choreiform movements slowed to dystonic movements with improved coordination and equilibrium. Untoward effects constituted of dizziness, ataxia, drowsiness and leg weakness. Marked improvement was observed in 3 patients.

Patton State Hospital
Patton, Calif.

2699 O'Reilly, P.O., & Reich, Genevieve. Lysergic acid and the alcoholic. Diseases of the Nervous System, 1962, **23**, 331-334.

LSD (200 µg p.o.) was administered to 33 chronic alcoholics, aged 21-59 years, directly before a 2-hour psychotherapy session. Objective questionnaires were completed by patients 1 day after the LSD interview. A 7-88 week period of followup indicated that 7 abstained completely, 10 improved, 10 were unchanged and 6 provided no available reports. Therefore, 17 patients derived benefit from the LSD experience and 16 did not. Apparently, the LSD experience is useful in treating chronic alcoholism.

Psychiatric Department
Union Hospital
Moose Jaw, Saskatchewan
Canada

2700 Khosbin, A., & Guyotat, J. Essais clinique avec le Ro 4-1575. [Clinical trials with RO 4-1575.] Annales Médico-Psychologiques, 1962, 120, **1**, 310-311.

Forty-one depressed patients were treated with 150-250 amitriptyline p.o. Twenty-seven percent improved markedly, 29% slightly and 44% showed no results. The product was more efficacious in women than in men (33% compared to 12.5%). Tolerance was excellent but transitory paraparesis, aggravation of a hemiparesis and confusion. However the drug was less efficiacious than imipramine.

[No address]

2701 Balatre, J., Berger, Cl., & Chirat, P. Etude clinique en milieu obstétrical d'un nouveau barbiturique: le 96 JD. [Obstetric study of a new barbiturate: JD 96.] Lyon Médical, 1962, **40**, 575-581.

5-Vinyl-5 (methylbutylmalonyl) urea - JD 96 - was employed clinically as a hypnotic in 50 patients. Half of the cases were women in good health before and after delivery, and the other half were women with disorders of pregnancies. It was not used as an analgesic in any case. Dosage was 1 or 2 100 mg tablets as a rule; rarely 100 mg suppositories were used. Results were excellent in 93% of cases and JD 96 was effective when phenothiazines, secobarbital or butobarbital were ineffective. The onset of drug effect took place at an average of 30 minutes with 1 tablet and in 20% of the cases sleep ensued in less than a quarter hour. Nightmares were very rare: 4%. No side effects were noted.

Service du Dr. Ed. Rochet
Hôpital de l'Hotel-Dieu
Lyon, France

2702 Robinson, J., McCabe, E., & Graves, Ch. Acepromazine. Un tranquillisant nouveau et très actif. [Acepromazine. A new extremely active tranquilizer.] Clinique, 1961, **56**, 593-594.

Acepromazine was given to 35 patients, including 17 schizophrenics. Average dosage was 100-200 mg i.v. on the 1st day continued as oral medication, 50 mg q.i.d. Seven cases showed excellent improvement, 10 good improvement, 9 fair results and 9 had poor reactions. No side effects were reported.

[No address]

2703 Ingvar, David, & Nilsson, Eric. Central nervous effects of neurolept-analgesia as induced by haloperidol and phenoperidine. Acta Anaesthesiologica Scandinavica, 1961, **5**, 85-88.

(100 mg i.v., i.m. or p.o. initially, then 10 mg p.o. q.i.d.) and 80 controls received placebo. Dose-response curves indicated that chlordiazepoxide was effective in alleviating the symptoms of acute alcoholism. In addition, 67 out-patients with postalcoholic tension state, aged 24-63 years, received chlordiazepoxide (10 mg b.i.d. to 25 mg q.i.d.) for 1 week-6 months. All except 5 reported relief from anxiety within 24 hours. No side effects were observed.

C. Dudley Saul Clinic
St. Luke's and Children's Medical Center
Philadelphia, Pa.

2706 Beck, D. Vegetative Untersuchungen, Therapie und Prognose der Erschöpfungsdepressionen. [Investigation of the autonomic system, therapy, and prognosis in exhaustion depressions.] Schweizer Archiv für Neurologie Neurochirurgie und Psychiatrie, 1962, 90, 370-391.

Twenty patients (18 female, 2 male) suffering from manifold autonomic-somatic disturbances, were tested by means of the Schelong cold pressor-and rewarming tests. Pathological results were obtained in all 20 cases; 18 patients displaying hyperfunction of the nervous system with sympathetic hypertonia, the remaining 2 demonstrating hyperfunction without exhaustion symptoms. In addition to psychotherapy, bedrest and insulin administration (4-12 U) for 10-30 days in combination with a thymoleptic drug, e.g., imipramine (at doses 3 x 30 mg i.m., and 3 x 25 mg i.m. respectively or oral administration of 3 x 30-90 mg and 10-50 mg respectively.) Cures were effected in 16 patients and improvement in 4. The exhaustion syndrome is generally due to chronic affective conflicts; it more frequently affects women and prognosis is good. A followup study of the patients revealed only 2 relapses.

Psychiatrische Universitätsklinik
Basel, Switzerland

2707 Lammers, H.J. Erfahrungen mit dem Psychopharmakon Truxal. [Experiences

with the psychiatric drug Truxal.] Therapie der Gegenwart, 1962, **101**, 310-319.

Chlorprothixene (Truxal) tablets were administered at doses of 50-100 mg t.i.d. to
118 patients consisting of 60 depressives,
33 schizophrenics, 12 psychopaths, 6 older
persons with paranoid psychoses or syndromes and 7 miscellaneous cases. Good
results were obtained in 52 cases, moderate to doubtful results in 27 cases and
failures in 31. Patients with endogenous
depressions responded well, as did excitability, restlessness and anxiety states.
Catatonics responded very poorly. Side
effects were generally mild, consisting of
tiredness, hyperhydrosis, nausea, dizziness, dry mouth and very slight extrapyramidal disturbances.

Psychiatrische Nervenklinik der Univ.
Giessen, Germany

2708 Niver, Edwin O. Carphenazine and
the extrapyramidal regulation of kinesthet-
ic function. Diseases of the Nervous System, 1962, **14**, 340-348.

Carphenazine (75-900 mg/day) was administered to 20 chronic parkinsonian patients
(duration of illness greater than 10 years),
for 6 months and to 20 other patients for
shorter periods of time. Results revealed
an increase in affective response away
from apathy, an improvement in quantity
and quality of communication, an increased
alertness and awareness of environment
and behavioral improvements. Side effects
constituted excessive sedation in patients
who initially manifested excessive lethargy.

Mental Health Institute
Clarinda, Iowa

2709 Wiehler, H. Zur Behandlung der
Depressionen mit Monoaminoxydasehem-
mern. [Treatment of depression with monoaminoxidase inhibitors.] Nervenarzt, 1962,
10, 462-466.

Fifty-two hospitalized patients were treated
with isocarboxizide (Marplan). Forty-eight
patients had depressions, 4 chronic
schizophrenia. The dosage was 3-8 tablets

reactive depression, aged 43-66 years, for
5-7 weeks. Control groups received placebos, and all groups received extensive
laboratory testing. Patients chosen at random were evaluated by means of the SRA
Non-Verbal and the Thurston Temperament Tests. Of the 17 receiving psychometric evaluation, results were 7 excellent, 6 good, 4 questionable and 0 negative. Of 9 with parkinsonism, 7 showed
poor responses and 2 did not change.
About 1/3 experienced drowsiness and
minor tremulousness during the 1st 10 days
of treatment. Symptoms disappeared upon
continuation of therapy. An additional 30-
day study was performed in which 9 patients with severe rigidity and tremor
received ethyltryptamine (15 mg t.i.d.).
Therapy was discontinued in 2 due to
marked increase in tremors and rigidity,
2 manifested no change, 1 became more
cheerful and the remaining 5 continued
to regimen despite deterioration of their
condition.

Department of Medicine
Oak Forest Hospital
Oak Forest, Ill.

2714 De la Fuente, Muniz, Ramón, &
Martinez Cid, Enrique. El G33040 (Insidon) en el tratamiento de las disfuncion-
es viscerales psicogenicas. [G 33040 (Insidon) in the treatment of psychogenic
visceral disfunctions.] Prensa Médica Méx-
icana, 1962, 5, 208-210.

Thirty-six patients, aged 23-62 years, were
treated with 50-200 mg piperazinoiminostilbene (Insidon) p.o., in 3 divided doses.
Duration of treatment was 3-18 weeks.
Conditions included gastritis, intestinitis,
circulatory and respiratory disorders, tension headache, etc. Aside from its anxiolytic effect, the drug has a regulatory
effect on visceral activity. Twenty-five
out of the 36 (64.1%) patients improved.
Five showed slight dry mouth, and 6 restlessness and increased anxiety in the 1st
3 days. Five showed slight drowsiness.
In 5 cases where the drug was intentionally withdrawn, symptoms reappeared; later after meprobamate and chlordiazepoxide
had been tried, piperazinoiminostilbene was
reinstituted and rapidly controlled symp-

toms.

Servicio de Psiquiatría
Hospital Español
Mexico City D.F., Mexico

2715 Hamilton, L. Dean, & Bennett, Jesse L. Acetophenazine for hyperactive geriatric patients. Geriatrics, 1962, 17, 596-601.

Acetophenazine (20-60 mg/day p.o.) or placebo waa administered on a double-blind basis to 27 hyperactive, psychotic men (19 organic brain disease with psychosis, 7 schizophrenia and 1 depression), mean age 71 years, for 3-8 weeks. Patients were rated by ward personnel on a scale based upon 13 target symptoms. Results showed that 13 (68%) showed a significant decrease in hyperactivity, 6 (31%) were mildly improved and 7 (37%) were moderately improved. Three were unchanged and 3 became worse. Controls showed 8 (25%) with significant improvement and 6 (75%) who failed to change appreciably. Maximal improvement began in 3-4 weeks. Giddiness and lethargy constituted the principle side effects in 37 and 26% respectively.

VA Hospital and University
Utah College of Medicine
Salt Lake City, Utah

2716 Neilson, Duncan R., & Neilson, Ronald P. Clinical evaluation of iproniazid in obstetrics. Western Journal of Surgery, Obstetrics and Gynecology, 1962, 70, 191-198.

Iproniazid (25 mg b.i.d. for 1 week, then 25 mg/day) was administered to 80 pregnant women (6 chronic recurrent depression, 5 postpartum psychosis, 51 constitutional fatigue syndromes with depression and 18 mixed emotional and behavioral disorders). Maintenance therapy varied from 12.5-37.5 mg/day for 5-90 days. All 6 with recurrent depression responded with gratifying results, as did those with postpartum psychosis. About 90-95% of those with constitutional fatigue syndrome manifested genuine improvement

The miscellaneous group showed 80% improvement overall. Side effects include hepatotoxicity, transitory jaundice, insomnia, hyperactivity and muscular twitching.

[No address]

2717 Batten, Charles T. Long-release barbiturate medication for relief of tension. Medical Times, 1962, 90, 1213-1218.

A sustained release capsule of pentobarbital (100-200 mg/day p.o.) was administered to 24 psychiatric patients, aged 25- 68 years, for 4-5 months. Overall results were optimal in the geriatric group of 9 elderly women with CBS. Clinic patients (3 emotionally unstable) were erratic in taking medication and unreliable in reporting results. The geriatric patients were far more manageable, with fewer complaints and less apprehension after phenobarbital administration. Of the private patients, 3 failed to improve, 1 showed relief of tension with persistent depression and 1 exhibited very gratifying overall improvement. Occasional drowsiness constituted the only side effect. Phenobarbital is apparently well suited for alleviation of transient tension.

Department of Psychiatry
Loma Linda University
Los Angeles Campus
Los Angeles, Calif.

2718 Broussolle, P. A propos de quatre années d'expérience de la prochlorpémazine en psychiatrie. [On four years of experience with prochlorpemazine in psychiatry.] In: Baruk, Henri, & Launay, Jacques [Eds.] Annales Moreau de Tours. Tome I. Mémoires récents sur la psychopharmacologie. -- Annals of Moreau de Tours. Volume I. Current memoirs in psychopharmacology. Paris: Presses Universitaires de France, 1962. Pp. 79-81.

In 4 years of clinical experimentation some 500 patients have been treated with prochlorpemazine; starting doses were 50-150 mg/day, increased to 600 mg/day p.o. Both the oral and i.m. routes were used,

& Launay, Jacques [Eds.] Annales Moreau de Tours. Tome I. Mémoires récents sur la psychopharmacologie. -- Annals of Moreau de Tours. Volume I. Current memoirs in psychopharmacology. Paris: Presses Universitaires de France, 1962. 89-98.

Experiments with progressively increasing doses of acepromazine are reviewed using pigeons, guinea pigs, mice and monkeys. Secondly, clinical trials with 30 patients (3 melancholic depression, 5 atypical schizophrenic depression and 22 cases of schizophrenia) are detailed. All dosages of acepromazine were 10-100 mg/day in 2 doses and treatment lasted 3 - 3½ months. The 3 cases of melancholia were worsened after 15 days to 3 weeks of treatment, necessitating the cessation of therapy. One case of atypical schizophrenic depression improved remarkably, while 3 did not improve and the 5th was worsened (appearance of excitation). Of the 22 schizophrenics 2 improved, 5 became worse with manifestations of aggression and impulsiveness. 1 became more apathetic and the remaining 15 did not change appreciably. Slight arterial hypotension and tachycardia were noted along with extrapyramidal signs. In relation to the blood picture, there was no significant modification though a slight increase in sedimentation rate and some slight leucocytosis. The drug is indicated for neurosis and anxiety, not major psychiatric conditions.

Société Moreau de Tours
Maison Nationale de Charenton
Paris, France

2721 Gurtler, J. & Goralsky, G. Essai thérapeutique du tartrate d'alimémazine (Théralène) portant sur 415 malades psychiatriques sur une période d'environ trois ans. [therapeutic trial of alimemazine tartrate (Theralene) in 415 psychiatric patients over a period of about three years.] In: Baruk, Henri, & Launay, Jacques [Eds.] Annales Moreau de Tours. Tome I, Mémoires récents sur la psychopharmacologie. -- Annals of Moreau de Tours. Volume I. Current memoirs in psychopharmacology. Paris: Presses Universitaires de France, 1962. Pp. 113-121.

Four-hundred-and-fifteen cases treated with alimemazine included 113 cases of melancholia, 71 neurosis, 67 schizophrenia and 68 cases of delirium. All patients were women. Parenteral administration was employed as well as the more usual use of tablets, syrup and suppositories. Dosage was progressively raised to 450 mg/day or 150 mg t.i.d. whereafter dosage was progressively diminished to 120-180 mg/day. Results (when 28 cases of senile dementia, oligophrenia and 12 cases of epilepsy were ommitted leaving 357 cases) were 25.9% cured, 34.7% failures.

Société Moreau de Tours
Maison Nationale de Charenton
Paris, France

2722 Gurtler, J. & Goralsky, G. Tracés électro-encéphalographiques au cours de traitements par le tartrate d'alimémazine. [Electroencephalographic tracings in the course of treatment with alimemazine tartrate.] In: Baruk, Henri, & Launay, Jacques [Eds.] Annales Moreau de Tours. Tome I. Mémoires récents sur la psychopharmacologie. -- Annals of Moreau de Tours. Volume I. Current memoirs in psychopharmacology. Paris: Presses Universitaires de France, 1962. Pp. 124-131.

Anomalies in EEG tracings have frequently been observed after 10-15 days of alimemazine treatment at 30-60 mg/day. Modifications consist of spontaneous dysrhythmic elements (often appearing as precursors to epileptogenic manifestations), typical spikes and sometimes a slowing in a rhythm. However towards the end of the treatment the tracing is often improved or even normal. Of 28 patients, 17 presented abnormal EEG's before treatment, and dysrhythmias remained in these cases after clinical cure. Alimemazine acts as a catalyzer for the accentuation of existing EEG abnormalities, but deviations lessened as treatment progressed and the drug does not appear to be a true epilepsy-inducing agent.

Société Moreau de Tours
Maison Nationale de Charenton
Paris, France

2723 Verdeau-Pailles, Jacqueline. Tolérrance locale et efficacité de la ppromazine. Comparaison avec la chlopromazine. [Local tolerance and efficacy of promazine. Comparison with chlorpromazine.] In: Baruk, Henri, & Launay, Jacques [Eds.] Annales Moreau de Tours. Tome I. Mémoires récents sur la psychopharmacologie. -- Annals of Moreau de Tours. Volume I. Current memoirs in psychopharmacology. Paris: Presses Universitaires de France, 1962. Pp. 132-135.

Twelve patients received 3 i.m. injections of promazine as a substitute for oral chlorpromazine therapy. One group received 75 mg/day promazine for 15 days, while another received 150 mg/day for 8 days. Efficacy at the 150 mg level of promazine was equivalent to that of 100 mg chlorpromazine p.o. Local and general tolerance for promazine was excellent. Slight tachycardia was frequently observed in patients on 150 mg/kg and 5 cases of rise in body temperature were noted.

Société Moreau de Tours
Maison Nationale de Charenton
Paris, France

2724 Fouks, Lainé, Pagot, & Ferrant. Note sur le G 22 355 (imipramine). [Note on G 22 355 (imipramine).] In: Baruk, Henri, & Launay, Jacques [Eds.] Annales Moreau de Tours. Volume I. Current memoirs in psychopharmacology. Paris: Presses Universitaires de France, 1962. Pp. 149-152.

Imipramine (i.m.) [dosage unspecified] produced appreciably good results in about 50% of 32 depression cases which were resistant to other therapies. Four patients were markedly aggravated by drug induced excitation and 1 of these suffered confusion. Marked improvement was noted in 9 cases of melancholia out of 21 and slight improvement in 9 others. Negative results were obtained in 10 cases of neurotic depression. Slight extrapyramidal reactions usually developed by the 2nd week.

Société Moreau de Tours
Maison Nationale de Charenton
Paris, France

Presses Universitaires de France, 1962.
Pp. 157-15

Indications for imipramine are discussed:
the melancholic type of depressive reaction,
manic depressive psychosis, presenile depression, etc. These remarks are accompanied by 6 case reports. The rapidity of
imipramine''s action, the common attain-
ment of approximately 50% success and side
effects such as parkinsonism are recorded.

Société Moreau de Tours
Maison Nationale de Charenton
Paris, France

2727 Baruk, H., Launay, J. Cournut, J.,
Vallée, A., & Tardy, C. Le problème
des indications thérapeutiques, des doses
et des incidents de traitement par l'imipramine après une expérience de 18 mois.
[The problem of therapeutic indications,
dosage and side-effects with imipramine
after an 18-month experience.] In: Baruk,
Henri, & Launay, Jacques [Eds.] Annales
Moreau de Tours. Tome I. Mémoires récents sur la psychopharmacologie. -- Annals of Moreau de Tours. Volume I. Current memoirs in psychopharmacology.
Paris: Presses Universitaires de France,
1962. Pp. 164-172.

Nineteen cases of anxiety, 14 asthenic syndrome, 10 erythismus, 9 cenesthesis (including depersonalization), 12 neurotics
with ideas of ruin, etc. with or without
delirium, 7 obsessional reaction and 8
treated with imipramine. Oral dosage was
begun with 25 mg once or twice a day,
raised to an individual optimum for each
case, usually 100-150 mg/day, modified in
cases of marked improvement to 50-75
mg/day. Cases intense intolerable dry
mouth necessitated interruption of treatment. Imipramine was often combined with
levomepromazine, alimemazine, meprobamate and other substances. Other imipramine side effects noted were drop in
arterial tension, slight leukocytosis, extrapyramidal reaction including hypotonia of
the arms, psychomotor tension and insomnia, etc. Results were considered sucessful
in 42 out of the 65 cases. Brief note was
also made of successful therapy with imipramine and chlordiazeposide in combina-

tion.

Société Moreau de Tours
Maison Nationale de Charenton
Paris, France

2728 Coirault, R. Une orientation thérapeutique nouvelle en neuropsychiatrie et en
pathologie générale. L'ester-diméthyl-
amino-éthylique de l'acide para-chloro-
phénoxy-acétique (A.N.P. 235). Psycho-
cortico-tonique régulateur des dctions hy-
pothalamo-hypophysaires et neuro-régula-
teur central. Action sur les troubles de la
conscience. Étude clinique biologique, élec-
tro-encéphalographique et psychométrique.
[New therapeutic orientation in neuropsychiatry and general pathology. The dime-
thylaminoethyl ester of parachlorophenoxy
acetic acid (ANP 235). Psychocorticotonic,
regulator of hypothalamohypophysio functions and central neuro-regulator. Action
on mental disorders. Clinical, biological,
electroencephalographic and psychometric
study.] In: Baruk, Henri, & Launay, Jacques
[Eds.] Annales Moreau de Tours. Tome I.
Mémoires récents sur la psychopharmacologie. -- Annals of Moreau de Tours.
Volume I. Current memoirs in psychopharmacology. Paris: Presses Universitaires de France, 1962. Pp. 173-183.

One-hundred- and-seventy-seven cases (76
cranial trauma, 29 endocrine disturbance
with hypothalamo-hypophyseal origin and
72 psychiatric cases - 35 cases of simple
neurosis, 22 depression, etc.) were treated
with centrophenoxine. Conventional oral
dosage was 400-800 mg/day. A dose as high
as 4 g/day was found nontoxic. Benton's
test and the Rorschach were used in evaluation along with EEG reports. Its effects
on anxiety-insomnia-fatigue were considered excellent and centrophenoxine augmented
lucidity and intellectualization. It had a
regulatory effect on the hypothalamo-hypophyseal axis, improving the general metabolism. It also had a possible effect on
the reticular system, providing improvement in hypertonic states. The agent is
considered as a psychocorticotonic and
central regulator.

Société Moreau de Tours
Maison Nationale de Charenton
Paris, France

2729 Launay, J., & Michelin, J. Action
de l'A.N.P. 235 (Lucidril) sur les états
confusionnels aigus et subaigus de l'éthyl-
isme chronique. [Action of ANP 235 (Lucidril) on acute and subacute confusional
states of chronic alcoholism.] In: Baruk,
Henri, & Launay, Jacques [Eds.] Annales
Moreau de Tours. Tome I. Mémoires récents sur la psychopharmacologie -- Annals
of Moreau de Tours. Volume I. Current
memoirs in psychopharmacology. Paris:
Presses Universitaires de France, 1962.
Pp. 157-163.

Ten cases of delirium tremens were treated
with centrophenoxine (usually 500 mg i.v.)
for 7-8 days followed by 250 i.m. for a
week or longer. This group was compared to
a group of 13 who did not receive centrophenoxine. Chlorpromazine, other tranquilizers and vitamins were also used. One
patient died of causes unrelated to drug
administration and the remaining 9 improved notably at about 48 hours, whereas
the group which was not treated with
centrophenoxine showed improvemtn at 4-5
days. Additionally 1 man in a state of
confusion, being treated with disulfiram
was successfully controlled with centrophenoxine.

Société Moreau de Tours
Maison Nationale de Charenton
Paris, France

2730 Fouks, Lainé, Mathis, Pagot, Ferrant, Delavalade, & Riou. Étude sur l'effet
du 2038 M.D. [Study of the effect of MD
2028.] In: Baruk, Henri, & Launay, Jacques
[Eds.] Annales Moreau de Tours. Tome I.
Mémoires récents sur la psychopharmacologie. -- Annals of Moreau de Tours.
Volume I. Current memoirs in psychopharmacology. Paris: Presses Universitaires de France, 1962. Pp. 194-223.

MD 2028 (fluomethoxylphenylpiperazine but-
yrophenone) has given best results in states
of acute agitation. MD 2028 is the best
available drug for psychiatric emergencies.
Several routes of administration are used,
the i.m. route being preferred. Sixty-nine
cases were treated, both psychiatric and
alcoholic states. Intravenously the agent
is used in 5 mg injections, up to 60 mg/day
Intramuscularly, 10-20 mg injections are

2732 Fouks, Lainé, Pagot, Mathis, Ferrant, Delavalade, & Riou. Rapport sur l'essai clinique de la phénelzine. [Report on a clinical trial with phenelzine.] In: Baruk, Henri, & Launay, Jacques [Eds.] Annales Moreau de Tours. Tome I. Mémoires récents sur la psychopharmacologie.--Annals of Moreau de Tours. Volume I. Current memoirs in psychopharmacology. Paris: Presses Universitaires de France, 1962. P. 234-242.

Phelelzine is an excellent thymoleptic with rapid and efficient action. Twenty-eight cases of neurotic depression, 28 manic-depressive psychotics, 25 chronic and involutional melancholia, 17 simple depression and 3 miscellaneous cases of mental illness were treated with 90 mg/day phenelzine given on waking, in the middle of the morning and at noon, for the first 10 days. In the next 10-15 days 60 mg was given each day. Fifty cases were studied encephalographically. Twenty of these cases showed no constant modification, while 30 did. Basic alpha rhythm was regularized and improved with increase in amplitude in 14 cases, but in 11 cases there was a drop in voltage with alpha waves more discontinuous and irregular. In a few cases alterations in the beta band were also noted. The drug not only alleviated depression but also favorably affected apathy. The only notable side effect was a frequency of hypotension.

Société Moreau de Tours
Maison Nationale de Charenton
Paris, France

2733 Baruk, H., & Richardeau. Essais de la phénelzine en thérapeutique clinique. [Trial of phenelzine in clinical therapeutics.] In: Baruk, Henri, & Launay [Eds.] Annales Moreau de Tours. Tome I. Mémoires récents sur la psychopharmacologie. Annals of Moreau de Tours. Volume I. Current memoirs in psychopharmacology. Paris: Presses Universitaires de France, 1962. Pp. 243-252.

Twenty-four women with mixed chronic

psychiatric conditions were treated orally with 15 mg phenelzine b.i.d. or t.i.d. Results were recorded as: 11 improvements, 4 no effect, 3 aggravations and 6 blood pressure or vasomotor disturbance. Results were considered particularly good in cases of obsessional states. Cardiovascular disturbances were frequent, i.e., a moderate bradychardia (60-70) repolarization with flattening of the T wave in a 3rd of the cases, and progressive severe hypotension with postural hypotension in all cases after the 25th day of treatment. In the 6 cases noted above this hypotension necessitated interruption of chemotherapy, i.e., difficulty in visual accomodation, weakness in the legs, fainting, etc. This hypotension is resistant to common analeptics and ephedrine. Also it was not modified by perlingual epinephrine. When neuroleptics were used with phenelzine in some cases while they did not potentiate the phenelzine hypotension, but they did favorably modify bradycardia due to phenelzine.

Société Moreau de Tours
Maison Nationale de Charenton
Paris, France

2734 Fouks, Ferrant, Lainé, Mathis, & Pagot. Rapport sur l'essai clinique de l'iproniazide en psychiatrie. [Report on a clinical trial of iproniazid in psychiatry.] In: Baruk, Henri, & Launay, Jacques [Eds.] Annales Moreau de Tours. Tome I. Mémoires récents sur la psychopharmacologie. -- Annals of Moreau de Tours. Volume I. Current memoirs in psychopharmacology. Paris: Presses Universitaires de France, 1962. Pp. 253-255.

Treatment of 88 patients was begun with 200 mg/day iproniazid rapidly reduced to 100 mg/day and even 25 mg/day. Iproniazid was in general combined with reserpine or chlorpromazine in the treatment of schizophrenics. The caseload included a proportion of depressives and many included a proportion of depressives and many elderly patients, some arteriopathic. Iproniazid is an energizer and a euphoriant, and appears indicated in various cases of depression. Some patients, including elderly ones, showed improved behavior, activity and intellectual ability. The most clear

lightly and 3 did not improve. One case of schizophrenia with anxiety improved slightly and another partially. Of 4 cases of obsession, 2 improved markedly and 1 partially; the other case was worsened. One patient with simple depression was cured. The last case, depersonalization, was very slightly improved.

Société Moreau de Tours
Maison Nationale de Charenton
Paris, France

2738 Fouks, Lainé, Périvier, Boucher, Matnis, Ferrant, & Riou. Rapport sur l'essai clinique du S. 186 (3,3-pentaméthylène-4-hydroxybutyrate de sodium). [Report on a clinical trial with S 186 (3, 3-pentamethylene-4-hydroxybutyrate sodium).] In: Baruk, Henri, & Launay, Jacques [Eds.] Annales Moreau de Tours. Tome I. Mémoires récents sur la psychopharmacologie. -- Annals of Moreau de Tours. Volume I. Current memoirs in psychopharmacology. Paris: Presses Universitaires de France, 1962. Pp.265-274.

For periods of 6 months, S 186 was used in depression, particularly senile depression. Results on 51 patients are presented; usual dosage was 25-150 mg/day. This central analeptic caused improvement in general tonus as well as cardiovascular tonus, improved attention and mentation. It is particularly recommended in cases of apathy.

Société Moreau de Tours
Maison Nationale de Charenton
Paris, France

2739 Coirault, R., Jarret, R., Girard, V., & Desclos, S. Intéret de la fixation thyroïdienne du radio-iode I 131 dans les troubles psychopathologiques. [The importance of thyroid fixation of radio-iodine, I^{131} in psychopathologic disorders.] In: Baruk, Henri, & Launay, Jacques [Eds.] Annales Moreau de Tours. Tome I. Mémoires récents sur la psychopharmacologie. -- Annals of Moreau de Tours. Volume I. Current memoirs in psychopharmacology. Paris: Presses Universitaires de France, 1962. Pp. 324-332.

One-hundred-and-fifty psychiatric patients were studied in regard to iodine fixation (25 μc I 131). Most patients suffered the triad anxiety-insomnia-fatigue. Iodine uptake was abnormal in 65% of the males and 36% of the females at 24 hours. The curve for psychiatric patients paralleled that for normal subjects but was higher, i.e., 50% fixation at the 6th hour reaching 60% fixation at the 24th hour.

Société Moreau de Tours
Maison Nationale de Charenton
Paris, France

2740 Coirault, R., Jarret, R., Girard V., Desclos de La Fouchais, S., Péchery, C. Cortico-surrénale et psychopathologie. Les dosages des corticoides et la thérapeutique cortico-surrénale. [The adrenal cortex and psychopathology. Assay of corticoids and cortico-adrenal therapy.] In: Baruk, Henri, & Launay, Jacques [Eds.] Annales Moreau de Tours. Tome I. Mémoires récents sur la psychopharmacologie. -- Annals of Moreau de Tours. Volume I. Current memoirs in psychopharmacology. Paris: Presses Universitaires de France, 1962. Pp. 333-341.

Psychoendocrinological factors were studied in 150 psychiatric patients and 600 general patients as controls, i.e., 11 oxysteroids and 17-ketohydroxysteroids. Variations in the urinary excretion of steroids was also studied following ECT, ACTH injection and insulin shock therapy. The excretion of 11-oxycorticosteroids by mental patients was less than that by general patients, and the excretion of 17-ketosteroids was much reduced in psychiatric cases. However in some cases of paranoid schizophrenia the excretion of 17-ketosteroids was elevated. Electrolyte balance, and the therapeutic use of ACTH, cortisone and triamcinolone was outlined.

Société Moreau de Tours
Maison Nationale de Charenton
Paris, France

2741 Coirault, R., Masbernard, A., Desclos de la Fouchais, S., & Mazingant, F. L'acide uridine-5-triphosphorique-

(U.T.P.). Thérapeutique majeure des atrophies musculaires (dystrophies musculaires, atrophies neurogènes). Influence sur les états de fatigue. Action neurostimulante. Controles biologiques et électrologiques. [Uridine-5-triphosphoric acid (UTP). Major therapy of muscular atrophies (muscular dystrophy, neurogenic atrophies). The influence on fatigue states. Neurostimulating action. Biological and electrologic control.] In: Baruk, Henri, & Launay, Jacques [Eds.] Annales Moreau de Tours. Tome I. Mémoires récents sur la psychopharmacologie. -- Annals of Moreau de Tours. Volume I. Current memoirs in psychopharmacology. Paris: Presses Universitaires de France, 1962. Pp. 342-348.

Nine cases of progressive muscular dystrophy, 1 myasthenia, 30 neurogenic muscular atrophy, 30 fatigue and 10 anxiety-insomnia-fatigue were treated with uridine-5-triphosphoric acid (UTP; 10-20 mg/day p.o.). The agent was ameliorative in muscular dystrophy, myasthenia, neurogenic muscular atrophy, and particularly efficacious in fatigue. No side effects were noted.

Société Moreau de Tours
Maison Nationale de Charenton
Paris, France

2742 Büssow, Hans. Vergleich der Wirkung zweier Glutarimide bei neuroleptischen Zuständen. [Comparison of the effect of 2 glutarimides in neuroleptic conditions.] Medicina Experimentalis, 1962, 6, 113-117.

A comparative investigation was carried out on 29 patients with acute or subacute endogenous psychoses, using Ba 12 408 (N-methyl-a-phenyl-a-ethylglutarimide) and glutethimide. All patients were pretreated with neuroleptic agents for 6-8 days; thereafter, either Ba 12 408 (100-200 mg t.i.d. or q.i.d.) or glutethimide (125-250 mg t.i.d. or q.i.d.) were administered in addition. Ba 12 408, which has no or only very slight anticholinergic effect, has no influence on mood changes in psychoses pretreated with neuroleptic agents; whereas glutethimide which has anticholinergic action is convincingly effective in bringing

(Taractan) for several weeks. The daily oral dosage varied from 30-120 mg during the 1st 1 or 2 weeks, and from 15-90 mg during the following 1 or 2 weeks. Headache and nausea improved so much that no additional therapy was necessary. Three patients developed minor allergic reactions and 3 patients did not respond.

Kantonsspital
Frauenfeld, Switzerland

2745 Meier, Paul J. Erfahrungen mit Neurocil in der Chirurgie. [Experiences with Neurocil in surgery.] Therapie der Gegenwart, 1962, 101, 322-325.

Levomepromazine (Neurocil; 0.025 gm i.m. or i.v.), a phenothiazine derivative, was used for the preparation of 163 patients for, mostly major, abdominal operations. It was administered once or twice, usually in combination with other drugs such as phenobarbital. The excellent sedating effect allowed considerable reduction in the use of analgesics. Nausea and vomiting were almost completely absent and blood pressure changes were minimal. A few older, arteriosclerotic patients responded with marked increase in blood pressure. Good results were also seen when levomepromazine was used in severely painful conditions.

Chirurgische Abteilung des St. Josef-
    Krankenhauses
Troisdorf/Siegkreis, Germany

2746 Gross, H., & Kaltenbäck, Elfriede. Sordinol R, ein neues Neuroleptikum der Thiaxanthenreihe. [Sordinol, a new neurolepticum of the thiaxanthene group.] Wiener Klinische Wochenschrift, 1962, 74, 549-554.

A chlorprothixene analogue (Sordinol) has been shown to produce in animals effects similar to those of chlorprothixene. It was used in the treatment of 139 hospitalized patients, 131 of them schizophrenics. Single oral or i.m. dosages varied from 5-75 mg, and daily dosages from 10-225 mg (average 30 mg). The drug was generally tolerated; minor local infiltrations occurred from time to time, sleepiness and tiredness frequently. Extrapyramidal side effects mixed with anticholinergic and/or antiadrenalergic effects, hypotonia and tachycardia were also seen rather often. Side effects were tolerable in most patients or could be controlled with additional medication. Blood counts, blood chemistry and urinalyses showed no pathological findings. The drug should be administered to hospitalized patients only. Fifty patients showed minor improvement; 35 others showed no improvement. The remaining 54 patients were released as cured. Among these were many who has not responded to other neuroleptic agents. The effect of Sordinol is considered superior to that of chlorperphenazine.

Heilabteilung für Männer der Heil-und
    Pflegeanstalt der Stadt Wien "Am
    Steinhof"
Vienna, Austria

2747 Gross, H., & Langner, E. Prophylaxe und Behandlung des medikamentös bedingten Parkinson-Syndroms mit Procyclidin-Hydrochlorid (Kemadrin[R]). [Prophylaxis and treatment of drug-induced Parkinson-syndrome with procyclidine-hydrochloride (Kemadrine[R].] Wiener Klinische Wochenschrift, 1962, 74, 569-570.

Procyclidine (Kemadrin) was used for the treatment of drug-induced postencephalitic parkinsonism. In comparison with atropine, its central effect is more pronounced, its peripheral effect 25 times weaker. Sixty-eight hospitalized and ambulatory patients were treated (5-15 mg t.i.d. p.o. and/or i.m.). A double-blind study was carried out with a group of 42 of these schizophrenic patients who had been treated previously with various neuroleptic agents. No effect was seen in 13 out of 14 patients who received the placebo. Good results were obtained in 19 out of 28 patients who had received procyclidine. The symptoms of the abulic-akinetic syndrome could be influenced very effectively in 95% of the patients. After disappearance or improvement of the akinetic syndrome, akathisia and akinesia could frequently be observed. These symptoms could be sufficiently improved with procyclidine in 43% (30-45 mg

out. At first, suppositories (30 mg) were used; the results were not satisfactory and 1 ml Pervetral (25 mg) or 1 ml of the placebo were administered. Pervetral was effective in 70%. The dosage was then increased according to age and condition (37.5-50 mg), and the results improved to 75-80%. In a further study, 21 patients with concussions (commotio cerebri) were treated with Pervetral. They received 25 mg at admission, regardless of whether vomiting had occurred or not. Nausea and retching could almost always be suppressed for 3-4 hours. Pervetral was well-tolerated, and has a sedating effect, potentiating the effect of analgesics.

Chirurgische Abteilung des Krankenhauses
Bethel
Bückeburg, Germany

2751 Thomas, Klaus. Suizidprophylaxe unter besonderer Berücksichtigung der pharmakopsychiatrischen Behandlung Lebensmüder. [Suicide prophylaxis with special consideration of the pharmaco-psychiatric treatment of depressed persons with suicidal tendencies.] Therapie der Gegenwart, 1962, 101, 319-321.

Suicides in Germany are almost as frequent as traffic deaths. This is a report on the activities of a medical agency which tries to cope with persons who want to take their own lives. It originated in 1956 in West-Berlin, and its telephones were used since that time by over 10,000 desperate and depressed persons. In cases of imminent suicide, hospitalization is attempted but often not possible. More often, the psychiatrists, physicians and social workers of the agency have to try to calm or treat the person in need. It was found to be an impossible task to cope with the anxieties, desperation, restlessness, affective tension and emotional lability without the help of drugs. A drug had to be found which was effective and could be used in visits without causing harmful side effects or severe hypnotic effects. The drug of choice was Phasein Forte (C.F. Boehringer, Mannheim), a combination of reserpine and orphenadrine. Twenty-five percent of all patients seen (2700 patients of whom 20% had endo-

genous and reactive depressions) received
Phasein Forte, alone or in combination
with reserpine or mephenamine (1st day:
1 tablet, increasing to 6-8 tablets; mg unspecified). After considerable improvement
in psychopathological symptoms, the daily
dosage was decreased by 1 tablet per week,
until a maintenance dosage of 3 tablets
daily was reached. Eighty-five percent of
patients who took the medication consistently were markedly improved, and in most
cases enabled to go on with their jobs.

Nismarckstrasse 66
Berlin-Steglitz, Germany

2752 Runyan, John W., Jr. Observations on
the use of phendimetrazine, a new anorexigenic agent in obese diabetics. Current
Therapeutic Research, 1962, 4, 270-275.

Sixty of an original 76 diabetic patients
completed a 3-month trial, 30 on phendimetrazine and 30 on placebo. The drug (35
mg tablets) was given 1/2 hour before each
meal, as was placebo. Patients were not in-
formed of the compounds anorexigenic properties and the suggestive element in weight
reduction was therefore minimized or eliminated. Phendimetrazine was found effective
with negligible side effects (transient nausea
in 5 and nervousness in 2). The weight loss
on drug was 2.7 pounds compared to 0.91
pounds on placebo. (No refs.)

University of Tennessee
Division of Medicine
Memphis, Tenn.

2753 Chemotherapy Review. The treatment of psychoneurotic depressed patients
with tranylcypromine/trifluoperazine,('Parstelin'). Report of a general practitioner
clinical trial conducted in Newcastle-on-
Tyne. Chemotherapy Review, 1962, 2, 255-
258.

Two-hundred-and-fifty-six patients suffering from depression with association of
psychoneurotic states were treated with
Parstelin (each tablet containing 1 mg trifluoperazine and 10 mg tranylcypromine).
One tablet was usually given in the morning
and early in the afternoon. On occasion 3

Ugarteche 2823
Buenos Aires, Argentina

2758 Duchastel, Yves. La methaqualone
(methyl-2-orthotolyl-3 quinozolone-4) HCl
Hypnotique non barbiturique de synthèse
(Etude clinique à "double inconnue" de 100
cas). [Methaqualone (methyl-2 orthotolyl-3
quinazolone-4) HCl Synthetic non-barbitu-
rate hypnotic ("double-blind" clinical study
of 100 cases).] Union Médicale du Canada,
1962, 91, 288-290.

One-hundred patients, hospitalized for insomnia, were given 150 mg methalaqualone
or placebo at night on a double-blind basis.
Eighty-seven % showed very good response
compared to 46 % obtained with placebo.
No physical side effects were noted.

Service de Neurologie
Hôtel-Dieu de Montréal
Montreal, Quebec
Canada

2759 Azima, H., Arthurs, Dorothy, Silver,
A., & Azima, Fern J. The effect of MP-809
in depressive states: a multi-blind study.
American Journal of Psychiatry, 1962, 119,
573-574.

MP-809, a tryptamine derivative, was investigated in 50 depressed patients and
compared to 2 other groups of 50 depressed
patients receiving inert and potent placebo
in a multiple-blind study. The chemical
formula is 4-methyl-α-methyl-tryptamine.
The average daily dose was about 60 mg
(20-100 mg) for an average period of 21 days
and the potent placebo dose (phenobarbital)
was 30 mg/day. Clinically MP-809 had a
significant (marked to moderate) antidepressant action in 52 % of all patients and
74.1 % of neurotic depressions. Side effect
were frequent but mild, consisting of fine
hand tremors in 10 patients, drowsiness in
8, weakness in 6, dizziness in 5, fatigue
in 4, nausea and vomiting in 5, generalized
pruritis in 2, diarrhea in 2 and ankle edema
in 1.

Department of Psychiatry
Psychopharmacology Section
Allan Memorial Institute
Montreal, Quebec, Canada

2760 Bonhour, Alberto, Jones, Blanca, &
Acebal, Enrique M. Experiencia clinica
con fenelzina. [Clinical experience with
phenelzine.] Prensa Médica Argentina,1962
49, 2336-2341.

Twenty patients with manic-depressive psychosis, 7 with reactive depression, 5 neurotic depression, 3 involutional depression
and 2 with depression emmerging in the
development of other psychoses were treated with 75 mg phenelzine/day in 32 cases
and 45 mg/day in 5 cases for 30-40 days.
Some dry mouth, orthostatic hypotension,
paresis of the leg, etc. was noted. Manic
depressives were treated with phenelzine
and ECT. Out of 21 mental patients with
manic psychosis, 12 remitted, 3 were improved and 6 showed no change of condition.
Out of 6 cases of reactive depression 3 were
in remission, 1 improved and 2 did not. Out
of 5 cases of neurotic depression, 3 were in
remission, and 2 had improved. With involutional depression 2 out of 3 were cured
while the other remained unchanged. With
psychotic depression neither of the 2 cases
improved. Global results were 20/37 remission, 6/37 improvement and 11 no
change.

Facultad of Medicina
Instituto de Clínica Psiquiátrica
Buenos Aires, Argentina

2761 Goldberg, Marshall. Thyroid impairment in chronic alcoholics. American Journal of Psychiatry, 1962, 119, 255-256.

Thyroid function was studied in 82 males and
18 females, aged 23-65 years, who were
confirmed alcoholics. One or more baseline PBI determinations, the rise in the
PBI 24 hours after 10 IU of thyrotropic
hormone i.m., electrometric recordings of
the Achilles tendon reflex by the Lawson
kinemometer and the tanned red-cell agglutination procedure for the detection of
circulating thyroglobulin antibodies were
made. Forty-five of the 100 chronic alcoholics tested were found to be thyroid
deficient to varying degrees, i.e., 47 considered euthyroid and the remaining 8 were
placed in a "borderline hypothyroid" category. Among 47 patients considered frank
or borderline hypothyroid and treated with
thyroid hormone, 16 were lost to followup

2765 Sampson, Patsy Hallock, Ray, Thomas S., Pugh, Lawrence A., & Clark, Mervin L. Picture recognition as an index of social sensitivity in chronic schizophrenia: the effects of chlorpromazine. Journal of Consulting Psychology, 1962, 20, 510-514.

Picture recognition data were collected from 72 chronic schizophrenic women on chlorpromazine or placebo. Their ages ranged from 28-53 years and they had been hospitalized a minimum of 8 years. Fifty-one were assigned to chlorpromazine and 21 to placebo. The treatments were administered double-blind for 10 weeks to a maximal dose of 800 mg chlorpromazine or 8 placebo capsules daily. A procedure involving recognition of pictures of self and others was devised and employed as a measure of social sensitivity, social stimulus value, and self acceptance. Chlorpromazine produces increased social awareness as measured by increases in both nonverbal (sorting) scores and verbal (naming) scores. It produces a greater acceptance of selfimage as reflected in increased frequency of acknowledgment of own photographs. However no effect of chlorpromazine on social stimulus value was found.

Cornell University
Ithica, N.Y.

2766 Horwitz, David, Fox, Samuel M. III, & Goldberg, Leon I. Effects of dopamine in man. Circulation Research, 1962, 10, 237-243.

Cardiovascular effects of dopamine in 11 normal volunteers and 2 patients undergoing diagnostic cardiac catheterizations were studied. Dopamine was prepared as a 1% solution in saline and administered i.v. Results of hemodynamic studies in 6 normal subjects indicated that dopamine increased cardiac output and stroke volume in all subjects. Arterial pressure also increased in all subjects with a predominant systolic pressure increment. Calculated vascular resistance decreased in 5 subjects and did not change in the other subject. Changes in heart rate were of small magnitude and were inconstant in direction. Left arterial pressure did not change in 2 patients at a time when substantial increments in cardia output were produced by dopamine. Comparison of the doses of dopamine and levarterenol calculated to produce equivalent increments in systolic pressure indicated that dopamine was 1/25 to 1/56 as potent as levarterenol in this respect.

National Heart Institute
Bethesda, Md.

2767 Dewar, Robert, & Ross, Hugo. The use and abuse of tranquillizing drugs for chronic mental patients. Canadian medical association Journal, 1962, 87, 1375-1377.

The behavior of 16 female hospitalized psychotic patients was measured while they received maintenance doses of chlorpromazine (average dose, 50 mg q.i.d.) and again while receiving identical doses of a placebo. The double-blind technique was employed. Nurses used a behavior rating scale to measure noisiness, personal cleanliness, interpersonal relations among patients, occupational activities, hostility, activity, cooperation, dress, eating and sleeping. Patients' behavior over a 6 week period of chlorpromazine administration was compared with behavior over an equal period of placebo administration. There was no evident difference in behavior in 90% of the cases. Among the others there was a slight trend towards improved behavior while the patients received placebo. Tranquilizing drugs are often used needlessly for chronic mental patients.

Psychology Department
McMaster University
Hamilton, Ontario
Canada

2768 Sibley, W.A., Tucker, H.J., & Randt, C.T. Quinacrine in the treatment of refractory petit-mal epilepsy. Canadian Medical Association Journal, 1962, 87, 6, [Abstract]

Thirty-three cases of petit-mal epilepsy were treated with atropine (Quinacrine) which successfully controlled seizures in 25 out of the 33. In 1 patient the seizures was suppressed for only 6 weeks, but in

Lancet, 1962, No. 7241, 1205-1208.

Haloperidol in a dose of 3 mg was combined with pethidine at usual clinical doses
in the management of labor in 350 women,
50 of whom were injected i.v. while the
remainder received haloperidol i.m. Sedation was deep after i.v. injection. The
evidence suggested slowing of labor with
a relatively high incidence of operative
overdose. Bradycardia and hypotension
occurred in some cases. Intravenous haloperidol is not advised for routine use in
labor, but it may be useful in a minority
of patients who need more sedation than
usual injected i.m., haloperidol proved a
safe and efficient complement to pethidine,
providing good "psychic sedation", not interfering with the course of labor or causing fetal depression. There were no extrapyramidal, cardiovascular or other side-
effects.

Department of Anesthetics
Royal Infirmary
Dundee, Great Britain

2774 Diggory, P.L.C., & Tomkinson, J.S.
Nausea and vomiting in pregnancy. A trial
of meclozine dihydrochloride with and without pyridoxine. Lancet, 1962, No. 7252,
370-372.

Of a random series of 100 pregnant women,
88 experienced nausea and vomiting; 73 had
taken some form of medication, a large
proportion treating themselves without any
medical advice. In 23% of the affected patients the onset of vomiting preceded the 1st
missed menstrual period and did not appear
entirely psychosomatic. Meclozine is effective in the treatment of these cases.
Twenty-five mg of meclozine was taken
every morning and 50 mg at night, or placebo. Some received meclozine plus pyridoxine with the same dosage of meclozine
used above, on a double-blind basis. Comparably good results were obtained with
both active medications: 28 out of 41 on
meclozine and 22 out of 35 on meclozine
plus pyridoxine.

Queen Charlotte's Maternity Hospital
London W. 6, Great Britain

2775 Bayliss, S.G., & Gilbertson, M.P
A trial of chlordiazepoxide in spastic children. Lancet, 1962, No. 7263, 995-996.

A double-blind, crossover trial with 41
spastic children was run in order to assess
the value of chlordiazepoxide; however only
29 children completed the trial (1 had to be
withdrawn because of side effects). Home
rating and school rating showed a significant difference, but the psychotherapy and
6-ball test scores were not significant,
which suggests that the improvement in the
other ratings was due mainly to behavioral
changes. Similar results could probably
have been achieved with a sedative. Nineteen
children did show signs of decreased spasticity or rigdity while receiving the drug,
but 10 of these became too relaxed, resulting in less control and poorer posture.
Side effects of drowsiness or increased
irritability and aggressiveness were also
troublesome, The dose of 0.75 mg/kg used
is probably close to the upper limit of the
tolerated dose.

Centre for Spastic Children
Chelsea, London, S.W. 3
Great Britain

2776 Aaronson, Herbert G., & Boger,
William P. Incontinence in the elderly: an
attempt at control. Journal of the American
Geriatric Society, 1962, 10, 626-632.

Forty incontinent female patients (CBS,
mental deficiency, involutional psychiatric
reaction, manic depression reaction-manic
type and schizophrenia) were given bedtime
administration of either 25 mg imipramine
or matching placebo. Each patient served
as their own control. Most patients were
past 60 years of age. No benefit was obtained from imipramine or placebo in relation to incontentence. Nevertheless the
moral of the patients was notably increased, apparently due to a program
which brought together the attendant,
nursing and medical personnel in a shared
therapeutic effort.

Arthur P. Noyes Research Department
Norristown State Hospital
Norristown, Penna.

able of causing phocomelia are reviewed.

Department of Pediatrics
University of Manitoba
Canada

2782 Easson, William M. Gasoline addiction in children. Pediatrics, 1962, 29, 250-254.

An 11-year-old and a 14-year-old boy, both mentally disturbed, were hospitalized because of gasoline sniffing. These boys were able to tolerate gasoline inhalation over prolonged periods, sometimes for several hours without physical discomfort which might indicate a degree of physical tolerance. No specific withdrawal reaction was noted.

Children's Service
Menninger Clinic
Topeka, Kan.

2783 Ling, George M., Dolman, C.L., & Boyd, John R. Drug-induced (thalidomide) malformations. Canadian Medical Association Journal, 1962, 87, 1259-1262.

Two cases of infants born with phocomelia, amelia and alimentary abnormalities are presented, where the mothers had received thalidomide in early pregnancies. The question is raised whether or not similar abnormalities might occur in comparable circumstances after the administration of other glutarimides currently in clinical use. Drug therapy should be kept at a minimum in pregnancy, particularly the first trimester.

Department of Pharmacology
Faculty of Medicine
University of British Columbia
Vancouver, British Columbia
Canada

2784 Le Van, Paul, & Bierman, Stanley M. Idiosyncratic drug eruption to Dilantin and trimethadione. Archives of Dermatology, 1962, 86, 254-256.

A 16-year-old boy developed a spontaneous

akinetic seizure and was placed on di-
phenlyhydantoin (Dilantin, 100 mg t.i.d.)
and 3 weeks later developed a pruritic
morbilliform eruption of his trunk, low-
grade fever, nausea and sore throat. Three
weeks later the patient was placed on
trimethadione, 300 mg t.i.d. and a month
later developed photophobia, butterfly facial
eruption, fever and malaise and was readmitted to the hospital. All antiepleptic
agents were withdrawn and the patient improved on 30 mg prednisone.

[No address]

2785 Pisciotta, Anthony V., & Kaldahl,
Joyce. Studies on agranulocytosis. IV. Effects of chlorpromazine on nucleic acid
synthesis of bone marrow cells in vitro.
Blood Journal of Hematology, 1962, 20,
364-376.

Studies were conducted on the bone marrow
of 27 random hospital patients who had
never received chlorpromazine and therefore were not known to be sensitive to
this drug. Also similar studies relating to
solutions of chlorpromazine on incorporation of H^3-thymidine and uridine were
performed on the bone marrow of 5 men
and 4 women who had had agranulocytosis
following treatment with chlorpromazine
and were now recovered. These results
were compared to those obtained from 10
persons who had been treated with comparable doses for more than 2 months
without developing agranulocytosis and 12
randomized hospital patients who had never
received chlorpromazine. When viable marrow cells were incubated with tritiated
thymidine and uridine, the cells became
radioactive as nucleic acid synthesis proceeded. Excessive concentrations of chlorpromazine partially inhibited the influx of
thymidine and uridine into granulocytes of
all patients who had had agranulocytosis
due to this drug, and of about 75% of
random hospital patients. This drug did
not effect nucleic acid synthesis in nine
individuals who had been treated with a
large amount of chlorpromazine, with no
alteration in their leukocyte count. A comparison of the effects of dilution of chlorpromazine upon influx of H^3-thymidine into
granulocytes showed significant dose-de-

amine, 3.0 mg/kg iproniazid, 35-37.5 mg/kg phenelzine, 1.2 g/kg alcohol, 15 mg chlordiazepoxide and 3 mg/kg diazepam. The action of chlordiazepoxide differed from that of the other drugs, probably through quantitative fear reduction. The method appears to be a step forward towards the goal of specifying the mechanism of abnormal behavior, and aid in the establishment of methods of reliable drug assessment.

University of Massachusetts
Amherst, Mass.

2789 Hoffer, A. Lack of potentiation by chlordiazepoxide (Librium) of depression or excitation due to alcohol. Canadian Medical Association Journal 1962, 87, 920-921.

A double-blind study was conducted comparing the interaction of 10 mg chlordiazepoxide for 1 day and 6 ounces of rye whiskey given over a 3-hour period in the evening of the same day. The comparison drug was a placebo. Four evening experiments were conducted using the same 6 normal subjects and 2 observers. At the end of the evening, the observers were unable to detect which subjects had had placebo or chlordiazepoxide. Therefore the recommended therapeutic dose of chlordiazepoxide did not potentiate what was considered a social quantity of alcohol.

Psychiatric Research Branch
University Hospital
Saskatoon, Saskatchewan
Canada

2790 Savage, R.D. The effect of reserpine on conditioned fear responses. British journal of Psychology, 1962, 53, 451-454.

Eight naive kids were placed in a harness with electrodes fastened to the right foreleg. The feared stimulation was an US of 10 volts inducing specific learning of a flexion response. A continuous 2-second electric shock was presented to the foreleg. Drug dosages (mg/lb) were 0.125 saline; 0.0375, 0.625 and 0.125 reserpine. Foreleg flexion and ambulation response showed that as the drug dosage increased the flexion scores increased ambulation decreased. This lowering of general activity could be related to drug effect on the limbic, hypothalamic and reticular systems, or a general decrease in motor facility because of depressant effect.

University of New England
Australia

2791 Ray, Oakley S., & Marrazzi, Amedeo S. Interaction of reinforcement schedule and dosage on response rate changes following drug administration. American Psychologist, 1962, 17, 397. [Abstract]

Food- or water-deprived rats were tested in a single session on both a fixed ration and a DRL schedule using separate levers and tones as discriminative stimuli. Amphetamine (0.25-4.0 mg/kg) was administered just before the start of the run. Three patterns of responding were obtained: at low doses response rates on both schedules increased; at moderate levels rates increased further on the DRL schedule and were depressed on the FR schedule; at higher doses rates on both schedules were depressed. The effects of amphetamine are dependent on both dose and behavioral procedure and all the above effects can be determined by 1 CNS effect that is dose dependent and results in a loss of control by the animal.

VA Research Laboratories in Neuropsychiatry
Pittsburgh, Pa.

2792 Oken, Donald, Grinker, Roy R., Heath, Helen A., Herz, Marvin, Korchin, Sheldon J., Sabshin, Melvin, & Schwartz, Neena B. Relation of physiological response to affect expression. Including studies of autonomic response specificity. Archives of General Psychiatry, 1962, 6, 336-351.

The physiological and psychological stress responses of 18 normal college students were studied with the primary purpose of testing the hypothesis that limitation of affective expression (lack of "discharge") under stress is associated with heightened physiological response. Two groups of 9

2795 Leaf, Russell C. Discriminative classical conditioning under curare can control
the performance of subsequently learned
avoidance responses. American Psychologist, 1962, 17, 398. [Abstract]

Dogs were completely immobilized by injections of d-tubocurarine. While paralyzed,
they were given discriminative fear conditioning to 2 tones; 1 tone was consistently
reinforced with shock presentations while
the other was never reinforced. After recovery from paralysis, subjects were never
reinforced. After recovery from paralysis,
subjects were given avoidance training in
which visual stimuli were used as conditioning stimuli. This was given in the
same apparatus in which classical conditioning occurred, or in a different apparatus.
Results obtained during extinction testing
showed consistent discriminative transfer
of both types of avoidance response in
both situations by all subjects.

University of Pennsylvania
Philadelphia 4, Pa.

2796 Gardner, Lucy, & McCollough, Celeste.
A reinvestigation of the dissociative effect
of curareform drugs. American Psychologist, 1962, 17, 398. [Abstract]

Recent experiments employing the curareform drug d-tubocurarine have produced
results contradictory to those reported for
earlier experiments which employed curareform drugs, with respect to their "dissociative" effect on transfer of learning
from drug to normal state and vice versa.
The present experiments support the data
on the dissociative effect of erythroidine
(which, pharmacologically, differs considerably from raw curare) and the failure
of d-tubocurarine to produce dissociation
(though pharmacologically very similar to
raw curare). Atropine blocked the erythroidine effect. Effects of the 2 curareform drugs on autonomic and striate muscle
conditioning were measured in both classical and avoidance conditioning situations.

Oberlin College
Oberlin, Ohio

See also 2579, 2586, 2619, 2621, 2642,
2650, 2765, 2767

2797 Necina, J. Antagonism between L-α-
methyl DOPA and reserpine. Life Sciences,
1962, 2, 301-303.

Female Wistar rats and female mice were
used in the following tests: cataleptic reaction, ptosis, pentetrazol tonic seizure
threshold, cholesterol level in adrenals and
adrenal ascorbic acid determination. One
group of animals was given 400 mg/kg
α-methyl DOPA i.p. followed 2 hours later
by 5 mg/kg reserpine i.p. The 2nd group
was given saline instead of α-methyl DOPA,
while in the 3rd group reserpine was replaced by saline. The 4th group was treated
twice with saline only. With reserpine only,
all animals showed marked ptosis and catalepsy, while in the α-methyl DOPA group
only a marked degree of ptosis was observed. The threshold of pentetrazol tonic
seizure was decreased in only the reserpine
treated group. An analogous inhibition of
reserpine effect was apparent in rats, where
α-methyl DOPA inhibited reserpine-induced
depletion of adrenal cholesterol and ascorbic acid completely.

Research Institute for Natural Drugs
U Elektry 8
Prague 9, Czechoslovakia

2798 Costa, E., Gessa, G.L., & Brodie,
B.B. Influence of hypothermia on chlorpromazine-induced changes in brain amine
levels. Life Sciences, 1962, 2, 315-319.

Chlorpromazine (20 mg/kg i.p.) administered to normal rats did not change the brain
content of 5HT and levarterenol, but as
described by others, markedly antagonized
reserpine in liberating animes from their
storage sites. As this dose of drug reduced
body temperature by about 8°C, role of
this hypothermia in blocking amine depletion through repetition of the studies in
rats maintained at an environmental temperature of 35°C was investigated. Chlorpromazine no longer produced hypothermia,
nor did it inhibit the reserpine-induced
drop in brain amines. Further evidence that
the inhibition of amine release was a hypothermic effect was obtained by studies of
the influence of chlorpromazine on amine
depletion elicited by SU 9064 and tetrabenazine, reversably-acting reserpinelike

Department of Pharmacology
Harvard Medical School
Boston, Mass.

2802 Wiseman, Ralph, Jr. The effect of acute and chronic administration of chlorpromazine on the I^{131} distribution in normal rats. Journal of Pharmacology and Experimental Therapy, 1962, 138, 269-276.

Adult male Sprague-Dawley rats were given 25 mg/kg chlorpromazine i.p., followed immediately by 30 mg/kg water by oral intubation to facilitate diuresis during the subsequent 6-hour test period. After 30 minutes animals were anesthetized and given ca 6 μc of sodium iodide-I^{131} i.v. Total urine and the thyroid gland tissue were assayed. In a 2nd series fasted rats were used. In chronic experiments rats received 1 mg/kg chlorpromazine daily and 6-hour I^{131} distributions were assayed at 35, 62 and 89 days. Blood pressure studies were made in an additional group of rats. After a single i.p. dose of 25 mg/kg of body weight of chlorpromazine in the rat a 40.3% decrease in the 6-hour I^{131} uptake by the thyroid was observed. Other changes encountered in these animals in 6 hours were a 92.7% decrease in urinary excretion of I^{131}, 29.7% increased retention of I^{131} in the body and 58.0% reduction in urine volume. Sixty-six hours after the last dose, the 6-hour I^{131} uptake was decreased 40.4%.

Radioisotope Service
VA Medical Teaching Group Hospital
Memphis, Tenn.

2803 Camponovo, Luis Emilio, & Langer, Salomon Z. Acción de la diethilamida del acido vanillinico sobre una cepa de ratones refractarios al estimulo audiogeno. [The action of vanilic acid diethylamide on a strain of rats refractory to audiogenic stimulus.] Prensa Médica Argentina, 1962, 49, 1414-1418.

Young C_3zH/Ep rats were divided into 4 groups and studied as followed: controls, 10 mg/kg, 20 mg/kg and 30 mg/kg s.c. vanilic acid diethylamide. They were exposed to audiogenic stimuli once a day f0r

5 days and graded: jumping, flight, convulsions, catatonia and death. The drug sensitized the animals in proportion to dose, as well as causing proportional decrease in the latency period responses. A death rate of ca. 75% was obtained with 30 mg/kg. The Z values obtained were: controls 0, 10 mg/kg 9.13, 20 mg/kg 36.25 and 30 mg/kg 39.47.

Instituto de Fisiologia
Buenos Aires, Argentina

2804 Drakontides, A.B., Schneider, J.A., & Funderburk, W.H. Some effects of sodium gamma-hydroxybutyrate on the central nervous system. Journal of Pharmacology and Experimental Therapy, 1962, 135, 275-284.

Behavioral studies in cats and mice and EEG investigations in cats indicate that sodium γ-hydroxybutyrate by i.v., i.p. and oral routes is a CNS depressant with a characteristic dos-dependent spectrum of activity, and a very low order of toxicity. In doses of 100 mg/kg and higher, decreased responsiveness to optic, acoustic and pain stimuli, drowsiness associated with ataxia, decreased spontaneous motor activity, muscular flaccidity and a state of detachment from environmental conditions were observed. In accord with the behavioral findings, EEG studies indicated slowing of electrical brain activity, decreased responsiveness of the reticular activating system to electrical stimuli, enhancement of thalamo-cortical recruitment and a trend toward prolongation of induced seizure activity of the limbic system. The effects of this drug could be readily differentiated from those of known sedatives, hypnotics and tranquilizers.

Department of Macrobiology
Medical Research Laboratories
Charles Pfizer & Co., Inc.
Groton, Conn.

2805 Wylie, David W., & Archer, S. Structure-activity relationships of 1-[(3-indolyl) alkyl]-4-arylpiperazines. A new series of tranquilizers. Journal of Medicine and Pharmaceutical Chemistry, 1962, 5, 932-943.

Compounds of a series of indolylalkylphenylpiperazines have been found active as CNS depressants (potentiation of hexobarbital anesthesia, head-withdrawal reflex, adrenergic blocking activity). The basic structure for CNS depressive activity was found to be:

Although these agents possess peripheral adrenolytic activity to the same degree as phenothiazines and benzodioxanes, no definite correlation could be found between various central activities and peripheral adrenolytic activity.

Departments of Pharmacology and Chemistry
Sterling-Winthrop Research Institute
Rensselaer, N.Y.

2806 Bonnycastle, D.D., Bonnycastle, M.F., & Anderson, E.G. The effect of a number of central depressant drugs upon brain 5-hydroxytryptamine levels in the rat. Journal of Pharmacology and Experimental Therapy 1962, 135, 17-20.

Male Sprague-Dawley rat cerebral 5HT content after the i.p. administration of drugs was bioassayed using heart tissue from commercial osters (Venus mercenaria). Coroborative fluorimetric determinations were also carried out. A variety of central depressant drugs, including sedatives (mostly barbiturates), hypnotics, analgesics, fixed and voltile anesthetics, during the course of their pharmacologic action result in a significant elevation of cerebral 5HT. Similar increases in brain 5HT have been detected following treatment of rats with pentobarbital, chloral hydrate, diphenylhydantoin and harmaline.

Department of Pharmacology
Seton Hall college of Medicine and Dentistry
Jersey City, N.J.

2807 Brodie, B.B., Gessa, G.L., & Costa, K. Association between reserpine syndrome and blockade of brain serotonin storage

of the two phenomena. Recovery, as urinary 5HIAA, of exogenous 5HIIA, 5HT and 5HPT is the same in control, nonhydrated rats and in rats given single or repeated doses of tap water, tap water plus ADH, or isotonic saline. The mechanism by which water or saline administration produces increased urinary excretion of 5HIAA is discussed.

Institute of Pharmacology
University of Parma
Parma, Italy

2809 James, J.A., Kimbell, Lewis, & Read, William T. Experimental salicylate intoxication I. Comparison of exchange transfusion, intermittent peritoneal lavage, and hemodialysis as means for removing salicylate. Pediatrics, 1962, *29*, 442-447.

Fasting dogs were given 125 mg/kg salicylate i.v. Following an equilibrium period (usually 1-2 hours), the selected procedure was begun under pentobarbital anesthesia and was continued for 4 hours, i.e., exchange transfusion, peritoneal lavage, memodialysis. All animals developed some hyperpnea following administration of salicylate, but other symptoms of intoxication did not appear. Hemodialysis with albumin was the most efficient method of removing salicylate, about 50% of the dose being removed during the 4-hour period. Exchange transfusion and peritoneal lavage were considerably less efficient. Peritoneal lavage with 5% albumin solution was more effective than lavage with an equal conventional dialysis solution, but absorption of albumin from the peritoneum took place unless addition dextrose was added to the solution. The amount of salicylate excreted in the urine sometimes exceeded that removed by peritoneal dialysis or exchange transfusion.

Department of Pediatrics
University of Texas Southwestern Medical
  School
Dallas, Texas

2810 Hilton, James G. A proposed mechanism for epinephrine potentiation by ganglionic blocking agents. American Journal of Physiology, 1962, *203*, 753-757.

The blood pressure responses elicited in dogs by the injection of 1.0, 5.0, and 10.0 μg/kg of epinephrine were studied before and after blockade of autonomic nervous activity by either ganglionic blocking agents or by total spinal anesthesia. After blockade, blood pressure levels of 100, 130 and 160 mm Hg were maintained by infusion of epinephrine. The pressor responses elicited were inversely related to the level of the maintained blood pressure and the maximal attained blood pressures did not change markedly with the various maintained blood pressures. In a series of animals treated with ganglionic blocking agents, (procaine or chlorisondamine dimethochloride), the maximal blood pressures were approximately the same as before and after blockade, but in the total spinal anesthetized animals these pressures were ea. 30 mm Hg lower after blockade. Autonomic blockade. Autonomic blockade produces an apparent potentiation of epinephrine pressor response not by sensitization of the reacting structures, but by lowering the level of catecholamines available to the receptor sites and shifting the dose-response curve to the left.

Department of Pharmacology
Marquette University
School of Medicine
Milwaukee, Wisc.

2811 Schain, R. J. Some effects of a monoamine oxidase inhibitor upon changes produced by centrally administered amines. British Journal Pharmacology & Chemotherapy 1961, 17, 261-266.

In cats treated with s.c. or i.p. pheniperzine, the effects of 5HT injected into the lateral cerebral ventricle were greatly intensified and prolonged; the effects of epinephrine were potentiated to a lesser degree. Those of levartenenol, dopamine and tryptamine were not intensified and were prolonged to only a slight degree.

National Institute for Medical Research
Mill Hill, London, N.W. 7
Great Britain

2812 Lee Peng, C. H., & Walsh, E. O'F.

Effects of morphine on uptake of glucose and synthesis of glycogen in muscle or normal and chronically morphinized rats. Nature, 1962, 196, 171.

In the search for the site of addicting action in hormonal systems, the affects of morphine in vitro on glucose uptake and glycogen synthesis rates in excized diaphragms from normal and chronically morphinized rats were studied using the experimental procedures of Gemmill (1940), Verzár & Wenner (1948) and others. In the absence of added morphine there is no significant difference between rates of glucose-uptake by tissue from normal and chronically morphinized rats, but the mean glycogen content of the diaphragms of morphinized subjects is somewhat higher than that of saline-injected controls. The effects of morphine on glycogenesis or glycogenolysis are secondary to direct effect on glucose uptake. Morphine does not influence the rates of oxygen consumption and has a negligible effect on lactate production in vitro by diaphragms from both normal and chronically morphinized rats.

Department of Biochemistry
University of Hong Kong,
China

2813 Soaje-Echagüe, E., & Lim, Robert K. S. Anticonvulsant acivity of some carbinylureas. Journal of Pharmacology & Experimental Therapeutics, 1962, 138, 224-248.

Three carbinylureas, MA-321 (1-methylcyclohexylurea), MA-337 (1-methylcyclopentylurea) and MA-367 (1-ethylcyclopentylurea) given orally have been found to have anticonvulsant properties in rats and dogs. They are comparable in potency to such anticonvulsants as trimethadione and diphenylhydantoin. All 3 also have sedative-hypnotic, antiemetic, but little or no hypotensive effects. MA-337 and MA-367 afford protection against both electroconvulsions and chemoconvulsions, resembling carbromal and phenobarbital in these respects. MA-337 is effective at a lower antielectroconvulsant dose than diphenylhydantoin, on both single and daily dosage, while MA-367 is effective at a lower antichemoconvulsant dose than trimethadione on single but

The adrenergic nature of neurohumoral transmission in the cat nictitating membrane following treatment with reserpine. Journal of Pharmacology & Experimental Therapeutics, 1962, 138, 301-308.

The influence of reserpine on tension development in the nictitating membrane following sympathetic nerve stimulation and exogenous catecholamine administration was investigated in cats. Tension development in response to nerve stimulation was decreased from ca. 9.68 g in controls to ca. 1.90 g in reserpinized preparations, indicating a decreased output of mediator. The effect of autonomic blocking agents was analyzed with regard to elucidating a cholinergic component in the neurally induced response of the nictitating membrane. Phenotolamine was virtually ineffective in inhibiting neurally evoked contractions of the reserpinized membrane. This lack of potency contrasted sharply to its marked blocking effect in normal animals. Methylatropine exerted no significant blocking effect on responses to nerve stimulation or catecholamine in either control or reserpinized preparations. Atropine in the range of $100\mu g/kg$ depressed both neurally and catecholamine induced responses in a nonspecific manner. β-TM-10 and bretylium abolished neurally induced responses in reserpinized animals. Cholinergic mechanism is not apparently involved in sympathetic transmission at the nictitating membrane.

Department of Pharmacology
State University of New York Downstate
    Medical Center
Brooklyn, N. Y.

2816 Walaszek, Edward J., & Chapman, John E. Bulbocapnine: an adrenergic and serotonin blocking agent. Journal of Pharmacology & Experimental Therapeutics, 1962, 138, 285-290.

Bulbocapnine was found to have an adrenergic blocking effect on cat and dog blood pressure. This antagonistic effect was also seen on the isolated rabbit ear and isolated rabbit jejunum but not on the carbachol-stimulated rat uterus. Bulbocapnine had no effect on responses to isoproterenol but potentiated the responses to vasopressin on dog and not on cat blood pressure. It is concluded that bulbocapnine is an α-adrenergic blocking agent and has no effect on β-adrenergic receptors. A 5HT antagonism by bulbocapnine was demonstrated on cat and dog blood pressure, isolated rabbit ear, isolated rabbit jejunum, and isolated rat uterus. The possible role of these antagonistic effects in the mechanism of experimental catatonia is briefly discussed.

Department of Pharmacology
Kansas University Medical Center
Kansas City, Kansas

2817 Mackintosh, J. H. Effect of strain and group size on the response of mice to "Seconal" anaesthesia. Nature 1962, 194, 1304.

In inbred mice of the CE and CBA strains, 5 weeks of age, were kept in groups of 30-50 for 1 week to allow acclimatization and were set up in experimental groups of 1,2 and 8 per cage. The animals were anesthetized 3 days after setting up the experiment and again a week later. Secobarbital (Seconal) was used i.p. and the dose was graded for body-weight in order to give a mean anesthetic time of ca. 20 min. A mouse was assumed anesthetized if it failed to give a righting reflex when placed on its back. The varients of the F_1 hybrids is considerably less than that of the parental stocks and secondly the strains themselves are different in their response, the CBA strain being more variable than the CE strain. The CE x CBA hybrid is more variable than the reciprocal cross and shows, as does the maternal strain, a high variation in groups of 8 animals that have been together for ten days, indicating some maternal effect. Thirdly the 2-per cage group is less variable than are the solitary animals or groups of 8-per cage.

UFAW Research Unit
Department of Medical Biochemistry and
 Pharmacology Medical School
Birmingham, 15, Great Britain

2818 Giarman, N. J., & Pepeu, G. Drug-induced changes in brain acetylcholine. British J. Pharmacol. 1962, 19, 226-234.

Benth. Part I. The anatomy of the leaf and stem. Journal of Pharmacy & Pharmacology, 1962, 14, 664-678.

Datura leichhardtii is readily distinguished from other species of the genus by its general morphology. Although similar to that of *D. stramonium*, the microscopy of the leaf differs in the length of the clothing trichomes and often in the form of the calcium oxalate crystals; it may be distinguished from other members of the Section Dutra, with the exception of *D. metel*, by the form and abundance of trichomes. *D. leichhardtii* differs from *D. metel* in possessing on the lamina of the leaf, glandular trichomes with uniseriate stalk and a single-celled head. The values of palisade ratio and stomatal index are within the same range as those of allied species.

University of Nottingham
Nottingham, Great Britain

2822 Mijan, Dominguez C. Estudio sobre la posibilidad de potenciación de los psicofarmacos por la procaina. [Study on the possibility of potenciating psychopharmaka with procaine.] Archivos Instituto Farmacología Experimental, 1962, 14, 91-129.

Imiprimine, hydroxyazide and chlorpromazine were studied in pentobarbital narcotized cats. Procaine (5-20 mg/kg) was used before treatment with the psychoactive drugs in order to ascertain possible potentiation. Imiprimine was potentiated by procaine, as was hydroxyzine, however chlorpromazine was not.

Instituto de Farmacología Experimental
Consejo Superior de Investigaciones
Cientificas
Madrid, Spain

2823 Nichols, John R. Addiction-prone and addiction-resistant rats. American psychologist, 1962, 17, 398. [Abstract]

When subjected to a previously reported procedure, some rats develop sustained opiate-directed behavior (are addiction prone), but others do not (are addiction resistant). Would the offspring of addiction-prone crosses and those of addiction-resistant crosses show behavior like that of their parents? The subjects, rats from previous experiments, were placed into ultra high, high, low, and ultra-low groups in terms of their morphine intake on relapse tests. The F_1 offspring of intra-group crosses were the experimental subjects. The offspring showed differences both in addiction proneness and in certain other variables.

[No address]

2824 Shimamoto, Takio, Ishioka, Tadao, & Fujita, Tsutomo. Antithrombotic effect of monamine oxidase inhibitor (Nialamide). Circulation Research, 1962, 10, 647-657.

Nialamide was compared with phenindione and warfarin for ability to prevent experimental thrombosis produced in rabbits. Rabbits were subjected to quantitative traumatization of the endothelial surface of the retroauricular artery and marginal ear vein. Pretreatment of the animals with 3-5 mg/kg nialamide, which did not prolong the 1 stage prothombin time (Quick), was much more effective in preventing thrombosis then either phenindione or warfarin, both of which prolonged the prothrombin time markedly. While 1.5 mg/kg nialamide was ineffective, concomitant application of subeffective doses of 150 mg phenindione and 1.5 mg nialamide was found effective. Nevertheless addition of larger amounts of phenindione did not enhance the antithrombotic effect of nialamide. Nialamide prevents the aggregation of platelets.

Department of Clinical Physiology and
 Medicine
Tokyo Medical and Dental University,
Tokyo, Japan

See also 2574, 2587, 2594, 2649, 2851, 2852, 2853, 2854, 2859

Apparently liver MAO activity changes more rapidly than that in the cerebellum. The liver-cerebellar type of correlation was not evident between the liver and other brain parts.

Institute of Psychiatric Research
Indiana University Medical Center
Indianapolis, Ind.

2827 Roa, P. Dante, Tews, J. K., & Stone, W. E. Anti-convulsive and neurochemical effects of amino-oxyacetic acid. Physiologist, 1962, 5, 204. [Abstract]

Aminooxyacetic acid (AOAA), which inhibits GABA conversion to succinic semialdehyde, was given i.v. to dogs for the recording of the cortical EEG activity and freezing of the brain in situ. A 20 mg/kg, AOAA has little effect on cortical activity while at higher doses there was some depression. Normally a dose of 20 mg/kg thiosemicarbazide or 15 mg/kg pentetrazol induced a severe seizure; a several-fold increase in the dose was required for this response after 20 mg/kg AOAA. Cerebral tissue was analyzed for 22 free amino acids and related substances by ion exchange chromatography, and for ammonia, glutamine and citrate. At various dosages AOAA induced large increases in brain GABA, ammonia, glutamine and tyrosine. Small increases in alanine and lysine and a decrease in aspartic acid. Convulsant doses of thiosemicarbazide alone induced a decrease in GABA and small increases in ammonia and alanine (observed during the seizure). With large doses of thiosemicarbazide after AOAA, the chemical pattern during the seizure was essentially the same as with AOAA alone. Hence the seizure cannot be attributed to low GABA or other observed chemical changes. Convulsant doses of pentetrazol alone induced small increases in ammonia; GABA did not decrease, and other constituents measured did not significantly change. With large doses of pentetrazol after AOAA, the chemical pattern during the seizure was like that with AOAA alone.

Department of Neurology and Physiology
University of Wisconsin
Madison, Wis.

2828 Cammarota, Hector E., & de Cam-
carota, Amalia C. La determinacion del
acido 5-hidroxiindolacetico en orina. Su
importancia en los casos de tumores car-
cinoides. (La serotonina y su metabolito.)
[Determination of 5-hydroxyindolacetic acid
in the urine. Its importance in cases of
carcinoid tumors (serotonin and its metabolite)] Prensa Médica Argentina, 1962,
49, 671-674.

The method of McFarlane et al. and the
method of Udenfriend et al. were used in
the assay of 24-hour urine samples for
5HIAA (daily average by the 1st method
6.3 mg compared with 5.9 mg). Results of
determinations from 28 patients suffering
from carcinomata were given, and these
tests advocated as of much use in this type
of case as in the study of mental patients.

Laboratorio Bioquimico Servicio de Cardio-
logía
Yerbal 2924
Buenos Aires, Argentina

2829 Ross, John J., Jr., Flanagan, Thomas
L., & Maass, Alfred R. In vitro metabolism
of 2-chloro-10-(3-dimethylaminopropyl)-
phenothiazine. III. Isolation and identification of metabolites. Journal of Medecine and
Pharmaceutical Chemistry. 1962, 5, 1035-
1041.

The metabolism of chlorpromazine by rat
and rabbit liver homogenates was studied
chromatographically using isotope techniques. Three metabolites of the -(N-methyl)-
C^{14} or S^{35} labeled drug were isolated and
identified as $C^{14}O_2$, $HO^{14}HO$ and 2-chloro-
10- (-3-methylaminopropyl)-phenothiazine-
S^{35}. The effects of various inhibitors upon
the oxidation of chlorpromazine -(N-methyl)-
C^{14} in the rat liver homogenate system
were also investigated.

Research and Development Division
Smith Kline & French Laboratories
Philadelphia 1, Pa.

2830 Axelrod, Julius. Enzymatic formation
of morphine and nicotine in a mammal.
Life Sciences, 1962, 2, 29-30.

Incubation of the soluble supernatant fraction of rabbit lung with 2-adenosylmethio-
nine-methyl-C^{14} and normorphine resulted
in a radioactive compound extractable with
isoamyl alcohol at pH 9.5 which acted
chromatographically as authentic morphine.
After elution with water this compound was
recrystallized and added to carrier morphine. The specific activity of morphine
did not decrease after 3 recrystallizations.
These observations were taken as evidence
that an enzyme in rabbit lung can transfer
the methyl group of S-adenosylmethione to
normorphine to form morphine. Similar
experiments were run with the following nor
compounds: norpethidine, norcodeine and
nornicotine. In all cases compounds were
obtained with the chromatographic properties of, respectively, pethidine, codeine and
nicotine.

NIMH
Bethesda, Md.

2831 Cession-Fossion, A., & Michaux, R.
Activités pharmacodynamiques comparées
de la 5-hydroxytryptamine et de la 5-
methoxytryptamine. [The comparison of the
pharmacodynamic activities of 5-hydroxy-
tryptamine and 5-methoxytryptamine.] Life
Sciences, 1962, 2, 483-486.

Carotid blood pressure was registered with
a manometer in anesthetized tracheoto-
mized rats. Injections were made into the
jugular vein. Cat nictitating membrane,
after preganglionic stimulation of the cervical sympathic nerve, was also used in assay.
Guinea pig ileum was also used as an
assay as a test material. Methylation of
5HT to 5 methoxytryptamine (5MT7 changes
little of its action on blood pressure in
the rat and cat, and its contractile action
on isolated ileum. Methylation slightly increases the potentiating action of 5HT on
the presynoptic orthosympathetic stimulation of the nictating membrane. Previous
large doses of 5MT (to a total of 180
$\mu g/kg$) do not influence the response of
rat blood pressure to 5HT. Some inhibitors of 5HT action have a similar effect
on 5MT response but at lower dosage levels.

Institut Léon Fredericq
Physiologie et Biochimie
Université de Liége
Liége, Belgium

having a strong basic group (guanidine or a quaternary annomium) separated from a benzene ring by 1 carbon atom appear to exert bretyliumlike effect; in contrast a strongly basic nitrogen separated from a ring by 2 carbons appears to elicit a guanethidinelike effect.

Laboratory of Chemical Pharmacology
National Heart Institute
Bethesda 14, Md.

2834 Desaty, D., O. Hadzija, S. Iskrić, D. Keglević, & S. Kveder. The synthesis of N-acetylserotonin. Biochimica Biophysica Acta, 1962, 62, 179-180.

Starting with 5-benzyloxytryptamine HCl, N-acetylserotonin was synthesized and identified using paper chromatography.

Tracer Laboratory
Institute "Ruder Boskovic"
Zagreb, Yugoslavia

2835 Robinson, Robert L., & Watts, Daniel T. Inhibition of adrenal secretion of epinephrine during infusion of catecholamines. American Journal of Physiology, 1962, 203, 713-716.

The effect of i.v. infusion of epinephrine or levartenenol on the secretion of epinephrine by the adrenal gland was studied in dogs. The epinephrine content of adrenal venous blood was assayed on the rat uterus, automatically stimulated. The infusion of epinephrine or levartenerol at a rate which produced an increase in blood pressure inhibited the output of epinephrine by the adrenal. If the rate of infusion of catecholamines was too slow to increase the blood pressure, or if the increase in blood pressure was prevented by a pressure compensator, secretion of epinephrine was not inhibited. A good correlation exists between the percent decrease in epinephrine secretion and the percent increase in blood pressure produced by infusion of catecholamines. The inhibition of epinephrine secretion during infusion of catecholamines is produced reflexly by the induced increase in blood pressure. In two experiments the aortic epinephrine concentration exceeded the adrenal venous epinephrine concentration during infusion of epinephrine, suggesting an uptake of epinephrine by the adrenal gland.

Department of Pharmacology
West Virginia University Medical Center
Morgantown, West Va.

2836 Brune, Guenter G., & Himwich, Harold E. Indole metabolites in schizophrenic patients. Archives of General Psychiatry, 1962, 62, 324-327.

Longitudinal studies of the urinary excretions of tryptamine and total indole-3-acetic acid as well as of behavior were made on 20 male schizophrenic patients. The average urinary output of tryptamine did not differ from normal values when all data were considered. There was only a slight elevation of total indole-3-acetic acid when compared with results obtained on normal subjects. For both indole derivatives, however, a wide range of variation was noted in individual patients. A striking correlation between excretion of tryptamine and total indole-3-acetic acid with the degree of psychotic activity was noted, both indoles attained increasingly high abnormal levels with increase in the severity of the psychosis. Also there was a reduction of indoles toward or to normal levels occuring with improvement in the mental state. Each of the 2 different biochemical patterns, 1 occurring with activation of the psychotic symptoms and the other with a reduction, retained its distinctive features whether or not reserpine was administered.

Thudichum Psychiatric Research
 Laboratory
Galesburg State Research Hospital
Galesburg, Ill.

2837 Fessel, W.J. Autoimmunity and mental illness. Archives of General Psychiatry, 1962, 62, 320-323.

Sera was subjected to the brain-latex test, the kidney-latex test, FII agglutination tests and analytical ultracentrifuge. Sera from 85 normal blood donors was obtained, and sera taken from 72 patients with acute mental disturbances within 24 hours of their admission. As well samples were obtained from 185 chronically psychotic patients from a state mental hospital; 28% of the acutely disturbed mentally ill patients had a serum substance, primarily protein, with reacted with a brain constituent. The incidence of such serum substances in chronically psychotic patients was 15%, in general hospital patients 11% and in blood donors 10%.

Langley Porter Neuropsychiatric Institute, San Francisco, Calif.

2838 Marks, B.H., Samorajski, T., & Webster, E.J. Radioautographic localization of norepinephrine-H^3 in the tissues of mice. Journal of Pharmacology and Experimental Therapeutics, 1962, 138, 376-381.

The radioautographic localization of levarterenol-H^3 in some tissues of mice has been described. In the 1st few minutes after injection, binding to storage sites was not prominent, but for some hours afterward, specific localization in sharply defined regions of tissues was noted. In the heart, long thin fibers, lying alongside myocardial cells, showed very intense labeling. In the spleen, short fibers in trabeculae and small "buttons" in splenic pulp appeared to be storage sites. In the small intestine, marked uptake of levarterenol was observed in polymorphic masses scattered throughout the regions of Auerbach's plexus, including those areas which could be demarcated as ganglia in this layer. In the kidney, storage of levarterenol was occasionally observed in fibers at the vascular pole of some glomeruli. In the adrenal, the medulla became heavily labeled, while the cortex demonstrated no storage of levarterenol. The sites of levarterenol storage in the tissues described were nerve endings of the sympathetic postganglionic system.

Ohio State University College of Medicine
Cleveland, Ohio

2839 Iversen, L.L., & Whitby, L.G. Retention of injected catechol amines by the mouse. British Journal of Pharmacology, 1962, 19, 355-364.

2841 Atkinson, R., & Wynne, N.A. A method
for the estimation of adrenaline and noradrenaline in urine. Journal of Pharmacy
and Pharmacology, 1962, 14, 794-797.

A method for the estimation of epinephrine
(adrenaline) and levarterenol (noradrenaline) in urine is described. The catecholamines are absorbed on aluminum oxide
and eluted with acid. The epinephrine and
levarterenol are estimated separately after
oxidation with maganese dioxide at different
pH values and converted to the trihydroxyindole derivative for fluorimetric estimation. A mean recover of 82% (± 5 %
S.D.) was obtained for total amines estimated as epinephrine, which recovery was
83 % (± 6 % S.D.), while levarterenol
recovery was 80 % (± 6 % S.D.). The
results were in good agreement with biological assay results.

Department of Pharmacy
Sunderland Technical College
Newcastle-on-Tyne
Great Britain

2842 Udenfriend, Sidney, Zaltzman-Niren-
berg, Perola. On the mechanism of the
norepinephrine release produced by a-
methyl-meta-tyrosine. Journal of Pharmacology and Experimental Therapeutics,
1962, 138, 194-199.

It has been shown that a-methyl-meta-
tyrosine (aMMT) must be decarboxylated
in order to bring about release of levarterenol (norepinephrine) from tissues.
a-Methyl-meta-tyramine and aramine, me-
te tabolic products of aMMT, are even more
potent with respect to levarterenol releasing activity. Thus aMMT, and no doubt
a-methyldopa, represent unique ways of
administering the corresponding pharmacologically active amines. Far less than
stoichiometric amounts of the a-methyl-
meta tyramines are required to bring about
and maintain depletion of levarterenol (compounds injected i.p. into guinea pigs).

Laboratory of Clinical Biochemistry
National Heart Institute
NIH
Bethesda, Md.

2843 Burack, W.R., & Draskóczy, P.R. The mode of secretion of catecholamines from the adrenal medulla. Journal of Pharmacology and Experimental Therapeutics, 1962, 138, 165-169.

The possibility that the heavy storage granules represent the sole immediate source of the catecholamines which are secreted by the adrenal medulla was tested in vivo. Rats were treated with tritiated DOPA of high specific activity so that labeled catecholamines were made and stored in the adrenal glands. The specific activity of the stored hormones was found to be the same as the specific activity of the hormones secreted into the adrenal vein. This finding supports the proposal that a degranulation mechanism operates and vitiates the proposition that a small but dynamic extragranular pool shunts freshly formed catecholamines past the granules directly into the blood. In the rat anesthetized with pentobarbital and subjected to laparotomy, the biological half-life of the catecholamines in the adrenal gland is 1 day, while others have found that under experimental conditions which involved no anesthesia or surgery, the life-life is 10 days.

Department of Pharmacology
Harvard Medical School
Boston, Mass.

2844 Moore, K.E., & Gosselin, R.E. Effects of 5-hydroxytryptamine on the anaerobic metabolism and phosphorylase activity of lamellibranch gill. Journal of Pharmacology and Experimental Therapeutics, 1962, 138, 145-152.

The effects of 5HT and certain other cilioactive agents were studied on the anaerobic metabolism of excised gills of the clam, *Modiolus demissus*. In these gills endogenous glycogen serves as a substrate and lactic acid is a product of anaerobic glycolysis. The rate of anaerobic glycolysis but not of glucose uptake is markedly stimulated by low concentrations of 5HT. At relatively high concentrations 5HTP and epinephrine stimulate while acetylcholine inhibits the rate of anaerobic lactic acid production. BOL blocks but LSD mimics the 5HT effects. The actions of 5HT on the carbohydrate metabolism of these gills cannot be ascribed to an activation of gill phosphorylase.

Department of Pharmacology and Toxicology
Dartmouth Medical School
Hanover, New Hamp.

2845 Alexander, George J., & Alexander, Rita B. Effect of Metrazol on isolated mammalian cells. II. Inhibition of synthesis of cholesterol. Biochemistry, 1962, 1, 783-788.

Mouse L cells grown in medium containing $4 \times 10^{-}M$ pentetrazol (Metrazol) had a lower sterol content than control cultures. Cells incubated in the presence of the drug with acetate-1 C^{14} incorporated 1/3 of the radioactivity normally incorporated. Cells grown in the presence of pentetrazol but incubated in drug-free media rapidly synthesized sterols of high specific activity. Rigorous analysis of the sterol fraction indicated that 79% of the radioactivity was present in cholesterol.

Department of Biochemistry
New York Psychiatric Institute
New York, N.Y.

2846 Eberhardt, H., Freundt, K.J., & Langbein, J.W. Der dünnschichtchromatographische Nachweis von Sclafmitteln als Reinsubstanzen und nach Körperpassage. [Thin-layer chromatography of hypnotic drugs as pure compounds and after passage through the body.] Arzneimittel-Forschung, 1962, 12, 1087-1089.

Twelve sedatives and hypnotic drugs, mostly barbiturates, were extracted from human urine (45 ml) with ether, washed, purified and dried. Chromatography was carried out with "Kieselgel C" (Merck-Germany), after addition of eosin (1:1000). Piperidine-petroleum ether (1:5) was used as solvent, Hg-I-NO3 as a developer and UV light for direct inspection. Rf values and data for identification of the pure drugs and their metabolites are presented. The density of spots allows estimation of urinary excre-

fonylation of phenothiazine and its 10-substituted derivatives. Journal of Organic Chemistry, 1962, 22, 1346-1351.

3-Methyl-, 3-phenyl-, and 3-p-tolylsulfonylphenothiazine were obtained from the reactions of phenothiazine or its 10-sulfonyl derivatives with the corresponding sulfonly chlorides in the presence of aluminum chloride. The same products also were obtained from the rearrangement of the corresponding 10-sulfonyl derivatives in the presence of aluminum chloride. 3-Methyl-sulfonylphenothiazine also was prepared by a Smiles rearrangement of 2'-formaamido -2-nitro -4-methylsulfonyldiphenyl sulfide.

Smith Kline and French Laboratories
Philadelphia, Pa.

2850 Sicuteri, F., Franchi, G., Michelacci, S., & Salmon, S. Aumento della escrezione urinaria dell'acido vanilmandelico - catabolita delle catecholamine - durante l'accesso emicranico. [Increase in the urinary excretion of vanilmandelic acid - catabolite of catecholamines - during migraine attacks.] Settimana Medica, 1962, 50, 13-16.

Ten patients, 6 women and 4 men, aged 34-56 years, were studied in relation to vanilmandelic acid excretion. No drugs were administered and coffee and chocolate prohibited. During attacks vanilmandelic acid excretion was elevated to as high as 12 mg/24 hours, and levels subsided to normal on recovery.

Clinica Medica dell'Università di Firenze
Florence, Italy

2851 Winthrop, Stanley O., Davis, M.A., Myers, G.S., Gavin, J.G., Thomas, R., & Barber, R. New psychotropic agents. Derivatives of dibenzo [a,d]-1,4-cycloheptadiene. Journal of Organic Chemistry, 1962, 27, 230-240.

A series of 5-dialkylaminoalkyl-5-hydroxy-dibenzo [a,d]-1,4-cycloheptadienes was prepared by alkylating dibenzo [a,d,[-1,4-cycloheptadien-5-ones with basically substituted Grignard reagents. The corresponding 5-dialkylaminoalkyl- and 5-dialkylidenedibenzo [a,d]-1,4-cycloheptadienes were also synthesized. Other alkylation procedures were adopted in instances where the Grignard method was unsuitable. Many of the compounds possess pharmacological activities characteristic of psychotropic agents. Some of the relationships between structure and activity are briefly mentioned. In general these compounds exhibited a spectrum of pharmacological activities characteristic of both tranquilizers and antidepressants. They reduced spontaneous motility, potentiated narcosis, caused hypothermia and were anticonvulsants.

Ayerst Research Laboratories
Montreal, Quebec
Canada

2852 Saito, Selichi, & May, Everette, L. Structures related to morphine. XXI. An alternative synthesis of diastereoisomeric 2'-hydroxy-2,5,9-trimethyl-6,7-benzomorphans. Journal of Organic Chemistry, 1962, 27, 1087-1089.

Cyclization of 2-(p-methoxybenzyl)-1,3,4-trimethyl-1,2,5,6-tetrahydropyridine with 48% hydrobromic acid leads to a mixture of diastereoisomeric benzomorphans IV and VI in a ratio of about 12:1, respectively (May and Ager 1959). The analgesic activity in mice of the lesser isomer (VI) was 7 times that of IV and 5 times that of morphine. Efforts to increase the yield of VI in the above mentioned ring closure have been unsuccessful and therefore attention was settled on the 9-methylcarbonyl (I; May and Kugita), the methoxy relative of which had previously been converted to 2,5,9-trimethyl-6,7-benzomorphan (May and Fry 1957) by catalytic hydrogenation of the corresponding 9-methylene derivative. By a similar sequence of reactions either IV or VI can be obtained depending on the medium used in the hydrogenation of the 9-methylene compound (II).

National Institute of Arthritis and
   Metabolic Diseases
NIH
Bethesda 14, Md.

Instituto Español de Fisiologia y Bioquímica
Barcelona, Spain

2858 Costa, E., Gessa, G.L., Kuntzman,
R., & Brodie, B.B. A differential action
of reserpine on brain dopamine stores in
rabbit. Life Sciences, 1962, 2, 599-604.

After the injection of 2 mg/kg with reserpine to New Zealand White adult rabbits,
5HT stores in the brainstem were depleted
for a period of 24-36 hours, and then rose
slowly so that at 80 hours there was a 50%
return of normal. Changes in brainstem
levarterenol closely paralleled those of
5HT. After 0.5 mg/kg reserpine i.v. at 90
minutes, the depletion of dopamine stores
in the carbate nucleus was almost complete
in all subjects. In contrast 5HT depletion
was variable, ranging from 40-80% of
normal. Large doses of reserpine deplete
the stores of all 3 amines, but dopamine
remains depleted long after the central
action of reserpine is terminated and the
ability of the brain to store 5HT and levarterenol is partially restored. Threshold
doses completely deplete dopamine stores,
but lower 5HT stores to a variable degree.
Central effects are not related to the
dopamine levels.

Laboratory of Chemical Pharmacology
NIH
Bethesda, Md.

2859 Creveling, Cyrus R., Levitt, Morton,
& Udenfried, Sidney. An alternative route
for biosynthesis of norepinephrine. Life
Science, 1962, 2, 523-526.

Studies with tyramine-2-C^{14} and norsyne-
phrine-3-H^3 were carried out in order to
investigate the occurence of the following
metabolic conversions:

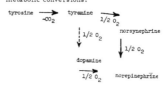

Biochemistry

Male rats were injected with the MAO
inhibitor iproniazid, 150 mg/kg i.p. at 48-
hour intervals. Twenty-four hours after the
1st dose of iproniazid, radioactive amine
was administered and the conversion of
tyramine and norsynephrine to levarterenol
(norepinephrine) and nonmetanephrine, establishing the route diagramed above.

National Heart Institute
Bethesda, Md.

See also   2588, 2609, 2621, 2622, 2645,
2677, 2785

ABBREVIATIONS

α-ketoglutarate	GABOB	γ-amino-β-hydroxybutyric acid
Zuckerman's Affect Adjective Check List	HD	hypnotic dose
adrenocorticotropic hormone	5HIAA	5-hydroxyindoleacetic acid
free choice	5HT	5-hydroxytryptamine
adenosinediphosphate	5HTP	5-hydroxytryptophane
morning		
American Medical Association	i.a.	intraarterial
Article	ibid.	in the same place
adenosinetriphosphate	i.e.	that is
	i.m.	intramuscular
British antiLewisite	IMPS	Lorr's Inpatient Multidimentional Psychiatric Scale
benzyl analogue of serotonin		
twice a day	i.p.	intraperitoneal
bromolysergic acid diethylamide	IPAT	Cattell's Institute for Personality & Ability Testing Anxiety Scale
blood urea nitrogen		
	I.Q.	intelligence quotient
Celsius scale	IU	international unit
about	i.v.	intravenous
conditioned avoidance response		
chronic brain syndrome	kg	kilogram
cubic centimeter	K_i	Michaelis constant for an inhibitor
convulsive dose	K_m	Michaelis constant for a substrate
centimeter		
square centimeter	lbs	pounds
cubic centimeter	LD	lethal dose
Centre National de la Recherche Scientifique	LSD	lysergide
central nervous system	μ	micron
catechol-o-methyl transferase	μc	microcurie
counts per second	μg	microgram
conditioned reflex (response)	μl	microliter
conditioned stimulus	μM	micromolar
Climbing Time Delay	mμ	millimicrons
	M	molar
dichlorodiphenyl trichloroethane	ma.	milliamperes
3, 4-dihydroxy-phenylalnine	MACC	Motility Affect Cooperation Communication
diphosphopyridineucleotide		
reduced diphosphopyridine-nucleotide	MAO	monoamine oxidase
	MAS	Taylor Manifest Anxiety Scale
	meq	milliequivalents
electrocardiogram	ml	milliliter
editor	mm	millimeter
effective dose	mm^a	square millimeter
ethylenediaminetetraacetic acid	MMPI	Minnesota Multiphasic Personality Inventory
electroencephalogram		
for example	MSRP	Multidimensional Scale for Rating Psychiatric Patients
electroretinogram		
and others		
and so forth	N	normal
	NEFA	nonesterified fatty acid
Fahrenheit scale	NIMH	National Institute of Mental Health
free fatty acid		
gram	p	probability
γ-aminobutyric acid	PAH	para-aminohippuric acid

PBI	protein-bound iodine	SRA
pH	negative logarithm of the hydrogen ion concentration	Suppl.
		TAT
P_i	inorganic phosphate	TH
P.M.	afternoon and evening	t.i.d.
p.o.	by mouth	TPN
ppm	parts per million	TPNH
PRP	Psychotic Reaction Profile	
		TSH
q.i.d.	four times a day	
		U
refs.	references	UR
R_f	ratio of the distance of dissolved substance to solvent distance	US
		USAF
RNA	ribonucleic acid	USDHEW
ru	rat unit	
		USP
s.c.	subcutaneous	USPHS
S.D.	standard deviation	
SGOT	serum glutamic oxaloacetic transaminase	UV
SGPT	serum glutamic pyruvic transaminase	VA
		viz.
sic	exactly as found	
SOSAI	Springfield Outpatient Symptom and Adjustment Index	WAIS
		WPRS

1120

Body image, LSD. 2787
Brain, amine levels, chlorpromazine, induced,
    2798
        hypothermia, 2798
    serotonin and reserpine, association,
    2807
Bretylium tosylate, methoxyvanilic acid,
    excretion, 2820
Bromide intoxication, 2669, 2780
Bulbocapnine, adrenergic and serotonin
    blocking, 2816
Butalbital, acetylsalicylic acid, caffeine
    and phenacetin combined, dysmenorrhea
    and premenstrual tension, 2681
Butyrylperazine compared with trifluopera-
    zine, schizophrenics, 2778

Carbinylureas, anticonvulsant activity, 2813
Cardiotonic agents, 2840
Carphenazine, parkinsonian patients, 2708
Catecholamine, excretion, adrenal medulla,
    2843
    retention, mouse, 2839
Catecholamines, epinephrine secretion, 2835
CB 1522, see acetopromazine
Central pressor effects, epinephrine and
    norepinephrine, 2587
Centrophenoxine, cranial trauma, 2728
    delirium tremens, 2729
    depression and neurosis, 2728
    endocrine disturbances, 2728
Cerebral palsy, chlordiazepoxide, 2686
Cerebral functions, and thinking, review,
    2656
    compared to computers, 2652
Children, epileptic, methetoin, 2712
        U 7524, 2769
    preoperative medication, 2661
    spastic, chlordiazepoxide, 2775
Chinese medicine, review, 2541
Classification, phenothiazines, 2648
    psychopharmacological agents, 2578
Chlordiazepoxide, alcohol consumption, 2789
    alcoholic withdrawal, 2705
    alcoholics, 2704
    anticonvulsant action, 2631
    anxiety-melancholia, 2737
    cerebral palsy, 2686
    combined with imipramine, 2727
    depression, 2737
    Huntington's chorea, 2698
    neuroses, alcoholic tremens, psycho-
    somatic disorders, 2675
    problem solving, 2788
    psychoneurotic patients, 2680

If you do not wish to continue receiving this publication, please check here ; tear off this label and return it to the address shown above. Your name will then be removed from

nopharmacology
STRACTS

vol. 2 no. 12

1962

?TMENT OF HEALTH, EDUCATION, AND WELFARE
Public Health Service

PSYCHOPHARMACOLOGY ABSTRACTS is a publication of the National Clearinghouse for Mental Health Information of the National Institute of Mental Health. It is a specialized information medium designed to assist the Institute in meeting its obligation to foster and support laboratory and clinical research into the nature and causes of mental disorders and methods of treatment and prevention. Specifically, this information service is designed to meet the needs of investigators in the field of psychopharmacology for rapid and comprehensive information about new developments and research results.

PSYCHOPHARMACOLOGY ABSTRACTS is distributed gratis to investigators doing research in psychopharmacology. It is not available on a subscription basis. Requests to receive the ABSTRACTS should be accompanied by a brief statement of the research interests and scientific specialty of the investigator. Requests to receive the ABSTRACTS, address changes, and other communications should be addressed to:

> Psychopharmacology Abstracts
> National Clearinghouse for Mental
>   Health Information
> National Institute of Mental Health
> Bethesda, Maryland 20014

U. S. DEPARTMENT OF HEALTH, EDUCATION, AND WELFARE
Public Health Service
National Institutes of Health
National Institute of Mental Health
Bethesda, Maryland 20014

PSYCHOPHARMACOLOGY ABSTRACTS

Volume 2, Number 12

large number of psychotropic agents (438
refs.)

Pharmacological Laboratory
Roche Products Limited
Welwyn Garden City, Hertfordshire
Great Britain

2861 Peigné, F. Les médicaments psycholeptiques. [Psycholeptic treatments.] France
Médicale, 1961, 1, 33-37.

Hypnotics, neuroleptics (or major tranquilizers) and tranquilizers (or minor tranquilizers)--all termed psycholeptics, are reviewed. The forms which are available in
France of chlorpromazine, levomepromazine,
acepromazine, methopromazine, prochlorpena-
zine, thiopropemazine, thioridazine, reserpine, alimemazine and aminopromazine are detailed. The major neuroleptics used at low
doses as tranquilizers are, principally,
chlorpromazine, reserpine, levomepromazine
and thioridazine. Miscellaneous tranquilizers listed are hydroxyzine, azacyclonol,
captodiame and meprobamate. The revolution
these agents have effected in the treatment
of psychoses is stressed. (No. refs.)

[No address]

2862 Masserman, Jules H., Kagen, Irving N.,
& Pauncz, Arpad. The neuroses. Progress in
Neurology and Psychiatry, 1962, 17, 450-462.

Etiology, communication and symbolism, developmental and clinical signs, prognosis
and therapy of the neuroses are reviewed.
The use of LSD and chlordiazepoxide as adjunctive to psychotherapy, improvement on
flupbenazine in patients suffering from
anxiety, the use of isocarboxazid in neurotic and psychotic depression, and the efficacy of Elavil (amitriptyline and perphenazine) in endogenous depression are noted.
(102 refs.)

[No address]

2863 Jost, F., & Geertz, V. W. Modernos trat-
amientos en psiquiatría alucinógenos: Psicosis por LSD [Modern treatments in psychiatry; hallucinogens: LSD psychosis.] Folia
Clinics Internacional, 1961, 11, 440-445.

The LSD experience (colored hallucinations,
loss of time sense, etc.) and the use of LSD
in postdelirium tremens patients, psychopaths
and schizophrenics is reviewed, with brief
mention of mescaline. (No refs.)

Neuropsychiatric Clinic
University of Innsbruck
Innsbruck, Austria

2864 Wikler, Abraham. Drug addiction. In:
Baker, A. B. [Ed.] Clinical Neurology. Volume II. Minnesota: Hoeber-Harper, 1962. Pp.
1054-1083.

The clinical features, pathology, diagnosis,
treatment, and rehabilitation of various
drug addictions are outlined. Opiates and
opioids, morphine, morphine mixtures and derivatives, synthetic analgesics (opioids),
barbiturates, meprobamate and intoxications
with marihuana, cocaine, amphetamine, and
mescaline are detailed in textbook fashion.
(142 refs.)

[No address]

2865 Hoeffler, Dennis F. Thalidomide. Journal of Pediatrics, 1962, 61, 483. [Letter]

A 40-year-old multipara with 2 normal children gave birth to a baby with typical tha-
lidomide-induced phocomelia. Her history revealed thalidomide ingestion during the 1st
trimester of pregnancy. Delivery took place
in the U.S.A., but the drug had been obtained during overseas assignment in West
Germany. (No refs.)

[No address]

2866 Taussig, Helen B. Phocomelia and thalidomide. American Journal of Obstetrics
and Gynecology, 1962, 84, 979. [Letter]

Phocomelia appears wherever thalidomide is
distributed, corroboration being found in
several hundred cases of phocomelia in the
British Commonwealth, 25 in Sweden, several
in Belgium, 5 in Italy, an epidemic in Brazil and numerous cases in Canada. Despite
polyneuritis with chronic drug use, thalidomide would probably have been marketed in
the U.S.A., had emphasis of its antiemetic
properties in pregnancy not been heavily
propounded in advertisements. The FDA did
not think the agent proven safe in pregnancy. (No refs.)

Department of Pediatrics
Johns Hopkins University
School of Medicine
Baltimore, Maryland

2867 New Medical Materia. UK-738. New
Medical Materia, 1962, 4, 41. [Editorial]

Grigyesi (Pownal, Me.) administered methylbenztropine (UK-738; 4-12 mg/day) to 84
patients with extrapyramidal disorders, 54
of whom had been receiving trihexyphenidyl
and benzatropine. Methylbenztropine appeared to be a weaker antiparkinsonian drug
than either of the controls, but its effectiveness against rigidity and lack of side
effects made it valuable as an addition to
the management of the 37 patients with parkinsonism. In 39 patients with athetosis,
6 with tremor and 2 with myoclonus, methylbenztropine exerted a clear therapeutic
effect in contrast to control drugs. (No
refs.)

The Hearst Corporation
1790 Broadway
New York 19, New York

2868 New Medical Materia. Dexedrine. New
Medical Materia, 1962, 4, 36. [Editorial]

Fish (Costa Mesa, Calif.) administered dexamphetamine (1 capsule/day or placebos) to
106 mentally retarded patients with speech
defects for 3 months. Only stutterers improved, and 5 of the 11 treated with dexamphetamine showed improvement as compared
with 1 of the 11 patients treated with placebos. Three stutterers improved so dramatically that their stuttering was controlled
to the point of obviation. Side effects included 2 with increased psychotic disturbances, 2 with increased athetosis and 2 with
excessive weight loss. (No refs.)

the most serious complication is acute liver
necrosis. MAO inhibitors available currently include iproniazid, phenelzine, isocarboxazid, pheniprazine , nialamide, and
tranycypromine. Theories for antianginal
and antihypertensive effects are elaborated.
(55 refs.)

Marquette University School of Medicine
Marquette, Illinois

2872 Bente, D. Remarks on modern German
psychiatry. Diseases of the Nervous System,
1962, 23, 32-35.

The University "Nervenklinik" at Erlangen
handles 1200 patients/year, usually on an
outpatient basis. Contemporary German psychiatry still derives from Kraepelin's
classifications although it has progressed
to include Gestalt psychology, phenomenology, Kretschmer's multidimensional diagnosis and therapy and, of course, Sigmund
Freud. Much emphasis has also been placed
upon ECT, insulin coma, chlorpromazine and
other psychotropic drugs. Psychopharmacology
will open new vistas in German psychiatry.
(No refs.)

Universitäts-Nervenklinik
Erlangen, Germany

2873 Fleck, Stephen. Residential treatment
of young schizophrenics. Connecticut Medicine, 1962, 26, 369-376.

At the Yale Psychiatric Institute, a private
44-bed intensive treatment, psychodynamically
oriented hospital, the treatment program may
be divided into 2 parts: intensive psychotherapy and the therapeutic community. In
addition, tranquilizing drugs are sometimes
used, particularly early in treatment. About
25% of the patients receive tranquilizers
and about 40% are on night sedation. Shock
therapy was being used with only 1 patient
in the last 2-2.5 years. Further, a program
of activities, athletics, occupational therapy, education, and work is available according to the needs of the individual patient.
Two-thirds of 85 schizophrenics discharged in
a recent 5-year period have adjusted with
some success. (28 refs.)

Yale University School of Medicine
New Haven, Conn.

2874 Geyer, Karl-Heinz. Über das Prinzip der therapeutischen Wirkungsumkehr psychotroper Substanzen. [The principle of reversal of therapeutic effect of psychoactive agents.] Therapie der Gegenwart, 1962, 6, 286-292.

Based on clinical and laboratory reports and the experience gained with 1 patient, specific conditions are discussed which may lead to a reversal of the expected effect of administered psychopharmacological agents, e.g. chlorpromazine and imipramine. The biologic reactions may be similar in spite of a pharmacologic antagonism (neuroleptic-thymoleptic); the direction of the therapeutic effect is determined by the individual initial mental stage of the patient rather than by the specificity of the psychotropic agent. The "toxic aggression" effect of the drug, and changes in customary dosages are factors which contribute to the occurrence of this reversal. (14 refs.)

Neurologische Abteilung der Städt. Krankenstalten
Aachen, Germany

2875 Petroff, Cottbus. Aus der internationalen Fachliteratur. Korsakow-Zeitschrift für Neuropathologie und Psychiatrie, 1962, Heft 1. [From the international medical literature. Korsakow-Journal for Neuropathology and Psychiatry, 1962, [No. 1.] Arzneimittel-Forschung, 1962, 12, 385-388.

After briefly summarizing German government directives for research in the field of neuropathology and psychiatry, the reviewer presents abstracts of 22 articles. Twelve papers deal with circulatory disturbances, mostly of the CNS, the remaining with different forms of psychoses and/or neuropsychiatric disorders. (12 refs.)

[No address]

2876 Grant, Quentin Rae. Psychopharmacology in childhood emotional and mental disorders. Journal of Pediatrics, 1962, 61, 626-637.

Psychopharmacologic agents provide symptomatic help without ameliorating underlying problems in childhood psychiatric distur-

bances. However, the amphetamines are advocated for ailments of organic or even mildly neurotic origin. Acute emergencies and severe emotional disorders respond optimally to phenothiazines like chlorpromazine. Reserpine is also widely applicable and efficacious. Mildly disturbed children may respond to meprobamate therapy in the behavioral disturbances. (75 refs.)

Department of Pediatrics and Psychiatry
Johns Hopkins University
Baltimore, Maryland

2877 Mandel, Arnold, Markham, Charles H., & Fowler, William. The use of Tofranil in the treatment of Parkinson's disease. Archives of Neurology, 1962, 6, 81; discussion 31-85.

Administration of imipramine (Tofranil; 250 mg/day) to patients with Parkinson's disease revealed mild benefit, no benefit, or in 6 with severe akinesia, considerable increase in activity. Of these, 3 showed considerable alleviation of depression while the rest exhibited only improvements in physical state. An extensive discussion is included. (No refs.)

[No address]

2878 Schmidt, Georg. Forensisch wichtige Fragen der Barbiturat-Ausscheidung im Harn. [Problems of forensic importance regarding the urinary barbiturate-excretion.] Arzneimittel-Forschung, 1962, 12, 1081-1085.

Intensity and course of action differs widely in various barbiturates. Therefore, conclusions concerning the effect may be drawn only if the drug has been specifically identified and quantitatively determined. The evaluation of small quantities of blood and urine for quantitative determination of barbiturates and their metabolites are complicated and time-consuming. Whenever possible the results should be checked by paper chromatography, spectrophotometry and crystaloptic methods. From the investigation of the urine important conclusions may be drawn

2881 German Medical Monthly. The occurrence of dopamine (3-hydroxytyramine) in the
central nervous system: its relationship to
parkinsonism. German Medical Monthly, 1962,
7, 344-346.

The physiological importance of dopamine for
the functioning of the extrapyramidal system
is suggested by the distribution of dopamine
in this system in animal experiments, and by
— the effect of L-DOPA on akinesia in parkinsonism, in which the neostriatum is depleted
of dopamine. Although of considerable theoretical interest, the therapeutic value of
L-DOPA in parkinsonian akinesis is not definitely established. Studies in changes in
dopamine, leverteranol and 5 HT in the brains
of patients who died of Parkinson's disease
and of postencephalic parkinsonism showed the
following: in the parts of the brain which
are normally rich in these amines, reduced
levels were found in cases of parkinsonism.
Dopamine was particularly reduced in the
caudate nucleus and the putamen, i.e., in
structures of the extrapyramidal motor system (41 refs.)

[No address]

2882 Bukiet, V. Embryopathies caused by
thalidomide. Concours Médicale, 1962, 84,
3999-4000.

The literature on thalidomide syndrome, with
an emphasis on German work, is reviewed.
(12 refs.)

[No address]

2883 Neuman, Maur. Psychotonics (Psycholeptics). Concours Médicale, 1962, 84, 4911-
4920.

Thymoleptics (MAO inhibitors, imiprimine)
psychotonics such as centrophenoxine, stimulants like the amphetamines and convulsive
central excitants such as bemegride are reviewed. Hormones, antigens and glucocortic-
oids are briefly noted. Criteria for the
choice of a psychotonic in the treatment of
ambulatory patients are outlined. (49 refs.)

[No address]

2884 Nature. Comparative neurochemistry.
Nature, 1962, 195, 443.

The 5th International Neurochemical Symposium was held at St. Wolfgang, Austria
during June 11-15, 1962 and the topic chosen was Comparative Neurochemistry. Available data on differences in structure, chemical composition, metabolism, enzymatic activity and drug and hormone effects on the
CNS of invertebrate and vertebrate species
were discussed on an interdisciplinary basis.
(No refs.)

McMillan & Co., Ltd.
St. Martin's Street
London, W.C. 2, Great Britain

2885 Nature. Addiction-producing drugs.
Nature, 1962, 195, 1154. [Editorial]

Continuing its work of notification, the
WHO Expert Committee on Addiction-producing
Drugs recommends in its 12th report exemp-
tion from the provisions of international
control for oxpheneridine, (-)-3-hydroxy-N-
propargyl-morphinan, methethoheptazine,
metheptazine, and 2 preparations of diphenoxylate, (Technical Report Series No. 229:
Pp. 16. Geneva, WHO), and 4 diphenoxylate
preparations. On the other hand, noracy-
methadol is considered to be an addiction-
producing drug comparable with morphine,
while nicocodine and the 4 compounds designated by the committee as methadone-inter-
mediate moramide-intermediate, pethidine-
intermediate-A and pethidine-intermediate-B
are all found to be convertible into addiction-producing drugs and therefore subject
to the relevant provisions of international
control. Concern is expressed about continuing traffic in heroin, which has been
more available than opium. The controls on
the illicit production of heroin and on
the traffic in this drug need to be enforced
more strictly. The Committee noted that the
Single Convention of Narcotic Drugs, drawn
up in 1961, affords the WHO the opportunity
to initiate the examination of dangerous
drugs and adapt the extent of control to
the degree of hazard to public health. (No
refs.)
McMillan & Co, Ltd.
St. Martin's Street
London, W.C. 2, Great Britain

effects, more stringent procedures governing the selection of physicians permitted to
experiment with new drugs, liberalization of
state abortion laws, limits to the number of
patients to be given experimental drugs, cooperation among government agencies in recording and classifying drug data, selection
of many more hospitals to engage in cooperative research on unfavorable side reactions,
crackdown on doctors suspected of rigging research on new drugs, creation of an impartial
committee of medical scientists to select re-
searchers for new drugs, compulsory use in
drug testing of pregnant animals, submittal
to FDA of all reports on the outcome of animal tests, termination of clinical testing
by FDA if doubts arise as to safety, federal
clearance for the importation of new drugs
by doctors and confiscation by the Post Office of unapproved drugs entering country.
(No refs.)

Hearst Corporation
1790 Broadway
New York 19, New York

2893 New Medical Materia. A concerted attack on narcotics, New Medical Materia, 1962,
4, 7. [Editorial]

Celebrezze's remarks at the 1st White House
Conference on narcotic and drug abuse clear-
ly underscore the tough, unyielding complex-
ities of narcotic addiction. New York
State's Metcalf-Volker law, the National
Council for the Prevention of Addiction to
Narcotics and recent federal legislation are
discussed. (No refs.)

Hearst Corporation
1790 Broadway
New York 19, New York

2894 New Medical Materia. The narcotics
problem is tough. New Medical Materia, 1962,
4 5-6. [Editorial]

The narcotics problem, involving 60,000
known addicts in the United States, is discussed in relation to reasons why society
wants the addict cured contrasted against
the addict's need to escape reality (91% relapse from cure), and the painful withdrawal
symptoms involved in cure. Pros and cons of
the "no compulsory treatment" and the

"compulsory treatment" are discussed. (No refs.)

Hearst Corporation
1790 Broadway
New York 19, New York

2895   Nature. Chemistry and mental disease.
Nature, 1962, 195, 439. [Editorial]

A symposium on "Chemistry and Mental Disease"
arranged by the Royal Institute of Chemistry,
the Chemical Society, and the Society of
Chemical Industry was held at the University
of Manchester on September 26, 1962. The
program included biochemical processes in
relation to mental disease (Todrick), inborn
metabolic errors and mental disease (Woolf),
pharmacologic assessment of psychotropic activity (Parkes), tranquilizers--structure
and activity relationships (Crowther), psy-
chostimulants--structure and activity (Young)
and values of modern drugs in psychiatric
practice (Jenner). (No refs.)

McMillan & Co., Ltd.
St. Martin's Street
London W.C. 2, Great Britain

2896   Medical World News. World experts
view thalidomide. International conclave
suggests drug's effect on the human embryo
could not have been predicted despite the
most thorough experimental testing. Medical World News, 1962, 3, 68, 70. [Editorial]

The consensus of opinion gathered from the
10th International Congress of Pediatrics in
Lisbon was that the thalidomide tragedy
could not have been avoided. However the
catastrophy revealed how poor the existing
warning system was. In Germany, the lay
press turned out to be the most efficient
warning system. Phocomelia is the most common malformation produced. (No refs.)

Medical World Publishing Co, Inc.
30 Rockefeller Plaza W.
New York 20, New York

2897   Laurent, J. M. Toxique et toxicomanie
peu connus, "le cath." [A little-known poison
and toxicomania, khat.] Annales Médico-
Psychologiques, 1962, 120, 2, 649-657.

stance P concentrations in whole brain and forebrain, as well as brainstem are given for some 26 species of animals. Relationship between organ function and tissue concentration of substance P in the intestines, CNS and degenerating nerve, and its postulated role as a transmitter substance of sensory nerves are detailed. The necessity of obtaining pure substance P preparations before attributing a central transmitter role to the substance is emphasized. (173 refs.)

Department of Pharmacology
University of Graz
Austria

2902 Abood, L. G., & Biel, J. H. Anticholinergic psychotomimetic agents. In: Pfeiffer, Carl C., & Smythies, John R. [Eds.] International Review of Neurobiology. Volume IV. London: Academic Press, Inc., 1962 Pp. 217-273.

A number of piperidyl glycolate esters have been found to produce hallucinations and other profound behavioral disturbances in humans. Emphasis is placed upon the structure-activity relationships of this class of agents and a possible mode of action on neuronal and other excitable systems. These agents may be classified into the following groups: Group I--esters of substituted glycolic acid derivatives and heterocyclic amino alcohols; Group II--esters of substituted glycolic acid derivatives and substituted piperazino alcohols; Group III--miscellaneous analogues of I and II. Gross effects in rats, sequential response in rats and behavioral effects in humans are reviewed. Neurological-autonomic (side effects) are listed. Psychological studies in humans have included comparisons to other agents such as LSD in various tests, e.g., MMPI, Jarvik Questionnaire, Clyde Mood Scale and the Rorschach Test. Phenothiazines and other tranquilizers, as well as d-tubocurarine, phenobarbital and other agents are antagonists to piperidyl glycolates (antagonism to hyperactivity in rats). Clinical studies with the glycolate esters and biochemical and electrophysiological studies with piperidyl glycolate, including effects on enzyme systems, metabolic effects in frog nerve and muscle, possible mechanism for biochemical effects, effects on contractile and excitable systems of frog sartorius muscle and the applicabil-

ity of piperidyl glycolates to studying biochemical, functional relationships are surveyed. (62 refs.)

Departments of Psychiatry and Biological
  Chemistry
University of Illinois
Chicago, Ill.

2903 Fletscher, A., Brossi, A., & Gey, K.F.
Benzoquinolizine derivatives--a new class of
monamine decreasing drugs with psychotropic
action. In Pfeiffer, Carl C., & Smythies,
John R. [Eds.] International Review of
Neurobiology. Volume IV. London: Academic Press Inc., 1962. Pp. 275-306.

Present knowledge on the chemistry, metabolism, biochemistry, pharmacology and clinical
effects of benzoquinolizines and the relationship between changes of monoamine metabolism and pharmacological action in relationship to the benzoquinolizine are reviewed.
Tetrabenazine (75-150 mg/day) is particularly
beneficial in relieving hallucinations and
paranoid symptoms of schizophrenia. It appears effective in euphoric hebephrenia
with superimposed mania and also has been
found beneficial in Huntington's chorea.
Side effects of tetrabenazine are generally
similar to those of reserpine, but rather
less severe. Several benzoquinolozines decrease 5HT and catecholamines contents preferentially in the brain. They are potent
but short acting. MAO inhibitors antagonize
or reverse several of these effects. Compounds discussed are given in the table below:

Code No.	Substitution	Formula
Ro 1-9288	2-Hydroxy-3-n-butyl-9,10 dimethoxy-	Va
Ro 1-9564	2-Hydroxy-3-ethyl-9,10-methylendioxy-	Va
Ro 1-9569	2-Oxo-3-isobutyl-9,10-dimethoxy- (= tetraben-zine, Nitoman)	IVb
Ro 1-9571	2-Hydroxy-3-isobutyl-9,10-dimethoxy-	Va
Ro 4-0786	2-Hydroxy-2-ethinyl-3-ethyl-9,10-dimethoxy	VIa
Ro 4-1284	2-Hydroxy-2-ethyl-3-iso-butyl-9,10-dimethoxy	VIa
Ro 4-1286	2-Hydroxy-2-ethyl-3-n-butyl-9,10-dimethoxy-	VIa

11

of hayatin, an alkaloid isolated from Cis-
sampelos pareira has been shown a potent
neuromuscular blocking agent. (167 refs.)

Central Drug Research Institute
Lucknow, India

2907 Rasková, Helena. Highlights of phar-
macology in Central Europe. In: Cutting,
Windsor C., Dreisbach, Robert H., & Elliott,
Henry W. [Eds.] Annual Review of Pharmacology
Volume II. Palo Alto: Annual Reviews, Inc.
1962. Pp. 31-36.

Pharmacological research in Czechoslovakia,
Hungary and Poland is reviewed under the
headings: CNS; pharmacology of the heart;
pharmacology of lipid metabolism; athero-
sclerosis; anticoagulants; antibiotics;
radiopharmacology, and information, non-
specific resistance and toxins. N-3-diethyl-
aminopropyl homacridine HCl, proheptadien,
chlorproheptatrien and chlorproheptadien
have antidepressant effects. 2-Piperidino-
methyltetralon-1 has major tranquilizing
properties; some of the β-amino-ketones
have anticonvulsant properties and potentiate the tranquilizing effect of reserpine
but antagonize its influence on electroshock.
A new drug, 1-piperidino-1-methyl-3-(ptolyl)-
propan-3-on has demonstrated interneuron-
depressing activity. Information on chronic
reserpine treatment and adaptation to external stimuli in dogs is presented. Chlorpromazine and other tranquilizers inhibit
in vitro oxidative phosphorylation and ATP
activity. The uncoupling effect of chlorpromazine is bound mainly to the subthal-
anic region, more specifically than the
barbiturates. Tranquilizing activity can
be predicted from in vitro experimentation.
The importance of chlorpromazine as a central antagonist of local anesthetics in
premedication has been emphasized. Long-
lasting increase of electrical activity
after a marked latency has been demonstrated
by injecting epinephrine levarterenol and
MAO inhibitors directly into the reticular
formation. Further information on phenothiazines and CR suppression is present. (86
refs.)

Department of Pharmacology
Charles University
Prague, Czechoslovakia

2908 Bain, J. A., & Mayer, S. E. Biochemical
mechanisms of drug action. In: Cutting,
Windsor C., Dreisbach, Robert H., & Elliott,
Henry W. [Eds.] Annual Review of Pharmacology.
Volume II. Palo Alto: Annual Reviews, Inc.,
1962. Pp. 37-66.

This review covers chlorpromazine effects on
d-amino acid oxidase, effects of chlorpromazine on mitochondral respiration and coupled
phosphorylation, barbiturates, ethyl alcohol,
salicylates, MAO inhibitors, GABA, vitamin
B6 and hydrazines, orally active hypoglycemic drugs, the effects of catecholamines
and adrenergic blocking agents, anticoagulants, carbonic anhydrase inhibitors, the
cytochemical effects of drugs and poisons
in the liver, including antihistaminics and
neuromuscular blocking agents, trialkyltins,
antibiotics, insecticides and antiparasitic
agents, protoveratrine and cocaine, and local anesthetics. (207 refs.)

Department of Pharmacology
Division of Basic Health Sciences
Emory University
Atlanta 22, Georgia

2909 Bloom, B. M. & Laubach, G. D. The
relationship between chemical structure
and pharmacological activity. In: Cutting,
Windsor C., Dreisbach, Robert H., & Elliott,
Henry W. [Eds.] Annual Review of Pharmacology. Volume II. Palo Alto: Annual Reviews, Inc., 1962. Pp. 67-108.

Structural parameters pertinent to biological interactions of drugs are reviewed.
The size, shape and electron distribution
of promazine and promethazine in relation
to Fisher-Hirschfelder-Taylor models, the
binding of 5HTP and DOPA to aromatic amino
acid decarboxylase, formulas of pethidine
analogues, absorption and distribution of
drugs, localization of drugs in tissues,
special transport mechanisms, metabolic
transformations, structure and actions at
receptors, Belleau's adrenergic receptor
model and other topics are elucidated. (249
refs.)

Medicinal Chemistry Department
Chas. Pfizer and Company Inc.
Medical Research Laboratories
Groton, Connecticut

sterone are reviewed. Within these frames
of reference, the effects of perphenazine,
nalorphine and morphine, ether and pentobarbital, reserpine, chlorpromazine, epinephrine and phenytoin are detailed. (326 refs)

Department of Anatomy and Brain Research
   Institute
University of California School of Medicine
Los Angeles, California

2915 Maickel, R. P., & Weissbach, H. Recent developments in chemical and biochemical assay techniques applicable in pharmacology. In: Cutting, Windsor C., Dreisbach,
Robert H., & Elliott, Henry W. [Eds.] Annual Review of Pharmacology. Volume II.
Palo Alto: Annual Reviews, Inc., 1962. Pp.
399-414.

Spectrophotofluorometry, gas chromatography
and new developments in radioisotope techniques are expounded. The basic components
of the spectrophotofluorometer are a high-
intensity xenon arc source which emits continuously throughout most of the UV and visible regions and 2 diffraction-grating mono-
chromators, 1 to separate monochromatic
light for excitation and a 2nd monochromator
at right angles to analyze the emitted fluorescence. A photomultiplier circuit measures the intensity of fluorescence. Its use
in the assay of tryptophan and its metabolites is detailed. The assay of 5HT and
related compounds (e.g., 5HIAA), is reviewed.
The applications of gas-liquid chromatography for steroids, amino acids and derivatives,
drugs and miscellaneous compounds (e.g., imipramine), tritium gas exposure labeling and
the application of liquid scintillation count-
ing techniques are explained. (119 refs.)

Laboratory of Chemical Pharmacology
National Heart Institute
NIH
Bethesda, Maryland

2916 Leake, Chauncey, D. Reviews of reviews. In: Cutting, Windsor, C., Dreisbach, Robert H., & Elliott, Henry W. [Eds.]
Annual Review of Pharmacology.Volume II.
Palo Alto: Annual Reviews, Inc., 1962. Pp.
415-430.

Review material is given on basic pharmacological problems, practical sociological
aspects of current pharmacology, pharmacological aspects of metabolism, chemical disin-
fection and chemotherapy of infectious diseases, autonomic drugs, CNS stimulants and
depressants, psychopharmacology, cardiovascular drugs, enzymes, proteins and hormones,
toxicology and miscellany. Analeptics have
been reviewed by Hahn (1960.) Sideman (1961)
surveyed 204 references on the clinical pharmacology of hypnotics and sedatives. Ecken-
hoff and Oech (1961) reviewed 262 contributions dealing with the effects of narcotics
and narcotic antagonists of respiration and
circulation in humans. Telford and Keats
(1961) reviewed narcotic and narcotic-an-
tagonist mixtures. Way and Adler (1960) reviewed 338 references bearing on the metabolic fate of morphine and its surrogates.
Callaway and Stone (1960) offered a critical
review of psychopharmacologic theory. The
placebo effect has been carefully analyzed by
Loranger, Prout and White (1961). Roth and
Barlow (1961) reviewed the penetration of
drugs into the brain, using autoradiography.
Bures (1960) has reviewed the spreading depression phenomenon following the local application of salt solutions to various parts
of the brain as 1st described by Leao. Impastato (1959) introduced a critical symposium on nialamide and Brill (1961) a symposium
on chlordiazepoxide. (91 refs.)

Laboratory of Chemical Pharmacology
National Heart Institute
NIH
Bethesda, Maryland

2917 Kapp, Frederic T., & Gottschalk, Louis
A. Drug therapy. Progress in Neurology and
Psychiatry, 1962, 17, 536-558.

Major tranquilizers, minor tranquilizers,
antidepressants and psychomotor stimulants
are detailed. Side effects and complications
of major tranquilizers are given. The evaluation of drugs for use in psychiatry is difficult and complicated. Preclinical data on
animals is often of little value in predicting the outcome of therapeutic trials in man.
Drug trials in hospitals are often made on
persons badly defeated in life, suffering rejection with no prospect of rehabilitation
into their former culture, while on the other
hand most outpatients have a world about them

with which they are interacting. These great
differences between in and outpatients make
a carryover of information of 1 type to the
other difficult and uncertain. Placebo effect is amplified. The control of abnormal
behavior and the lessening of symptoms by
major tranquilizers is not great enough;
better answers about mental illness will be
found when psychopharmacology considers man
in all his relationships. (290 refs.)

[No address]

2918 Ulett, George A., Smith, Kathleen, &
Biddy, Ralph. Shock treatment. Progress in
Neurology and Psychiatry, 1962, 17, 559-571.

Techniques of ECT, complications, selection
of patients and mode of action are reviewed.
Tranquilizers appear to be about equally effective to ECT in most cases of manic and
schizophrenic reactions. Reserpine combined
with ECT is contraindicated, but the combination of ECT with the phenothiazines appears
safe, except with massive doses. No conclu-
sive statement can be made on the value of
antidepressants versus ECT, however the combination of ECT with antidepressant is apparently safe. It does not appear that any
of the antidepressants available can wholly
replace ECT in the treatment of the more severe hospitalized depressions. There is as
well a 3-21 day delay in antidepressant treatment allowing a period of time in which suicide may occur. (195 refs.)

[No address]

2922 Baker, Walter W. Pharmacology of the
central nervous system. Progress in Neurology and Psychology, 1962, 17,101-127.

Chlorpromazine and the phenothiazine derivatives, reserpine and related alkaloids, miscellaneous tranquilizing agents, depressants
and analeptics, CNS stimulants, imipramine,
MAO inhibitors, convulsants, cholinergics,
catecholamines and 5HT, GABA, psychotomimetics, analgesic and anesthetic agents and
anticonvulsants are reviewed. As well, drugs
used in hyperkinetic disorders, antiparkinsonian drugs, muscle relaxants and neuromuscular blockers are outlined. (279 refs.)

[No address]

2926 Shore, Parkhurst A. Release of serotonin and catecholamines by drugs. Pharmacological Reviews, 1962, 14, 531-550.

The following topics are discussed: agents
releasing both serotonin and catecholamines
(reserpine, benzoquinolizines, decarboxylase
inhibitors and related agents and other a-
gents), procedures modifying the ability of
agents to release amines (MAO inhibitors,
chlorpromazine and stress), agents affecting mainly catecholamines in peripheral tissues (guanethidine and related compounds and
tyramine and other noncatechol sympathomimetic amines), and agents which block the uptake of catecholamines by peripheral tissues. (111 refs.)

Department of Pharmacology
University of Texas Southwestern Medical
  School
Dallas, Texas

2927 Delgado, Jaime N. & Worrell, Lee F.
Drug Notes,, Psychopharmacologic, antidiabetic agents; anabolic steroid reviewed.
Texas State Journal of Medicine, 1962, 58,
431-432.

Chlorprothixene (Taractan) leads to tranquilization without depression and may be
therefore used in cases of agitated depression. It is better tolerated than the phenothiazines and favored for outpatient use.
It is indicated in moderate to severe emotional disorders, especially agitated states.
It is reported relatively free from severe
toxic effects. (No refs.)

College of Pharmacy
University of Texas
Austin, Texas

2928 Texas State Journal of Medicine. Up-
john withdraws Monase from market. Texas
State Journal of Medicine, 1962, 58, 372.
[Editorial]

The Upjohn Company has announced the withdrawal of its product etryptamine (Monase)
from the market because of the occasional
development of agranulocytosis. It was 1st
marketed in June 1961 and used in the

treatment of depression. (No refs.)

Texas Medical Association
1801 N. Lamar Blvd.
Austin, Texas

2929 Killam, Eva King. Drug action on the
brain-stem reticular formation. Pharmacological Reviews, 1962, 14, 175-223.

Major topics reviewed are: fundamental considerations of structure and function of
the brainstem reticular formation (anatomi-
cal investigations, afferent connections,
special neural aggregations for autonomic
integration and efferent connections--the
functional role of the reticular formation
in CNS regulation), methodological considerations in drug research, the influence of
drugs on the reticular formation (chemical
mediators, sedative-anesthetic agents, phenothiazines and Rauwolfia alkaloids, miscellaneous sedatives, muscle relaxants, stimulants, psychotomimetics and miscellaneous
centrally active compounds (opioids, anticonvulsants, antiparkinsonian agents). (44
refs.)

Department of Pharmacology
Stanford University School of Medicine
Palo Alto, California

2930 Silvette, H., Hoff, E. C., Larson, P.
S., & Haag, H. B. The actions of nicotine
on central nervous system functions. Pharmacological Reviews, 1962, 14, 137-173.

The effects of nicotine on spontaneous activity, CR's learning, higher cerebral functions (sensorimotor functions, brain potentials, tremor, convusions, nicotine paralysis
and catelepsy), medullary functions (vomiting,
respiration and vasomotor functions), cerebellar functions and spinal functions are
reviewed. (184 refs.)

Departments of Pharmacology and Neurological
  Science
Medical College of Virginia
Richmond, Va.

2931 Weiss, Bernard, & Laties, Victor G.
Enhancement of human performance by caffeine
and the amphetamines. Pharmacological Re-

2936 Hastings, Donald W. Depression. Journal Lancet, 1962, 82, 9-11.

In a discussion of evaluation, physicians' attitude, family attitudes and therapy in depression, ECT, is cited as the backbone of treatment. Reports in the literature appear conflicting in relation to the value of antidepressants. With suitable outpatients, usually the physician preferred 1 or another of these drugs and gives it a therapeutic trial for a minimum of 2 weeks. If there is little or no change for the better after 2 weeks "try one of the others." (No refs.)

Department of Psychiatry
University of Minnesota
Minneapolis, Minnesota

2937 Journal of Iowa Medical Society. Sadove says addicts shouldn't be regarded as criminals. Journal of Iowa Medical Society, 1962, 52, 38. [Editorial]

Max S. Sadove deplores the practice of regarding drug addicts as criminals when they are really peaceful, nonbelligerent individuals (except when in need of a fix). In Great Britain addicts can register at a regional clinic and receive a plethora of legally prescribed drugs. Americans should emulate this example and provide narcotics (by controlled prescription, of course) for those so addicted. These unfortunate derelicts should also be regarded as human beings who desperately require our understanding. (No refs.)

Iowa State Medical Society
529 36th St.
Des Moines 12, Iowa

2938 Journal of Iowa Medical Society. Drug treatment for mental patients. Journal of Iowa Medical Society, 1962, 52, 48. [Editorial]

A film short entitled "No Man Is a Stranger" (Audio-Visual Department, Schering Corp., 1011 Morris Avenue, Union, N. J.) deals with the history and treatment of mental disorders in Haiti. Minimal hospitalization and maximal reliance on drug therapy are emphasized. Patients receiving main-

tenance therapy are soon able to resume pro-
ductive activity. (No refs.)

Iowa State Medical Society
529 36th Street
Des Moines 12. Iowa

2939 Chemotherapy. Progress in imipramine
therapy. Depressive states, combination
therapy. Chemotherapy, 1962, 2, 183-184.
[Editorial]

Imipramine has proven to be efficacious in
ameliorating depressive states according to
Blair, Kiloh and Ball's double-blind studies.
Succinct resumes of all work provide relevant
information as regards dosage, duration, results and side effects. (3 refs.)

[No address]

2940 Chemotherapy. Amitriptyline: a new
tranquilizer and antidepressive. Chemotherapy, 1962, 2, 182. [Abstract]

A review of amitriptyline cites work by Freed,
Dorfman, Barsa and Saunders to emphasize the
fact depressed patients respond dramatically
to amitriptyline therapy with only minimal
side effects. Salient facts are presented
from several studies. (No refs.)

[No address]

2941 Kris, Else B. Post-hospital care of
patients in their community. Current Therapeutic Research, 1962, 4, 200-205.

Tranquilizers like triflupromazine or fluphenazine, sometimes combined with antidepressants, are frequently used in maintain-
ance therapy of released chronic patients.
General procedures, pharmacotherapy, the day
hospital, employment, and the patient and
the community are discussed. (No refs.)

Department of Mental Hygiene
State of New York
New York, New York

these patients died with a temperature of
109° F. It seems that any MAO inhibitor
yields the same results: phenelzine (Nardil),
nialamide (Niamid), tranylcypromine (Parnate),
iproniazid (Marsilid), isocarboxazid (Marplan), and a mixture of trifluoperazine and
tranylcypromine. All these MAO inhibitors
produced untoward effects when given with
imipramine. Brodie's hypothesis that 5HT
may be the neutral transmitter in place of
acetylcholine in the brain and the suggestion that levarterenol is active as a neu-
rotransmitter is noted. Marazzi's views on
5HT blocking at the transcallosal synapse,
as well as other information on neurotrans-
mitters were elucidated in the discussion.
(19 refs.)

[No address]

2948 Alonso Jimeno, S. Psicofarmacos.
[Psychopharmaka.] Medicina, 1962, 30, 133-
140.

The classification of psychoactive drugs,
after Delay, is given in the scheme below:

Psycholeptics
    Hypnotics or hypnosedatives
        Barbiturates
    Neuroleptics
        Haloperidol
        Chlorprothixene, etc.
    Tranquilizers
        Phenothiazine derivatives
        Chlorpromazine
        Mephenesin
        Rauwolfia alkaloids
        Captodiame
        Hydroxyzine
        Chlordiazepoxide
        Benactyzine
        Meprobamate
Psychoanaleptics
    Psychotonics
        Amphetamines
        Centrophenoxine
    Thymoleptics
        Imipramine
        MAO inhibitors
Psychodysleptics
    Old
        Alcohol
        Marihuana
        Ergot

Modern
　　Mescaline
　　LSD
　　Harmine, harmaline
　　5HT and epinephrine metabolites

[No address]

2949 Médecine et Hygiène. Psycholeptiques
[Psycholeptics.] Médecine et Hygiène, 1962,
No. 5402, 212-213.

This chart gives commercial names, chemical
description, structure, mode of action, and
CNS effects, as well as neurological and psychiatric indications, side effects, and par-
ticulars for the antidepressants nialamide,
iproniazide, pivazide, phenelzine, tranylcypromine, imipramine, amitriptyline, phenpro-
bamate, troxazine, and mephenoxalone. (No
refs.)

[No address]

2950 Greene, Raymond. Thalidomide and congential abnormalities. Lancet, No. 7253,
452.

Regardless of the thalidomide tragedy, it
has often been demonstrated that animal experiments cannot obviate risk. Clinical
testing of new drugs must continue and some
risk must be expected or we must do without
new drugs. (No refs.)

[No address]

2951 Cleghorn, R. A., Moll, A. E., & Roberts,
C. A. [Eds.]. Third World Congress of Psy-
chiatry Proceedings. Volume I. Toronto/
Montreal: University of Toronto Press and
McGill University Press, 1962. Pp. 1-746.

This volume of papers of the Third World
Congress of Psychiatry held in Montreal, 4-
10 June, 1961 contains papers ranging through
the entire gamut of psychiatry. Child and
family psychiatry, concepts and methods, mental hospitals, neurophysiology, physical
therapy, psychopathology, psychotherapy,
social psychiatry, aftercare, communication,
community mental health, alcohol and drug
dependency, electroencephalography, genetics,

urated. In studies on phenothiazines in the
treatment of schizophrenics there is still
doubt as to whether results are due to pharmacological action alone, to a patient-phar-
macology interaction or to a patient-pharma-
cology-milieu interaction. Further there is
a real problem in distinguishing side effects
from psychiatric symptoms, e.g., insomnia.
More should be learned about the role of psychoactive agents in the treatment of the elderly, about the length of time the drug
should be administered and about combinations of chemotherapy with other major treatment methods such as psychotherapy. (12 refs.)

VA Hospital
Perry Point, Maryland

2956 Lopez-Ibor, J. El sintoma "clave" en
el tratamiento de las depressiones. [The
key symptom in the treatment of depression.]
In: Cleghorn, R. A., Moll, A..E., & Roberts,
C. A. Third World Congress of Psychiatry
Proceedings. Volume I. Toronto/Montreal:
University of Toronto Press and McGill
University Press, 1962. Pp. 165-169.

The efficacy of a drug can be assessed by
observing its capacity to reduce, alter or
eliminate target symptoms (behavioral, somatic, and experiential symptoms). In en-
-dogenous depression, the central symptom is
vital sadness, which is an expression of
alteration in vitality. The rate of remission with imipramine obtained in Spain is
about 69%. (No refs.)

[No address]

2957 Lewis, Nolan D., Tobin, Joseph M.
Boyle, Daniel, & Caton, John. Psychopharma-
cological research in an outpatient setting.
In: Cleghorn, R. A., Moll, A. E., & Roberts,
C. A. Third World Congress of Psychiatry
Proceedings. Volume I. Toronto/Montreal:
University of Toronto Press and McGill Uni-
versity Press, 1962. Pp. 374-379.

Parameters involved in multi-physician
double-blind crossover psychopharmacologic
research in an outpatient setting are detailed. The patient's attitude towards participation in such a study appears to be
the most challenging area of investigation
and suggests the need for the development

of test techniques more refined than those used to date. For example, drug reactors will respond differently to the same agent or similar agents at different points of time. The comparison of new with standard drugs is preferred if the pharmacological profile of the agent is comparable. While side effects have not generally been a major cause for drug discontinuation, behavioral toxicity, i.e., the patient's acting out of aggressive impulses, has occasionally presented problems. A double-blind study of 4 drugs (chlordiazepoxide, meprobamate, perphenazine and thioridazine) is detailed with an emphasis on variables. (16 refs.)

Bureau of Research in Neurology and
    Psychiatry
Princeton, N. J.

2958 Fort, Joel. The use and abuse of alcohol and narcotics around the world. In: Cleghorn, R. A., Moll, A. E.,& Roberts, C. A. Third World Congress of Psychiatry Proceedings. Volume I. Toronto/Montreal: University of Toronto Press and McGill University Press, 1962. Pp. 393-401.

Ten percent of the French population of 45 million suffers from alcoholism. This means that 1 out of every 4 or 5 adult men plus a considerably smaller number of women are alcoholics. Normal consumption is up to 4-5 liters/day for the average male. Cirrhosis and secondary psychiatric problems are the main consequences with accidents and drunken driving running close behind. Twenty-five percent of male and 10% of female admissions to state hospitals have alcoholic psychosis, a total of 30,000 admissions per year. Treatment programs involve vitamins, disulfiram, tranquilizers, and sometimes psychotherapy. In contrast France has an almost negligible narcotic addiction problem, about 1,000 individuals. However France is involved in the narcotics traffic of heroin from Lebanon for dissemination to Italy and the United States. Alcoholism in the United States is second only to France, i.e., 3% or 5 million alcoholics. The loss per year in accidents, absenteeism and job loss is approximately $1 billion. Narcotics addiction is a far smaller problem affecting 50-100 thousand Americans. Hong Kong has the highest known incidence of narcotics addiction, ca. 10% of its 4-4.5 billion Chinese using opium or

should be prescribed only in special situations. Phenothiazines such as chlorpromazine are an exception and may be prescribed without risk of excessive self-medication or addiction. The antidepressants such as MAO inhibitors are often helpful in those alcoholics who drink to relieve depression or its equivalents. These drugs are not habit forming but the amphetamines are and should be avoided in the treatment of alcoholism. (5 refs.)

University of Washington and Shadel Hospital
Seattle, Washington

2963 Arlen, Harold W. The treatment and rehabilitation of drug addiction. In: Cleghorn, R.A., Moll, A. E., & Roberts, C. A. Third World Congress of Psychiatry Proceedings. Volume I. Toronto/Montreal: University of Toronto Press and McGill University Press, 1962. Pp. 431-435.

Drug addict rehabilitation as practiced in California is detailed. The necessity of institutionalizing patients during the initial days of treatment for drug addiction to accomplish withdrawal from physiological dependence has achieved the status of a "sine qua non." The rehabilitation of the drug addict is essentially the same as the rehabilitation of any patient whose compromised ego strength has rendered him particularly vulnerable to the stresses of life. The 1959 Narcotic Treatment Control Project of the California Department of Correction is reviewed. (No refs.)

South California Parole Outpatient Clinic
Beverly Hills, California

2964 Hurst, Lewis A. Research implications of converging advances in psychiatric genetics and the pharmacology of psychotropic drugs. In: Cleghorn, R. A., Moll, A. E., & Roberts, C. A. Third World Congress of Psychiatry Proceedings. Volume I. Toronto/Montreal: University of Toronto Press and McGill University Press, 1962. Pp. 538-542.

The comparison of the mechanisms of antidepressants shows that 2 types of antidepressants (MAO inhibitors and imipramine), despite

fundamental differences in chemical structure
and numerous differences in their detailed
chemical effects, nevertheless a similar influence on 5HT and catecholamines, strength-
ening the view that these are the significant chemical entities involved in the therapeutic action of both types of drugs. This
comparison pinpoints the search for the etiological enzyme block postulated by genetic
evidence on the field of 5HT, catecholamines
and their progenitors. Enzyme chemistry,
neurochemistry, and neuropsychopharmacology,
including the advent of the psychotomimetic
and psychotropic drugs are briefly noted.
Psychiatric genetics and neuropsychopharmacology are brought to a more defined focus
by consideration on the specificity of action for the depressive states vis-à-vis
schizophrenia of the mentioned antidepressants
and the similarity of clinical outcome in
depression with either MAO inhibitors and
imipramine. (11 refs.)

University of Witwatersrand
Johannesburg, South Africa

2965 Sankar, D. V. Siva, Gold, Eleanor,
Phipps, Edward, & Sankar, D. Barbara. Bio-
chemical studies on schizophrenic children.
In: Cleghorn, R. A., Moll, A. E., & Roberts,
C. A. Third World Congress of Psychiatry
Proceedings. Volume I. Toronto/Montreal:
University of Toronto Press and McGill Uni-
versity Press, 1962. Pp. 610-613.

The biochemistry of schizophrenic and autistic children is reviewed with emphasis on
the excretion of total aromatic amines and
total indole compounds. Absence of galactosemia in autistic children is noted. The
study of 5HT uptake by platelets is altered
not only in childhood schizophrenia but also
in adults subsequent to the administration
of tranylcypromine and chlorpromazine. A
5HT analogue may be produced in schizophrenia which passes through the same metabolic
sites as 5HT does. Thus it is possible that
a study of 5HT level and uptake in platelets
may throw more light on the biochemistry of
schizophrenia. (19 refs.)

Creedmoor State Hospital
Jamaica, New York

2966 Batt, J. C. Review of endocrinological
investigations at St. Ebba's hospital. In:

weeks with the aid of one of the energizing
drugs. Drugs do not combat disease directly
but act to correct a disturbance of psychic
function created by disease and offer only
symptomatic therapy, i.e., no drug is currently available that can undo the dynamic
disturbance in family relations that lies at
the basis of every neurosis and nonorganic
psychosis. However, when dynamic forces become sufficiently strong to cripple ego functions, they can be attenuated by pharma-
ceutic means. (18 refs.)

[No address]

2970 Feer Hans. Vergleich der klinischen
eigenschaften von drei phenothiazin-ähnlich-
en substanzen. [Comparison of the clinical
effects of three phenothiazine derivatives.]
In: Cleghorn, R. A., Moll, A. E., & Roberts,
C. A. Third World Congress of Psychiatry
Proceedings. Volume II. Toronto/Montreal:
University of Toronto Press and McGill University Press, 1962. Pp. 964-966.

The chemistry of chlorpromazine, chlorprothixene, amitriptyline, and imipramine is
described rather extensively. Therapeutic
and side effects are discussed in very general terms. Chlorpromazine is considered
the drug of choice for treatment of schizophrenic psychoses; the other drugs, especially
chlorprothixene and amitriptyline have mainly antidepressive effects. (2 refs.)

Psychiatrische Universitätsklinik
Basel, Switzerland

2971 Berthier, Ch. Les neuroleptiques sé-
datifs en thérapeutique psychiatrique. [Se-
dative neuroleptics in psychiatric therapy.]
In: Cleghorn, R. A., Moll, A.E., & Roberts,
C. A. Third World Congress of Psychiatry
Proceedings. Volume II. Toronto/Montreal:
University of Toronto Press and McGill
University Press, 1962. Pp. 973-976.

The pharmacology and indications for levomepromazine, cyamepromazine, alimemazine,
thioridazine, chlorprothixene, prothipendyl
and combinations are reviewed. (No refs.)

Domité Lyonnais de Recherches Thérapeutiques
  en Psychiatrie
Bron, France

2972 Levy, Sol. A new approach to the treat-
ment of depressive reactions. In: Cleghorn,
R. A., Moll, A. E. & Roberts, C. A. Third
World Congress of Psychiatry Proceedings.
Volume II. Toronto/Montreal: University of
Toronto Press and McGill University Press,
1962. Pp. 1357-1361.

The roles of psychopharmaka, ECT and psychotherapy in depression are discussed.
Generally pharmacology is aimed at certain
target symptoms, while convulsive therapy
attacks the depression per se. Psychotherapy
in depression is a rather complex problem
and includes difficulty in rapport, difficulty
with potential suicidal dangers, and etc.
Tranylcypromine is found reliable in the
treatment of mild depressions not endangered
by suicidal risks. Imipramine is a well-
tried agent and chlordiazepoxide is of use
in mild depressions of recent origin. The
successful use of sedatives for the suppression of insomnia, including thalidomide, is
noted. (10 refs.)

[No address]

2973 Medical World News. New boost for 'GP
psychiatry.' Medical World News, 1962, 3,
27. [Editorial]

Diazepam and chlordiazepoxide were reviewed
in regard to clinical efficacy in anxiety
and depression at the San Francisco Symposium on Neuropsychotropic Drugs. (No refs.)

Medical World Publishing Co, Inc.
30 Rockefeller Plaza W.
New York 20, New York

2974 Chemotherapy Review. Orphenadrine
hydrochloride. Drug of choice in neuroleptic parkinsonism. Chemotherapy Review, 1962,
2, 139 & 155. [Editorial]

Success was obtained in alleviating neuroleptic parkinsonism with orphenadrine, which
has also proved efficacious in ameliorating
schizophrenic dejection and listlessness in
conjunction with phenothiazines. Depressive
states were also responsive to orphenadrine
therapy. The combination of orphenadrine
and thioproperazine is considered as being
superior to ECT. (No refs.)

(Archivos de Criminología Neuro-Psiquiatría y Disciplinas Conexas 1951) were treated with thiopropazate. Partial remission was obtained in 13%, social remission in 60% and failure in 25%. (1 ref.)

[No address]

2978 Sulé Sagarra, J. Psicosis maniaco-depresivas. [Manic depressive psychosis.] Revista de Psiquiatría y Psicología Media, 1962, 5, 644-666.

This is an abbreviated version of a work by the same name appearing in Tratado de Psiquiatría under the auspices of the Catedra de Psiquiatría de Barcelona, couched along the lines of Kleist (1959), following Kraepelin's (1918) system. In relation to treatment, ECT is preferred to pentetrazole shock. The usefulness of psychoactive drugs is stressed, especially imipramine. Promazine, methazine, perizine, and others including haloperidol, neuroleptics, MAO inhibitors, and tranquilizers are also useful in the treatment of endogenous psychosis. Neuroleptics are frequently of use in manic states. (46 refs.)

Instituto Pedro Mata de Reus
    Neuropsiquiatra
Hospital Clínico de Barcelona
Barcelona, Spain

2979 Von Planta, Peter. Sur l'emploi clinique des inhibiteurs de la monoamine-oxydase dans l'angine de poitrine. [The clinical use of MAO inhibitors in angina pectoris.] Médecine et Hygiène, 1962, No. 541, 223-225.

Iproniazid, phenipratine, isocarboxazid, phenelzine, nialamide and pivazid are discussed in relation to ambulatory patients with angina pectoris, particularily those with a neurotic, anxious, or depressive component. The psychostimulant and analgesic effect, dilitation of coronary arteries, diminution of oxygen consumption, accumulation of lactic acid, antithrombotic effect and the prevention of myocardial necrosis are reviewed. The most important side effects are lowering of blood pressure, most often orthostatic, hepatotoxicity, the possibility of cardiac insufficiency, and

the possible appearance of psychomotor excitation and manic states. (No refs.)

Laboratory Hoffmann La Roche
Basel, Switzerland

2980 Giberti, F. Problemi metodologica ed aspetti teorico-practicidella moderna psicofarmacologia. [Methological problems and theoretic-practical aspects of modern psychopharmacology.] Sistema Nervosa, 1962, 14, 437-453.

The classification of psychotropic drugs, general trends, ethics and methods of study and evaluation in clinical research, including the placebo problem and the question of quantitation in psychopharmacology are discussed (77 refs.)

Clinica delle Malattie Nervose e Mentali
Università Genova
Genoa, Italy

2931 Kolb, Lawrence. Drug addiction: A medical problem. Springfield: Charles C Thomas, 1962, Pp. 1-183.

The purpose of this book is to point out understanding of the addiction phenomenon and the development of programs of control and treatment which are compatible with the interest of the whole society. The chapter titles are: a perspective on drug addiction; drug addiction and crime; types and characteristics of cases of medically induced addiction; juvenile addiction; the struggle for cure and conscious reasons for relapse; pleasure and deterioration from narcotic addiction; effects of addiction of health; treatment of narcotic addiction; highlights in the history of addiction; propaganda about addiction, its cause, nature and effect and solution of addiction problem. (129 refs.)

NIMH
Bethesda, Maryland

2932 Welsh, Ashton L. Side effects of anti-obesity drugs. Springfield: Charles C Thomas, 1962, Pp. 1-243.

Obesity and its problems are reviewed. Side

effects and the role of central stimulating
appetite distractors, i.e., amphetamine, methamphetamine, phenylpropanolamine, phenmetrazine, phentermine, and diethylpropoin, are
detailed. Sedatives and tranquilizers, bulk
producers, dietaries and thyroxine, and sodium liothyronine are discussed at length.
Management of a patient's obesity problem
should include accurate diagnosis, psychologic
directions, recommendation of a balance, low-
calorie diet, selection and prescription of
accepted medications, and supervision of the
weight-reducing program. (301 refs.)

University of Cincinnati
College of Medicine
Cincinnati, Ohio

2983 Hoffer, A. Niacin therapy in psychiatry.
Springfield: Charles C Thomas, 1962, Pp. 1-
165.

Information on the role of nicotinic acid
therapy, especially in inhibiting senile mental changes and in reversing some of the changes produced by lysergide and adrenolutin are
reviewed. Sixty case histories are included
in the appendix. Nicotinic acid as a vitamin, its toxicity, nicotinic acid and nicotinamide as sedatives, their use in the
treatment of schizophrenia and in confusional and drug-induced psychoses are detailed.
A double-blind trial is described including
82 patients of various diagnoses treated 33
days with nicotinic acid or placebo. They
were given the Weyburn Assessment Scale before and at various periods after treatment.
Nicotinic acid or nicotinamide as 3 g/day or
more, materially improved the recovery rate.
Patients who were discharged as improved tended to remain better and had fewer remissions
if they continued taking nicotinic acid or
its amide. (122 refs.)

Psychiatric Services Branch
Department of Public Health
Saskatoon, Saskatchewan, Canada

2984 Kalow, Werner. Pharmacogenetics. Here-
dity and the response to drugs. Philadelphia:
W. B. Saunders Co., 1962, Pp. 1-231.

This book discusses drug resistance in micro-
organisms, drug responses of somatic cells in

11

synaptic neurohumoral role contributed to
5HT (serotonin). Through intracarotid arterial injection in the anesthetized cat, the
cerebral actions of iproniazid, isoniazide,
and pheniprazine were studied. Influence on
trancallosally evoked cortical potentials was
used as the index of synaptic transmission,
accomplished by denervation of the carotid
sinus and by-passing the lesion. Cerebral
concentration of MAO inhibitors, MAO activity,
5HT concentration and the ability of cerebral
synapsy to transmit test impulses were assayed.
Results allow the following hypotheses: a)
augmentation of the existing distortion of
synaptic equilibrium in the direction of inhibition of extending inhibition to sites
that result in release phenomena or secondary
activation; b) counteraction of excessive excitation due to existing distorted cerebral
synaptic neurohumoral equilibrium by the inhibitory action of the locally accumulated
5HT, and c) an action unrelated to the MAO
inhibitory effects of these antidepressants.
These 3 alternatives are not necessarily exclusive, since they may apply to 3 different
forms of mental disturbance whose underlying
mechanism is characterized in 1 case by excessive synaptic inhibition, in another by
excessive synaptic excitation, and in a 3rd
by some as yet unclear mechanism. (15 refs.)

VA Hospital
Pittsburgh, Pennsylvania

2989 Schaefer, H. Anasthesie und Narkose in
der Praxis (II). [The theory of anesthesia
(II).] Therapiewoche, 1962, 24, 1053-1054.

Various theories are reviewed relating to the
effects of narcotic agents on the cell membranes, on the CNS as seen in the EEG, and
on rise and fall of blood pressure. It is
postulated that anesthesia, in all probability, causes the suspension of function of a
desynchronized, activating, reticulo-thalamo-
cortical system. Anesthesia is also regarded a psychophysical occurrence which abolishes the characteristics of pain (analgo-
thymia). At least some narcotics intensify
the depth of anesthesia by effecting the
lowering of blood pressure. (No refs.)

Physiologische Institut
Universität Heidelberg
Heidelburg, Germany

2990 Van Eck, C. R. Ritsema Die Behendlung
chronischer Schmerzzustände in der ärztlichen.
[The treatment of chronic pain in the medical
practice.] Therapiewoche, 1962, 24, 1055-
1057.

The need for extensive diagnostic investigations at the onset of treatment for pain is
emphasized. Chronic painful conditions as
rheumatism, arthritis, neuralgia, are different from the pains of the terminal cancer
patient. The 1st group has to learn to live
with pain; the complaints can be reduced
with medication, diet, and good health habits.
For the 2nd group, the necessity for evaluation of the environmental conditions is
stressed. The author has not used morphine,
or morphine derivatives, in the treatment of
this type of condition for years. Acetylsalicylic acid is the preferred analgesic,
and its efficacy is close to that of morphine,
while the analgesic efficacy of a placebo is
approximately 50%. The combination of acetylsalicylic acid, phenacetin, and codeine
is highly recommended because it is one of
the most effective combinations. In the case
of existing addiction to hypnotic agents,
incomplete withdrawal and intensive occupational therapy are recommended. The prescription of tranquilizers is contraindicated, except for occasional psychological
crises, or during the last days of life.
(14 refs.)

Institut für Anästhesiologie
Reichs-Universität
Groningen, The Netherlands

2991 Therapiewoche. Thrombosegefährdung
durch Barbiturate. [Barbiturate effect on
thrombosis.] Therapiewoche, 1962, 16, 692.
[Editorial]

Poumailloux has pointed out that barbiturates are able to influence the long-term
therapy with anticoagulants by raising the
prothrombin level. The prothrombin level
may be elevated to such a degree that it may,
in turn, cause occurrence of thrombosis or
embolism. The use of barbiturates during
anticoagulant therapy should therefore be
avoided; if unavoidable, the barbiturates
should be administered regularly and the
dosage of the anticoagulant increased, in
order to counteract the prothrombin level.

well as ethyl alcohol and phenothiazine derivatives are noted. (16 refs.)

[No address]

2994 Médecine et Hygiène. Narcotiques en
injection: danger! A propos de l'Estil.
[Injectable narcotics: Danger! On Estil.]
Médecine et Hygiène, 1962, No. 542, 262.
[Editorial]

Estil, produced by the Dr. Rudolf Reiss
Chemische Werke, Berlin, was taken off the
market at the end of February 1962, after a
17-year-old man lost his fingers by ampu-
tation following gangrene and the death of
a woman from renal insufficiency following
Estil. The narcotic might have been the
cause of death. (No refs.)

22, rue Michell-du-Crest
Geneva, Switzerland

2995 Sirbu, Aurelia, Simulescu, Eugenia, &
Stolla, Nicolae. Cu privire la medictia
psihotropa. [On psychotropic drugs.] Viata
Medicala, 1962, 9, 538-590.

The advent of psychotropic drugs in 1952
and Delay's classification are outlined.
Chlorpromazine, reserpine, levomepromazine,
imipramine, meprobamate and other drugs are
reviewed. (27 refs.)

[No address]

2996 Médecine et Hygiène. Psycholeptiques
VII et VIII. [Psycholeptiques VII and VIII.]
Médecine et Hygiène, 1962, No. 536, 116-117.

Details relative to phenothiazine derivatives; i.e., commercial names, generic
names, structure, CNS effects, neurologic
indications, psychiatric indications, side
effects and peculiarities are presented.
(No refs.)

22, rue Michell-du-Crest
Geneva, Switzerland

2997 Médecine et Hygiène. Psycholeptiques
IX. [Psycholeptiques IX.] Médecine et Hygiène, 1962, No. 537,145.

Details relative to rauwolfia alkoloids, giving commercial names, generic names, structure, CNS effects, neurologic indications,
psychiatric indications. side effects and
peculiarities are presented.(No refs.)

22, rue Michell-du-Crest
Geneva, Switzerland

2998 Medical World News. Sedative stirs
up a new storm. Medical World News, 1962,
26-27, [Editorial]

New means must be found for avoiding the
possibility of a tragedy in the future.
Present drug testing procedures could not
have predicted thalidomide's teratogenic
effects. Duttmacher (Planned Parenthood
Federation of America) stated that U.S.
abortion laws make no provision for the
child. There is no legal sanction for therapeutic abortion, but even in the absence
of legal precedent, therapeutic abortions
are being carried out in many U.S. Hospitals,
possibly 75% of non-Catholic hospitals and
40% of Catholic hospitals. Laws have not
kept up with medicine. (No refs.)

[No address]

2999 Medical World News. Drug safety
rules proposed: thalidomide issue. Medical World News, 1962, 3, 22-23. [Editorial]

Proposed FDA rules would require manufacturers to supply the government with a detailed summary of all preclinical tests including animal studies, and prove that "it
is reasonably safe" to begin clinical
trials. If in a trial a "substantial doubt"
about safety develops, a pharmaceutical
house must stop the trial, notify FDA and
recall all drug stocks. FDA itself can ban
or halt clinical trials. (No refs.)

[No address]

3000 Guyotat, J. Association de la pharma-
cotherapie a la psychotherapie dans le
traitement de nevroses. [Combination of
pharmacotherapy and psychotherapy in the

treatment of neuroses.] Medicina Experimentalis, 1962, 7, 87-99.

The function of neuroleptics is to break
through a circle of stereotyped attitudes to
the psychiatrist or to overcome the effects
of an acute attack. Psychoanaleptics like
imipramine or MAO inhibitors can aid in
externalizing the patient's self-aggression
into aggressive attitudes vis-à-vis the psychiatrist. Psycholeptics will frequently re-
inforce a long-standing attitude of despair,
in which case MAO inhibitors will aid in
attaining a breakthrough. Neuroleptics can
also aid in the application of analytic
techniques employed in teaching the patient
to face reality. Working hypotheses are
needed in order that (e.g. suppression of
agitation by thioproperazine) may be more
effectively employed for therapeutic ends.
Neurotic depressions are treated primarily
by imipramine-meprobamate-chlorpromazine
combinations. (No refs.)

Hopitaux Psychiatriques
Université de Lyon
Lyon, France

3001 Pogády, J., & Grígelová, M. Systém
otvorených dverí v psychiatrickom ústav-
níctve a ataraktika. [Open door policy in
psychiatric institutions and ataractics.]
Ceskoslovenská Psychiatrie, 1962, 58, 238-
244.

Statistics are given from 1955-1961, with
notes on the influence of psychiatric drugs,
for the 160-bed female ward of the Regional
Psychiatric Hospital of Pezinok. In 1955
the ward was closed. Classical shock treatment and an extensive occupational therapy
program were in vogue. By 1958 while the
ward was still closed, intensive occupational therapy and treatment with tranquilizers
were current, shock treatment receding into
the background. In 1960-1961 the open door
system was introduced with concurrent rehabilitation on a wide scale and intensive psychopharmacotherapy. Study was made of verbal,
physical and interpersonal aggression, the
number of escapes, suicide attempts and suicides. The incidence of these parameters was
lower in 1960 than in 1955. Verbal and physical aggression were considerably lower in
1960 compared to 1958. Verbal aggression

3007 Kranzdorf, Charles D. Early recognition
and management of depressions. California
Clinician, 1962, 58, 237-239.

In view of the suicide factor the early recognition and management of depression are urgent matters. There are essentially 3 appro-
ches: 1) psychotherapy, 2) chemotherapy and
3) shock therapy. Among available antidepressants, the phenylethylamines, MAO inhibitors
and imipramine have had extensive clinical use.
In view of rapid onset of action tranylcypromine is recommended. The role of the general
practitioner is stressed. (2 refs.)

Department of Psychosomatic Medicine
California College of Medicine
Los Angeles, California

3008 Cooper, Peter. Psycho-pharmacology:
restrospect and prospect. Chemotherapy Review,
1962, 2, 164-167.

Reserpine and chlorpromazine 1st were used to
alleviate mental illness 10 years ago. The
advent of the phenothiazines represents the
1st great class of major antipsychotic drugs.
Chlorpromazine has proved remarkably effective
in manic psychoses, schizophrenia, senile
agitation and anxiety. Phenothiazine derivatives display a marked propensity to provoke
extrapyramidal reactions. Haloperidol appears far more effective than chlorpromazine.
Other useful drugs include chlorprothixene,
imipramine, and iproniazid, MAO inhibitors,
isocarboxazid, phenelzine, etc. The milder
tranquilizers include meprobamate and chlordiazepoxide. Model psychoses may be induced
with LSD, psilocybin and mescaline. (58 refs.)

[No address]

3009 Cameron, Dale C. Narcotic drug addiction.
American Journal of Psychiatry, 1962, 119,
793-794.

With respect to narcotic addiction, the AMA
and National Research Council support follow-
up and rehabilitation procedures following
complete drug withdrawal, compulsory civil
commitment of drug addicts for treatment in
a drug-free environment, augmentation of addict rehabilitation under continuing civil
commitments, research on prevention and treat-

ment of addiction and dissemination of fac-
tual information on narcotic addiction. Treatment of drug addicts is a medical problem.
Drug addiction in the US is a symptom of an
underlying personality or emotional problem
which precedes deleterious psychological,
physiological and pathological changes. It
is exceedingly difficult to achieve successful
drug withdrawal in the absence of a drug-free
environment. (No refs.)

[No address]

3010 Cooper, Peter. Drugs affecting the
nervous system. Chemotherapy Review, 1962,
2, 100-102.

New psychoactive drugs include methohexital
(an anesthetic), dichloralphenazone (a nonbarbiturate sleeping preparation), phenmetrazine and amphetamine (for weight reduction),
methylphenidate, vanillic acid diethylamide,
trifluoperazine and thioridazine (thioridazine proved excellent for those who could
not tolerate chlorpromazine), levomepromazine, Deprol (meprobamate and benactyzine),
hydroxyzine, trimethobenzamide (an antiemetic)
and triflupromazine (also used as an antiemetic). (No refs.)

[No address]

3011 Rassegna Internazionale. Novità per gli
schizofrenici. [New information on schizophrenia.] Rassegna Internazionale, 1962, 42,
1336-1337. [Editorial]

The efficacy of haloperidol and triperidol in
the treatment of schizophrenia is briefly noted. The former is useful in the reduction
of agitation and aggressiveness; the latter
improves catatonia, negativism and various
states of indifference. (No refs.)

[No address]

3012 Pfeiffer, Carl C., & Smythies, John R.
[Eds.] International Review of Neurobiology.
Volume IV. London: Academic Press, Inc.,
1962. Pp. 1-388.

This book covers the nature of spreading depression in neural networks; the organizational
aspects of some subcortical motor areas; the
biochemical and neurophysiological development of the brain in the prenatal period;
substance P--a polypeptide of possibly physiological significance, especially within the
nervous system; anticholinergic psychomimetic
agents; benzoquinolizine derivatives--a new
class of MAO decreasing drugs with psychotropic action, and the effect of adrenochrome
and adrenolutin on animal behavior and human
psychology. (854 refs.)

New Jersey Psychiatric Institute
Princeton, New Jersey

3013 Molhant, M. Le role et l'importance des
nouveaux médicaments psychotropes dans le
traitement des psycho-névroses. [The role
and importance of the new psychotropic drugs
in the treatment of psychoneuroses.] Presse
Médicale, 1962, 70, 377-379.

Psychotropic drugs fall into 2 major classes,
psychosedatives including the tranquilizers:
phenothiazine derivatives, rauwolfia alkaloids
thioxanthenes, butyrophenones and thiophenyl-
pyridilamines, and the psychostimulants; including a) antidepressants, such as MAO inhibitors, imipramine, amitriptyline, etc., b)
psychotonics e.g., amphetamine. A 3rd group
includes the psychodyleptics (mescaline, atropine, lysergide, etc.). Their effects are
purely symptomatic and their action is selective, varying from 1 person to another. No
exact correlation can be established between
dosage and clinical effects. They are poly-
valent, with undesirable side effects at certain doses and liable to cause visceral compli
cations. Psychodysleptics must be considered
purely as adjuncts. (8 refs.)

[No address]

3014 Kagan, G. 'Librium' in anxiety and depressive states seen in general practice. Chemotherapy Review, 1962, 2, 231-232.

Eighty-one women and 29 men whose main complaint were anxiety and depression often associated with domestic difficulties were treated with chlordiazepoxide (Librium) for 4-6 weeks. The majority were given 20 mg chlordiazepoxide t.i.d. for the 1st week and if improvement was apparent, the dose was reduced to 10 mg t.i.d. Complete relief of symptoms was obtained in 62, marked improvement in 31, moderate improvement in 11 and little or no improvement in 5. Additionally about 15 children whose main complaint was bed wetting was treated with 5 mg b.i.d., many showing considerable improvement. A few patients complained of nausea, dizziness or drowsiness in the first few days of treatment.

Leek, Staffordshire
Great Britain

3015 Van Rhijn, C.H. An evaluation of means of a controlled group. Psychiatria, Neurologia, Neurochirurgia, 1962, 65, 117-128.

Fifty patients treated with thioridazine (Melleril) were observed for an average of 6 months: 22 chronic defective schizophrenics, 15 patients suffering from schizoid psychoses and 13 miscellaneous cases. Dosage ranged to 900 mg/day. Seventeen were markedly improved and 16 improved. Percentages of "good effect" on symptoms were: 50 paranoiac, 33 delusionary, 22 hallucinatory, 20 catatonic, 25 restless, 36 confused, 22 aggressive, 40 manic, 60 depressed and 50 anxious. Best results were obtained with patients with paranoid reactions. Catatonia reacted the least. Some slight drowsiness and paleness was noted.

Mental Hospital "Brinkgreven"
Deventer, The Netherlands

3016 Wells, B.G. The treatment of psychoneurotic patients with "Amylozine" (trifluoperazine/amylobarbitone). Chemotherapy Review, 1962, 2, 21-22.

Fifty-six anxiety depressive states were treated with from 2 to 6 capsules of Amylozine [(trifluoperazine and amobarbital) dosage unspecified] results were excellent in 42 cases, good in 6, fair in 2 and poor in 5. Side effects were few: heartburn was recorded in 1 patient and 2 patients who consumed small amounts of alcohol while on drug said that the effect of the drink was enormously increased. Alcohol should be forbidden to those on Amylozine until further experience is obtained.

[No address]

3017 Mossberg, Sanford M., Bloom, Alan, Berkowitz, Jess, & Ross, George. Serum enzyme activities following morphine. A study of transaminase and alkaline phosphatase levels in normal persons and those with gallbladder disease. Archives of Internal Medicine, 1962, 108, 429-437.

Of 48 individuals with no known gallbladder disease, none exhibited an increase of SGOT or serum alkaline phosphatase activities following morphine administration. Significant morphine-induced SGOT elevations occurred in 5 of 6 cholecystectomized patients, in 1 of 2 with radiographically nonfunctioning gallbladders, and in none of 4 with demonstrable stones and radiographically functioning gallbladders. Serum alkaline phosphatase was concomitantly increased in 2 patients with cholecystectomy and in 1 with a nonfunctioning gallbladder. Transaminase increments were from 2 1/2 to 65 times control values while serum alkaline phosphatase increases did not exceed 3 times control values. Increased SGOT values must be viewed with caution in patients with combination of (a) suspected myocardial infarction, (b) normal of equivocal EKG, (c) biliary tract disease, and (d) prior narcotic administration. Biliary obstruction per se may provoke an elevation of SGOT and serum alkaline phosphatase activities. Functioning gallbladder acts as a safety-valve, reducing the effective intraductal pressure following biliary obstruction.

Department of Medicine
Montefiore Hospital
New York, N.Y.

3018 Hankoff, Leon D., Rudorfer, Leon, &
Paley, Herbert M. A reference study of atarax-
ics. A two-week double blind outpatient evaluation. Journal of New Drugs, 1962, 3, 173-178.

The capsules, given t.i.d., contained 200 mg
meprobamate, 50 mg chlorpromazine, 10 mg chlordiazepoxide or placebo. One-hundred-and-
thirty-four outpatients treated were divided
into 2 groups: schizophrenic and nonschizophrenic. The chief criterion was manifest
anxiety, as measured by a 4 point scale. The
Affect Adjective Check List was also used. In
relation to untoward effects, chlorpromazine
showed the highest incidences of reported
somatic discomfort with 48%, in contrast to
29.6% with chlordiazepoxide, 16.6% with
placebo and 11.1% with meprobamate. Signs of
motor retardation were particularly high with
chlorpromazine, seen in 10 out of 25 patients.
Meprobamate used at the dosage of 600 mg/day,
half the usual dosage, was no more effective
than placebo. At conventional dosages both
chlordiazepoxide and chlorpromazine showed a
profile of drug activity which included global
psychiatric improvement, reduction of manifest
anxiety, fewer subjective patient responses
indicative of anxiety, higher dropout rate
(originally started with 174 patients), and a
higher incidence of somatic side reactions.

Department of Psychiatry
State University of New York
Downstate Medical Center
Brooklyn, N.Y.

3019 Michaux, Leon, Duche, D., & Perpiniotis.
Etude pharmacodynamique, clinique et thera-
peutique du G 22.355 en pedo-psychiatrie.
[Therapeutic and clinical pharmacodynamic study
of G 22.355 in child psychiatry]. Third World
Congress of Psychiatry Proceedings. Volume II.
Toronto/Montreal: University of Toronto Press
and McGill University Press, 1962. Pp. 927-929.

Imipramine in 25 mg p.o. or i.m. doses was
used in 13 children, 9-16 years of age, for an
average period of 6 weeks. Five had depression, 4 obsessional syndrome and 4 miscellaneous states. The dosage was progressively increased to a maximum of 75 mg, rarely
100 mg/day. Good results were obtained in 4
cases of depression, 3 cases of obsessional
syndrome, 1 case of tic and 1 hysterical-type
reaction. Slight improvement was obtained in
3 cases: 1 atypical depression, 2 obsessional
syndrome. No improvement was obtained in 1

case of inhibition. EEG surveillance was
maintained throughout. Tolerance was excellent.
[No address]

3020 Rothman, Theodore, Grayson, Harry, &
Ferguson, James. A comparative investigation of
isocarboxazid and imipramine in depressive syn-
dromes: autonomic measures. In: Cleghorn, R.A.,
Moll, A.E., & Roberts, C.A. Third World Congress
Psychiatry Proceedings. Volume II. Toronto/Montr
University of Toronto Press and McGill Universit
Press, 1962. Pp. 937-941.

Sixty-four male depressives, aged 30-60 years,
most showing suicidal tendencies were treated wi
isocarboxazid, imipramine or placebo. There wer
23 cases of schizophrenia, 4 were schizoaffectiv
25 had endogenous or manic depression, 7 had
personality disorders and 5 had psychoneuroses.
Isocarboxazid was given in an initial dose of 40
mg daily reduced to 20 mg; imipramine was given
initially at 100 mg daily and gradually reduced
to 50 mg; the placebo was administered 3 times a
day and eventually reduced to once a day. The
patients were placed on their treatment regimen
for a period of 10 weeks. Laboratory tests,
tests of autonomic function, EEG's, MSRPP, a
battery of psychological tests and scales, facial
photographs of the patient smiling and reposed,
the Rothman's Symptom Check List and other tests
were applied. An $\bar{A}$ score was derived by combini
weighted standard scores of 7 measurements: viz,
salivary output; sublingual temperature, heart
period while reclining, diastolic blood pressure
while reclining; palmar skin conductance while reclining; palmar skin conductance while straining
and a ratio of palmar conductance measured while
reclining to that measured while straining. For
unselected populations the $\bar{A}$ is distributed norma
and this mean is defined as "autonomic balance."
Patients with depressive syndromes have $\bar{A}$
scores indicating that the direction of movement is towards the sympathetic branch of the
autonomic nervous system. Those patients
treated with a drug show: a) isocarboxazid
as an $\bar{A}$ score showing a parasympathetic directior
b) placebo showed less parasympathetic dominance than isocarboxazid; c) imipramine shows
sympathetic dominance. Patients treated with
placebo showed measurable change. There
is a correlation between the parasympathetic
dominance as shown by the $\bar{A}$ scores which
cuts through treatment procedures when
improvement occurs. Global evaluations may

Fourteen chronic schizophrenic women received 10 mg of reserpine as a single dose and 2 days later the only sign of an altered brain milieu was the miosis. They then received 120 μg of LSD and showed prolonged and toxic reactions: marked tremor and akathisia in the majority; and in 1, an oculogyric crisis. Each felt the drug was less pleasant than her control LSD and that the effects lasted longer. With the exception of pupil size, tolerance developed normally. LSD and related psychotomimetics appeared to effect both the level and distribution of biogenic amines in the brain and the alteration of normal rates of binding and release leads to different behavioral, autonomic and chemical response to such drugs.

Yale University School of Medicine
New Haven, Conn.

3023 Gamna, G., Gobbi, L., Ferrio, L., Rivolta, A., Gandiglio, G., & Vercellino, F. Contributo clinoco, elettroencefalografico e biologico allo studio della psilocibina [Clinical, EEG and biological contribution to the study of psilocybin.] Sistema Nervoso, 1962, 14, 389-408.

Five nondeteriorated chronic paranoid schizophrenics and 5 affective depressive psychosis cases were given 2 and 8 mg doses of psilocybin respectively, p.o. for 10 days. Eleven volunteers, including 1 normal subject (male medical student) and 10 females of various psychiatric diagnoses were given i.v. doses of 3-9 mg psilocybin. In the 1st experiment psychothymic changes were noted ranging from excitation to psychonudism with, generally, aggravation of the EEG. Most subjects showed almost constant mydriasis, tardycardia, and irregular pressor effects, with the manifestation of some elation. The normal subject saw kaleidoscopic colored hallucinations. Variations in alpha wave rhythm were noted in some subjects, along with psychomotor unrest. Psilocybin is of value in revealing psychopathological structures and personalities.

Ospedali Psichiatrici Provinciali di Torino
Torino, Italy

3024 Jacquin, Maurice. Etude du Tofranil
10 en psychiatrie gerontologique. [Study
of Tofranil in gerontological psychiatry.]
Strasbourg Medicale, 1962, 13, 790-793.

Thirty-four patients in the following
categories were studied: female, aged 60
years or over, chronic psychotics in advanced
stages of their illness, showing some signs
of depression associated with other psychiatric symptoms. Usual daily dosage was 20 mg
imipramine (Tofranil). In some cases, 3
weeks after beginning of treatment, it was
raised to 10 mg t.i.d., and maintained for
over 5 months. Good results were obtained
in 12 (35%) of these patients, thus encouraging the use of higher dosages.

Hôpital Psychiatrique de Hoerdt
(Bas-Rhin), France

3025 Janke, Von W., & Schmatzer, Elisabeth.
Experimentalpsychologische Untersuchungen
zur Wirkung einer Prothipendyl-Cyclobarbital-
Calcium-Kombination im Vergleich zu Cyclo-
barbital-Calcium und Placebo. [Experimen-
tal psychological studies on the effects
of a prothipendyl-cyclobarbital-calcium
combination in comparison with cyclobarbital
and placebos.] Arzneimittel-Forschung,
1962, 12, 1031-1036.

The effects of Itridal were evaluated in 2
series of tests, each comprised of 5 males
and 5 females, 20-30 years of age, to
determine depth of sleep, performance
capacity, and subjective sensations. Each
of 3 dosage regimens was administered before
sleep: 2 tablets consisting of either
Itridal (40 mg prothipendyl and 200 mg
cyclobarbital calcium), cyclobarbital
calcium (400 mg), or placebo. Depth of
sleep (determined from movements during
sleep) was equal for both drugs but differed from placebo in that the depth of
sleep was increased over a period of several
hours. Psychological and psychomotor
tests showed marked differences between
Itridal and cyclobarbital calcium. Following cyclobarbital, impairment of performance
was observed in reaction time and psychomotor coordination. Itridal did not differ
from placebo in this respect.

Institut für Psychologie
Universitat Marburg/Lahn
Marburg/Lahn, Germany

3026 Smith e Incas, Jaime, Frazier,
Robert L., & Patterson, Ralph M. The
treatment of depression with meprobamate-
benactyzine (Deprol). Evaluation of a
"sliding scale" method of dose selection.
Journal of the National Medical Association, 1962, 54, 472-475.

Deprol (400 mg meprobamate and 1 mg
benactyzine) 4-10 tablets/day p.o. was
administered to 62 depressive patients,
aged 17-77 years, for 7 weeks to 10 months.
Positive results ranged from good to
excellent in all patients. Dosage adjustment was based upon initial response, with
a sliding scale of dosage selection recommended. Remission was generally observed
in 9-12 days.

Orient State Institute
Columbus, Ohio

3027 Gratton, L., Houde, L., Lafontaine,
R., & Fournier, G. "Syndromes hypermoteurs
et trifluoperazine". [Hypermotor syndromes
and trifluoperazine.] Canadian Psychiatric
Association Journal, 1961, 6, 257-260.

Thirty-three boys, aged 7-12 years, were
divided into 3 groups of 11 for study
purposes: administration of the Bender-
Gestalt, Goodenough, and Draw-a-Tree tests
in relation to the effects of trifluoperazine on ego functions and ego structura-
tion in hypermotor syndrome. One group
was given trifluoperazine, the 2nd group,
placebo, and 3rd group, no medication.
Trifluoperazine and placebo were prescribed
at a dose of 0.5 mg/10 lbs of body weight/
day. The doses were increased when needed
after 2 weeks, at a ratio of 0.25 mg/10
lbs. The tests were repeated after 2
months, and the children were seen regularly for 5-10 minutes once a week; a complete
observation form was filled out every 2
weeks by the nurses and psychiatrists.
Poor results were obtained in Group I, but
this was found to be due to the drug's
opposite effects on 2 types of hyperkinetic
children. In graphs with the level of
motor activity on the ordinate and days of
treatment on the abscissa, "Type I children"
showed a curve with wide fluctuations.
Children of this type showed corresponding
variations in motor activity with apparently

and meprobamate. Imipramine and prochlorperazine were both found to produce a significant reduction in histamine wheal formation
in chronic schizophrenics.

Research Facility
Rockland State Hospital
Orangeburg, N.Y.

3030 Mariategui, Jaview, & Ramirez del
Villar, E. Tratamiento de los cuadros de-
presivos con amitriptilina. [Treatment of depressive cases with amitriptyline.] Revista
de Neuro-Psiquiatría, 1962, 25, 281-290.

Thirty-four cases of depression were treated
with amitriptyline for 3-5 months. Usual dosage
was 60-90 mg/day i.m. or 75 mg/day p.o. initially. Dosage was progressively raised to the
average level of 100-200 mg/day. Complete remission was achieved in 35.3%, improvement in 29.4%
and slight improvement in 20.6%. No change was
observed in 8.8% and worsening, a swing towards
mania, occurred in 5.9%. The drug is particularly beneficial in cases of endogenous depression.
Its anxiolytic effect is stressed.

[No address]

3031 Cornil, J., Ajzenberg, D., & Mans, J.
Contribution à l'étude du syndrome secondaire des
neuroleptiques. Son traitement pare le chlorhydrate d'orphenadrine. [Contribution to the study
of neuroleptic syndrome; its treatment with orphenadrine.] Gazette Médicale de France, 1961,
68, 2583-2585.

Orphenadrine (Disipal) was found useful in controlling neuroleptic-induced extrapyramidal
disorder in 41 out of 56 patients. The case load
included 20 men and 36 women. Fifty milligram
tablets were used and dosage progressively increased, beginning with 100 mg/day reaching a
maximal dose of 800 mg/day, most often optimal
at 200-300 mg/day. In 16 cases there was a favorable potentiation of the neuroleptic effect (14 on
chlorpromazine and 2 on levomepromazine).

[No address]

3032 Gelinet, M.M. Étude biologique et
clinique d'un anorexigène: la diethylaminopro-
phénone retard. [Clinical and biological study
of an anorexigen: slow-release diethylamino-
propiophenone.] Gazette Médical de France, 1962,
69, 821-823.

9

Derfon tablets (0.025 g diethylpropion) were given t.i.d. or q.i.d. to over 11 obese patients, 12-74 years of age. Diethylpropion was perfectly tolerated in spite of coexisting diseases such as diabetes, psychiatric disturbances, etc. and was compatible with other medications given these patients. Results were consistently good in relation to weight loss, on the average, 4 kg a month and 1-1.5 kg in 8 days. However 3 failures were recorded. No significant changes in urinary metabolites were noted except for a slight increase in glomerular filtration.

College de Médecine des Hôpitaux de Paris
Centre d'Endocrinologie
Hôpital Laennec
Paris, France

3033 Schenker, Victor J., Marjerrison, Gordon, Schlachet, Peter, Feedman, N., Hankoff, L.D., & Engelhardt, D.M. Monoamine oxidase inhibition and antidepressive correlates. In: Cleghorn, R.A., Moll, A.E., & Roberts, C.A. Third World Congress of Psychiatry Proceedings. Volume I. Toronto/Montreal: University of Toronto Press and McGill University Press, 1962. Pp. 642-649.

Nineteen male patients (reactive depression, involutional psychosis, psychoneurosis, schizophrenia with depression) were randomly assigned to pheniprazine (12 mg orally each day at 10 A.M.) or placebo. MAO inhibition was assessed spectrophotofluorometrically by increase of urinary tryptamine. The Abbreviated Depression scale of the MMPI, the Clyde Mood Scale, Digit Symbol test, perseveration tests, Wechsler Memory Scale, time estimation, tapping test, work association tests and WAIS vocabulary as well as the Bender Visual-Motor Gestalt Test, the TAT, Rosenzweig Picture Frustation test, childhood memories and the Rorschach test were used in evaluation. The inhibitor produced a distinct effect in the alleviation of depressive symptomology which could be objectively described in psychiatric testing, and the drug induced alleviation could be correlated with biochemical response to the drug. Lack of clinical

improvement showed a lower index of MAO inhibition.

State University of New York
College of Medicine
Downstate Medical Center
Brooklyn, N.Y.

3034 Resnick, Oscar, Krus, Donald, Raskin, Milton, Rivera, Milagros, & Freeman, Harry. The effect of pretreatment with monoamine oxidase inhibitors on reserpine action in normal subjects and in schizophrenic patients In: Cleghorn, R.A., Moll, A.E., & Roberts, C.A. Third World Congress of Psychiatry Proceedings. Volume I. Toronto/Montreal: University of Toronto Press and McGill University Press, 1962. Pp. 638-642.

Six normal male subjects were given 1.25 mg reserpine i.m. and 2 days later were put on 20-50 mg isocarboxazid for 2 weeks. On the 14th day they received another 1.25 mg reserpine injection. One hour after administration of reserpine, flushing, a feeling of warmth, a "big-head" feeling, headache, nasal congestion and sniffles, bronchial constriction, miosis, bloodshot eyes, gastritis, and lowered blood pressure were noted. Mild sedation usually was noticed about 2 hours after the injection. The same dose, given after 2 weeks of isocarboxazid therapy, produced the same effects, but they were much more pronounced and prolonged. This was especially true for sedation and tranquilization. The level of apparent eye horizon was raised in all cases. One subject, a very good bowler, complained that his score was very low while on isocarboxazid. Reserpine alone has a biphasic effect on the apparent eye horizon--a rise followed by a fall. Ten weeks after these trials 3 subjects were placed on nialamide, 100 mg/day. On the 14th day the subjects received the same 1.25 mg reserpine dose i.m. Nialamide did not raise the apparent eye horizon, but produced a biphasic response. Also, there was no lowering of blood pressure, and in 2 subjects systolic blood pressure actually rose. Nialamide, unlike isocarboxazid, may have produced a rise in the concentration of both 5HT and catecholamine centrally and peripherally. Four schizophrenics received 150 mg iproniazid

aggression score was worked out equal to
"aggression score"/"aggression inward score
plus aggression score." As the percentage
rises, more tendency toward aggressive
expression is indicated. The MMPI correlated satisfactorily with the checklist
measures of percent aggression. Reserpine
cases showed an increased tendency toward
aggression, while placebo cases showed a
slight shift toward more inhibition and
anger-dominance. Reserpine causes patients
to show moderation in behavioral organization in the direction of a greater dominance of aggressive, and perhaps generally
alloplastic, behavior. If reserpine causes
a shift towards freer aggressivity, it
follows that a patient whose symptoms
already betray an anger-dominance should
not be considered as improving and is
probably getting worse. However, a patient
who shows a premedication adjustment of
inhibition and anger-intype symptoms should
be considered improving if he moves towards
freer drive expression. In the reserpine
group 71% of the initially low percent
aggression cases were drug-successes compared
to only 27% of the initial high scores.
The direction of success was reversed in
the placebo group. Of the patients given
placebo only, 14% of those initially low
were successful drug cases while 57% of
those scoring high were in this category.
Improvement on reserpine could be predicted
in 72% of cases while for placebo the
prediction accuracy was only 26%.

University of North Carolina
Chapel Hill, N.C.

3037 Jus, Andrzej. Conditioned reflex
experimental research in the evaluation of
action of some psychotropic drugs. In:
Cleghorn, R.A., Moll, A.E., & Roberts, C.A.
Third World Congress of Psychiatry Proceedings.
Volume I. Toronto/Montreal: University of
Toronto Press and McGill University Press,
1962. Pp. 151-155.

Observations were carried out on 202 patients
comprised of 167 schizophrenics, 8 manic-
depressives, 15 patients with involutional
psychosis, 5 with posttraumatic psychosis
and 7 with psychoneurosis. The following
methods of treatment were applied: insulin
coma - 85 patients, chlorpromazine - 35
patients, reserpine - 18 patients,

thioproperazine - 20 patients, haloperidol -
5 patients, benactyzine - 3 patients and
nialamide - 33 patients. Polygraphic
reactivity studies were applied to 136 of
these patients with simultaneous observation of UR's and CR's in the ECG, neurogram
and electrodermogram (psychogalvanic
reactions). Hypoglycemia was also assessed.
Numerous remarks are made on CR experiments
in the course of pharmacological treatment.
In some psychoses, but not all, the appearance of a CR is a very sensitive indicator
which can presage an improvement long before
it may be seen clinically. For instance in
states of catatonic stupor during treatment by insulin coma or by neuroleptics,
the appearance by conditioned alpha blocking
with acoustic stimuli as CS and light as
reinforcement can be observed. This conditioning appeared in patients who improved
clinically only later.

Academy of Medicine
Warsaw, Poland

3038   Brune, Guenter G., Pscheidt, Gordon
R., & Himwich, Harold E. Correlations
between the behaviour of patients with
mental disturbances and effects of psycho-
active drugs on some urinary products.
In: Cleghorn, R.A., Moll, A.E., & Roberts,
C.A. Third World Congress of Psychiatry
Proceedings. Volume I. Toronto/Montreal:
University of Toronto Press and McGill
University Press, 1962. Pp. 111-117.

Behavioral changes wrought by therapeutic
doses of reserpine and isocarboxazid on 12
patients (9 schizophrenia and 3 mental deficiency) were studied in relation to
changes in 5HT and levarterenol metabolism.
Twenty-four hour urine specimens were
collected for each patient and the following
indole metabolites were measured: 5HIAA,
total 3-indoleacetic acid and tryptamine.
Levarterenol and epinephrine were also
assayed. Four schedules were used: placebo,
4 mg reserpine/day or 30 mg isocarboxazid/
day, 4 mg reserpine plus 30 mg isocarbox-
azid/day followed by a placebo. Patients
were kept on a constant-intake protein diet,
i.e., tryptophan intake was kept constant,
during the 47-day observation period. A
close relationship between the degree of
psychotic behavior and the amounts of indole
metabolites eliminated in the urine existed.

Schedule were used in evaluation. After
administration of thyroid medication [un-
specified], most of the abnormal behavioral
symptoms (irritability, lethargy) decreased
or disappeared, and the patients returned
to a state of general well being. They
achieved a significantly higher score on
the Block Design Test after treatment, but
the time required to carry out the task was
not affected. The patients' memory for
digits improved, retention for digits back-
wards being mainly affected. Temperament
tests showed that they were more capable
of taking the initiative, that they had
a more even disposition, were less irritated,
could concentrate better and were more
cooperative. However, the changes were not
statistically significant and this appears
to indicate that interviews were more reliable than the testing data.

Memorial Sloan Ketering Cancer Center
New York

3042 Véziris, C.D. Données récentes sur
la ménopause. [Recent data on menopause.]
In: Baruk, Henri, & Launay, Jacques [Eds.]
Annales Moreau de Tours. Tome I. Mémoires
récents sur la psychopharmacologie. - Annals
of Moreau de Tours. Volume I. Current
memoirs in psychopharmacology. Paris:
Presses Universitaires de France, 1962.
Pp. 353-366.

Menopausal patients were examined for FSH
excretion levels. Of women recently past
menopause, 30 had normal FSH levels while
15 had higher than normal levels. Seven
out of 104 women who had passed menopause
for about a year and a half had normal
levels while the rest showed higher than
normal FSH levels. Treatment with di-
enestrol and similar products was beneficial, alleviating stress in some cases and
and causing a diminution in histamine and
acetylcholine levels.

[No address]

3043 Contini, Paolo. Esperienze geriatriche
con un nuovo neurostimolante: l'1-fenil-2-
pirrolidinopentano. [Geriatric experience with
a new neurostimulant: 1 phenyl-2-pirrolidine-
opentane.] Settimana Medica, 1962, 50, 815-
823.

Dillescno (10 mg 1-phenyl-2-pirrolidine
pentane combined with vitamins) was given to
23 patients, 60 years and older, 1 tablet
t.i.d., usually for 10-20 days. Patients
fell into 2 categories: arteriosclerotic,
general asthenia in acute convalence patients,
and chronic depression. Eight patients
showed improvement and 10 slight improvement.
The drug seems to be a suitable psychotonic
for the aged and tolerance has been excellent.

Istituto de Gerontologia
Università degli Studi di Firenze
Florence, Italy

3044 Goldman, Milton S. Experience with
antidepressants in general practice. Journal
of the Florida Medical Association, 1962,
45, 727-729.

Isocarboxazid was given to a random series of
65 outpatients, all females, with the following diagnoses: endogenous depression, agitated depressive reactions, reactive depressions, postmenopausal involutional depressions and manic depressive in the depressed
phase. Four also complained of angina pectoris. All received 10 mg t. i. d. for the
1st week, reduced to 10 mg in the morning
and at bedtime thereafter. Excellent to
good results were obtained in 82%, and 92%
showed excellent, good or fair results.
Three out of the 5 failures were in the endogenous depression group (38 cases). The
response in 20 out of 21 patients with postmenopausal depression was good to excellent.
Minor side effects were nausea (5 mild, 2
severe), anorexia (3 mild) and insomnia
(8 mild and 1 severe).

1680 Meridian Avenue
Miami Beach, Fla.

for 7-14 days. Complete or marked relief of
itching was observed in 85% with Diperm and
59% with trimeprazine. No antipruritic
effect was apparent in 6% with Diperm and
30% with trimeprazine. Minor side effects,
primarily mild drowsiness, occurred in 10%
of both drug groups. The Diperm repeat-
action tablet, at a dosage of 1 tablet b.i.d.
appears to be an effective and generally
well tolerated preparation for the oral
treatment of itching.

Division of Dermatology
Department of Medicine
Georgetown University School of Medicine
Washington, D.C.

3050 Fullerton, A.G., Boardman, R.H.,
Bethell, M.S., & Conway, Stella. Neurotic
and mild psychotic depression: combined
drug treatment of the target-symptom.
Chemotherapy Review, 1962, 2, 38-40.

The initial dose of Parstelin (1 mg trifluoperazine and 10 mg tranylcypromine) generally
was 1 tablet t.i.d., and if tolerated, it
was gradually increased. Maximal daily
dosage reached 6 tablets per day. Of the
60 patients treated for mild depression,
43 (70%) benefited satisfactorily and 17
(30%) either received minimal benefit or
none. Faintness, drowsiness, blurred
vision, urgency of micturition and diminished libido (3 males), sudden severe
occipital headache in 11 patients and mild
parkinsonism in 1 patient on 6 tablets a
day were listed as side effects.

Gerrison Hospital
Dorchester
Dorset, Great Britain

3051 Dorison, Ezra E., & Blackman, Sheldon.
Imipramine in the treatment of adult enuretics.
American Journal of Psychiatry, 1962, 119, 474.

Thirty soldiers, aged 17-23 years, referred
to a clinic because of enuresis were studied
in a double-blind trial where 50 mg impramine was given to half the subjects at bed
time, while the other half received a placebo.
After 2 weeks, of the 15 subjects in the
medication group, 6 reported improvement.
Eleven of the 15 in the placebo group

reported improvement. None of the 30 subjects reported any worsening of their condition.

Mental Hygiene Consultation Service
Fort Knox, Ky.

3052 Letailleur, Maurice, Monnerie, Rene, Colas, Yves, & Vinyes. Chlorpromazine et gestation. [Chlorpromazine and gestation.] In: Baruk, Henri, & Launay, Jacques [Eds.] Annales Moreau de Tours. Tome I. Mémoires recents sur la psychopharmacologie. Annals of Moreau de Tours. Volume I. Current memoirs in psychopharmacology. Paris: Presses Universitaires de France, 1962. Pp. 367-373.

A 22-year-old woman suffering from hallucinations was given various psychiatric treatment including ECT, trihexyphenidyl, and chlorpromazine over a period of some 4 years. She received no less than 150 mg/day chlorpromazine throughout most of a pregnancy. She delivered a female child weighing 4.06 kg under normal circumstances. The child was normal, and psychological and psychomotor development was in no way unusual. The placenta showed a chlorpromazine recovery level of 2.5 mg/kg/ while no chlorpromazine was detectable in the umbilical cord (sensitivity of method ca 0.5 mg/liter).

Clinique de Neuropsychiatrie de
Clermont-de-l'Oise
Clermont-de-l'Oise, France

3053 Bruyn, G.W. Thiopropazate dihydrochloride (Dartal) in the treatment of Huntington's chorea. Psychiatria, Neurologia, Neurochirurgia, 1962, 65, 430-438.

Choreatic hyperkinesia were reduced in 1, markedly reduced in 2 and practically eliminated in another out of 4 patients suffering from Huntington's chorea who received 2-20 mg thiopropazate t.i.d. Findings relating to urinary excretion of copper and amino acids as well as serum ceruloplasmin were essentially normal in all patients with the exception of a slightly raised amino acid excretion in 1 (no

significance). Both thiopropazate and perphenazine are considered drugs of choice in Huntington's chorea.

Neurological Department
Institute of Neurological Sciences
University Hospital
Leyden, The Netherlands

3054 Musaph, Herman, & Van Loggem, Manuel. Research of chlordiazepoxide (Librium) into normal subjects and neurotics with pathological itching states. Psychiatria, Neurologia, Neurochirurgia, 1962, 65, 402-423.

Twenty neurotic patients, treated for pathologic itching, and 25 normal persons were tested before and after 10 mg chlordiazepoxide p.o. Ten patients were studied on a double-blind basis. The assessment test used was the Van Loggem test (4 picture representing love and sexuality, loneliness, aggression, and social contact with many people). Chlordiazepoxide may make patients more indifferent, anxiolytic effects resulting from a socalled "declutch" mechanism. The drug caused improvement of basic mood and decrease in fear. No strikking differences were found between normals and neurotics. While not a specific antipruritic drug, it may break through a vicious cycle and allow better psychotherapy

[No address]

3055 Horne, P.M., & Forrest, A.D. Pilot trial of I.C.I. 31397. A new mono-amine oxidase inhibitor. Scottish Medical Journal, 1962, 7, 224-229.

In a pilot study, α-methylbenzylhydrazine (I.C.I. 31397; 3-20 mg/day) was administered to 24 depressive patients aged 24-72 years for 10 days to 12 weeks. Evaluation by psychiatric assessment and a 3-point rating scale at 2 weeks revealed 62.5% patient improvement, with optimal dosage lying between 10-30 mg/day. Abnormal cephalin chloesterol flocculation tests were manifested by 2 patients during treatment, a fact which suggests

nervous system. Indian Journal of Medical
Research, 1962, 50, 46-60.

Asarone and β-asareon, recently isolated active
principles of Acornus calamus, are psychoactive
drugs. Asarone and β-asarone (50 mg/kg i.p.)
prolonged sleeping time in mice induced by pentobarbital (40 mg/kg i.p.) hexobarbital (100 mg/kg
i.p.), or ethanol (3g/kg i.p.). Lysergide (1 μg/kg
i.p.) and iproniazid (150 mg/kg i.p., t.i.d.)
failed to influence the hypnotic potentiating
property of asarone and β-asarone (50 mg/kg i.p.).
Both asarone and β-asarone produced significant
reduction in the rectal temperature of 80 mice.
Neither asarone nor β-asarone exhibited analgesic
activity. β-asarone appeared to facilitate
electroshock while asarone revealed a slight protective influence. Asarone (25-50 mg/kg i.p.)
effectively protected mice against 70 mg/kg pentetrazol s.c. conclusions, while β-asarone enhanced pentetrazol toxicity. Picrotoxin (2 mg/kg s.c.)
convulsions were facilitated by both drugs, while
strychnine (0.3 mg/kg s.c.) convulsions were not
influenced by either drug. Neither drug induced
ataxia. Both agents exerted a taming influence
on hostile cats as indicated by Norton and de Beer's
"sociability" scores. β-Asarone specifically
blocked CAR's in rats. Asarone produced comparable
results at lower dosages.

Department of Pharmacology
S.M.S. Medical College
Jaipur, India

3059 Theodorides, M.M. Essai du bromométhylate
de alpha-pyrrolidinopropionyl-phénothiazine (Diaspasmyl) en pédiatrie. [A test of α-pyrrolidinopropionyl phenothiazine bromomethylate (Diaspasmyl)
in pediatrics.] Journal de Médecine de Bordeaux,
1962, 139, 459-464.

α-Pyrrolidinopropionyl phenothiazine (Diaspasmyl)
was administered to a group of 23 infants who
suffered from vomiting (12 otorhinolaryngeal or
bronchial cases, 9 gastroenteritis cases, and 2
pyloric stenosis cases), either orally (2-2.5 mg/
kg), rectally (1-3 mg/kg) or s.c. (1-2 mg/kg.
Mean duration of the therapy was 3 days. Cessation of the vomiting was attained in 20 cases,
the other 3 failures consisting of the 2 stenosis
cases and 1 case of intolerance. In addition,
12 successes were noted in all 12 cases of
children 1-6 years old suffering from vomiting accompanying meningitis, or rhinopharyngeal
or other disorders. Doses were 1-2 mg/kg orally,
0.5-1 mg/kg s.c., or 0.6 mg/kg i.v. Finally,

the drug was administered to 5 children suffering from acute dyspneic conditions, and in
all cases the dyspnea was reduced clearly and
rapidly.

[No address]

3060 Knoll, W. Gibt es neue Möglichkeiten
der pharmakopsychiatrischen Behandlung? [Are
there new possibilities in pharmacopsychiatric
treatment?] Therapiewoche, 1962, 14, 545-547.

Sixty-seven female subjects were treated with
Vesitan, a combination of thiopropazate and
chlorphencyclane (1st 3 days: 1.5 cc i.m.,
t.i.d. or q.i.d.; thereafter, 2 tablets t.i.d.;
after 3 weeks only 1 tablet t.i.d. or q.i.d.)
The patients were hospitalized for catatonic
conditions of excitement, hebephrenia, paranoid psychoses and symptomatic psychoses
accompanying carcinoma, and for conditions of
restlessnes caused by arteriosclerosis. With
the exception of a few cases, all patients
had been ill for several years. In spite of
these unfavorable conditions, 41 patients
were so much improved that they could be discharged. Thirty-five out of these 41 were
exclusively treated with Vesitan. The other
6 patients received Vesitan combined with ECT
or with MAO inhibitors. Twelve psychotic
patients, hospitalized for years, were improved and could be transferred from the
violent ward. Nine patients showed no improvement; 4 showed increased restlessness
and the medication had to be discontinued.
Best results were seen in those schizophrenic
processes where restlessness, anxiety, tension
and delusions were factors. Side effects
were minimal.

Psychiatrische Landeskrankhaus
Emmendingen/Bd, Germany

3061 Gore, Charles P., & McComisky, James G.
A study of the comparative effectiveness of
Librium, amylobarbitone, and a placebo in
the treatment of tension and anxiety states.
In: Cleghorn, R.A., Moll, A.E., & Roberts,
C.A. Third World Congress of Psychiatry
Proceedings. Volume II. Toronto/Montreal:
University of Toronto Press and McGill Univer-
sity Press, 1962. Pp. 979-982.

Initially chlordiazepoxide (Librium) was
given to 50 patients who complained of tension

the patients were treated with chlorpromazine-
insulin and regained weight. After weight has
y been restored psychotherapy may be needed to
- complete the cure, particularly in the anxiety-
hysteria type of anorexia nervosa. The relapse
rate was about 50% and these were readmitted within
6 months of leaving hospital. When early treatment
is directed to restoring lost weight, the prognosis
is less gloomy than many investigators would believe.

St. Thomas' Hospital
London, Great Britain

:

3064 Gabriel, Arthur N. A psychobiologic
s. approach to the treatment of tics. In: Cleghorn,
R.A., Moll, A.E., & Roberts, C.A. Third World
Congress of Psychiatry.Proceedings. Volume II.
Toronto/Montreal: University of Toronto Press
and McGill University Press, 1962. Pp. 1050-1052.

Five cases are presented in which tics were
successfully treated with psychopharmacologic
agents (meprobamate up to 3,200 mg/day, chlorpromazine up to 800 mg/day and 4,000 mg/day, 200 mg
imipramine/day) even in a treatment situation
that concerns itself primarily with psychological
factors.

[No address]

3065 Denham, John. Experimental approach to the
treatment of schizophrenia. In: Cleghorn, R.A.,
Moll, A.E., & Roberts, C.A. Third World Congress
of Psychiatry Proceedings. Volume II. Toronto/
Montreal: University of Toronto Press and McGill
University Press, 1962. Pp. 1094-1096.

Chronic schizophrenics received 0.1 mg epinephrine
and on the following day 10 mg mecholyl before,
during, and after treatment with thioproperazine
[dosage unspecified] on 3 separate occasions.
The reactivity to epinephrine before treatment
was found within normal limits in two-thirds of
the patients while in the remainder it was
reduced and short-lasting. Reactions to mecholyl
were slight and short-lasting or absent in all
patients. During thioproperazine treatment reactions were found excessive and abnormally prolonged. On completion of treatment, when there
was no further evidence of autonomic disturbance
attributable to the drug, repetition of tests
showed no change to epinephrine in those patients
whose reading had been normal before treatment,
but the rise of systolic blood pressure was
increased in those with previously reduced

reactivity. Retested with mecholyl, 50% of
the patients showed no change in pretreatment
values and the rest exhibited increase and
prolongation of reaction. Significantly the
latter group showed more marked psychiatric
improvement. Other tests were conducted with
5HT, α-methyldopa, and LSD. A return towards
normal values was observed and found correlated
with psychiatric improvement.

Long Grove Hospital
Epsom, Great Britain

3066 Bigelow, Newton, Ozersngin, Feyzi,
Schneider, Jacob, & Sainz, A. Carphenazine
in the treatment of chronic schizophrenia.
In: Cleghorn, R.A., Moll, A.E., & Roberts, C.
A . Third World Congress of Psychiatry
Proceedings. Volume II. Toronto/Montreal:
University of Toronto Press and McGill Univer-
sity Press, 1962. Pp. 1102-1105.

Eight-hundred-and-nine patients on carphenazine were studied, using largely the Marcy
Psychiatric Rating Scale. The research design
excluded immediate and latent placebo reactors. Placebos, mepazine, and fluphenazine
groups were used as controls. Carphenazine
was found to be specially valuable in chronic
schizophrenia and particularly against 1
specific modality named "hypodynamic" where
it produced twice as many remissions as
fluphenazine and 10 times as many as mepazine.
The study of carphenazine aided in isolating
this schizophrenic modality. The pharmacology
indicates that the principal action is within
the cortical and subcortical cerebral cells,
with little action on the basal ganglia,
hypothalamus and reticular system. Carphenazine induces few and mild extrapyramidal
reactions and only scattered hypotensive
effects. It does produce a centrocerebral
reaction called provisionally an "atypical
central nervous system reaction", which
appears quite different from the tremulous or
dystonic extrapyramidal syndromes usually
seen, even with the same drug. The principal
side effect of carphenazine is drowsiness and
toxic reactions were not observed. Caffeine
has been found to be a rapid and effective
antidote.

Marcy State Hospital
Marcy, N.Y.

Six patients with longstanding neurotic illnesses
were given 3-5 mg phencyclidine (Sernyl) by slow
i.v. injection. After treatment patients were
asked to write down their experiences under the
drug and later these were discussed within a
normal psychotherapy interview. Marked abreactions
occurred on 1 or more occasions as significant
episodes in the past were remembered. Patients
talked little throughout the interview but repetition of words or phrases was common. Feelings
of bodily change were often followed by a description of childhood fantasies. One obsessional
patient felt that he obtained more benefit from
8 phencyclidine interviews than from 14 previous
LSD interviews. Unlike LSD, phencyclidine caused
diminution in obsessional rituals for several
hours after injection. When the drug became available in oral form, 8 more patients were studied.
Five mg were given 1 hour before the interview and
then the dose was increased at subsequent interviews to 7.5-10 mg. The drug was helpful in
promoting a free flow of emotionally charged
material, though in 2 patients the drug produced
marked thought bloc, clinically similar to that
seen in schizophrenia.

Bethlem Royal and Maudsley Hospitals
Beckenham, Kent
Great Britain

3072 Jean-Yves, & Achallé, Pierre. L'utilisation du R. 381-R. 382 dans les états confusionnels
éthyliques ou post-traumatiques, et la désintoxi-
cation alcoolique. [The use of R. 381-R. 382 in
alcoholic or posttraumatic states of confusion,
and in alcoholic cures.] Annales Médico-Psychologiques, 1962, 120, 101-104.

Phenmethrazine (R. 381-382) usually in doses of
6 tablets was successful in combating confusional
states induced by alcoholism or occurring after
traumas. In addition, it was used in connection
with standard cures in 100 cases of alcoholism.
Whereas formerly, states of confusion appeared
with a frequency of 10%, addition of phenmetrazine
to the course of treatment prevented the occurrence of such states. Also, its tonic effects
counterbalance the lowered tonus and depressive
reactions formerly exhibited by some patients.

Centre Psychothérapique,
La Charité-sur-Loire
Nièvre, France

3073 Borenstein, P., Dabbah, M., Blés, G.,
Roussel, A., & Rosemberger, Mme. Etude clinique de l'ethylbenzatropine (U.K. 738 ou
tropéthydryline), correcteur des syndromes
extra-pyramidaux dus aux neuroleptiques. [A
clinical study of ethylbenztropin (U.K. 738
or tropethydrylin) an antiparkinsonian agent.]
Annales Medico-Psychologiques, 1962, 120,
2, 281-288.

Ethylbenztropin was administered to 65 patients
displaying predominantly extrapyramidal syndromes (excito-tonic seizures and parkinsonism)
following treatment with thioproperazine,
haloperidol, and other neuroleptics. The
drug was administered either orally (2 mg
and 5 mg tablets) or i.p. (1 mg or 5 mg
ampoules) at doses up to 30 mg. Cure was
effected in 53%, and results were excellent
in 30%, moderate in 4%, fair in 7% and
negative in 7%. Side effects were mydriasis,
other visual disorders, dry mouth, asthenia,
somnolence and autonomic disturbances.
Tolerance was excellent.

Hôpital Psychiatrique
Villejuif, France

3074 Leube, H. Über die Behandlung der
Schizophrenie mit einem neuen Psychopharmakon.
[The treatment of schizophrenia with a new
psychopharmacologic agent.] Therapiewoche,
1962, 16, 688-692.

Fluphenazine was used for the treatment of 95
male schizophrenics, aged 21-73 years. The
duration of treatment during hospitalization
was 32-168 days; it is strongly recommended
that treatment for ambulatory patients be
continued for several more weeks or months.
The total amount administered during hospitalization ranged from 84-1170 mg; the daily
dosage from 3 mg (1 mg t.i.d.) to 12 mg.
Fluphenazine was generally administered orally
in the form of tablets or drops, in severe
cases with psychotic symptoms i.m. (1-3 mg
per injection). Of the 95 patients under
study, 62 had acute schizophrenia, and 33
cronic schizophrenia. The best results were
seen in cases of acute schizophrenia in which
symptoms of paranoia and hallucinationw were
coupled with anxiety and helpness. The
therapeutic effect in chronic schizophrenia
was mostly limited to effect on symptoms.
It was sometimes necessary to give supporting

subjectively even after 3-5 days. Side effects
were not observed.

Psychiatrische-Neurologische Universität
Vienna, Austria

3078 Schwarz, H. Therapeutische Erfahrungen mit
Nialamid. [Therapeutic experiences with nialamide.]
In: Cleghorn, R.A., Moll, A.E., & Roberts, C.A.
Third World Congress of Psychiatry Proceedings.
Volume II. Toronto/Montreal: University of Toronto
Press, 1962. Pp. 1405-1406.

Two separate investigations using nialamide were
carried out. In the first study, 174 patients
were treated for an average of 40 days (1-3
tablets t.i.d.). The patients were suffering from
depressions of various genesis, as well as from
epilepsy and schizophrenia. Good therapeutic
results were seen in endogenous and involutional
depressions and less favorable results in schizophrenia. The tolerance was good. In the second
double-blind study, 157 patients were treated
for a period of 2-3 months. Good results were
seen in 68 patients; 67.3% of these were seen in
psychopathic patients, and in those suffering
from epilepsy; depressions during aging, and
endogenous and symptomatic depression. Good results were seen in patients with arteriosclerotic
dementia, imbecility, atrophic brain processes,
and schizophrenia (40-50%). Of 36 cases in the
placebo group 9 appeared improved, though 4 of
these patients had received additional medication. Fifty-three patients showed no change.
The following results with regard to dosage were
observed: of 42 patients which had received 50
to 150 mg daily, 69.2% showed good results; of
46 patients with an average dosage of 100-300 mg,
56.3% good results; of 33 patients with an
average daily dosage of 150-450 mg, 40% good
results. Best results may be achieved with 100-
200 mg/day, while higher doses might be necessary for individual cases but may lead to increased agitation. Administration of higher
dosages did not speed up onset of effect.

Pfälzische Nervenklinik,
Landeck über Landeau/Pfalz
Germany

3079 Tweedy, P.S. A clinical trial of
heptabarbitone (Medomin). Gerontologia Clinica, 1962, 4, 276-280.

A double-blind trial was used in which 0.2 g
butobarbital (2 tablets) were compared with
0.4 g (2 tablets) of heptabarbital (Medomin).
Each patient tested was given the drugs on
successive nights or on the 1st and 3rd
nights without any sedative on the intervening
night. With 31 patients, 60-90 years of age,
no difference was found between them in
regard to effectiveness of sedation; the incidence of confusional states was much the
same for both.

St. Thomas' Hospital
Stockport, Cheshire
Great Britain

3080 Wittenborn, J.R., Plante, Marc, Burgess,
Frances, and Maurer, Helen. A comparison of
imipramine, electro convulsive therapy and
placebo in the treatment of depressions.
Journal of Nervous and Mental Diseases, 1962,
135, 131-137.

The efficacy of imipramine, ECT and a placebo
was compared in the treatment of newly-ad-
mitted, female depressives. None of the
patients appeared to be schizophrenic or
addicts. The placebo and imipramine were
indistinguishable and the dosage (which did
not exceed 200 mg/day) was determined by the
physician in charge of the patient. Assignment of patient to treatment groups was pre-
determined on a random basis: Patients were
observed, tested, and rated before assignment
to groups, when they were ready to go home,
or at end of ten weeks. Tests and ratings
represented criteria for the major characteristics of depression. Using the method of
analysis of cavariance, an adjustment posttreatment mean for each treatment group was
found, and comparison of these means indicated the relative efficacy of the treatment.
The imipramine group was found to be superior
to the placebo group with respect to symptoms
of anxiety and depression, subjective depression as revealed by the MMPI, and the
"friendly" score on the Clyde Mood Scale.
The imipramine group showed a much shorter
latency than the ECT group on the Standard
Interview. The ECT group was superior to
the placebo group with respect to the

to extrapyramidal reaction, amenable to antiparkinsonian drugs and the combination to
psychotonics. No mortality has been observed
in spite of massive ingestion by patients attempting suicide.

Hôpital de Saint-Venant
Saint-Venant, France

3084 Lindsley, Ogden R. Direct measurement
and functional definition of vocal hallucinatory
symptoms in chronic psychosis. In: Cleghorn,
R.A., Moll, A.E., & Roberts, C.A. Third World
Congress of Psychiatry Proceedings. Volume II.
Toronto/Montreal: University of Toronto Press
and McGill University Press, 1962. Pp. 983-986.

Chlordiazepoxide was considered the most effective drug currently available in the treatment
of tension and/or anxiety states. Over 30
thousand hours of data were collected from 80
adult chronic psychotics. Patients sat in a
small 6 x 6 foot experimental room containing a
chair on 1 wall, a small plunger, and delivery
tray. The operation of this plunger (a free
operant response) could be made to deliver automatically various reinforcers to the patient on
different schedules of intermittent reinforcement.
The nature of these reinforcing events, (e.g.,
food, candy, money) determines the class of motivation that is being investigated. The different rates of plunger responses are recorded on
cumulative response recorders and indicate the
patient's current interest in and ability to work
for different reinforcers. Both manual non-
sympathetic responses and vocal sympathetic responses of overtly hallucinating patients were
directly and simultaneously recorded. Vocal
hallucinatory symptoms, and possibly all psychotic symptoms, are defined in terms of their
functional rather than topographical or bizarre
properties. Vocal symptoms appeared to have the
following functional properties: (1) an abnormally high degree of nonmechanical competition
with strongly reinforced nonsymptomatic behavior;
(2) the ability to be elicited by hidden stimuli
of incomplete topography in the appropriate modality; (3) an abnormally long after-discharge
from such elicitation, and (4) independence of
their environmental consequences or direct reinforcement.

Harvard Medical School
Boston, Mass

3085 Mall, G. Some observations on the
aetiology and therapy of endogenous de-
pressions. In: Cleghorn, R.A., Moll, A.E.,
& Roberts, C.A. Third World Congress of
Psychiatry Proceedings. Volume II. Toronto/
Montreal: University of Toronto Press and
McGill University Press, 1962. Pp. 1402-1404.

The treatment of periodic depressions (post-
menstrual period or in the puerperium, i.e.,
women 22-38 years of age; 35 patients) with
estradiol combined with testosterone [dosage
unspecified] resulted in radical fading of
the depressions; phenothiazines, meprobamate,
and imipramine were not particularly effective when not supported by hormone therapy.
Depot-testosterone treatment of male psychotic
depressives with 250-500 mg/ month and in
obstinate cases in combination with chorio-
gonadotropin (24-40,000 μ/month) results
frequently but not always in a satisfactory
remission. The short term use of ACTH and
the use of deoxycorticosterone with antidepressants such as chlordiazepoxide and MAO
inhibitors like isocarboxazid, opium, or
haloperidol was also discussed. Depressions
in women in menopause and old age, have
responded to depot-testosterone (250 mg/
month) combined with 3 mg estradiol.

Pfälzische, Nervenklinik
Landeck uber Landau/Pfalz
Germany

3086 Billig, Otto, & Adams, Robert W., Jr.
Middle-age depressions. In: Cleghorn, R.A.,
Moll, A.E., & Roberts, C.A. Third World
Congress of Psychiatry Proceedings. Volume
II. Toronto/Montreal: University of Toronto
Press and McGill University Press, 1962.
Pp. 1406-1409.

In a series of 100 consecutive patients seen
for psychiatric evaluation in connection
with application for total and permanent
disability, 90 patients fell into the 40-60
age group. Most of the claims were initially
on physical disability; psychiatric evaluation was obtained when physical symptoms
appeared largely functional. Sixty-four out
of 90 patients were males. The diagnosis
of chronic anxiety was made in 18 males and
19 females. The next diagnostic group was
organic brain syndrome with cerebral arteriosclerosis (15 males). Ten patients were
schizophrenic and 5 were diagnosed as manic

10 mg optional; phenelzine maximal 60 mg with
another 15 mg optional; imipramine, minimal 150
mg with another 37.5 mg optional. Dosages
reached maximal in the 3rd week of treatment.
ECT, modified by suxamethonium, was given with
a minimal of 9 treatments (3 weekly for 3 weeks)
with further treatments based on clinical
judgment. The full treatment period for all was
limited to 8 weeks, though patients could be
discharged at any time after 4 weeks of treatment. Psychoneurotic depressive reactions show
marked improvement and no failures, whereas
patients in the psychotic groups show 25-50%
treatment failures. While all treatments work
well for psychoneurotic depressive reaction, ECT
proves somewhat more effective in affective
psychoses. MAO inhibitors show a more gradual
response in the 1st 3 weeks than ECT and imipramine,
but the improvement rate remains steadier throughout the 8-week period. ECT and imipramine show
maximal change in the first 3 weeks, with subsequent slowing in improvement rate.

Mental Health Center
74 Fernwood Road
Boston, Mass.

3090 DeVerbizier, J., Guillon, A., & Benkhoucha,
M. A propos de cures d'amaigrissement par le
8.228 R.P. en milieu hospitalier psychiatrique.
[Antiobesity treatment with RP 8-228 in a
psychiatric hospital environment.] Toulouse
Médical, 1961, 63, 437-443.

Eighteen paranoid patients (16 women and 2 men),
were treated for overweight with levophacetoperane
(5 and 20 mg tablets, 20-120 mg/day, usually in 3
doses an hour before meals). Treatment lasted
about 5 months, with a range of 1-19 months. The
agent had a clear anorexic effect in 11 cases,
moderate action in 2 cases and no appetite suppressing effect in 5 cases. One bedridden
women was able to go back to normal routines in
the hospital after a weight loss of 26 kilos.
Tolerance was excellent and side effects occurred
in only 2 cases: epigastric cramps in 1 and
generalized fatigue in the other.

Société de Neurologie et Psychiatrie
  de Toulouse et du Sud-Ouest
Toulouse, France

3091 Gayral, L. Resultat de cent traitements par imipramine (Tofranil). [The result
of 100 treatments with imipramine (Tofranil)]
Toulouse Médical, 1961, 63, 435-437.

One-hundred patients suffering from anxiety-
melancholia were treated with 100-250 mg/day
imipramine, p.o. or i.m. Twenty-six percent
were cured, 29% showed no change, 25% were
found intolerant necessitating the cessation
of medication, 17% improved temporarily, and
3% showed improvement but also intolerance
necessitating discontinuation of imipramine.
Side effects were as follows: 1 case of
polyneuritis, 3 erythrodermic eruption, 2
confusion, 5 excitation and insomnia, 1
ataxia with trembling and anxiety, 2 stupor
and 9 cases of gastrointestinal upset with
autonomic disturbances, nausea and hypotension. Results could be restated as 33%
good, 33% poor, and 33% intolerance.

[No address]

3092. Chanoit, P., & Vallée, A. L'emploi
de la thioridazine en psychiatrie. Réflexions
critiques d'une expérience clinique.
[Thioridazine in psychiatry. Critical re-
flections on clinical experience.] Annales
Médico-Psychologiques, 1962, 120, 104-109.

Thioridazine was administered in tablet
form to 55 patients, in doses of 50-300 mg
per day. Good results were obtained in 24
cases, moderately good in 14, poor results
in 7, no effect in 8, and aggravation in 2.
Persons under 60 responded to treatment
better than the older patients. Better
results were obtained in acute than in chronic
conditions. The drug is principally indicated in anxiety, depression, schizophrenia,
chronic deliriums, and alcoholic neuroses.
Thioridazine was extremely well tolerated
and very simple to administer.

[No address]

3093 Mellien, G. Klinische Erfahrungen mit
Tryptizol. [Clinical experience with Tryptizol (amitriptyline).] Therapiewoche, 1962,
22, 999-1003.

Amitriptyline was used in the treatment of
58 hospitalized patients, aged 18 to 72,
suffering from severe depressions of various

Complete medical and psychiatric examinations were performed on 26 hyperthyroid patients. The Clyde Mood Scale was administered to 16 of them. Large doses of triiodothyronine (300 μg/day for 3 days) were administered to 11 normal subjects and changes in affect were determined according to the Clyde Mood Scale. The predominant symptomatology of thyrotoxic patients is affectively determined and the presence or absence of symptoms correlates well with Clyde Mood Scale scores. The administration of thyroid hormone produced depression, decreases friendliness, and increases jitteriness in normal subjects.

[No address]

3098 Bartholomew, Allen A. An evaluation of tranylcypromine ("Parnate") in the treatment of depression. Medical Journal of Australia, 1962, 149, 655-661.

A double-blind study of tranylcypromine was made of 84 depressive outpatients (6-week trial). The initial dose was 10 mg t.i.d.; it was doubled after 2 weeks if neither patient of a pair showed any improvement. Side effects were mild and those causing cessation of treatment were hypomania (if it may be called a side effect), dependent edema, impotence, nausea and vomiting. Global results showed tranylcypromine superior to placebo. However tranylcypromine did not significantly differ from placebo in either endogenous or involutional depression. In the case of reactive depression the drug was superior. Improvement, when it occurs, should be evident after about 2 weeks of treatment.

Alexandra Clinic
Department of Mental Hygiene
Victoria, Australia

3099 Richardeau, N., & Asfar, M. Spasmes de la face et du cou a caractère extrapyramidal après 36 ans d'évolution d'une psychose périodique. Action thérapeutique contre les spasmes du majeptil. (Presentation de malades). [Spasms of the face and neck, extrapyramidal in character, after a 36 year period of recurrent psychosis. Therapeutic action of thioproperazine (Majeptil) against spasms. (A case history).] Annales Médico-Psychologique, 1962, no. 1, 71-77.

A 66-year-old woman, who had suffered from
encephalitis 36 years previously and had
been under treatment for 35 years for a
recurrent psychosis of a marked agitational
type, suddenly developed uncoordinated
spasms, primarily of the face and the neck
which also affected the general musculature.
Extrapyramidal hypertonia, due to chlorpromazine administration, was believed the
cause. Treatment with thioproperazine, in
doses of 15 mg twice weekly, for several
months suppressed extrapyramidal manifestations. Cessation of thioproperazine
therapy was followed by reappearance of
symptoms.

Service du Professeur Baruk
Saint-Maurice (Seine),
Paris, France

3100 Sila, Basri, Mowrer, Marie, Ulett,
George, & Johnson, Margaret. The differentiation of psychiatric patients by EEG
changes after sodium pentothal. Progress
in Neurology and Psychiatry, 1962, 17,
191-199; discussion 199-203.

Thirty-nine schizophrenics and 19 psychotic
depressive cases were studied before and
after thiopental (Pentothal). After 5
minutes of resting EEG recording, 100 mg
thiopental was injected i.v. in 5-7 seconds.
The drug was reinjected twice more at 2-
minute intervals, giving a total of 300 mg
in a 4-minute period. Patients were observed until EEG tracings returned to premedication levels. Both groups of mental
patients had similar basic resting EEG's.
Thiopental produced an increase in EEG
activity frequencies, particularly in the
β range. There was a significant difference in the reaction of the 2 groups with
a quantitatively greater EEG response in
the schizophrenic subjects. When a group
of 24 patients was carefully selected from
a larger group and dichotomized on the
basis of symptoms typical for schizophrenia
or depression, and with little or no over-
lapping, no significant difference in
response between the 2 groups of patients
was found. In the discussion Goldman
reviews thiopental-activation studies in
about 2,000 patients.

[No address]

high stimulation, in which an auditory stimulus
was presented constantly; low or high escape in
which an auditory stimulus was presented from
which the subject could escape, and control,
which had no such collateral stimulus. The
control and low escape groups performed the same.
The high escape group performed better than the
control group, and the 2 stimulation groups did
worse than the control. For the post-experimental
condition, the medium stimulation of the low
escape group was found worse than the others which
were not different from each other. Improvement
in the psychomotor performance of chronic schizophrenics presented with an intense stimulus
characterized as aversive was a function of reinforcement rather than solely as an increase in
the level of arousal.

University of Rochester
Rochester, N.Y.

3105 Bennett, Ivan F. The constellation of
depression: its treatment with nortriptyline.
II. Clinical evaluation of nortriptyline.
Journal of Nervous and Mental Disease, 1962,
135, 59-68.

Nortriptyline was proven a safe and effective
antidepressant in a trial with 75 patients
represented by both outpatients and hospitalized groups and including psychotic, psychoneurotic, geriatric, neurologic and psychosomatic cases. Side effects were few and mild,
e.g., 16% dry mouth, 16% drowsiness, 12% increased psychomotor activity and 12% dizziness.
Dosage was 25 mg nortriptyline b.i.d. to q.i.d.
Global clinical improvement was 37%. In relation
to target symptoms, improvement was 82% for depression, 70% for hostility and 74% for anxiety.

Lilly Laboratory for Clinical Research
Marion County General Hospital
Indianapolis, Ind.

3106 Gradillas Regodon, Vicente. Observaciones
sobre el tratamiento de esquizofrenicos cronicos
con fluorclorpromacina. [Observations on the
treatment of chronic schizophrenics with triflupromazine.] Medicina, 1962, 30, 97-99.

A double-blind study was conducted with 50
chronic schizophrenics, hospitalized for over 10
years, 25 on triflupromazine and 25 on placebo.
Triflupromazine dosage was 200 mg/day for 3
months. Side effects consisted of edema,

anorexia, hypokinesis, trembling, unrest, rapidly alleviated with promazine injections. Some improvement especially in relation to deliriums or hallucinations was obtained, without real effect on the schizophrenic disease process. A practical rule is to begin with a drug such as chlorpromazine or reserpine, and if favorable results are not obtained to switch to another product.

Hospital Psiquiatrico de Leganes
Leganes, Spain

3107 Rondepierre, J.J., Ropert, R., & Azoulay, J. Sur l'utilisation clinique en neuro-psychiatrie du chlorhydrate d'éthyl-3-(méthyl-2'-diméthylamino-3'-propyl) 10 phénothiazine (6484 RP) nouveau neuroleptique phénothiazin-ique. [On the clinical employment in neuro-psychiatry of ethyl-3-(methyl-2'-dimethyl-amino-3'-propyl) 10 phenothiazine HCl (RP 6484), a new phenothiazine neuroleptic.] Presse Medicale, 1962, 70, 1342-1344.

Ethotrimeprazine was administered to 42 hospi-talized and 26 ambulatory patients, suffering from delirious psychoses, schizophrenia, melancholia, depression, etc., at 40-400 mg doses for the hospitalized group, and 20-100 for ambulatory patients. Neuroleptic effects obtained were similar to those of chlorpro-mazine or levomepromazine, while the side effects noted with the latter drug were absent. Tolerance was excellent. The drug does not have any inherent antidepressant action, and its combination with imipramine results in synergistic action.

[No address]

3108 Priest, R.G., & Forrest, A.C. Nethalide. The Lancet, 1962, No. 7253, 451.

No direct evidence of psychopharmacological effect for nethalide has been established. A 200 mg single oral dose was given to 5 normal volunteers who reported: 2 no effects, 1 fatigue, and 2 noted giddiness. One female depressed patient was given 200 mg t.i.d. for 7 days with no effect. This patient later improved with 15 mg phenelzine t.i.d. A manic depressive female in a depressive phase was given 50 mg nethalide i.v. with no effect; the same was true for a schizophrenic

designated as endogenous depression. This
appears to concern the value of classical
psychiatric nosology and indicates that investigations into the affects of the drug
among adult relatives opens up new possibilities
for clinical research.

Psychiatrische Universitätsklinik
Burgholzli, Zurich
Switzerland

3113 Busfield, Bernard L., Jr., Wechsler, Henry,
& Barnum, William J. A physiological correlate
of diagnosis and treatment outcome in depression.
In: Cleghorn, R.A., Moll, A.E., & Roberts, C.A.
Third World Congress of Psychiatry Proceedings.
Volume II. Toronto/Montreal: University of
Toronto Press and McGill University Press, 1962.
Pp. 1367-1371.

One-hundred nine severely depressed adult inpatients in three different hospitals were
treated for a 4-8 week period with either isocarboxazid (20 mg/day, up to 50 mg/day), chlorphenoxamine (30 mg/day), imipramine (75 mg/day,
increased to 185 mg/day) or ECT (3 treatments/
week for a minimum of 3 weeks). After selection,
each patient underwent a 5-day pretreatment
clinical assessment which included determination
of salivation rate by the Peck technique. Perceptual complaint of dry mouth, diagnosis,
assessment of severity of depression, and determination of improvment were carried out independently of salivation collection by different psychiatrists. Patients with reactive
(endogenous) depression had significantly higher
rates of salivation compared with those with
nonreactive (endogenous) depression, including
involutional and manic-depressive cases. Female
depressed (more often endogenous in diagnosis)
salivate at significantly lower rates than male
counterparts. Salivation rates do not vary with
severity of depression in any diagnostic groups.
There is no correlation of perception of dry
mouth with diagnostic category, nor actual
measured physiological hyposalivation. Thirty-
one patients who improved on antidepressant
medications have significantly higher pretreatment salivations as compared with 37 patients
who did not improve. The salivation rate provides a possible criterion for judging success
in treatment on a specific biological basis.
Analysis of age, sex, diagnosis, and initial

Clinical Studies
Abstract 3114

severity of depression showed that none de-
cisively alters this relation of salivation
rate to improvement.

74 Fenwood Rd.
Boston 15, Mass.

SEE ALSO: 2873, 2877, 2917, 2918, 2924,
2925, 2932, 2941, 2955, 2956, 2957, 2962,
2963, 2967, 2968, 2969, 2970, 2971, 2972,
2973, 2974, 2975, 2977, 2978, 2979, 2983,
2985, 2987, 2990, 3000, 3001, 3006, 3013,
3117, 3118, 3122, 3125, 3137, 3195.

3114 Kaplan, Stanley M., Kravetz, B. Stuart,
& Ross, W. Donald. The effects of imipramine
on the depressive components of medical
disorders. In: Cleghorn, R.A., Moll, A.E.,
& Roberts, C.A. Third World Congress of
Psychiatry Proceedings. Volume II. Toronto/
Montreal: University of Toronto Press and
McGill University Press, 1962. Pp. 1362-1367.

Forty-nine patients, 18 men and 31 women,
aged 20-50 years, were treated with 75-500
mg imipramine/day. Observational approaches
included double-blind, single-blind and
open observations. Patients were selected
for evidence of overt depression, evidence
of experiencing object loss and indication
that the patient's adaptive measures had
failed and the responsive was rather passi-
vity, helplessness, and restlessness.
Greater interaction with the environment,
decreased depression and decreased physical
manifestations of disease were noted.
Some beneficial results were obtained in 42
out of the 49 patients.

Dept. of Psychiatry
University of Cincinnati
Cincinnati 29, Ohio

ml. or higher. Thirty-eight patients
showed symptoms of acute bromide intoxication; in 48 others, a subacute reaction was
observed. In 52 cases, the cause was due
to self-medication with proprietary bromi-
reide preparations and in 32 cases, patients
had taken a mixture prescribed by a doctor
or a pharmacist. In the remaining 44 cases,
the source of bromide was doubtful. In 2
experiments observed, serum bromide levels
were proportional to the ingested daily
dose. Bromides in any form no longer de-
serve a place in the pharmacopaeia and, by
the same token, the sale of proprietary
preparations should be restricted. (9 refs.)

University of Sydney
Sydney, Australia

3118 Hodgkinson, Robert. A study of the
clinical effects of Catha edulis (khat,
miraa) in Kenya. Medical Journal of Australia, 1962, 1, 884-886.

Khat is widely used in Abyssinia, Arabia
and East Africa, being an important article
of commerce in these areas. It is alleged
to be a habituating drug. Continuous chewing over a long period is said to lead to a
loss of a sense of reality. Users become
listless. No increase in crime is associated with its use. The experience of a
European where Khat appeared to be a stimulant causing euphoria, mental stimulation,
and anorexia is described. Ten African
volunteers were studied; a 20 mm. rise in
systolic blood pressure and slight increase
in pulse rate were noted. Then a study
using 30 male African volunteers was made
of preference for Khat, 15 mg. sustained-
release capsules of dexamphetamine or placebo. No preference was demonstrated between Khat and dexamphetamine, but both were
preferred to a placebo. No effect of Khat
is described which cannot be attributed to
an amphetaminelike drug. Alles et al.(1961)
indicate that the active principle of Catha
edulis is dextro-nor-pseudo-ephedrine. (No
refs.)

Department of Clinical Investigation
Parke, Davis and Co.
Ann Arbor, Mich.

3119 Friis, Thorkild. Eksperimentelle undersogelser under fenacetinindgift til mennesker. [Experimental examinations after the administration of phenacetin in man.] Nordisk Medicin, 1962, 67, 755.

Sixteen phenacetin-habituated patients with renal insufficiency and 22 cases without renal insufficiency, 11 nonhabituated patients with insufficiency and a fourth group with insufficiency were given phenacetin and determinations of erythrocyte stability were made. The second group had a markedly low erythrocyte stability while the other groups showed normal times. Because impure phenacetin contains acetate-4-chloranilide (0.1%), trials were run with pure and impure phenacetin or nothing in 15 patients. In 9, the time was markedly shortened after pure or impure phenacetin, while it was normal when no phenacetin was given. In 4, time was slightly shortened after impure phenacetin and in 2, normal but markedly shortened after common phenacetin. Phenacetin has a similar effect but not as marked as the impure substance.

[No address]

3120 Hojman, D., Lemberg, A., De Palol, J., & Rubin, B. Estudio experimental de la acción de la iproniazida sobre hígado, miocardio y cerebro. [Experimental studies of the action of iproniazid on liver, heart, and brain.] Revista Clínica Española, 1962, 87, 91-94.

In acute toxicity studies, rabbits received 450 mg/kg iproniazid i. v.; in chronic studies the daily dose was 12 mg/kg p. o. for 30 days. No mortality was noted in the first hour after 450 mg/kg i. v. doses. No pathologic histochemical or histopathological changes in liver or brain were noted. Changes observed included an increase in the number of cases of chronic angiocholitis, lower sinusoidal blood circulation, greater frequency of hydropic degeneration, reduction of chondrioma, and of RNA and of glycogen in hepatocytes. (16 refs.)

Cátedra de Toxicología Facultad de Ciencias Médicas
Universidad de Buenos Aires
Buenos Aires, Argentina

3121 Jenkins, Margaret Q. Poisoning of the month. Journal of the South Carolina Medical Association, 1962, 58, 400. [Editorial]

Two boys, ages 4 and 6 years, were admitted in coma following a gasoline sniffing episode. Administration of oxygen resulted in return to consciousness whereupon an extensive history of gasoline sniffing was revealed. (No refs.)

[No address]

3122 Nayrac, P., Lorrain, A., & Arnott, C. Modifications apportées par le traitement à la sémeiologie des psychoses maniacodépressives. [Modifications in the symptomatology of manic-depressive psychoses brought about by drug therapy.] Lille Médical, 1962, 7, 209-211.

Administration of conventional doses of imipramine to cases of melancholia may completely alleviate the patient's anxiety, confusion, and hypomania. However, confusion may increase at doses higher than 200 mg/day. Hypomania may result independent of the dose, occasionally leading to the mistaken belief that the patient has been cured whereas subsequently suicide may be attempted; i. e., psychotonics are capable of camouflaging the underlying psychosis. Haloperidol, used in the treatment of psychomotor excitation in manic states (at doses of 15-20 mg/day) may trigger, after a period of calmness, excitomotor convulsions which then must be treated with chlorpromazine. Subsequently the patient appears to be in a confused-agitated state. In other patients, an extrapyramidal syndrome appears in which hypertonia is predominant. But psychomotor agitation and logorrhea are suppressed in time, without the underlying condition being affected, and the patient's family is likely to remove him from the institution prematurely. (No refs.)

[No address]

3123 Loiseau, P., Bargues, R., Planques, L., & Cohadon, S. Accidents nerveus dus aux hydantoïnes: aspec électroencephalograph-ique. [Neurologic side effects due to hydantoins: electroencephalic aspects.] Révue Neurologique, 1962, 106, 171-176.

Following some accidental changes in the method of manufacture of melantoin, a drug which had hitherto been innocuous, the drug began to trigger some intolerance reactions in some epileptic patients. The factor common to all 4 cases is that of disorganization, but the manner of disorganization is not specific with respect to either patient or drug. Some evidence of intoxication was present however. Cessation of use of the drug resulted in a return of the EEG tracings to a stable and conventional form. (No refs.)

[No address]

3124 Michon, P., Larcan, A., Huriet, C., & Calamai, M. Hépatite mortelle au cours d'un traitement par l'iproniazide. [A hepatitis fatality in the course of iproniazid therapy.] Bulletin et Mémoires de la Société Médicale des Hôpitaux de Paris, 1962, 113, 21-23.

Over a 63-day period, a depressed woman, 39 years old, received a total of about 6 g. iproniazid. The first symptoms consisted of nausea, and vomiting, then icterus followed by coma, and eventually death. The autopsy findings were in agreement with those of both viral hepatitis and iproniazid hepatitis. (No refs.)

[No address]

3125 Faure, Henri. Sur les effets activateurs d'un psychotonique en neuro-psychiatrie infantile. Le problème du risque thérapeutique. [On the activating effects of a psychotonic in pediatric neuropsychiatry. The problem of the therapeutic risk.] Annales Médico-Psychologiques, 1962, 120, 87-90.

Phacetoperane administration in a pediatric clinic resulted in 4 types of reactions: psychic disequilibrium involving cyclical anxiety, and capable of being favorably influenced by levomepromazine; appearance or reactivation of latent conflict with accentuation of prepsychotic or preneurotic personality traits; fluctuations in psychometric output during medication, but with evidence of the intellectual capacities of the child being observable; diminution or extinction of the scholastic efficiency during medication, but appearance of a new higher level of scholastic efficiency after a period of latency following cessation of the drug. The third phase, i. e., regression to infantile behavior, is frequently marked by violent nightmares and quasihallucinatory pictures of ravishing monsters. Cathartic psychotherapy is aided by the expression of the experiences with the aid of drawings.

Hôpital Psychiatrique
Bonnevat, France

3126 Frankel, Jerome J. Hepatic and renal damage with azotemia associated with iproniazid administration. American Journal of Gastroenterology, 1962, 37, 64-69.

A 63-year-old male executive, who had been on long-term anticoagulant therapy because of myocardial infarction had been receiving 10 mg iproniazid/day for 3 months which was increased to 30 mg/day for 5 months. Estimated total intake of iproniazid was 5,480 mg. The patient developed profound azotemia superimposed upon hepatic dysfunction. Complete recovery of both renal and hepatic functions ensued in 33 days of hospitalization. (8 refs.)

Michael Reese Hospital
Department of Medicine
Chicago, Ill.

3127 Trueta, J., & Agerholm, Margaret. Thalidomide-damaged infants. Lancet, 1962, No. 7253, 452.

Request is made that cases of congenital limb defect in Britain should be registered as soon as possible after birth with the Nuffield Department of Orthopedic Surgery, Oxford. All cases will be given a code number and personal details withheld. Cooperation of all organizations, official and voluntary, are welcomed and it is hoped that this move will provide information on the numbers involved. (No refs.)

Nuffield Department of Orthopedic Surgery
Oxford, Great Britain

3128 Dijkhuis, F. J., Hagenbeek, J. H., Bekker, V. V., van Creveld, S., de Monchy, C., & de Jonge, G. A. Thalidomide and congential abnormalities. Lancet, 1962, No. 7253, 452.

A warning was sent out by The Netherlands medical authorities in November, 1961 relating to discontinuation of thalidomide, sold as Softenon, Noctosediv, and Enterosediv. Up to June 27, 1962, 12 cases of malformations in children attributed to thalidomide had been reported, which is limited in view of a population of about 11 million. (No refs.)

Committee of the Dutch Pediatric Society
The Hague, The Netherlands

3129 Rüttner, J. R., Rondez, R., & Maier, C. Chlorpromazin-Ikterus, eine Form der cholostatischen Hepatose. [Chlorpromazine-icterus, a form of choleostatic hepatosis.] Deutsche Medizinische Wochenschrift, 1962, 87, 1107-1110.

Fourteen cases of icterus which appeared 5-23 days after administration of chlorpromazine (50-8200 mg. total intake) are reported. Four patients died in connection with pyelonephritis (2), heart failure (1), and nephrosis with uremia (1); the others recovered. One or more liver biopsies were performed in 10 patients. The histopathological hepatic changes observed in biopsy and autopsy material were relatively minor. All cases showed bile thrombi in the biliary capillaries. Formation of thrombi was never pronounced. Liver cells were enlarged, showed loss of glycogen, and sometimes increased lipid content. They contained various amounts of bile in form of droplets or drops. Occasionally, cell necrosis occurred. The hepatic reticuloendothelial cells may also contain bile. No signs of inflammation,

and no accumulation of bile in bile ducts were noted. (9 refs.)

Histopathologsiches Institut
Universität Zürich
Zürich, Switzerland

3130 Fisher, Hyman W. Coma due to a combination of barbiturates, scopolamine and dihydroergotamine. Journal of the Medical Society of New Jersey, 1962, 59, 500-502.

A 20-year-old woman ingested 99 tablets of Plexonal (45 mg barbital, 15 mg phenobarbital, 25 mg isobutylallylbarbiturate, 0.08 mg scopolamine and 0.16 mg dihydroergotamine per tablet) after which she was in coma 5 days. This amount is 25 times the hypnotic dose. The course was complicated by convulsions, airway obstruction, phlebitis, bronchopneumonia, anemia, kypokalemia, and hematuria due to anticoagulants. No abnormal physical residuals were observed. (No refs.)

121 East Northfield Road
Livingston, N. J.

3131 Koutsky, Carl D., Mulvahill, John E., & Orbuch, Martin W. Danger of depression associated with Rauwolfia therapy. Lancet, 1962, No. 82, 346-349.

Rauwolfia drugs induced depression in 8 hypertensive patients, ages 32-70 years, 6 of whom had compulsive personalities and 4 psychotic depression. Onset of depression varied from 2 weeks to 10 months after initiation of Rauwolfia therapy. Rauwolfia compounds utilized included reserpine, Rauwolfia, and alseroxylon. Tranylcypromine and trifluoperazine [dosages unspecified] were administered to combat depression. The use of Rauwolfia drugs should be avoided in depression prone patients. (8 refs.)

University of Minnesota Medical School
Minneapolis, Minnesota

SEE ALSO 2865, 2866, 2887, 2899, 2934, 2935, 2942, 2943, 2947, 2950, 2976, 2982, 2994, 3003, 3095, 3099.

3132 Molinengo, L. Profil psicofarma-
cologico del meprobamato. [Psychopharma-
cologic profile of meprobamate.] Archivio
Italiano di Scienza Farmacologia, 1962,
12, 118-129.

Rats were studied with the following
schedules: (1) concurrent variable ratio
avoidance schedules, (2) guided extinction
and (3) simple extinction. The meprobamate
dosages, which were administered 1/2 hour
before trials, were 0.08, 0.16, 0.24, and
0.32 g/kg. Food motivation was reduced by
meprobamate in females more than in males.
Meprobamate interfered with right-left discrimination in both sexes. CARs were modified only at the highest doses. Meprobamate produced irreversible modifications
in behavior in some cases.

Instituto di Farmacologia e Terapia
  Sperimentale
Università di Torino
Torino, Italy

3133 Waller, Marcus B., & Waller,
Patricia F. Effects of chlorpromazine on
appetitive and aversive components of a
multiple schedule. Journal of the Experimental Analysis of Behavior, 1962, 5,
259-264.

Chlorpromazine (30-225 mg sustained released
capsules or 25-150 mg b.i.d., p.o.) was administered to 2 male beagles 2 hours before
presentation of a multiple schedule (S)
with approach-avoidance components (flashing light coupled with food or shock).
Chlorpromazine exerted no differential depressing effect. Response rates at low
dosages increased slightly on the food reinforced components, while rates on avoidance components remained relatively unchanged. Higher doses resulted in equally depressed response in all components.

Department of Pharmacology
Harvard Medical School
Cambridge, Mass.

3134 Zimmerman, J., & Schuster, C.R.
Spaced responding in multiple DRL schedules.
Journal of Experimental Analysis of Behavior,
1962, 5, 497-504.

Rats were able to adjust to 2 different

temporal requirements within several multiple DRL schedules of reinforcement and a
slight induction between pairs of components
was found. Initial administration of 1
mg/kg amphetamine differentially disrupted
spaced responding in the components of a
multiple DRL 36 DRL 18 schedule, but did
not eliminate discrimination between the
components. After maximal drug effects,
the chronic administration of 0.6 mg/kg
amphetamine was accompanied by a progressive recovery of behavior towards the characteristics of saline control.

Indiana University Medical Center
Indianapolis, Ind.

3135 Janssen, Paul A.J., Niemegeers, Carlos
J.E., & Verbruggen, Frank J. A propos d'une
methode d'investigation de substances sus-
ceptibles de modifier le comportement
agressif inné du rat blanc vis-à-vis de la
souris blanche. [On a method for the investigation of substances able to modify innate
aggressive behavior in the white rat against
white mice.] Psychopharmacologia, 1962,
3, 114-123.

Killer rats were selected among male Wistar
rats for persistent killing of mice. Three
dosage levels of drugs were tested s.c.:
160, 80, 40, etc. mg/kg. The dose of an
agent inhibiting or abolishing aggressivity
in 50% of killer rats (ED 50 in mg/kg s.c.)
was calculated by probit analysis (Siegel
1956). In a series of about 300 compounds,
none were specifically inhibitory for either
aggressiveness or voracity (tendency to de-
vour the victim), without severe catatonia
or some other severe behavioral effect.
Chlorpromazine, haloperidol, triperidol,
haloanisone, perphenazine, morphine, meprobamate, chlordiasepoxide, amphetamine, and
hydroxyzine were among the agents tested.
In contrast to Karli's (1959) results,
hydroxyzine did not modify aggressivity.

Research Laboratorium Dr. C. Janssen
Beerse, Belgium

3136 Flexner, J.B., Flexner, L.B., Stellar,
E., de la Haba, G., & Roberts, R.B. Inhibition of protein synthesis in brain and
learning and memory following Puromycin.
Journal of Neurochemistry, 1962, 9, 595-605.

Young adult albino mice were used in a study
of cerebral protein synthesis following an
antibiotic, Puromycin, given s.c. At various times after Puromycin administration,
0.1 ml of C 14 valine 4 µc/30 g mouse was
injected s.c. Intraventricular and combined
intracerebral and s.c. injections of Puromycin were also used. Behavior was tested
in a 2-compartment hurdle box (grid shock
causing the animal to leap the hurdle into
the "safe" compartment) and in a Y-maze.
Injections of Puromycin suppressed the incorporation of radioactive valine into the
protein of several areas of the brain by
83% on the average. This apparent degree
of inhibition of protein synthesis, maintained for various periods of time, was
without effect on the learning and retention of simple or discrimination avoidance
responses. Inhibition of valine incorporation into protein was raised to 95% by combining s.c. and intracerebral injections
with Puromycin. However, animals so treated
showed disorientation incompatible with
learning or memory.

Department of Anatomy
University of Pennsylvania
Philadelphia 4, Pa.

3137 Diethelm, Oskar. Psychotherapeutic
interviews and alcohol intoxication.
Quarterly Journal of Studies on Alcohol,
1962, 23, 243-251.

Psychotherapeutic interviews were taped on
6 occasions for 45 minutes in 23 alcoholics
who received saline or 60-70 cc of 95%
ethanol i.v. over a period of 18-22 minutes
Blood alcohol levels ranged from 168-190
mg/100 cc after 20 minutes and from 144-122
mg/100 cc after 45 minutes. In 2, blood
levels reached 248 mg/100 cc. Toxic behavior varied widely, and was also elicited by
placebo infusions in some instances. During
the initial 8-10 minutes of acute intoxication, patients spoke with considerable freedom. Revelation of much repressed material
was accompanied by subsequent amnesic

episodes pertaining to mention of this
material.

Department of Psychiatry
Cornell University Medical College
Ithaca, N.Y.

3138 Wallgren, Henrik, & Sinikka
Savolainen. The effect of ethyl alcohol on
a conditioned avoidance response in rats.
Acta Pharmacologica et Toxicologica, 1962,
19, 59-67.

Rats were given 0.4 mg alcohol and the
effect of CARs were studied in a 2-compart-
ment shutter box (using electric shocks
from a grid floor). Reaction time and
number of responses only after shock increased after administration of alcohol,
however the CAR was rather insensitive.
Major impairment of CARs was only observed
when there were overt signs of motor incoordination. After administration of 3 mg/g
alcohol outside training sessions every other
day for 20 days, dimunition of alcohol effect
was observed, apparently due to increased
tolerance.

Research Laboratories
State Alcohol Monopoly
Helsinki, Finland

3139 Jacob, J. Action analgésique et
effets psychotropes de la morphine.
[Analgesic action and psychotropic effects
of morphine.] Thérapie, 1962, 17, 507-518.

In rats, 25 and 50 mg/kg s.c. morphine de-
presses the avoidance reaction and prolongs
exhaustion time in the forced-swim test.
At 5 mg/kg maze reaction time is slowed,
but errors do not increase significantly
until a dose of 25 mg/kg s.c. is reached.
The CARs are inhibited at hypoalgesic doses
of 7-10 mg/kg.

Institut Pasteur
Paris, France

3140 Faidherbe, J., Richelle, M., & Schlag, J. Nonconsumption of the reinforcer under drug action. Journal of the Experimental Analysis of Behavior, 1962, 5, 521-524.

After 5 cats were trained to respond to an auditory stimulus (buzzer) coupled with reinforcement (milk), they experienced alternate sessions in which they received 2 mg methylphenidate s.c. or no drug. On 1 occasion, 2 cats received 6 mg methylphenidate, although they failed to consume the reinforcer (milk). Under normal conditions these 2 animals never ignored the reinforcer. Reinforcement, however, was not essential to produce drug response.

Université de Liège
Liege, Belgium

3141 Sadowski, B., & Longo, V.G. Electroencephalographic and behavioural correlates of an instrumental reward conditioned response in rabbits. A physiological and pharmacological study. Electroencephalography and Clinical Neurophysiology, 1962, 14, 465-476.

Male rabbits with chronically implanted electrodes in the hippocampus and thalamus were trained to pull a ring for a food reward at the sound of a buzzer. When the CS was presented the most striking changes were seen in the hippocampal lead in which the synchronous waves increased in amplitude and frequency up to 9 c/seconds. In the period of satiation high amplitude slow waves at 2-3 c/second, intermingled with spindles in the anterior cortex. During the eating period masticatory waves appeared, particularly in the anterior cortex. The CR was very sensitive to cholinergic drugs. Small doses of scopolamine (0.1 mg/kg) abolished but did not interfere with food intake. Eserine restored the performance of the test as well as EEG activation patterns. Chlorpromazine and imipramine exerted a blocking effect only in doses which produced motor disturbances. Amphetamine had 2 effects: in lower doses it facilitated the CR and with higher doses pulling of the ring occurred unaccompanied by feeding. LSD had a similar effect to that of amphetamine in prolonging the performance of the CR. The appearance of masticatory waves was inhibited by scopolamine, chlorpromazine and imipramine, i.e., by "synchronizing" drugs, as well as by LSD. Amphetamine on the other hand facilitated these waves.

Laboratorio di Chimica Terapeutica
Istituto Superiore di Sanità
Rome, Italy

3142 Dureman, Ingmar, & Scholander, Torkel. Studies in the psychosensory pupillary reflex. II. Habituation after unilateral local application of a sympathicolytic agent. Journal of Psychosomatic Research, 1962, 6, 55-57.

Thirty-five healthy students, aged 21-23 years, were seated in a comfortable chair in a semi-sound proof room fixating a blinking red light. Pupillograms (psychosensory pupillary reflex) were recorded with a movie camera. After the adaptation period the subjects were exposed to 30 white noise stimuli, given through the earphones. The maximal phasic reaction curve followed the tonicity curve, except primarily for the 1st 3 stimuli. Here the tonicity curve shows a slow recruitment reaching a maximal level at the 3rd stimulus while the maximal phasic reaction curve is near its maximum by the 1st stimulus and starts declining at the 2nd, suggesting 3 components: tonic activation (prestimulus area), the maximal area of phasic reaction (maximal poststimulus area) and the amplitude of phasic reaction (equal to the difference between maximal post - and prestimulus areas.)

Department of Psychiatry
University of Uppsala
Uppsala, Sweden

3143 DiMascio, Alberto, Rinkel, Max, & Leiberman, James. Personality and psychotomimetic drugs. In: Cleghorn, R.A., Moll, A.E., & Roberts, C.A. Third World Congress of Psychiatry Proceedings. Volume II. Toronto/Montreal: University of Toronto Press and McGill University Press, 1962, Pp. 933-936.

In a double-blind study, 0.07 mg LSD, 500 mg mescaline, 10 mg psilocybin or placebos were given to 18 college students. Nine

Behavioral Studies
Abstract 3144

"athletic type" (Type A) and 9 "asthetic" SEE ALSO: 2931,3104, 3180, 3181, 3186.
(Type B) had been selected through MMPI test-
ing. Before the ingestion of the drugs,
psychomotor tasks, learning and mental functioning tests, psychological observations,
measures of mood changes and changes in
anxiety levels, and the presence or absence
of somatic complaints were recorded. Two-
and-a-half hours after drug ingestion the
battery of 16 tests and psychiatric interviews were repeated. In general, psilocybin
tended to produce fewer and milder changes
than those of LSD or mescaline. Mescaline
produced the most marked alterations. The
reactions were a joint function of the drugs
administered and personality of the subject;
asthetic individuals showed predominantly
intellectual and mental alterations, while
athletic individuals responded with euphoria
and physiological changes.

Psychopharmacology Research Laboratory
Massachusetts Mental Health Research Corp.
Boston, Mass.

3144 Schachter, Stanley, & Wheeler, Ladd.
Epinephrine, chlorpromazine, and amusement.
Journal of Abnormal and Social Psychology,
1962, 65, 121-128.

In order to conceal the purpose of the study
and the nature of the injection, subjects
were told that injections related to the
effects of vitamin and vision. Fourteen odd
minutes of a slapstick comedy were shown to
male college students and evaluation made
as to how amusing the film was considered.
The 3 injections used were: epinephrine
0.5 cm of a 1:1000 solution s.c., 25 mg
chlorpromazine i.m. or placebo s.c. Physical
effects were also reported. Epinephrine
subjects were more amused than were placebo
subjects who, in turn, were more amused than
chlorpromazine subjects.

Columbia University
New York, N. Y.

3147 Gessa, G. L., Costa, E., Kuntsman, R., & Brodie, B. B. Evidence that the loss of brain catecholamine stores due to blockade of storage does not cause sedation. Life Sciences, 1962, 2, 441-452.

Levarterenol and 5HT were assayed in mice, rabbits and rats after various treatments with α-methyl-metatyrosine, (αMMT), α-methyl-metatyramine and α-methyl-β-hydroxyl-meta-tyramine. The injection of 100 mg/kg αMMT i.v. produced a small transient decline of 5HT and a complete depletion of levarterenol in brainstems of rabbits which lasted 11 days or more. Doses as low as 10 mg/kg almost completely depleted brain levarterenol stores without affecting those of 5HT. None of the animals showed sedation. The action of αMMT was far less prolonged in mice than in rabbits. Measurements of αMMT amines in rat heart were made. The effects of αMMT and its metabolites on the heart provided confirming evidence against the view that levarterenol is displaced by αMMT-yramines. After hydroxy-MMTA, levarterenol (1 µg/g) is completely depleted when the level of αMMT-yramines is less than 0.05 µg. Inhibition of catecholamine storage by itself does not cause sedation.

Laboratory of Chemical Pharmacology
NIH
Bethesda, Maryland

3148 Gupta, S. S., Gupta, J. C., & Agarwala, V. Hepato-toxic effects of hydantoin derivatives used in epilepsy. Current Medical Practice, 1962, 6, 57-62.

Of 4 groups, of male rats, 1 received no drugs, 1 diphenylhydantoin, 1 phethenglate for 10 weeks. All drugs were administered intragastrically, 10 mg/kg. After sacrifice, liver secretions were fixed and studied for evidence of hepatotoxicity. Controls revealed no pathological changes. Diphenyl-hydantoin-treated animals showed definite areas of focal necrosis in 40%, although alleviation was marked in rats receiving concomitant high protein diets. Phethenglate produced patchy, centrilobular and hemorrhagic necrosis, which was again diminished with a high protein diet. Hepatic damage was observed in all animals treated with hydantoin derivatives. Hepatotoxic effects may be minimized, however, by concomitant administration of a high protein diet.

Gandhi Medical College
Bhopal, India

3149 Stern, Jack, & Ward, Arthur A., Jr.
Supraspinal and drug modulation of the alpha
motor system. Relation of supraspinal and
drug modulation to parkinsonism. Archives
of Neurology, 1962, 6, 404-414.

The modulating effects of supraspinal stimulation and drug administration (pentobarbital,
30 mg/kg, curare or atropine) on the alpha
fraction of the motor system were monitored
by monosynaptic testing in 49 cats. Facilitation of the alpha motor system is evoked by
stimulation of contralateral or homolateral
globus pallidus. Alpha facilitation evoked
by ventrolateral thalamic or pallidal stimulation is abolished or reversed by barbiturates. Chlorpromazine (1.5-5 mg/kg i.v.)
markedly augments alpha motor discharge in
intact alpha preparations.

Division of Neurosurgery
University of Washington School of Medicine
Seattle, Washington

3150 Zilberstein, R. Michel. Reserpine and
serotonin-estrogen interactions on the uterus
of the rat. Life Sciences, 1962, 2, 281-283.

Various doses of 5HT and reserpine were administered s.c. daily for 4 days to 24-25
day old Harvard rats and concomitantly they
received daily injections of 0.1 μg estradiol. Autopsy was performed 24 hours after
the last set of injections. Estrogen enhanced the effects of reserpine and 5HT. In
spite of the fact that food and water were
freely available the reserpine-treated group
suffered from inanition;   the heightened
response to estrogen may be due to the phenomenon described by Jailer (1948), i.e.,
to starvation-induced interference with the
normal hepatic detoxification of steroid
hormones. Increased sensitivity of the uterus of the estrogen-treated rat to 5HT and
heightened uterine response to estrogen in
the 5HT-treated animal were parallel.

RFD #2
Manchester, Connecticut

thidine, 89, 78 and 49. Sympathetic blocking agents were used and the experiment repeated. Guanethidine releases levarterenol
in sympathetic nerve endings by an action
which seems different from reserpine, acting
oppositely to bretylium and activates the
process involved in the normal release of
levarterenol by nerve impulses.

Laboratory of Chemical Pharmacology
National Heart Institute
NIH
Bethesda, Maryland

3153 Kreppel, E. Zur Differenzierung zwis-
chen zentraler und ganglionärer pharmako-
dynamischer Dämpfung des Sympathicus. [A
method for differentiation between central
and ganglionic pharmacodynamic inhibitors of
the sympathicus.] Medicina Experimentalis,
1962, 7, 223-231.

Spontaneous electrical activity was registered from the sympathetic fibers of the
hilus of the left kidney of anesthetized
cats. Both vagi had been cut and the carotid sinus eliminated. Narcotin (3 mg/kg i.v.)
and Phentanyl (10 mg/kg i.v.) produced reduction and cessation, respectively, of the
electrical activity. Activity reappeared
after asphyxia which stimulates central sympathetic centers. The electrical response
at the hilus seen after stimulation of the
brachial plexus was not affected by these
drugs, while ganglionic blocking agents a-
bolish spontaneous response as well as that
induced by asphyxia and plexus stimulation.

Pharmakologische Institut
Rheinische Friedrich Wilhelms-Universität
Bonn, Germany

3154 Kuhn, H. F., & Friebel, H. Die Ausscheidung von Codein und Codeinmetaboliten
im Harn codeingewöhnter Ratten und Meerschweinchen. [Urinary excretion of codeine and codeine metabolites of rats and guinea pigs
made tolerant to codeine.] Medicina Experimentalis 7, 1962, 255-261.

Rats and guinea pigs received codeine s.c.
1-3 times daily for 6-9 weeks in increasing
amounts, up to 3-5 times the LD 50. Free
and bound codeine, morphine, norcodeine and

normorphine were identified in the urine.
Amounts of codeine and codeine metabolites,
and the ratio freebound codeine were different in the 2 species. Amounts excreted were
dependent only on the administered dosage
and were not affected by the duration of treatment.

Pharmakologische Institut
Universität Bonn
Bonn, Germany

3155 Estler, C. J., Heim, F., & Strubelt,
O. Sauerstoffverbrauch, Körpertemperatur,
Futteraufnahme und Metabolitgehalt des Ge-
hirns weisser Mäuse nach Reserpin [Oxygen
and food consumption, body temperature, and
content of brain metabolites of white mice
after reserpine administration.] Medicina
Experimentalis, 1962, 6, 395-401.

Reserpine (1 μg/g/s.c.) administered to mice
maintained at 24°C reduced oxygen, food consumption and body temperature, while raising
the glycogen and ATP content of the brain.
It reduced brain phosphocreatine and coenzyme A levels but did not affect lactate and
ADP content. Most of these changes are
found more pronounced at 18°C.

Pharmakologische Institut
Universität Erlangen-Nürnberg
Erlangen, Germany

3156 Arora, R. B., Singh, M., & Kanta, Chan-
dra. Tranquilizing activity of jatamansone--
a sesquiterpene from Nardostachys jatamansi.
Life Sciences, 1962, 2, 225-228.

The i.p. injection of an alcoholic extract of
root and rhizomes of Nardostachys jatamansi
in mice showed demonstrable sedative action
at 40 mg/kg and above while the ID_{50} of this
extract was 975 mg/kg. The average fall in
mean rectal temperature of mice injected i.p.
with 10, 30, 100, 300, 1000 mg/kg of jatamansi was 1.5, 5.2, 6.3, 10.6 and 12.6°C respectively. For the study of hypnotic potentiation, 1, 3, 10, 30 and 100 mg/kg jatamansone
was injected i.p. into mice, followed by a
standard dose of 35 mg/kg pentobarbital i.p.
Maximal potentiation and hypnosis (assessed
by the righting reflex) was achieved when
35 mg/kg phentobarbital was given 3 hours

after 100 mg/kg jatamansone. Antiapomorphine effect was studied in dogs and 100 mg/kg jatamansone i.p. reduced emisis by 75%. Hostile monkeys were given 100 mg/kg jatamansone i.p., which provided a 75% reduction in excitement, defensive and aggressive hostilities, while sociability and contentment increased by 80%. The i.p. LD 50 in mice is 580 + 6 mg/kg.

Department of Pharmacology
All-India Institute of Medical Sciences
New Delhi 16, India

3157 Pittman, James A. Antithyroid activity of a tranquilizer. New England Journal of Medicine, 1962, 267, 861-864.

Amphenidone possessed antithyroid activity when administered in large doses (0.6 or 1% of the diet by weight) to rats. Goiters developed in the rats and accumulation of I^{131} in the thyroid gland was depressed. Its action is mediated by a block in the thyroidal organic binding of iodide similar to that induced by drugs such as thiourea. The discharge of thyroidal I^{131} in dogs showed that while it was more rapidly accumulated it was not retained and leaked out quickly so that the 24-hour uptake approximated 0. Radioiodide uptake in 7 psychiatric patients after a single dose of 1200 mg showed no change in thyroidal function.

VA Hospital
Birmingham, Alabama

3158 Roath, S., Elves, M. W., & Israëls, M. C. G. Effect of thalidomide on leucocyte cultures. Lancet, 1962, No. 7250, 812-813.

Leukocytes from healthy individuals were treated in vitro as follows: controls, 50 µg/ml thalidomide, 25 µg/ml thalidomide, 150 µg/ml phenobarbital and 50 µg/ml glutethimide. Differential counts were made after 72 hours incubation. Inhibition of the cells was demonstrated only with thalidomide. Results support the suggestion of Hinter (1962) that thalidomide may be a potential antimitotic agent and also indicate that the effects of all new agents on normal cell cultures might be part of a screening program to which these drugs should be subjected.

as predominantly direct acting. 2) Tyramine-like amines were less effective after pre-treatment with reserpine; the maxima of their dose-response curves were depressed, and this reduction of their maximal response was correlated with the reduction of the response of the nictitating membrane to nerve stimulation. Therefore they may be regarded as predominantly indirect acting. 3) Pretreatment with reserpine shifted the dose-response curves of several amines to the right without affecting their maxima (ephedrine, m-tyramine, etc.). These amines have both direct and indirect actions, and seem to represent a gradual transition from the 1st to the 2nd group rather than a distinct 3rd group. Five pairs of meta-OH and para-OH analogues were studied; all 5 meta-OH compounds had more pronounced direct effects than the para-OH analogues. The position of the phenolic hydroxyl group is of greater importance and the presence or absence of the alcoholic hydroxyl group in the -position of less importance than hitherto assumed.

Department of Pharmacology
Harvard Medical School
Boston, Massachusetts

3161 Roos, Björn-Erik, & Werdinius, Bengt. Effect of reserpine on the level of 5-hydroxy-indoleacetic acid in brain. Life Sciences, 1962, 2, 105-107.

Reserpine (2-5 mg/kg) was injected i.v. into rabbits which were killed at 2-48-hour intervals. Analysis of 5HIAA was performed on 2 or 3 pooled brainstems; 5HT was also analyzed. Two hours after the injection of reserpine the value of 5HT in the brainstem had decreased 3% of the normal, while the corresponding value of 5HIAA had decreased 38% above normal. This high level was still found 12 hours after the injection, but after 24 hours the value of 5HIAA was again normal. The increase of 5HIAA values seems to reflect the release of 5HT induced by the drug.

Department of Pharmacology
University of Goteborg, Sweden

3162 Dereymaeker, A., Theenwissen-Lesuisse, F., Buu-Hoï, N.P., & Lapière, C. L'anoxie cérébrale expérimentale; effet protecteur des dérivés di l'acide p-chlorophénoxyacétique. [Experimental cerebral anoxia; protective effect of p-chlorophenoxyacetic acid derivatives.] Medicina Experimentalis, 1962, 239-244.

p-Chlorophenoxyacetic acid and 14 of its derivatives were tested for their efficacy in combating nitrogen-induced anoxia in rabbits. Nitrogen was introduced into a Plexiglas box at the rate of 5 liters/minute and the onset of anoxia measured by EEG. The effectiveness of the substances was measured by the activity quotient, i.e., the ratio of pre-and post--perfusion times before the onset of anoxia occurred. p-Chlorophenoxyacetic acid, its bromine and fluorine analogues, and the dimethylaminoethylester are equal to or more effective than the acid proper, while the remaining derivatives are inactive or toxic. Modification of respiratory rate does not occur with these compounds.

Institut de Neurologie
Université de Louvain
Louvain, France

3163 Lamarche, Guy, & Patoine, Jean-Guy. Propriétés convulsives du diéthylamide de l'acide vanillique. Note préliminaire. [Convulsive properties of vanillic acid diethylamide. Preliminary note.] Laval Médical, 1962, 33, 571-575.

Intract curarized cats and encéphale isolé preparations were used in the study of vanillic acid diethylamide (EEG & ECG; average convulsive dose 8 mg/kg up to 40 mg/kg). The compound has marked convulsive properties at doses lower than those usually used with pentetrazol. The convulsive dose varies from animal to animal. Vanillic acid diethylamide acts at all levels of the CNS and produces neuronal hypersynchrony in the brain. Predominance of action at any 1 level has not been demonstrated. Cortical convulsive crises resemble those of pentetrazol, however the frequency of discharges is usually lower.

Départment de Physiologie
Universite Laval
Québec, Canada

3164 Gordonoff, T. Über die analgetischen
Wirkungen von Monoaminoxydase-Hemmern. [On
the analgesic action of monoaminoxydase inhibitors.] Medicina Experimentalis, 1962, 7,
201-204.

Iproniazid, bromide, nialamide and phenelzine
were tested for their analgesic properties in
rabbits by the Gordonoff method (1962), and
in rats by the Wolff, Hardy and Goudell method. Doses were 25 mg/100 g iproniazide p.
o. (rats only) and 50 mg/kg p.o. for all 4
substances in the rabbit experiments. In addition rabbits also received 0.1 mg pyrido-
stigmine s.c. Analgesic effects were significant, especially in the rabbits. Under oral
administration, analgesia sets in after 20-
40 minutes and lasts for 100-120 minutes.
The analgesic effect is however too weak to
explain improvement noted in angina pectoris
patients when these drugs are administered
in terms of MAO activity, and is probably
due to psychopharmacologic action.

Laboratorium von Prof. Gordonoff
Medizinische Fakultät der Universität
Bern, Switzerland

3165 Gisset, G. W., & Lewis, G. P. A spectrum of pharmacological activity in some biologically active peptides. British Journal
of Pharmacology, 1962, 19, 168-182.

The actions of bradykinin, angiotension, oxytocin, vasopressin and substance P were examined on isolated smooth muscle preparations
and in vivo. Isolated rat uterus and guinea
pig ileum can be used to distinguish between
oxytocin and bradykinin, and isolated rat
colon and hen rectal cecum are almost specific test preparations for substance P.
All the peptides were active on peripheral
blood vessels, bradykinin, substance P and
oxytocin causing vasodilation and vasopressin and angiotensin vasoconstriction; bradykinin, substance P and angiotension also
caused an increase in capillary permeability
in guinea pigs. Only bradykinin and substance
P were active in low concentrations in producing pain when applied to an exposed blis-
ter base. These two peptides were also active in causing bronchoconstriction. Oxytocin and vasopressin were the only peptides which
have milk-ejecting (lactating guinea pig) and
antidiuretic activity (rat) which could be
dissociated from cardiovascular effects. A
possible function for substance P is based

on its vascular and permeability effects.

National Institute for Medical Research
Mill Hill
London N.W. 7
Great Britain

3166 Carissimi, M., Grasso, I., Grumelli,E.,
Milla, E., & Ravenna, F. Nuovi barbiturici
alogenati. [New halogenated barbiturates.]
Farmaco, 1962, 17, 390-413.

Two series of new barbiturate derivatives
have been prepared, whose general formula is:

When R is ethyl or allyl, X in the 4 position
can be any halogen, however in 2' and 3'
position X can only be chlorine. Acute toxicity
and hypnotic properties were studied in mice.
Halogen derivatives appeared to have a greater
muscle relaxing effect than the parent compounds and they show some effectiveness in
protection against electroshock convulsions.

Laboratori Richerche Maggioni & Co.
Milan, Italy

3167 Efron, D. H. Reserpine toxicity and
"nonspecific stress." Life Sciences, 1962,
2, 561-564.

Increased toxicity of reserpine in adrenalectomized rats is unrelated to the lack of a
pituitary-adrenocortical response and cannot be attributed to a "nonspecific stress."
Normal, adrenalectomized and hypophysectomized
male Sprague-Dawley rats were used and LD 50's
(mg/kg iv. reserpine) established at 26.4,
18.6 and 0.28 which indicate that the toxicity in adrenalectomized animals is about 100
times greater in intact animals, while in
hypophysectomized rats it is only about 1.4
times greater than in intact animals. Increase
reserpine toxicity in adrenalectomized rats is
related to the absolute lack of certain adrenal steroids which in some way may condition
the nervous system to the effect of the drug.

Laboratory of Chemical Pharmacology
National Heart Institute
Bethesda 14, Maryland

3168 George, Robert, Haslett, Wilford L, & Jenden, Donald J. The central action of a metabolite of tremorine. Life Sciences, 1962, 2, 361-363.

The central actions of oxotremorine are described following injection of 50-250 mg/kg into laboratory animals including chickens, pigeons, mice, rats, guinea pigs, rabbits, cats, dogs and monkeys. As it has a marked parasympathomimetic effect when administered alone, it was found desirable to premedicate the animals with methantheline or atropine methylbromide. Tremor, ataxia and spasticity always follows the administration of oxotremorine, which are immediate in mice, rats, and rabbits following i.v. injection. Cats and monkeys, in particular, become markedly excited, pacing, jumping and circling around. This is followed by a ragelike state lasting 20-40 minutes. When rage gradually subsides it is followed by a pronounced fear or withdrawal reaction. Some effects suggested the possibility of hallucinatoric experiences. Evidence for CNS action is obvious. Intraventricular injection of a small dose in rabbits produced pronounced tremor. Also transection of the spinal cord in rats at T6 or L1 abolished tremor only below the level of the section. Thirdly, ablation of the midbrain tegmentum prevents tremor in rats while removal of structures rostral to this area did not alter the normal response.

Department of Pharmacology
University of California Medical Center
  and Brain Research Institute
Los Angeles, California

3169 Scott, George T. Suppression of melancoyte dispersion in the frog by psychic energizers. Nature, 1962, 193, 552-554. Varying amounts of amphetamine and methylphenidate were injected i.p. into light-adapted frogs. The degree of melanocte exposure was observed microscopically in the web of the foot and a notation made according to the Hogben and Slome melanphore scale (1931). The percentage of pigment dispersion caused by the drugs was determined by comparison with controls. Similar experiments were carried out with MAO inhibitors (pheniprazine, phenelzine and iproniazid), as well as antidepressants (pipradol, isocarboxazid, nialamide and imipramine). Amphetamine is a potent dispersion suppressor.

Of the MAO inhibitors, pheniprazine was most active, phenelzine intermediate and iproniazid least active.

Department of Biology
Oberlin College
Oberlin, Ohio

3170 Day, M.D., & Rand, M. J. Antagonism of guanethidine by dexamphetamine and other related sympathomimetic amines. Journal of Pharmacy and Pharmacology, 1962, 541-549.

Chloralozed dogs and cats were injected or infused with drugs into a suitable vein. Sympathetic responses were elicited either directly, by stimulating the cervical sympathetic nerve and recording the contractions of the nictitating membrane, or reflexly, by bilateral occlusion of the carotid arteries or by electrical stimulation of the central end of a divided vagus nerve and recording the effects on blood pressure. Dexamphetamine and certain other reacting sympathomimetic amines prevent or reverse the sympathetic nerve blocking action of guanethidine. Levarterenol and dopamine do not antagonize the blocking action of guanethidine. The possession of a reliable and rapidly acting antagonist of bretylium and guanethidine such as dextroamphetamine may extend their use to patients with occlusive vascular disease in whom unpredictable falls in blood pressure are dangerous.

Department of Pharmacology
School of Pharmacy
University on London
Brunswick Square
London, W.C. 1, Great Britain

3171 Dobkin, Allen B., Israel, Jacob S., Criswick, V. Guy. Prolongation of thiopental anaesthesia with hydroxyzine, SA 97, thiethylperazine, and thioridazine. Canadian Anaestiological Society Journal, 1962, 9, 342-346.

Four series of crossover experiments were carried out on dogs to establish prolongation of thiopental induced sleep (20 mg/kg thiopental i.v., followed immediately by i.v. injection of the test drug). Percentage increases were: 5 mg/kg hydroxyzine plus 44%, 5 mg/kg SA 97 plus 50%, 0.5 mg/kg thiethylperazine plus 60% and 0.5 thioridazine plus 107%. Hydroxyzine caused prolongation of thiopental sleep but inconsistently, whereas the other 3 drugs invariably delayed recovery.

Department of Anesthesiology
Upstate Medical Center
Syracuse, N. Y.

3172 Perlès, R., & Benda, Ph. Pharmacologie de quelques γ butyrolactones a`action centrale. [The pharmacology of some γ-butyrolactones with central action.] In: Baruk, Henri, & Launay, Jacques [Eds.] Annales Moreau de Tours. Tome I. Mémoires récents sur la psychopharmacologie. --Annals of Moreau de Tours. Volume I. Current memories in psychopharmacology. Paris: Presses Universitaires de France, 1962. Pp. 374-378.

γ-Butyrolactone at 300-700 mg/kg i.p. causes sleep with loss of the righting reflex in rats for several hours. Onset of action is rapid, i.e., hypnotic effects noted at 10 minutes. At 300-600 mg/kg i.m. in pigeons loss of muscle tonus is noted at 1-3 minutes, lasting 1-2 hours. In rabbits ca. 500 mg/kg γ-butyrolactone i.v. causes an immediate hypnotic effect. Pharmacologic information is presented on α-bromobutyrolactone and 2-dichlorobutyrolactone. These compounds are readily water soluble and may be administered in the form of an emulsion. The action of α-hydroxy-ββ-dimethyl-γ-butyrolactone in pigeons, rabbits and rats (rat i.p. LD 50 700-1200 mg/kg) is discussed.

[No address]

3173 Ernst, A. M. Phenomena of the hypokinetic rigid type caused by O-methylation of copamine in the para-position. Nature, 1962, No. 4811, 178-179.

Carlsson (1958) showed that practically all dopamine in the mammalian brain is found in the caudate-and entiform nucleus and that reserpine depletes dopamine from the corpus striatum producing parkinsonism which can be counteracted by DOPA the precursor of dopamine. There is a striking similarity in the chemical structure of dopamine compared to bulbocapnine, papaverine and the drugs laudanosine and lauianine: For example,

lauianine in cats causes a hypokinetic rigid syndrome combined with tremors. Only 1 of the 2 OH groups of the dopamine-ring (I) were changed into OCH_3 groups, Moreover, mescaline (VI) with 3 OCH_3 groups causes a similar hypokinetic syndrome.

Pharmacological Institute
University of Utrecht
Utrecht, The Netherlands

3174 Palomo Salas, T. Études expérimentales et histopathologiques de l'imipramine. [Experimental and histopathologic studies of imipramine] In: Baruk, Henri, & Launay, Jacques [Eds.] Annales Moreau de Tours. Tome I. Mémoires récents sur la psychopharmacologie Annals of Moreau de Tours. Volume I. Current memories in psychopharmacology. Paris: Presses Universitaries de France, 1962. Pp. 148

Experimentation with fish, guinea pigs, pigeons, cats, mice, rabbits and monkeys was pursued on an acute or chronic basis using imipramin [dosage unspecified]. Pyridoxine neutralized spasms in fish and epileptiform crises in monkeys. Animals sacrificed after chronic intoxication showed diffuse cerebral lesions, including cortical and central nuclear sclerosis. These leisons were observed even in cases where clinical signs were not apparent. In contrast few or slight lesions were noted in a monkey killed in a major seizure by the acute injection of imipramine.

Société Moreau de Tours
Maison Nationale de Charenton
Paris, France

3175 Baruk, H., Launay, J., & Perlès, R. Expérimentation animale du G 22 355 (Imipramine) chez le singe. [Animal experimentation with G 22 355 (Imipramine) in the monkey. In: Baruk, Henri, & Launay, Jacques [Eds.] Annales Moreau de Tours. Tome I. Mémoires récents sur la psychopharmacologie. --Annals Moreau de Tours. Volume I. Current memories in psychopharmacology. Paris: Presses universitaires de France, 1962. Pp. 144-147.

Imipramine was used in increasing doses (7-40 mg/kg i.m.) in monkeys in order to study psychomotor behavior. Up to 30 mg/kg, a phase of excitation with hyperactivity and

occurred, while no neurological disturbances
of the extrapyramidal type were noted. With
the combination, imipramine's psychomotor
exciting properties were inhibited but its
extrapyramidal disorder-inducing faculties
were not affected by alimemazine. Psychomotor and neurological disturbances are unrelated phenomena.

Société Moreau de Tours
Maison Nationale de Charenton
Paris, France

3178 Schenker, Anne C., Schenker, Victor J.,
& Kissin, Benjamin. Aberrations in the pul-
monary respiratory pattern in alcoholics and
the acute effects of ethyl alcohol and chlor-
promazine upon such patterns. In: Cleghorn,
R. A., Moll, A. E., & Roberts, C. A. Third
World Congress of Psychiatry Proceedings.
Volume I. Toronto/Montreal: University of
Toronto Press and McGill University Press,
1962. Pp. 389-396.

In many alcoholics there is a consistent inability to complete expiratory excursions in
the manner requisite for an even baseline on
the spirogram. Spirograms were recorded on
101 male alcoholic patients, aged 20-56 years
and in 20 nonalcoholic subjects, aged 22-55
years. The alcoholic population was comprised
of 56 chronic alcoholic inpatients, 22 alcoholic outpatients and 23 abstainers who volun-
teered. In acute tests 1 mg/kg of absolute
alcohol was given p.o. and led to an apparent
alleviation of respiratory irregularity. Parallel tests were run with 4 patients using 25
mg chlorpromazine i.m. Analogously, improvement in respiratory irregularity occurred in
3 of these 4 patients. While there is no
evidence to indicate that respiratory irregularity is specific to alcoholism, the spirogram method described is suggested as a testing procedure for assay of drug effects.

Downstate Medical Center
Brooklyn, New York

3179 Stokes, Peter E., & Lasley, Betty.
Blood alcohol-kinetics in humans as influ-
enced by thyroid administration or by induced
changes in carbohydrate metabolism. In:
Cleghorn, R. A., Moll, A. E., & Roberts,
C. A. Third World Congress of Psychiatry

Proceedings. Volume I. Toronto/Montreal:
University of Toronto Press and McGill University Press, 1962. Pp. 385-389.

A series of 91 studies was performed on 26
patients selected from psychiatric wards.
Some were diagnosed as chronic alcoholics
while others had occasional excessive alcohol
ingestion associated with their mental problems. The effect of glucose, insulin and
thyroid analogues on blood alcohol disappearance curves were studied. Tests were performed in the fasting state starting in the
morning, once or twice a week. The effect of
insulin on blood alcohol levels in man is unpredictable, generally small and often absent. Hyper- or hypoglycemia increased blood
epinephrine or cortisone do not per se produce any effect on blood alcohol. Triiodothyronine and its propionic and acetic acid derivatives given in pharmacologic doses have
no significant effect on blood alcohol curves
under the controlled conditions of these
studies during the 4-6 hour periods of observation after their administration. There is
no striking reproductive clinical effect of
insulin, hyperglycemic or thyroid substances
on the return to sobriety in the intoxicated
persons studied.

Payne Whitney Psychiatric Clinic
New York, New York

3180 Werboff, Jack, & Gottlieb, Jacques S.
Behavioural effects of prenatal administra-
tion of psychotropic drugs. In: Cleghorn,
R. A., Moll, A. E., & Roberts, C. A. Third
World Congress of Psychiatry Proceedings.
Volume II. Toronto/Montreal University of
Toronto Press and McGill University Press,
1962, Pp. 921-924.

Reserpine, iproniazid, 5 HTP,
BAS and distilled water as a control were
administered i.p. during the 2nd trimester of
gestation from days 8 through 14 to rats. Prenatal treatment had no effect on measures
of motor maturation or learning ability. There
were changes or reduced weight gain, increased
activity and emotionality on the open field
test and increased susceptibility to audiogenic seizures (bell alone or pentetrazol and
bell). Apparently the psychotropic drugs altered the histochemical action of focalized
CNS areas (hypothalamus and reticular for-

mation) to produce a relatively long-lasting functional improvement or detrimental
change in behavior. Increased pharmacological technology will one day be able to produce psychotropic drugs with great specificity in site and mode of action so that we
might be able to control or improve intellectual or emotional patterns by alteration
of the prenatal environment.

Lafayette Clinic
Detroit, Michigan

3181 Heise, George A., & McConnell, Howard.
Differences between chlordiazepoxide-type
and chlorpromazine-type action in "trace"
avoidance. In: Cleghorn, R. A., Moll, A. E.,
& Roberts, C. A. Third World Congress of
Psychiatry Proceedings. Volume II. Toronto/
Montreal: University of Toronto Press and
McGill University Press, 1962. Pp. 917-921.

Chlordiazepoxide (i.p.), meprobamate (i.p.),
phenobarbital(s.c.) chlorpromazine (s.c.)
and pentobarbital (s.c.) were administered
to rats. Rats were trained to respond during the initial noise in "trace" classical
avoidance trials consisting of 3 events in
sequence: 5 seconds of noise, 5 seconds of
silence, 5 seconds of noise and shock (scare
boxes containing a lever, loud speaker and
a grid scrambler circuit for shocking--auto-
matic recording with an Esterline-Angus
Operations Recorder. The dose-response curve
and the dose ratios for failure to respond
during the 3 events in the trial differentiated between chlordiazepoxide-type compounds,
chlorpromazine-type compounds and hypnotics.
The distinctive action of chlordiazepoxide-
type compounds in trace classical avoidance
is interpreted as a shift in latency distribution rather than as a specific block
of a secondary CR. The chlordiazepoxide-
type compounds in trace avoidance produced
the effects reported for chlorpromazine-type
compounds in Maffi's (1959) secondary CR
situation, while chlorpromazine-type compound
in the secondary CR situation.

Hoffman-LaRoche, Inc.
Nutley, New Jersey

having an edemagenic effect on nerve cells
producing intense excitation and causing
plasma potassium loss. Chlorpromazine-imipramine was nontoxic, though the edemagenic
action of imipramine was still present.
Chlorpromazine lessened excitation due to
imipramine.

Clinica Psichiatrica dell'Università di Milano
Milan, Italy

3184 Sanz Gadea, R. Accion de la clorproma-
cina sobre la vitamina C en orina de rata y
cobaya. [Action of chlorpromazine on vitamin
C in the urine of the rat and guinea pig.]
Archivo Instituto Farmacologia Experimental,
1962, 26, 61-64.

Guinea pigs were given 300 mg/kg vitamin C/
day and rats 100 mg/kg/day along with chlorpromazine as follows: 5, 10 and 20 mg/kg/
day for guinea pigs and 3, 6 and 8 mg/kg/
day for rats. Only vitamin C was administered for the 1st 10 days followed by its
combination with chlorpromazine for the ensuing 10 days. In guinea pigs, chlorpromazine vitamin C excretion was reduced by 40,
46 and 77% in accordance with increasing
chlorpromazine dosage. The relevant figures
in rats were 21. 23 and 30%.

Instituto de Farmacologia Experimental
Madrid, Spain

3185 Baruk, H., Launay, J., Bergès, & Perlès,
R. Action expérimentale de la serotonine sur
le comportement psychomoteur du Singe. Antag-
onisme et synergie avec les neuroleptiques
et le L.S.D. 25. [Experimental action of
serotonin on the psychomotor behavior of the
monkey. Antagonism and synergism with neuroleptics and LSD 25.] In: Baruk, Henri, &
Launay, Jacques [Eds.] Annales Moreau de
Tours. Tome I. Memoires récents sur la psychopharmacologie.--Annals of Moreau de Tours.
Volume I. Current memoires in psychopharmacology. Paris: Presses Universitaires de
France, 1962. Pp. 275-290.

Intramuscular and i.p. doses of 5HT (5-1000
mg/kg) were used in monkeys. Also doses of
5HT were combined with chlorpromazine and
LSD. 5HT did not cause complete experimental
catatonia, but induced flaccidity and diminution of initiative in monkeys with exhibition
of inquietude, instability and pathetic

attitudes reminescent to phenomena observable in precatatonic periods. The combinations 5HT-chlorpromazine and 5HT-reserpine showed that 5HT inhibited chlorpromazine effects and increased reserpine effects. 5HT counteracted LSD psychomotor effects. Present knowledge still appears insufficient for proper elucidation of pathogenetic mechanisms of action in regard to these substances.

Société Moreau de Tours
Maison Nationale de Charenton
Paris, France

3186 Baruk, H., & Launay, J. Expérimentation psychopharmacologique de la chlordiazépoxide (R.O. 5-0690) chez le Singe. [Psychopharmacologic experimentation with chlordiazepoxide (RO 5-0690) in the monkey.] In: Baruk, Henri, & Launay, Jacques [Eds.] Annales Moreau de Tours. Tome I. Mémoires récents sur la psychopharmacologie. --Annals of Moreau de Tours. Volume I. Current memoires in psychopharmacology. Paris: Presses Universitaires de France, 1962, Pp. 256-259.

Progressive doses of chlordiazepoxide (20-100 mg/kg i.m.) were given to 5 monkeys. Sedative action with slowing of spontaneous activity and a tendency to immobility was noted without catalepsy at 20 mg/kg. Neurological difficulties with incoordination and marked drowsiness was noted at 50 mg/kg, and these manifestations were exaggerated at 75-100 mg/kg, e.g., incoordination in jumping. Chlordiazepoxide appeared only slightly toxic and interest was expressed in its suppression of aggressiveness and fear reactions.

Laboratoire de Psychopharmacologie Expérimentale
Etablissement National de Saint-Maurice
Saint-Maurice, France

3187 Bagdon, R. E. Experimental and clinical toxicology of Librium, a tranquilizing agent. In: Cleghorn, R. A., Moll, A. E., & Roberts, C. A. Third World Congress of Psychiatry Proceedings. Volume II. Toronto/Montreal: University of Toronto Press and McGill University Press, 1962. Pp. 915-917.

Chlordiazepoxide toxicity tests were conducted in rats, chickens, dogs (liver function tests), guinea pigs (copulatory reflex) and rabbits

(ovulation). Some rats received amounts 600 times the usual clinical daily dose of 0.5 mg/kg prescribed for man; in these measurements where rats received the drug continuously over the entire life span, chlordiazepoxide was revealed to be an innocuous substance. In dogs 20-60 mg/kg/day produced mild to moderate sedation and animals which received 80 mg/kg displayed gastrointestinal disturbances, some ataxia, and marked sedation and hypnosis for ca. 4-6 hours after each dose. Tests in rabbits and guinea pigs showed the compound devoid of endocrine influence. Additionally suicide attempts with amounts ranging to 1630 mg are reviewed; here toxic reactions were limited to slight ataxia and drowsiness.

Hoffman-LaRoche Inc.
Nutley, N. J.

3188 Schmidt, Joachim & Matthies, Hansjürgen. Über einen zentralen Serotonin-Noradrenalin-Antagonismus. [Central antagonism between serotonin and levarterenol.] Acta Biologica et Medica Germanica, 1961, 7, 107-109.

Experiments with mice showed that the marked potentiating effect on hexobarbital anesthesia (100 mg/kg i.p.) obtained when either 5HT (100nM) or levarterenol (50 nM) was injected into the forebrain alone was abolished and even reversed when the 2 drugs were injected together. Thus, the potentiating effect of 5HT could be reversed by 0.5 nM levarterenol, as well as by dopamine, while the potentiating effect of levarterenol was abolished by 40 nM 5HT. The analeptic effect of injections of 5HT into the hindbrain could also be abolished by simultaneous injection of levarterenol or dopamine, but the reverse in this case was not true.

Pharmakologische Institut
Medizinische Akademie Magdeburg
Magdeburg, Germany

3189 Mouquin, M., & Milovanovich, J. B. Contribution a l'étude clinique et expérimentale en cardiologie de la nialamide ou (pyridinyl 4) 1-phenyl 8-dioxo 1, 6-triaza 2, 3, 7-octane. [Clinical and experimental use of nialamide (pyridinyl-4) 1-phenyl-8-dioxo-1, 6-triaza-2, 3, 7-octane) in cardiology.] Presse Médicale, 1962, 70, 1189-1192.

Nialamide action was investigation on isolated rabbit ventricles and guinea pig hearts. At concentrations of 10-50 mg/100 cc of the perfusion liquid, it has a negative inotropic and chronotropic action, and at sufficiently high concentrations (200 mg/100 cc) will cause complete stoppage. Epinephrine is antagonistic to this action. Of 127 cases of coronary angina treated with nialamide, an attenuation of the spasms up to the point where the patients were able to resume light work was recorded in 103 cases, failure was noted in 16; 3 had died because of infarcts and 5 other infarct patients were saved. Side effects include abdominal distension, postprandial tachycardia, paroxysmal tachycardias and constipation all requiring use of adjunct drugs. Tolerance was good; only 2 cases reacted unfavorably to the dose used.

Hôpital Broussais-La Charité
Paris 14, France

3190 Türker, Kazim, & Akcasu, Alaeddin. The effect of morphine on 5HT content of cat's brain. New Istanbul Contribution to Clinical Science, 1962, 5, 89-97.

The 5HT level in cat brain is 2.63 to 0.553 γ/g in the diencephalon and 0.8 to 0.55 γ/g in the frontal lobes. Morphine (1-6 mg/kg s.c.) induced 5HT depletion in the frontal lobes and, to a lesser extent, in the diencephalon. With 1 mg/kg morphine, a sharp decrease in 5HT level was evident, whereas less depletion occurred with 3-6 mg/kg doses. Diencephalon 5HT levels were 1/3 that in normal preparations 24 hours after morphine administration, whereas frontal lobe levels were approximately normal. No linear relationship was observed between dose and depletion. No direct correlation could be determined between morphine effects and 5HT level.

Department of Pharmacology and Therapeutic Clinic
University of Istanbul
Istanbul, Turkey

3191 Baruk, H., & Launay, J. Expérimentation psychopharmacologique animale du S. 1544 (phénelzine). [Animal psychopharmacologic experimentation with S 1544 (phenelzine).] In: Baruk, Henri, & Launay, Jacques [Eds.] Annales Moreau de Tours. Tome I. Mémoires récents sur la psychopharmacologie. --Annals of Moreau de Tours. Volume I. Current memoirs in psychopharmacology. Paris: Presses Universitaires de France, 1962. Pp. 229-233.

The pharmacology of phenelzine in dogs, cats and particularly monkeys, guinea pigs, mice and pigeons is outlined. Psychomotor excitation with hyperactivity and hypersensitivity to stimuli is evident at low doses (10-120 mg/kg). In mice the i.p. ID_{50} is 168 mg/kg compared to an oral ID_{50} of 156 mg/kg. At high doses hypotonia, motor incoordination and ataxia are evident sometimes associated with generalized epileptic crises. It is less epileptogenic than imipramine.

Société Moreau de Tours
Maison Nationale de Charenton
Paris, France

SEE ALSO 2909, 2910, 2911, 2912, 2913, 2914, 2922, 2929, 2930, 2953, 3038, 3081, 3136, 3141

3192 Gessa, G. L., Costa, E., Kuntzman, R., & Brodie, B. B. On the mechanism of norepinephrine release by α-methyl-metatyrosine. Life Sciences, 1962, 2, 353-360.

Various test substances were injected i.p. or i.v. into Sprague Dawley rats and levarterenol (norepinephrine) levels were determined according to Shore & Olin (1958). After injection of 400 mg/kg α-methyl-metatyrosine (αMMT), the stores of levarterenol in brain and heart depleted for a period of more than 24 hours. αMMT reached a peak in the brain within 1 hour and thereafter its level fell rapidly so that in 5 hours it was no longer detectable. To determine the part played by αMMT in releasing levarterenol, rats were pretreated with the decarboxylase inhibitors, NSD 1034 or NSD 1024 and then injected with αMMT. After this pretreatment, αMMT is not converted to the corresponding amine and does not release levarterenol in heart and brain. αMMT acts only through the decarboxylation product.

Laboratory of Chemical Pharmacology
National Heart Institute
Bethesda, Maryland

3193 Brodie, B. B., Kuntzman, R., Hirsch, C. W., & Costa, E. Effects of decarboxylase inhibition on the biosynthesis of brain monoamines. Life Sciences, 1962, 2, 81-84.

Even after 5HTP/DOPA decarboxylase in brain is almost completely blocked, 5HT and dopamine are still formed. Therefore, inhibition of this enzyme does not seem to offer a promising approach in the search for agents that block the formation of monoamines. Male NIH general-purpose mice were treated with N-(3-hydroxybenzyl)-N-methylhydrazine (NSD 1034) injected into the tail vein (6.25-200 mg/kg). To block MAO, the inhibitor N-methyl-N-benzylpropynylamine was injected i.p. in doses of 100 mg/kg. Doses of NSD 1034 (6.25-mg/kg) which inhibited decarboxylase by 75% had no effect on the rise of 5 HT and dopamine after blockade of MAO; with doses that blocked the enzyme almost completely, the levels of 5 HT and dopamine still rose by 50%.

Laboratory of Chemical Pharmacology
National Heart Institute
Bethesda, Md.

3194 Street, Harold V. The rapid separation of drugs and poisons by high temperature reversed phase paper chromatography. 2. Phenothiazine tranquillizers and imipramine. Acta Pharmacologica et Toxicologica, 1962, 19, 312-324.

Rapid separation of 8 phenothiazine tranquilizers and imipramine occurs during reversed-phase chromatography with aqueous solvents on ester-impregnated paper at temperatures between 85-95°C. The effects of R_f values of a) type and amount of ester, b) pH and concentration of solvent and c) different temperatures have been studied. A modified Marquis reagent and other developing reagents containing concentrated sulphuric acid are described for direct use on the ester-impregnated paper. Time required for ascending chromatography is 20 minutes and for circular chromatography 40 minutes. Blood and urine extracts were sampled.

Department of Forensic Medicine
University of Edinburgh
Edinburgh, Scotland

3195 Berry, Helen K. Use of micromethod for phenylalanine in management of phenylketonuric patients. Clinical Chemistry, 1962, 8, 172-173.

Blood is collected in capillary tubes and sealed. The tubes are centrifuged and then the sera from several tubes combined. In a small conical test tube, 0.20 ml 95% ethanol is added to 0.050 ml serum (or plasma) to precipitate protein. The supernatant is drawn into a 50-μl pipet and carefully applied to filter paper. Quantitative estimations of phenylalanine in serum can be made by comparing the density of ninhydrin color obtained (solvent butanol-ethanol-water;

70-20-20) with known amounts of phenylalanine. The sera from normal and phenylketonuric individuals can be differentiated visually.

Children's Hospital Research Foundation
Cincinnati 29, Ohio

3196 Horita, A., & Weber, L. J. Dephosphorylation of psilocybin in the intact mouse. Toxicology and Applied Pharmacology, 1962, 4, 730-737.

Male mice were injected i.p. with 100 mg/kg psilocybin or 72 mg/kg psilocin (equimolar amounts- 0.35 mM/kg). The administration of psilocybin results in the accumulation of its 4-hydroxy analogue, psilocin in the kidney, liver and brain. Highest concentrations in kidney and liver were found within 10 - 20 minutes and brain levels reached a peak at 25-30 minutes after administration of psilocybin. Behavioral effects, characterized by piloerection, exophthalmos and motor incoordination, closely followed the increase in brain levels of psilocin. In mice pretreated with large doses of sodium β-glycerophosphate, a substrate of alkaline phosphatase, the administration of psilocybin resulted in much lower increases of tissue psilocin levels and behavioral effects were attenuated. The accumulation of tissue psilocin after administration of psilocin did not differ significantly in control or β-glycerophosphate-pretreated mice. Correspondingly, no difference in intensity of behavioral effects was noted. Evidence is presented for the rapid dephosphorization of psilocybin in the intact mouse and its CNS effects are exerted only after its transformation to its analogue psilocin.

Department of Pharmacology
School of Medicine
University of Washington
Seattle, Wash.

3197 Wilson, Irwin, B., & Alexander, J. Acetylcholinesterase: reversible inhibitors, substrate inhibition. Journal of Biological Chemistry, 1962, 237, 1323-1326.

Kinetic measurements show that reversible inhibitors of acetylcholinesterase have a noncompetitive component. The correct explanation of substrate inhibition is that the dealkalation of the acetyl enzyme is prevented by a binding of a molecule of acetylcholine. These findings are consistent with deduction arising from the intermediate formation of an acetyl enzyme in enzymic hydrolysis, as it should be possible to inhibit the dealkalation and this introduces the non-competitive component. Reversible inhibitors are shown to inhibit the hydrolysis of methylcarbamyl enzymes, a reaction analogous to the hydrolysis of acetyl enzyme. Acetylcholine inhibits the hydrolysis of the methylcarbamyl enzyme and, therefore, would be expected to inhibit the hydrolysis of the acetyl enzyme. This would produce substrate inhibition.

Department of Neurology
College of Physicians and Surgeons
Columbia University
New York, N.Y.

3198 Huszak, I., & Durko, I. The metabolism of the indole compounds in schizophrenia. In: Cleghorn, R. A., & Roberts, C. A. Third World Congress of Psychiatry Proceedings. Volume I. Toronto/Montreal: University of Toronto Press and McGill University Press, 1962. Pp. 674-676.

The urinary excretion of 5HIAA by schizophrenic patients and normal subjects using the colorimetric method of Udenfriend et al. (1955) was studied with and without tryptophan loads. When tryptophan loads were applied the number of chromatographic spots did not increase in either schizophrenics or controls and the 5HIAA spot did not enlarge. However in controls the spots corresponding to indoleacetic acid (not 5HIAA) got larger on the days when tryptophan loading was applied, while in the schizophrenics the tryptophan load scarcely influenced the indoleacetic acid excretion. In about 2/3rds of the urines from schizophrenics, a moderately intense pink spot could be detected at 0.07-0.10 Rf values with Ehrlich reagent which was soluble in ethanol and not observed in the controls. The spectrum of this material was found between 210-220 mμ with a maximum at about 205 mμ, which suggests an indole compound.

[No address]

3199 Jackim, Eugene, & Wortis, Joseph.
Metabolic abnormalities in mongolism: respi-
ratory activity and triiodothyronine uptake
of erythrocytes. In: Cleghorn, R.A., Moll, A.E.,
& Roberts, C.A. Third World Congress of Psy-
chiatry Proceedings. Volume I. Toronto/
Montreal: University of Toronto Press and
McGill University Press, 1962. Pp. 667-670.

Mongoloid erythrocytes tended to show high
oxygen-sugar uptake values as measured manometrically; they also showed a slightly increased lactic acid output and a reduced ability to convert inorganic phosphorus to organic
phosphate. The mean phosphorylation-oxidation
ratio in mongoloids was 0.077 compared with
0.131 in normal controls. Standard radio-
iodated triiodothyronine was used in the in
vitro REC uptake test of Hamolsky, Golodetz
and Freedberg (1957). Twenty-three control
individuals and 22 mongoloids were used as
erythrocyte donors. Triiodothyronine uptake
increase was consistent and significant for
the mongoloids. The mean for the control
groups was 50.4 while for the mongoloid group
22.9. Qualitatively both the mongoloid and
control sera appeared to bind thyroxine in
both the albumin and globulin fractions. Increased triiodothyronine uptake by mongoloid
erythrocytes probably is due to an abnormality
in serum fraction that binds thyroid hormone
and not to the erythrocytes per se. The test
is based on a competitive uptake of triiodothyronine between several serum proteins and
the erythrocytes. Electrophoresis did not
show either a quantitative or a qualitative
abnormality in 1 or more of the mongoloid serum fractions.

Jewish Hospital of Brooklyn
Brooklyn, N. Y.

3200 Haddad, R. K., & Rabe, Ausma. An ana-
phylactic test for abnormal antigen(s) in
schizophrenics' serum. In: Cleghorn, R.A., Moll,
A.E., & Roberts, C.A. Third World Congress of
Psychiatry Proceedings. Volume I. Toronto/
Montreal: University of Toronto Press and
McGill University Press, 1962. Pp. 658-661.

Malis and Rybas (1959) reported an abnormal
factor in the serum of chronic schizophrenics
discovered through challenge to sensitized
guinea pigs. This report corroborates their
work. The volume, route and time sequence of

glycoprotein content of the CSF dropped. Whether the accumulation of hexoses and hexosamine precursors bound to protein with a failure of accumulation of neuraminic acid (derivative) represents some form of enzymatic block in biosynthesis, and whether the correlation of this disturbance might be accompanied by clinical improvement is a question for further study.

Neurochemical Research Laboratory
Department of Psychiatry
Harvard Medical School
Cambridge, Mass.

3202 Heath, Robert G., Leach, Byron E., & Byers, Lawrence W. Taraxein: recent developments in processing and identification. In: Cleghorn, R. A., Moll, A. E., & Roberts, C. A. Third World Congress of Psychiatry Proceedings. Volume I. Toronto/Montreal: University of Toronto Press and McGill University Press, 1962, Pp. 619-624.

Three possible compounds are referred to: taraxein, a small molecule, taraxein binding protein (TAR B.P.) and taraxeinogen, a small molecule plus a protein. Standard assay was made with rhesus monkeys prepared with chronically implanted electrodes in subcortical structures. The fraction tested is rapidly injected i.v. into the monkey. If the fraction contains taraxein, the monkey developed catatonia and typical EEG changes, unlike the shocklike reaction with stupor waves seen on the injection of either normal or schizophrenic serum. Fractionation of taraxeinogen (protein) included chloroform-alcohol extraction, chloroform-alcohol followed by DEAE cellulose chromatography, DEAE cellulose batch and chromatographic column, batch DEAE cellulose treatment followed by extraction with various phosphate buffers and phosphate buffer fractionation. Fractionation for taraxein (small molecule) involved the following 5 variations: serum pretreated at pH 2 and precipitated with alcohol; serum pretreated at pH 2, incubated with trypsin for 2 minutes followed by alcohol precipitation; pretreated serum at pH 2 and incubated with trypsin for 20 minutes; pretreated serum at pH 2, incubated with trypsin for 3 minutes followed by Retardion column, and pretreated serum at pH 2, incubation with trypsin for 20 minutes followed by Retardion column.

Views are presented on the relation between the protein molecule and the small molecular substance as they relate to the fluctuating symptomatology of schizophrenia.

Tulane University School of Medicine
New Orleans, La.

3203 Fischer, Roland & Griffin, Frances. Biochemical-genetic factors of taste-polymorphism and their relation to salivary thyroid metabolism in health and mental retardation. In: Cleghorn, R. A., Moll, A. E., & Roberts, C. A. Third World Congress of Psychiatry Proceedings. Volume I. Toronto/Montreal: University of Toronto Press and McGill University Press, 1962. Pp. 542-547.

The distributions of quinine and 6-n-propylthiouracil taste-thresholds for 37 parents of mongoloids and 48 normal subjects were established. At least one of the parents in each couple or, in twelve out of eighteen pairs of parents of mongoloids, both parents are very high quinine tasters.

Colombus Psychiatric Institute and Hospital
Colombus, Ohio

3204 Smith, W. James, & Kirshner, Norman. Mechanism of 3,4-dihydroxyphenylethylamine-α-hydroxylase. Journal of Biological Chemistry, 1962, 237, 1890-1891.

3,4-Dihydroxyphenylethylamine-β-C^{14}, H^3 was converted to levarterenol α-C^{14}, H^3 by beef adrenal chromaffin granules and by an enzyme isolated from the banana plant (dopamine hydroxylase). The H^3:C^{14} ratio of the isolated 3,4-dihydroxyphenlethylamine indicating that an α,β-dehydrogenation-hydration mechanism is not involved in the conversion of 3,4-dihydroxyphenylethylamine to levarterenol.

Department of Biochemistry
Duke University Medical Center
Durham, N. C.

3205 Gyermek, Laszlo, & Bindler, Elliot.
Action of indole alkylamines and amidines on
the inferior mesenteric ganglion of the cat.
Journal of Pharmacology and Experimental
Therapeutics, 1962, 138, 159-164.

Several indole compounds related to 5HT were
found to have marked action on the inferior
mesenteric ganglia of the cat. Methylation
of the terminal N atom of 5HT maintained or
increased ganglionic stimulation dependent
upon the number of methyl substituents. N-
Dimethylation of tryptamine definitely increased ganglionic stimulant potency as compared to the weak activity of tryptamine.
The stimulant action of some of the N methylated compounds (bufotenidine, N,N,N-tri-
methyltryptamine) was, however, not 5HT-like,
but rather of the cholinergic type. N,N-
Diethyl and di-n-propyl derivatives of tryptamine and N,N-dipropyl 5HT were considerably
weaker than the corresponding N,N-dimethyl
compounds. Methylation of the 5OH group of
5HT or altering its ethylamine chain by methyl substitution, or both, brought about marked
loss of ganglionic stimulant and blocking
potencies. 4- and 6-hydroxy indole alkylamines were inactive on the inferior mesenteric ganglion as compared to 5HT and bufo-
tenine. Introduction of an amidine group in
the molecules of tryptamine and 5HT resulted
in compounds which primarily blocked the action of 5HT. Marked divergence between the
ganglionic and smooth muscle stimulant actions
of these agents was demonstrated.

Geigy Research Laboratories
Ardsley, N. Y.

3206 Koella, Werner P., & Schaeppi, Ulrich.
The reaction of the isolated cat iris to
serotonin. Journal of Pharmacology and Experimental Therapeutics, 1962, 138, 154-158.

The effect of 5HT (serotonin) and a number
of other substances was tested on the isolated intact cat iris and on the isolated
iris sphincter and dilator muscle. The reaction of the pupillary opening on the intact
iris was recorded by means of a photoelectric
technique. The reaction of the isolated
muscles was measured by means of ("isometric")
mechanoelectric transducers. The isolated
iris reacted to 5HT with miosis. Concentrations of 0.3 μg/ml of Ringer solution were
effective. The pupillary constriction and
ensuing dilation lasted up to 15 or more minutes. Two-peak patterns occurred often with
larger doses. 5HT treatment desensitized
the preparation to later injections of 5HT.
The isolated constrictor muscle reacted to
5HT with contraction and the dilator strip,
with relaxation often followed by contraction
when larger doses were used. Epinephrine
and levarterenol induced dilation of the pupil. Levarterenol led to contraction of the
dilator muscle. Atropine had only small influence on 5HT reactions but in moderate
doses eliminated acetylcholine effects on
the intact iris and the constrictor muscle
completely.

Laboratory of Neurophysiology
Worcester Foundation for Experimental
  Biology
Shrewsbury, Mass.

3207 Abbs, E. T. The acute sensitization
of tissues by choline 2,6-xylyl ether (TM 10),
bretylium and guanethidine. Life Sciences,
1962, 2, 99-103.

The effect of TM 10 (the bromide), bretylium
tosylate and guanethidine as well as epinephrine and levarterenol were studied in vitro
on O-methyl transferase derived from rat and
cat livers. Supernatants containing both
O-methyl transferase and a methionine-activat-
ing enzyme were prepared. Concentrations of
test drugs varied from 25 g/ml to 1.25 mg/ml.
Recovery of synthetic metanephrine added to
incubation mixtures containing inactivated
enzyme varied from 46.5 - 57%, but was constant in any one experiment. Pyrogallol was
used as a reference substance. TM 10 (choline
2: 6-xylyl ether bromide), bretylium tosylate,
guanethidine sulphate have been shown to have
no significant effect in vitro on the activity of COMT from rat and cat liver, using
epinephrine and levarterenol as substrates.
The sensitization to epinephrine and levarterenol which these drugs produce in vivo
is unlikely to be due to inhibition of the
biotransformation of the amines by O-methyl
transferase.

Department of Pharmacology
University of Leeds
Leeds, Great Britain

3208 Gheorghiu, P., Schwartz, Rita, Stroescu, V., & Popescu, E. Influentarea compozitiei proteice a creierului prin clorpromazină. [The influence of chlorpromazine on the protein composition of the brain.] Studii si Cercetari Fiziologe, 1962, 7, 361-366.

Rats were treated with 1-50 mg/kg chlorpromazine s.c. for 15 days and sacrificed. Trichloracetic acid precipitates of brain tissue were hydrolized and the amino acids analyzed, using descending paper chromatography (ninhydrin). Chlorpromazine induced an increase in the amounts of glutamic acid and alanine. In view of the importance of glutamine and GABA, it is possible that at the central action of chlorpromazine is related to an increase in the amount of glutamic acid available in the brain.

Institutul de Fiziolojie Normalai si
    Patolojica "D. Danielopolu"
Academiei R. P. R.
Bucharest, Romania

3209 Whittaker, V. P. Sub-cellular distribution of 5-hydroxytryptamine in guinea pig brain. Nature, 1962, 195, 1100.

5HT in guinea pig brain is localized in the presynaptic vesicle containing nerve-ending fraction, and the dense type of storage particle found in the duodenum does not occur in this brain. These conclusions were reached by Whittaker in 1959, but disputed by Inouye, Kataoka and Shinagawa (1962). The latter workers inferred that previous 5HT assays had been interfered with by substance P. However, substance P was probably present at the low threshold concentrations, is relatively inactive with rat fundus strip, and the work has been corroborated by Baker (1959) and others.

Biochemistry Department
Agricultural Research Council
Institute of Animal Physiology
Babraham College
Cambridge, Great Britain

3210 Briseid Jensen, Kjell, & Vennerőd, Anne Marie. Pharmacological and chromatographic differentiation between a secondary kinin from human urine and brandykinin. Acta Pharmacologica et Toxicologica, 1962, 19, 337-334.

Biological effects of urinary kinin and bradykinin were studied on stimulation of the isolated rat uterus, isolated guinea pig uterus, relaxation of isolated rat duodenum and rat blood depressor effect. Chromatographic study of urines was made using the method of Briseid, Jensen & Vennerőd (1962) and a secondary kinin not identical to brandykinin was demonstrated. Rat uterus, guinea pig ileum, or rat blood pressure tests distinguished between the substances, but parallel assays with rat uterus and rat duodenum failed to discriminate.

Biological Department
Pharmaceutical Institute
University of Oslo
Oslo, Norway

3211 Creveling, Cyrus R., Daly, John W., Witkop, Bernhard, & Udenfriend, Sidney. Substrates and inhibitors of dopamine-β-oxidase. Biochimica et Biophysica Acta, 1962, 64, 125-134.

Dopamine-β-oxidase not only affects the hydroxylation of dopamine to levarterenol, but accepts as substrates a wide variety of phenethylamine derivatives such as epinine, m-tyramine and their branched -methyl derivatives, m-methoxytyramine, which is converted to normetanephrine, 3,5-dimethoxytyramine, and to some extent even mescaline. The fact that many well-known sympathomimetic drugs are good substrates for the enzyme raises the possibility that compounds such as amphetamine, paredrinol, paradrine and α-methyl-m-tyramine owe some of their activity to the corresponding metabolites which are all derivatives of ephedrine. The nonspecificity of dopamine-β-oxidase prompted a search for competitive or specific inhibitors. Benzylhydrazine, isosteric with phenethylamine, inhibited the enzyme strongly at concentrations of 10^{-5}M.

NIH
Bethesda, Md.

3212 Suwa, N., Yamashita, I., Ishikane, M., Owada, H., Shinohara, S., & Nakazawa, A. Fluctuations of the autonomic and endocrine functions in mental disorders. In: Cleghorn, R. A., Moll, A. E., & Roberts, C. A. Third World Congress of Psychiatry Proceedings. Volume II. Toronto/Montreal: University of Toronto Press and McGill University Press, 1962. Pp. 839-841.

Day by day estimations of some indices of autonomic and endocrine functions were made on about 50 mixed patients for several weeks to 6 months. BMR, adrenocortical function (circulating eosinophils, urinary 17-ketosteroids, 17-hydroxy-ketosteroids and uropepsin), gonadal function indicated by estrogen and pregnandiol were estimated. Seven case histories are given. Conclusions drawn were: changes in autonomic and endocrine functions are not strictly parallel to emotional changes, but are related; changes in these indices are not specifically related to a disease entity; these biological changes represent attempts at maintaining homeostasis; when homeostasis cannot be preserved as in deteriorated schizophrenics, fluctuations in this function are extreme, and longitudinal observation will aid in integrating contradictory results so far reported by those investigators holding different viewpoints.

Hokkaido, Japan

3213 Kaelbling, Rudolf, Craig, James B., & Passamanick, Benjamin. The association of hepatic porphyria with mental illness -- the screening of 2,500 psychiatric patients for urinary porphobilinogen. In: Cleghorn, R.A., Moll, A. E., & Roberts, C. A. Third World Congress of Psychiatry Proceedings. Volume I. Toronto/Montreal: University of Toronto Press and McGill University Press, 1962. Pp. 624-630.

This study was performed in a 125-bed intensive-treatment hospital. During a 46-month period the Watson-Schwartz test was performed on 2,126 consecutive admissions. Repeat Watson-Schwartz tests were made routinely on readmission of former patients. Of the total 2,500 psychiatric patients examined for porphobilinogenuria, 626 were readmissions. Porphobilinogenuria was considered to mean that Ehrlich-aldehyde reacting substances were found in the urine of all probands and the purple color which was developed was assumed but not proven due to porphobilinogen. Only 12 of the 35 probands had a clinical picture of acute intermittent porphyria. Nine more were considered to have latent porphyria, 13 secondary porphobilinogenuria and 1 mixed porphyria. Rates of selected clinical manifestations found in probands and controls as well as exposure to possible precipitating factors with comparisons of probands and controls was made. Possible precipitating agents were: chronic alcoholism, addiction to barbiturates, addiction to narcotics, sulfonamid treatments and estrogen treatments. Routine Watson-Schwartz test for all psychiatric patients is advocated.

Tulane University School of Medicine
New Orleans, La.

3214 Jensen, Knud, & Osterman, Einar. Glutamic-oxalacetic transaminase in cerebrospinal fluid in patients with cerebral atrophy. In: Cleghorn, R. A., Moll, A. E., & Roberts, C. A. Third World Congress of Psychiatry Proceedings. Volume I. Toronto/Montreal: University of Toronto Press and McGill University Press, 1962. Pp. 607-609.

Fifty controls and 46 patients, including 34 cases of presenile dementia and others (e.g., manic-depressive psychosis and schizophrenia), were tested for GOT content in the CSF. In the 34 cases of presenile dementia the average age was 59.4 years. The duration of the disease was 1-12 years. In 44 cases, cerebral apathy was demonstrated by pneumoencephalography and in 2 cases by autopsy. In cerebral atrophy, the value in Karmen Units was 11.7, s=3.56. In 1 patient an increased GOT content in the CSF was noted while no pneumoencephalographic alterations indicating cerebral atrophy were found. However, when pneumoencephalography was repeated after a 1/2 year, signs of central atrophy were found. In the diagnosis of cerebral atrophy, the determination of CSF GOT content is a valuable aid.

State Mental Hospital
Risskov, Denmark

3215 Yamashita, M. Histopathological stud-
ies of the brain tissues of four patients of
alcohol delirium. In: Cleghorn, R. A.,
Moll, A. E., & Roberts, C. A. Third World
Congress of Psychiatry Proceedings. Volume
I. Toronto/Montreal: University of Toronto
Press and McGill University Press, 1962.
Pp. 396-398.

Histopathologic signs in 4 patients (alcoholic delirium) were relatively acute changes
in the diencephalon and the mesencephalon.
Examination of blood vessels, especially
capillaries and precapillaries revealed endothelial hypertrophy. Neuronophagia, small
necrotic lesions and changes in blood vessels
in the thalamus, hypothalamus, central nucleus, semilunar nucleus, periventricular
gray matter, mammillary body, quadrigeminal
bodies and reticular nucleus are evident.
The pathogenesis of delirium is considered
due to indirect and relatively acute malnu-
trition and circulatory disturbance in the
cerebral blood vessels in chronic alcoholism.
Hallucinations in alcoholic delirium is ele-
mentary, simple, real and sensory, and shows
diencephalic microorganic characteristics.
This type of hallucination is termed diencephalic hallucination.

Osaka Kaisei Hospital
Kitakti, Osaka
Japan

3216 Kinross-Wright, John, & Ragland, James
B. Clinical pharmacology of some newer phe-
nothiazine analogues. In: Cleghorn, R. A.,
Moll, A. E., & Roberts, C. A. Third World
Congress of Psychiatry Procsedings. Volume
II. Toronto/Montreal: University of Toronto
Press and McGill University Press, 1962.
Pp. 901-905.

Determination of blood drug levels with
tranquilizers should offer at least some
help in evaluating their relative merits.
Endeavor in this area has been relatively
unrewarding and possibly current studies at
the cellular level will be more rewarding.
Notes are presented on 4 psychochemical
series: phenothiazines, iminodibenzyls,
thioxanthenes and dibenzocycloheptanes.
Imipramine, chlorprothixene, TX 35, amitriptyline, cyclobenzaprine, cyproheptadine and
other agents are discussed. A method for

the determination of phenothiazines based
on fluorescence when the compounds are oxidized in acetic acid is described. Fluorescence measurements are made in a spectrophotofluorometer following basic extraction
of the drugs from blood or other samples
with heptane, which is then extracted with
acetic acid; this allows determination of
blood concentrations down to ca.1 $\mu g/ml$ whole
blood, and sometimes even lower concentrations, e.g., 0.05 $\mu g/ml$ blood thioridazine.
All work in this area indicates that blood
levels in no way reflect tissue concentrations which are of paramount importance in
evaluation. In rats, tissue levels of thioridazine, trifluoperazine and chlorpromazine
after i.p. injection lead to the following:
1) all 3 drugs are very rapidly taken up
since intracellular concentrations exceed
blood levels in 2 minutes; 2) highest concentrations are invariably found in the lungs
and liver, as much as 20 times those in other
tissues (brain tissue usually has one of the
lowest concentrations); 3) levels of thioridazine in brain appear to be consistently
lower than those of the other 2 drugs relative
to other tissues; 4) thioridazine shows little
variation in concentration in different brain
areas other than a very small but consistent
excess in the thalamus and hypothalamus, and
5) ultracentrifugal fractionation of brain
homogenates has shown that thioridazine is
restricted to the microsomal fraction and is
not found in other particulates or in the
supernatant.

Baylor University College of Medicine
Waco, Texas

3217 Rey, J. H. A study in the relationship
of hormones, brain activity, and behaviour in
women suffering from mental illness. In:
Cleghorn, R. A., Moll, A. E., & Roberts, C.A.
Third World Congress of Psychiatry Proceedings.
Volume II. Toronto/Montreal: University of
Toronto Press and McGill University Press,
1962. Pp. 830-832.

Fluctuations in mood, onset of depression
and/or schizodepressive episodes were related

to the menstrual cycle and excretion of 17-ketosteroids and rise in the cornification index in 4 women.

Maudsley Hospital
Camberwell, London
Great Britain

3218 Sourkes, Theodore L., Murphy, Gerard F., & Chavez-Lara, Beatriz. Experimental and clinical studies of anti-decarboxylases. In: Cleghorn, R. A., Moll, A. E., & Roberts, C. A. Third World Congress of Psychiatry Proceedings. Volume I. Toronto/Montreal : University of Toronto Press and McGill University Press, 1962, Pp. 649-653.

The excretion of α-methyldopa and a metabolite α-methyldopamine was followed in 3 normal males and 10 psychiatric patients. The drug was administered both i.m. and p.o. in acute and chronic experiments, e.g., 0.75-10 g/day. Only when smaller amounts of α-methyldopa were administered could both the amino acid and its amines be determined in the urine. α-Methyldopa did not significantly change behavior or thinking in the patients, however there are good reasons for retaining an interest in antidecarboxylases as possibly useful agents in clinical medicine aside from α-methyldopa's antihypertensive action.

Worcester Foundation for Experimental
  Biology
Shrewsbury, Mass.

3219 Bodur, Hatice, Alatas, Sevda, Sisli, Ceyhan, & Sisli, Tomris. A study on protein-bound hexoses during insulin coma. New Istanbul Contribution to Clinical Science. 1962, 5, 79-88.

Total protein, serum albumin and globulin, and the amount of protein bound hexoses were determined and the amount of hexoses in protein calculated during and after insulin coma of 19 schizophrenics. The amount of insulin used was 100-540 U. No significant differences were detected in the parameters studied.

Departments of Biochemistry and Psychiatry
Faculty of Medicine
University of Istanbul
Istanbul, Turkey

3220 Briggs, Michael H., & Harvey, Natalie. Urinary metabolites of aromatic amino acids in schizophrenia. Life Sciences, 1962, 2, 61-64.

The urinary metabolites of 15 schizophrenic patients, 12 non-schizophrenic psychiatric patients and 18 normal subjects were studied. An abnormality in tyrosin metabolism is indicated in schizophrenia. The metabolic abnormality is explained as a partial inhibition of p-hydroxyphenylpyruvate oxidase due to suboptimal amounts of escorbate.

Victoria University
Wellington, New Zealand

3221 Antebi, R. N., & King, J. Serum enzyme activity in chronic schizophrenia. Journal of Mental Science, 1962, 108, 75-78.

Twenty-six cases of chronic schizophrenia, including 15 females, were assayed for the following serum enzymes. The serum activities of 9 enzymes, SGOT, SGPT, lactate dehydrogenase (LDH), malate dehydrogenase (MDH), isocitrate dehydrogenase (ICD), pseudocholinesterase (pCE), aldolase (ALD), alkaline phosphatase (ALP) and leucine aminopeptidase (LAP) were measured. Two cases, 1 in remission, showed simultaneous elevated pCE and ALP activity; 1 patient had concomitantly elevated ALP and ICD levels and another ALP and LAP activities. One patient had a high ALP level and 3 had elevated pCE activity. No symptoms of other disease were evident in any of these patients showing abnormal enzyme levels and it is difficult to offer an explanation of these findings as there was no correlation between serum enzyme abnormality and clinical state or age. Estimation of any of the enzymes studied holds no diagnostic value in chronic schizophrenia.

Moorhaven Hospital
Ivybridge, Devon
Great Britain

3222 Levine, Walter G., & Peisach, J. Studies on the substrate specificity of ceruloplasmin. Biochimica et Biophysica Acta, 1962, 63, 528-529.

For each substrate, V_{max} expressed as μl O_2 consumer per h per μg ceruloplasmin CU, was plotted semilogarithmically against the sum of Hammett sigma values for all ring substituents. The more reactive compounds are those with the more highly negative sigma values. Thus a reaction rate of 835 was obtained for p-phenylenediamine with a total sigma value of -1.320, while m-phenylenediamine, with a total sigma value of -0.322 gave a reaction rate of only 39. Compounds having substituents with high positive sigma values showed little or no activity. Although o-phenylenediamine was readily oxidized, 4-nitro-o-phenylenediamine did not react. Similarly, the reaction rate with hydroquinone was 285, while 2,5-dihydroxybenzoic acid, the carboxyl analogue, showed only very slight activity. An increased ring electron density in the substrate is associated with increased activity with ceruloplasmin and it is apparent the enzyme binding may not be through the amine or phenolic groups, but instead directly to the ring, or more specifically, to the π electrons of the ring.

Department of Pharmacology
Albert Einstein College of Medicine
Yeshiva University
New York, N. Y.

3223 Long, R. F., & Lessin, A. W. Inhibition of 5-hydroxytryptamine uptake by platelets in vitro and in vivo. Biochemical Journal, 1962, 82, 5P. [Abstract]

A large number of organic bases inhibited uptake of 5HT by ox blood platelets in vitro, in platelet enriched plasma. Inhibition was competitive and could be reversed by washing the platelets. Active compounds included chlorpromazine, chlorprothixene, imipramine, cocaine, ibogaine, α-methyltryptamine, harmaline, amphetamine, benzylhydrazine, pheniprazine. Benactyzine, caffeine, mescaline, salicylic acid, N-benzyl-N-methylpropyne, pentobarbital, dimethylaniline and iproniazide were only slightly active or were inactive. 5-Hydroxy-α-methyltryptamine was taken up by ox platelets the same as 5HT, and this uptake inhibited competitively by α-methyltryptamine. Concentrations for 50% inhibition of uptake by imipramine ranged from 8×10^{-7}M using human platelets, to 4×10^{-5}M using bovine platelets. Cat platelets were the most sensitive to the inhibitory action of methyltryptamine, 50% inhibition of uptake occurring at 3×10^{-6}M whereas to produce equivalent inhibition using guinea pig platelets, a concentration of more than 10^{-4}M was required. In these studies 5HT was estimated fluorimetrically.

Research Department
Roche Products Ltd.
Welwyn Garden City, Hertfordshire
Great Britain

3224 Ruscak, M. Changes in the level of ᵞ-aminobutyric acid (GABA) in the ischaemic brain of rats following application of some stimuli evoking spreading EEG depression. Physiologia Bohemoslovenica, 1962, 11, 192-198.

In rats, stimuli evoking spreading EEG depression lead to a significant increase in brain GABA content only if bilaterial ligature of the carotid arteries was performed concomitantly. The ligature itself however did not affect brain GABA nor the ratio of glutamic acid to GABA in the course of 30 minutes. Local application of 0.3 M and 3M KCl onto the brain as well as mechanical stimuli caused a significant rise in GABA content of the brain cortex. Following 30 minutes applications of 0.3 M KCl, GABA content increased by 41.6%, after 30 minutes application of 3 M KCl by 65.1% and after mechanical stimulation by 31.1% as compared with the GABA content in the hemispheres of control rats. A tracheal ligature of 150 seconds duration also led to an increase of GABA in the cortex by 88.5%. Since the brain GABA content was raised even after stimuli which do not evoke spreading EEG depression, the increase of GABA in the ischemic brain is not specific for EEG depression. This increase in GABA is considered the result of increased utilization of free amino acids in the brain, GABA's formation being increased and its oxidation slowed.

Institute of Experimental Medicine
Slovak Academy of Sciences
Bratislava, Czechoslovakia

3225 Michaux, R. Action catatonigene de la
5-methoxytryptamine. [Catatonic action of
5-methoxytryptamine.] Life Sciences, 1962,
2, 617-619.

Intracisternal injections of 25 and 50 μg
5-methoxytryptamine and 50 μg 5HT were made
in rats. 5-Methoxytryptamine caused intense
catalepsy which decreased slowly so that 72
hours after injection, psychomotor inertia
was still evident. 5HT rats showed the same
symptoms but 48 hours later animals recovered
spontaneous activity. The i.p. injection of
700-1400 μg 5-methoxytryptamine to 140 g rats
does not effect their behavior. Methylation
of the indole OH 5HT does not suppress its
catatonic action; methylation lengthens the
action of the drug.

Université de Liège
Département de Biochimie
Laboratoire des Isotopes
Liege, Belgium

3226 Bernheimer, H., Birkmayer, W., &
Hornykiewicz, O. Verhalten der Monoaminoxydase im Gehirn des Menschen nach Therapie
mit Monoaminoxydase-Hemmern. [Monoamino-
oxydase in the human brain after therapy with
monoaminoxydase-inhibitors.] Wiener Klinische
Wochenschrift, 1962, 77, 558-559.

Determination of MAO activity were carried
out in the nucleus caudatus, cortex cerebri
and renal cortices of deceased normal humans,
patients with Parkinson's disease, and patients with Parkinson's disease who had been
pre-treated with MAO inhibitors. The manometric method was used. High enzyme activity
could be measured in the tissues of "normal"
controls and "untreated" patients with Parkinson's disease. No significant differences
were observed in these 2 groups. In pretreated Parkinson patients, MAO in the kidney
was inhibited to a high degree and brain MAO
was completely inhibited.

Pharmakologische Institut
Universität Wien
Vienna, Austria

3227 Kveder, S., Iskric, Sonja, & Keglevic,
Dina. 5-Hydroxytryptophol: a metabolite of
5-hydroxytryptamine in rats. Biochemical
Journal, 1962, 85, 447-449.

Radioactive 5HT (2.26 μc/mg) was injected i.p.
into rats (2.9 mg/100 g). A phenolic eluate
from urine was subjected to paper chromotography
and autoradiographs studied. A radioactive
area with R_f 0.25 was eluted and rechromato-
graphed, resolving into individual peaks with
R_f 0.22 and 0.476. The latter, metabolite C,
was eluted again and hydrolized for further
identifications. 5-Hydroxytryptophol was
identified as 5HT metabolite. Then the metabolism of 1'-N-acetyl-5-hydroxytryptamine
and 5-hydroxytryptophol in rat-liver slices
was studied. The former compound remained
mainly unchanged (80-90%), whereas 60-70% of
5-hydroxytryptophol was metabolized, being
partly oxidized to 5HIAA and partly conjugated.
1'-N-Acetyl-5-hydroxytryptamine and 5-hydroxy-
tryptophol were chromatographically indistinguishable but only the latter was shown to
be a metabolite of 5HT. A scheme for the
metabolism of 5HT is suggested above. A
major metabolite of 5HT excreted in rat urine
is a 5-hydroxytryptophol-O-glucuronide. The
chemical synthesis of 5-hydroxytryptophol is
described.

Tracer Laboratory
Institute Rudjer Boxkovic
Zagreb, Yugoslavia

3228 Marquillo, Carlos L., Esperbén, Maria
T., & Lasalvia, Eduardo. Variation of pyruvic
acid in enzymatic inhibition of monoamine
oxidase. Chemotherapia, 1962, 4, 580-585.

Blood and urine specimens from 10 normal subjects were analyzed to determine pyruvate and
lactate variations before and after administration of nialamide (100 mg/day), Tersavid (1-
pivaliol-2-benzyl-hydrazine, 45 mg/day) and
Nardelzine (fenelzine-beta-phenylethylhydrazine,
45 mg/day). All patients showed sizeable
increases in pyruvate blood and urine levels,
i.e., the MAO inhibiting properties of the
drugs resulted in the increased pyruvate
levels.

Departamento de Investigación Clinica
Hospital Pasteur
Montevideo, Uruguay

3229 Mall, G. Sur la toxicité de la bile
et du sérum chez les épileptiques et les
schizophrènes. [On the toxicity of bile and
serum from epileptics and schizophrenics.]
In: Baruk, Henri, & Launay, Jacques (Eds.)
Annales Moreau de Tours. Tome I. Mémoires
reconts sur la psychopharmacologie. [Annals
of Moreau de Tours. Volume I. Current
memoires in psychopharmacology.] Paris:
Presses Universitaires de France, 1962.
Pp. 349-352.

Bile from normal subjects and schizophrenics
was injected into mice (1 ml i.p.) in order
to determine sedative, cataleptic and lethal
effects. With control bile mortality was
10.9% compared to 43% for schizophrenic bile.
No catatonia occurred in mice treated with
normal bile, while 17% became catatonic with
experimental bile. With control bile 89.1%
were asymptomatic compared to 41% for schizophrenic bile. Serum samples from 46 healthy
controls and 41 epileptics were hydrolyzed
and 1 ml aliquots injected i.p. into mice.
Fresh serum was mixed with 2% trypsin in a
proportion of 4:1 and incubated for 16 hours
at 37°C before use. Results below apply to
epileptic sera taken in the attack phase.
Mortality was 40.4% for epileptic sera and
11.7% for control sera.

Société Moreau de Tours
Maison Nationale de Charenton
Paris, France

3230 Zmorski, Tadeusz. Aktywność fosfatazy
zasadowej w surowicy krwi w przebiegu
leczenia schizofrenii chlorpromazyną. [The
activity of alkaline phosphatase in plasma
during treatment of schizophrenia with
chlorpromazine.] Roczniki Akademii Medycznej
im. Juliana Marchlewskiego w Białymstoku,
1961, 7, 57-63.

Alkaline phosphatase activity in the plasma
of 49 schizophrenics (26 men and 23 women),
under prolonged chlorpromazine treatment,
was assayed. The highest daily dose of
chlorpromazine averaged 327 mg and was given
for 36 days. On the average treatment lasted
77 days. Determinations of phosphatase activity were made at 7 day intervals,
Bodansky's method being employed. The activity of phosphatase was found unchanged
in 36 patients, slightly increased in 10

(an average of 0.7 Bodansky U), and decreased
in 3 (0.5-1.0 Bodansky U). Apart from a
moderate increase in blood sedimentation rate,
no side effects were observed. While no liver
damage was indicated by alkaline phosphatase
testing, great care is advocated in the administration of chlorpromazine, and liver
function should be assayed before and after
treatment.

Klinika Psychiatrycznej Akademii Medycznej
Białystok, Poland

SEE ALSO: 2881, 2884, 2901, 2908, 2915,
2926, 2954, 2965, 2966, 2986, 2988, 3017,
3021, 3029, 3147, 3173.

ABBREVIATIONS

α-KG	α-ketoglutarate	GABOB	γ-amino-β-hydroxybutyric acid
AACL	Zuckerman's Affect Adjective Check List	HD	hypnotic dose
ACTH	adrenocorticotropic hormone	5HIAA	5-hydroxyindoleacetic acid
ad lib.	free choice	5HT	5-hydroxytryptamine
ADP	adenosinediphosphate	5HTP	5-hydroxytryptophane
A.M.	morning		
AMA	American Medical Association	i.a.	intraarterial
Art.	Article	ibid.	in the same place
ATP	adenosinetriphosphate	i.e.	that is
		i.m.	intramuscular
BAL	British antiLewisite	IMPS	Lorr's Inpatient Multidimentional Psychiatric Scale
BAS	benzyl analogue of serotonin		
b.i.d.	twice a day	i.p.	intraperitoneal
BOL	bromolysergic acid diethylamide	IPAT	Cattell's Institute for Personality & Ability Testing Anxiety Scale
BUN	blood urea nitrogen		
		I.Q.	intelligence quotient
C	Celsius scale	IU	international unit
ca.	about	i.v.	intravenous
CAR	conditioned avoidance response		
CBS	chronic brain syndrome	kg	kilogram
cc	cubic centimeter	K_i	Michaelis constant for an inhibitor
CD	convulsive dose	K_m	Michaelis constant for a substrate
cm	centimeter		
cm^2	square centimeter	lbs	pounds
cm^3	cubic centimeter	LD	lethal dose
C.N.R.S.	Centre National de la Recherche Scientifique	LSD	lysergide
CNS	central nervous system	μ	micron
COMT	catechol-o-methyl transferase	μc	microcurie
cps	counts per second	μg	microgram
CR	conditioned reflex (response)	μl	microliter
CS	conditioned stimulus	μM	micromolar
CTD	Climbing Time Delay	mμ	millimicrons
		M	molar
DDT	dichlorodiphenyl trichloroethane	ma.	milliamperes
DOPA	3, 4-dihydroxy-phenylalnine	MACC	Motility Affect Cooperation Communication
DPH	diphosphopyridineucleotide		
DPNH	reduced diphosphopyridine-nucleotide	MAO	monoamine oxidase
		MAS	Taylor Manifest Anxiety Scale
		meq	milliequivalents
ECG	electrocardiogram	ml	milliliter
Ed.	editor	mm	millimeter
ED	effective dose	mm^2	square millimeter
EDTA	ethylenediaminetetraacetic acid	MMPI	Minnesota Multiphasic Personality Inventory
EEG	electroencephalogram		
e.g.	for example	MSRP	Multidimensional Scale for Rating Psychiatric Patients
ERG	electroretinogram		
et al.	and others		
etc.	and so forth	N	normal
		NEFA	nonesterified fatty acid
F	Fahrenheit scale	NIMH	National Institute of Mental Health
FFA	free fatty acid		
g	gram	p	probability
GABA	γ-aminobutyric acid	PAH	para-aminohippuric acid

1228

PBI	protein-bound iodine	SRA	Science Research Associates
pH	negative logarithm of the hydrogen ion concentration	Suppl.	supplement
		TAT	Thematic Apperception Test
P_i	inorganic phosphate	TH	thyroid hormone
P.M.	afternoon and evening	t.i.d.	thrice a day
p.o.	by mouth	TPN	triphosphopyridinenucleotide
ppm	parts per million	TPNH	reduced triphosphopyridine-nucleotide
PRP	Psychotic Reaction Profile		
		TSH	thyroid-stimulating hormone
q.i.d.	four times a day		
		U	unit
refs.	references	UR	unconditioned response
R_f	ratio of the distance of dissolved substance to solvent distance	US	unconditioned stimulus
		USAF	United States Air Force
RNA	ribonucleic acid	USDHEW	United States Department of Health, Education, and Welfare
ru	rat unit		
		USP	United States Pharmacopoeia
s.c.	subcutaneous	USPHS	United States Public Health Service
S.D.	standard deviation		
SGOT	serum glutamic oxaloacetic transaminase	UV	ultraviolet
SGPT	serum glutamic pyruvic transaminase	VA	Veterans Administration
		viz.	namely
sic	exactly as found		
SOSAI	Springfield Outpatient Symptom and Adjustment Index	WAIS	Wechsler Adult Intelligence Scale
		WPRS	Wechsler Psychiatric Rating Scale

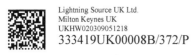

Lightning Source UK Ltd.
Milton Keynes UK
UKHW020309051218
333419UK00008B/372/P

9 780332 747873